Preventive management of children with congenital anomalies and syndromes

This unique source of reference and clinical guidance provides health professionals with an invaluable, structured approach to the preventive care of children with congenital anomalies. Over 120 disorders ranging from cerebral palsy to Down syndrome are discussed. For each disorder there is an introductory summary of key information, followed by more detailed listing of general pediatric and speciality concerns, all structured to provide an integrated approach to patient care. For 30 common disorders, preventive management checklists are provided: these checklists provide an ongoing record of the child's medical complications and progress and they are designed to be copied or printed and placed in the medical record.

The text provides details of medical complications and preventive recommendations, supported by more than 500 references. The introductory chapters provide an overview of the approach to genetic/metabolic disease and developmental disabilities, and a useful glossary is also included.

Golder N. Wilson is Mary McDermott Cook Distinguished Professor of Pediatric Genetics and Director, Division of Genetics and Metabolism, Department of Pediatrics, University of Texas Southwestern Medical Center, Dallas, Texas. He has 20 years experience in an academic center running programs in genetic/metabolic disease and birth defects.

W. Carl Cooley is Medical Director, Crotched Mountain Rehabilitation Center, Greenfield, New Hampshire, and Associate Professor of Pediatrics, Dartmouth–Hitchcock Medical Center, Hanover, New Hampshire. He has an equivalent experience in an academic center running programs in developmental pediatrics. Both men have children with disabilities and are active on boards and in parent groups targeted towards children with special needs.

ement
hital
nes

ITEMS MAY ALSO
BE RENEWED
BY PHONE

 CAMBRIDGE
UNIVERSITY PRESS

PUBLISHED BY THE PRESS SYNDICATE OF THE UNIVERSITY OF CAMBRIDGE
The Pitt Building, Trumpington Street, Cambridge, United Kingdom

CAMBRIDGE UNIVERSITY PRESS
The Edinburgh Building, Cambridge CB2 2RU, UK   http://www.cup.cam.ac.uk
40 West 20th Street, New York, NY 10011–4211, USA   http://www.cup.org
10 Stamford Road, Oakleigh, Melbourne 3166, Australia
Ruiz de Alarcón 13, 28014 Madrid, Spain

£45

Purchasers of the book may wish to photocopy the checklists for use with their patients. This is acceptable to the publisher, who, nevertheless, disclaims any responsibility for the consequences of any such use of this material in clinical practice. It is not necessary to write to Cambridge University Press for permission to make individual photocopies. This permission does not extend to making multiple copies for use by others, or for resale.

First published 2000

Printed in the United Kingdom at the University Press, Cambridge

Typeface Minion 10.5/14pt   *System* QuarkXPress™   [s E]

A catalogue record for this book is available from the British Library

Library of Congress Cataloguing in Publication data
Wilson, Golder.
Preventive management of children with congenital anomalies and
syndromes / Golder N. Wilson, W. Carl Cooley.
p.   cm.
Includes index.
ISBN 0 521 77673 2 (pbk.)
1. Genetic disorders in children – Complications – Prevention.
2. Developmental disabilities – Complications – Prevention.
I. Cooley, W. Carl (William Carl), 1947– . II. Title.
[DNLM: 1. Abnormalities – therapy. 2. Abnormalities – diagnosis.
QS 675 W748p 2000]
RJ47.3.W55 2000
618.92′0042–dc21
DNLM/DLC   99-40520 CIP

ISBN 0 521 77673 2 paperback

Every effort has been made in preparing this book to provide accurate and up-to-date information which is in accord with accepted standards and practice at the time of publication. Nevertheless, the authors, editors and publisher can make no warranties that the information contained herein is totally free from error, not least because clinical standards are constantly changing through research and regulation. The authors, editors and publisher therefore disclaim all liability for direct or consequential damages resulting from the use of material contained in this book. Readers are strongly advised to pay careful attention to information provided by the manufacturer of any drugs or equipment that they plan to use.

Advisory Board

Pediatric Genetics:

John C. Carey, M.D., M.P.H.

Professor of Pediatrics

Chief, Division of Medical Genetics

University of Utah Health Sciences Center

James W. Hanson, M.D.

Senior Advisor for Medical Genetics

Division of Cancer Control and Population Sciences

Acting Chief

Clinical and Genetic Epidemiology Research Branch

Epidemiology and Genetics Program

National Cancer Institute

National Institutes of Health

Development Pediatrics:

Michael E. Msall, M.D.

Director, Child Development Center

Rhode Island Hospital

Professor of Pediatrics and Human Development

Brown University

General Pediatrics:

Joel B. Steinberg, M.D.

Professor of Pediatrics

University of Texas Southwestern Medical Center

Medical Director, Children's Hospital of Dallas

For Shamus Wilson and his wonderful pediatrician,
Suzanne LeBel Corrigan, M.D.

GNW

For my wife, Seddon Savage, who is, among other more
important things, the best physician I know.

WCC

Contents

Preface   *page* xi
How to use this book   xi
Which disorders are included?   xii
Rationale for preventive guidelines   xii
Types of preventive guidelines   xiii
Validation of preventive management guidelines   xiv
Acknowledgments   xv

Glossary of genetic and molecular terms   xxi

Part I   Approach to the child with special needs

1   Approach to the child with genetic disease   3
         Categories of genetic disease   3
         Approach to genetic counseling   6
         Diagnostic approach to the child with congenital anomalies   8
         Diagnostic approach to the child with metabolic disease   12
         The laboratory diagnosis of genetic/metabolic disease   15

2   Approach to the child with a developmental disability   19
         Definitions and epidemiology   20
         Recognizing developmental differences in a primary care setting   22
         Chronic condition management in primary care   27
         Supporting the families of children with disabilities   28

3   Approach to preventive management for children with disabilities   31
         General considerations in preventive medicine   31
         Defining the effectiveness of preventive measures   36
         Designing a preventive care plan for the child with disability   40

Part II   **The management of selected single congenital anomalies and associations**

4	Congenital anomalies associated with developmental disability	49
	Cerebral palsy and congenital brain defects	49
	Hydrocephalus	58
	Spina Bifida	62
5	Single anomalies, sequences, and associations	79
	Single anomalies and sequences	79
	Associations	85
	VATER association	86
	CHARGE association	91
6	Teratogenic syndromes	103
	Less common syndromes	103
	Fetal alcohol syndrome	110
	Fetal hydantoin syndrome	115
	Diabetic embryopathy	118

Part III   **Chromosomal syndrome**

7	Autosomal syndromes	135
	Less common aneuploidies	135
	Trisomy 13/18	142
	Down syndrome	146
8	Sex chromosome aneuploidy and X-linked mental retardation syndromes	161
	Sex chromosome aneuploidy	161
	Turner syndrome	161
	Klinefelter syndrome	167
	Less common sex chromosome aneuploidies	169
	X-linked mental retardation syndromes	171
	The fragile X syndrome	174
9	Chromosome microdeletion syndromes	191
	Rare contiguous gene deletion syndromes	191
	Williams syndrome	195
	Prader–Willi syndrome	198
	Shprintzen syndrome and the Del(22q) spectrum	203

Part IV   **Syndromes remarkable for altered growth**

10	Syndromes with proportionate growth failure as a primary feature	221
	Rarer disorders	222
	Noonan syndrome	228
	Brachmann–de Lange syndrome	232
11	Syndromes with disproportionate growth failure (Dwarfism)	245
	Less common skeletal dysplasias	245
	Achondroplasia	253
	Osteogenesis imperfecta	256
12	Overgrowth syndromes	269
	Less common growth disorders	269
	Beckwith–Wiedemann syndrome	273
	Sotos syndrome	277
13	Hamartosis syndromes	289
	Less common syndromes	289
	Neurofibromatosis-1	298
	Tuberous sclerosis	302

Part V   **Management of craniofacial syndromes**

14	Craniosynostosis syndromes	317
	Less common syndromes	318
	Saethre–Chotzen syndrome	323
15	Branchial arch and face/limb syndromes	331
	Branchial arch syndromes	331
	Goldenhar syndrome and related defects	336
	Face/limb syndromes	340

Part VI   **Management of connective tissue and integumentary syndromes**

16	Connective tissue disorders	355
	Rarer connective tissue disorders	357
	Marfan syndrome	362
	Ehlers–Danlos syndrome, types IV, VI, and VII	366
	Ehlers–Danlos syndrome types I–III	367

17	Integumentary syndromes	379
	Ectodermal dysplasias	379
	Other pigmentary disorders	385
	Disorders with telangiectasias	389
	Disorders with radiation sensitivity and/or rapid aging	391

Part VII   The management of neurologic and neurodegenerative syndromes

18	Neurologic syndromes including the arthrogryposes	395
	Pain insensitivity syndromes	395
	Syndromes with brain anomalies	398
	Syndromes with congenital contractures (arthrogryposes)	400
	Arthrogryposis syndromes	404

Part VIII   Management of neurodegenerative metabolic disorders

19	Organellar and miscellaneous neurodegenerative disorders	413
	Lysosomal enzyme deficiencies	414
	Lysosomal diseases: Lipidoses and mucolipidoses (oligosaccharidoses)	414
	Lysosomal diseases: mucopolysaccharidoses	420
	Mitochondrial disorders	425
	Peroxisomal diseases	430
	Miscellaneous metabolic disorders	434

20	Metabolic dysplasias susceptible to dietary treatment	445
	Disorders of carbohydrate metabolism	446
	Glycogen storage diseases	449
	Disorders of amino acid metabolism	453

	References	463
	Index	527

Colour plates between pp. 230 and 231

Preface

How to use this book

This book is designed as a reference in which health professionals can access possible complications and design preventive management for common congenital anomalies or syndromes. Over 120 disorders are discussed, and 30 are described in detail with flow sheets that summarize preventive care considerations (see sample checklist). These preventive management checklists are intended for copying and placement in the medical record. By checking off the appropriate boxes as shown, the practitioner can assemble an ongoing record of screening, examination, and referral/counseling measures.

The standardized text entries for each disorder are organized by terminology, etiology, differential diagnosis, genetic/family counseling, complications, preventive management, validation of checklist guidelines, and, where available, specialized growth charts. Clinically oriented references are included to facilitate decisions about particular interventions. It is envisioned that most users will turn to the book with a specific disorder in mind and focus on the relevant management suggestions. A detailed table of contents and index are available for this purpose.

Another use of the book is to read more broadly about the approach to children with developmental disabilities and genetic disease. Because of rapid progress in the field of medical genetics, certain terms or concepts encountered in the chapters may be unfamiliar. For this reason, introductory chapters on the approach to genetic disease and developmental disabilities have been provided (Part I, Chapters 1 and 2). These sections review basic characteristics of the diseases and the specialized tests that are available for diagnosis. These facts allow pediatricians and family practitioners to be informed participants in the management of congenital disorders. A glossary is also appended to aid with specialized terminology. Other books include more extensive discussion of genetic/developmental principles and of particular birth defect/syndrome disorders (Jones, 1997; Gorlin et al., 1990).

Which disorders are included?

The more common congenital anomalies and syndromes were selected for detailed discussion, with emphasis on those requiring chronic management due to mental and physical disability. To qualify as a "more common" disorder, an estimated incidence above 1 in 25,000 births was required, since that number makes it probable that the disorder will come to the attention of the average pediatric practitioner. If the disorder is rarely encountered by practitioners or if there are limited strategies for preventive care, then the discussion is limited to a few paragraphs without the inclusion of a checklist. Sample, blank checklists are appended to this preface so that practitioners can tailor them for rarer disorders.

It should be noted that hydrocephalus and spina bifida are isolated anomalies rather than syndromes, and that cerebral palsy is a functional description of brain injury or developmental anomaly. However, their congenital origin and requirements for chronic management justify coverage in this book. It is expected that the developmental pediatrician will provide specialty expertise for the latter disorders, while the pediatric geneticist will be more actively involved with patients having malformation syndromes.

Some common metabolic disorders are also discussed in the book, although it is recommended that metabolic specialists be continuously involved in their care. The frequent laboratory measurements and dietary modifications required by acute metabolic disorders are not adequately conveyed by a checklist approach, but the occurrence of developmental disabilities in many of these children justifies attention to preventive management in other areas. Checklists are definitely useful for some chronic metabolic conditions, exemplified by the mucopolysaccharidoses discussed in Chapter 19.

Rationale for preventive guidelines

For those interested in the rationale for particular management guidelines, reading of Chapter 3 is recommended. The central rationale is that each syndrome or anomaly places the patient at higher risk for particular complications as compared to the general population; preventive screening or evaluation for these complications is then justified by criteria of efficiency (selection of high-risk patients) and ethics (improved quality of life). This strategy of ameliorating complications is one of secondary or tertiary rather than primary prevention, since few congenital disorders can be prevented or cured (see Chapter 3). A list of complications is the basis for preventive management guidelines, and is rendered in a standard format on part 1 of each checklist. General complications are listed first (e.g., increased mortality, feeding problems), followed by a standard sequence of organ systems and body regions. The Committee on Genetics, American Academy of Pediatrics (1994, 1995a, 1995b, 1995c, 1996a, 1996b) has published consensus recommendations for the health care supervision of children with Down syndrome, Turner syndrome, achondroplasia, neurofibromatosis-1, fragile X syndrome, and Marfan syndrome. These recommendations are certainly followed in this book, and their spirit is extrapolated to 25 other common disorders for which consensus guidelines are not yet formulated.

Although there is a clear rationale for alerting practitioners to the complications of a disorder, the nature and timing of intervention often requires clinical judgment. Some children with severe dysfunction may benefit more from palliative care than the inconveniences of medical intervention. Decisions about screening measures become particularly difficult when anesthesia is required (e.g., brain imaging), or when a positive result has controversial significance (e.g., cervical spine radiographs for atlantoaxial instability in Down syndrome). Such recommendations are often footnoted in the checklists, with the reminder that clinical judgment must always be used.

Types of preventive guidelines

The sample checklist, parts 2–4 includes general pediatric recommendations in the first column, drawn from the guidelines in Bright Futures (Greene, 1994) and updated with a current immunization schedule. The next three columns list recommendations for the specific anomaly or syndrome, grouped by screening (e.g., laboratory tests, imaging studies), evaluation (e.g., alertness for particular signs or symptoms), and referral/counseling (e.g., specialty evaluations, counseling services). The presence of general pediatric and disease-specific guidelines on the same flow sheet provides the practitioner with a comprehensive, on-going summary of patient care.

"Family Support" appears frequently in the referral/counseling column. This is a prompt to the primary care physician to inquire about the general impact of the child's condition on family life. Questions should routinely be raised about specific family stresses, school issues, the status of siblings, access to information, contact with other families affected by the same condition, and financial pressures. Eligibility for benefits such as Medicaid, Supplemental Security Income (SSI), Title V, and respite care should be considered and followed with appropriate referrals. Some families may need to consider the financial planning issues related to income taxes, trusts, and estate planning when individuals with developmental disabilities are involved. Many states have family support programs for families of children with disabilities which may include the services of a family support coordinator. All eligible families should be referred to such programs. Birthdays, the anniversaries of a diagnosis, and life transition (preschool to elementary school; school to work/adult life) are particularly difficult times for families during which extra support may be needed.

Included in family support are links to disease-specific family support groups that can be invaluable in sharing experience with social and medical concerns. Many of these are listed on the checklists, part 1. The Exceptional Parent Magazine annual guide (http://www.eparent.com) and the Alliance of Genetic Support Groups (http://www.medhelp.org/geneticalliance/), and the Association for Retarded Citizens (ARC, http://www.arc.org) provide good sources for American and Canadian groups, while the searchUK function (http://www.searchuk.com) can find links to many groups in the United Kingdom. The ARC and Family Village (http://familyvillage.wisc.edu/) websites are also excellent sources of information about disabilities.

Validation of preventive management guidelines

Having stated that the preventive management guidelines are based on disease complications, it must again be emphasized that the invasiveness and frequency of preventive screening may be subject to dispute. Decisions between recommended screening (e.g., echocardiography) versus evaluation of symptoms (e.g., auscultation for cardiac murmurs) are often difficult, and practitioners should bear in mind that guidelines promoted by professional organizations such as the American Academy of Pediatrics are available for only a few disorders. Certainly practitioners should feel free to modify the guidelines based on their experience and style.

To offer greater breadth of perspective, the recommendations have been reviewed by members of an editorial advisory board: Drs. John Carey and James Hanson in medical genetics, Dr. Michael Msall in developmental pediatrics, and Dr. Joel Steinberg in general pediatrics. Dr. Steinberg has the added perspective of being in a pediatric practice for many years before becoming Medical Director at Children's Medical Center of Dallas. Clearly there is much work to do regarding disease natural history and outcome before these preventive recommendations acquire the force of scientific validation. Even the Down syndrome management guidelines, endorsed by several authorities (Rubin and Crocker, 1988; Cooley and Graham, 1991; Carey, 1992; Committee on Genetics of the American Academy of Pediatrics, 1994), remain to be justified by controlled studies.

In summary, this book should be used to enhance the health care of patients with congenital anomalies and syndromes by considering preventive management guidelines. It is certainly not intended to impose unwanted advice on experienced physicians or to add new burdens to the already busy routines of those involved in patient care. However, anyone observing the improved outcomes for patients with

Down syndrome over the past few decades must award some merit to preventive management. While congenital disorders are often incurable, preventive care offers a satisfying opportunity for health professionals to enhance the quality of life of children with developmental or genetic disorders.

Acknowledgments

The authors wish to thank the advisory board for their many suggestions regarding the format and content of preventive management checklists.

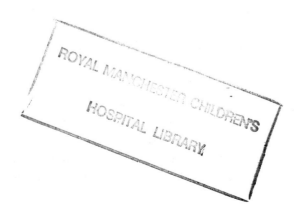

Preventive Management of

Clinical diagnosis:
Incidence:
Laboratory diagnosis:
Genetics:
Key management issues:
Growth charts:
Parent groups:
Basis for management recommendations:

Summary of clinical concerns

General	Life cycle	
	Learning	
	Behavior	
	Growth	
Facial	Face	
	Eye	
	Ear	
	Nose	
	Mouth	
Surface	Neck/trunk	
	Epidermal	
Skeletal	Cranial	
	Axial	
	Limbs	
Internal	Digestive	
	Pulmonary	
	Circulatory	
	Endocrine	
	RES	
	Excretory	
	Genital	
Neural	CNS	
	Motor	
	Sensory	

RES, reticuloendothelial system, **bold**: frequency > 20%

Key references

Syndrome

Preventive medical checklist (0–1yr)

Patient   **Birth Date** / /   **Number**

Pediatric	Screen		Evaluate		Refer/Counsel	
Neonatal		❑		❑		❑
/ /		❑		❑		❑
Newborn screen ❑ HB ❑		❑		❑		❑
1 month		❑		❑	Family support[4]	❑
/ /		❑		❑		❑
				❑		❑
2 months		❑		❑	Early intervention[3,5]	❑
/ /		❑		❑		❑
HB[1] ❑ *Hib* ❑ *DTaP, IPV* ❑ *RV* ❑				❑		❑
4 months		❑		❑	Early intervention[3,5]	❑
/ /		❑		❑		❑
HB[1] ❑ *Hib* ❑ *DTaP, IPV* ❑ *RV* ❑				❑		❑
6 months		❑		❑	Family support[4]	❑
/ /		❑		❑		❑
Hib ❑ *OPV[1]* ❑ *DTaP* ❑ *RV* ❑				❑		❑
9 months		❑		❑		❑
/ /		❑		❑		❑
OPV[1] ❑		❑				❑
1 year	Hearing, vision[2]	❑		❑	Family support[4]	❑
/ /		❑		❑	Early intervention[5]	❑
HB ❑ *Hib[1]* ❑ *OPV[1]* ❑ *MMR[1]* ❑ *Var[1]* ❑				❑		❑

Clinical concerns for _____ **syndrome, ages 0–1 year**

Guidelines for the neonatal period should be undertaken *at whatever age* the diagnosis is made; DTaP, acellular DTP; IPV, inactivated poliovirus; RV, rotavirus; Var, varicella;[1]alternative timing; [2]by practitioner; [3]as dictated by clinical findings; [4]parent group, family/sib, financial, and behavioral issues as discussed in the preface; [5]including developmental monitoring and motor/speech therapy.

Syndrome

Preventive medical checklist (15m–6yrs)

Patient		Birth Date / /	Number	

Pediatric	Screen	Evaluate	Refer/Counsel	
15 months	❑	❑	Family support[4]	❑
/ /	❑	❑	Early intervention[5]	❑
Hib[1] ❑ *MMR[1]* ❑ *DTaP, OPV[1]* ❑ *Varicella[1]* ❑	❑	❑		
18 months	❑	❑		❑
/ /	❑	❑		❑
DTaP, OPV[1] ❑ *Varicella[1]* ❑ *Influenza[3]* ❑	❑	❑		❑
2 years	❑	❑	Family support[4]	❑
/ /	❑	❑		❑
Influenza[3] ❑ *Pneumovax[3]* ❑ *Dentist* ❑	❑	❑		❑
3 years	❑	❑	Family support[4]	❑
/ /	❑	❑	Preschool transition[3,5]	❑
Influenza[3] ❑ *Pneumovax[3]* ❑ *Dentist* ❑	❑	❑		❑
4 years	❑	❑	Family support[4]	❑
/ /	❑	❑	Preschool program[3,5]	❑
Influenza[3] ❑ *Pneumovax[3]* ❑ *Dentist* ❑	❑	❑		❑
5 years	❑	❑	Preschool program[3,5]	❑
/ /	❑	❑	School transition	❑
DTaP, OPV[1] ❑ *MMR[1]* ❑	❑	❑		❑
		❑		
6 years	Hearing, vision[2] ❑	❑	Family support[4]	❑
/ /	❑	❑		❑
DTaP, OPV[1] ❑ *MMR[1]* ❑ *Dentist* ❑	❑	❑		❑

Clinical concerns for _____, ages 1–6 years

Guidelines for prior ages should be undertaken *at the time of diagnosis*; [1]alternative timing; [2]by practitioner; [3]as dictated by clinical findings; [4]parent group, family/sib, financial, and behavioral issues as discussed in the preface; [5]including developmental monitoring and motor/speech therapy.

Syndrome

Preventive medical checklist (6+ yrs)

Patient		Birth Date / /		Number	

Pediatric	Screen	Evaluate	Refer/Counsel	
8 years	❑	❑	Family support[4]	❑
/ /	❑	❑	School options	❑
Dentist ❑	❑	❑		❑
10 years	❑	❑		❑
/ /	❑	❑		❑
	❑	❑		❑
12 years	❑	❑	Family support[4]	❑
/ /	❑	❑	School options	❑
Td[1], MMR, Var ❑	❑	❑		❑
CBC ❑ *Dentist* ❑				
Scoliosis ❑				
Cholesterol ❑				
14 years	❑	❑		❑
/ /	❑	❑		❑
CBC ❑ *Dentist* ❑	❑	❑		❑
Cholesterol ❑				
Breast CA ❑				
Testicular CA ❑				
16 years	❑	❑	Vocational planning[3]	❑
/ /	❑	❑		❑
Td[1] ❑ *CBC* ❑	❑	❑		❑
Cholesterol ❑				
Sexual[5] ❑				
Dentist ❑				
18 years	❑	❑	Vocational planning[3]	❑
/ /	❑	❑		❑
CBC ❑ *Sexual[5]* ❑	❑	❑		❑
Cholesterol ❑				
Scoliosis ❑				
20 years[6]	Hearing, vision[2] ❑	❑	Family support[4]	❑
/ /	❑	❑		❑
CBC ❑ *Sexual[5]* ❑		❑		❑
Cholesterol ❑				
Dentist ❑				

Clinical concerns for _____ syndrome, ages 6+ years

Guidelines for prior ages should be undertaken *at the time of diagnosis*; Td, tetanus/diphtheria; Var, varicella; [1]alternative timing; [2]by practitioner; [3]as dictated by clinical findings; [4]parent group, family/sib, financial, and behavioral issues as discussed in the preface; [5]birth control, STD screening if sexually active; [6]repeat every decade.

Glossary of genetic and molecular terms

These brief definitions should be supplemented by consulting the texts recommended in the Preface.

Acrocentric chromosome: Chromosome with small short (p) arms as opposed to metacentric chromosomes with approximately equal short and long (q) arms.

Allele: Alternative gene structure (e.g., S and A alleles of the β-globin gene).

Agenesis: Absence of a part of the body caused by an absent anlage.

Aneuploidy: Abnormal chromosome number that is not an even multiple of the haploid karyotype, i.e., 47,XX,+21 or 90,XX.

Anlage, primordium, blastema: Embryonic precursor to a tissue, organ or region.

Anomaly: Any deviation from the expected or average type in structure, form and/or function which is interpreted as abnormal.

Anticipation: Worsening of phenotype with subsequent generations.

Aplasia: The absence of a body part resulting from a failure of the anlage to develop.

ASO: Allele-specific oligonucleotides used for DNA diagnosis.

Association: Any non-random occurrence in one or more individuals of several morphologic defects not identified as a sequence or syndrome. Associations represent the idiopathic occurrence of multiple congenital anomalies.

Atavism: A developmental state that is normal in phylogenetic ancestors, but abnormal in their descendants.

Atrophy: Decrease in a normally developed mass of tissue(s) or organ(s) due to decrease in cell size and/or cell number.

Base pairs (bp): Adenine-Thymine (A-T) or Guanine-Cytosine (G-C) pairing in DNA; also the basic unit for DNA strand length.

Blastogenesis: Stages of development from karyogamy and the first cell division to the end of gastrulation (stage 12, days 27–28).

Candidate gene: A gene implicated in pathogenesis based on protein function, chromosomal location, or sequence homology.

Chromosomal rearrangements: Aberration where chromosomes are broken and rejoined as opposed to numerical excess or deficiency.

Chromosome painting: Use of repetitive DNA FISH probes to fluoresce entire chromosomes or chromosome regions.

Contiguous gene deletions: Deletion encompassing neighboring genes to produce a composite phenotype.

Cross-over: Breakage and reunion of chromosomes that realign parental loci.

Cytogenetic notation: Formal nomenclature describing karyotypes and chromosome location, i.e.:

　　47,XY+11: Extra chromosome 11 (Trisomy 11)

　　45,XY-11: Absent chromosome 11 (Monosomy 11)

　　46,XY,11q-: Terminal deletion of chromosome 11

　　46,XY,11q+: Extra material of unknown origin on 11q

　　46,XY,del(11p11p13): Interstitial deletion between bands p11 and p13 of chromosome 11

　　46,XY,dup(3q): Extra material derived from the long arm of chromosome 3.

Dysmorphogenesis: Abnormal development leading to abnormal shape of one or more body parts (dysmorphology).

DNA cloning: Isolation of a DNA segment by insertion into a simple genome (plasmid, bacteriophage) and production of multiple copies.

DNA diagnostic techniques: Use of DNA modifying enzymes, hybridization, and size separation technologies for diagnosis of identity, genetic disease, or predisposition.

DNA hybridization: Rejoining (reannealing) of complementary DNA or RNA stands.

DNA marker: DNA segment, often anonymous, that exhibits sufficient sequence variation to be useful in genetic linkage and DNA diagnosis.

DNA sequence: Order of nucleotides in a DNA segment, usually displayed from the 5′-triphosphate (5′ end) to the 3′-hydroxyl (3′ end) nucleotides.

Empiric risks: Recurrence risk based on epidemiologic survey of affected families.

Exon: Portion of gene that encodes protein.

First degree relative: Those with 50% of genes in common (child, parent, sibs).

FISH: Fluorescent in situ hybridization, a technique by which fluorochromes are attached to DNA probes and hybridized with cytogenetic or cell preparations.

Functional cloning: Isolation of gene segments based on gene function, i.e. using antibodies to a characterized protein or expression assays where traits are deleted or restored to cultured cells.

Gene map: Order of genes within a chromosome or entire genome.

Genetic heterogeneity: Multiple loci where mutations can produce a similar phenotype, such as autosomal dominant or X-linked Charcot–Marie–Tooth disease.

Genetic mapping: Use of genetic linkage to produce a relative gene order based on recombination distances (centimorgans = approximately 1 megabase).

Genome: Complete set of genes (DNA) in an organism.

Genomic DNA: DNA isolated from an organism or tissue, containing transcription signals and introns that will be absent from cDNA.

Genomics: The study of function and disease based on gene structure and organization.

Genotype: Genetic constitution, often with reference to particular alleles at a locus.

Germinal mosaicism: Mosaicism within the germ line, whereby a fraction of eggs or sperm may contain a particular mutation or chromosome aberration.

Heteroplasmy: Different mitochondrial genomes in the same cell, a mechanism by which the proportions of altered mitochondria may increase in specific tissues to cause disease.

Heterozygote: Individual with different alleles at a locus.

Homeobox: A DNA sequence shared by several Drosophila segmentation genes.

Homeotic mutations: Mutations altering segment identity in Drosophila. In a broader sense, a developmental switch analogous to that replacing one homologous insect segment with another.

HOX, hox: Gene clusters in humans and mice that exhibit homology to the structure and expression of Drosophila homeotic loci.

Hyperplasia: Overdevelopment of an organism, organ or tissue resulting from a decreased or increased number of cells.

Hypertrophy: Increase in size of cells, tissue or organ.

Hypoplasia: Underdevelopment and overdevelopment of an organism, organ or tissue resulting from a decreased or increased number of cells.

Hypotrophy: Decrease in size of cells, tissue or organ.

IGF: Insulin-like growth factor.

Incomplete penetrance: Absence of phenotypic expression in a person known from a pedigree to have an abnormal genotype.

Interstitial deletions: Chromosomal deletion removing regions between termini.

Isochromosomes: Duplicate long or short chromosome arms that result in deficiency – i.e., Turner syndrome patients with i(Xq) are monosomic for Xp.

Karyotype: A standard number and arrangement of chromosomes as obtained from human blood or tissue specimens. A normal karyotype is 46,XX for females and 46,XY for males.

Kilobases (kb): Unit of DNA/RNA length = 1000 bp; megabase = 1 million bp.

L1CAM: L1 cell adhesion molecule implicated in X-linked hydrocephalus.

Linkage: The tendency for neighboring genes to segregate together in families.

Locus: Unique location of a gene on a chromosome.

Major anomaly: Anomaly with cosmetic or surgical consequences.

Malformation: A morphologic defect of an organ, or larger region of the body, resulting from an intrinsically abnormal developmental process.

Maternal inheritance: Inheritance mechanisms that exhibit maternal transmission based on abnormal mitochondria or maternal RNAs.

Meiosis: The process of germ cell division that randomly allots one chromosome of each pair to gametes.

Mendelian inheritance: The classical autosomal dominant, autosomal recessive, and X-linked inheritance mechanisms derived from Mendel's observations in peas.

Microdeletions: Chromosome deletions requiring prometaphase banding for visualization.

Minor anomaly: Anomaly of no medical but considerable diagnostic significance.

Mitosis: The process of somatic cell division that produces identical genomes in daughter cells.

Morphogenesis: A developmental process that includes the stages of blastogenesis and organogenesis.

Morphology: Discipline of zoology that concerns itself at once with the form, formation and transformation of living beings.

Mosaicism: Variation in DNA sequence or chromosome constitution among different cells of an organism.

Multifactorial determination: Dependence of traits on multiple genes plus the environment.

Multipoint linkage: Linkage analysis that examines multiple traits or markers in a pedigree and orders them relative to one another.

Normal variant: Deviation from expected or average type in structure, form or function that is more frequent (arbitrarily >4% of population) and more innocuous than an anomaly.

Obligate carrier: Carrier deduced by pedigree structure.

Oligonucleotide: Short nucleotide sequence often obtained by chemical synthesis.

Organogenesis: A developmental process that extends from late stage 13 (day 28) until the end of stage 23 (day 56) when the major organs and body parts are formed.

Paired box: A DNA sequence motif found in the paired gene of the fruit fly.

PAX: Genes in mice and humans containing paired boxes.

PCR: Polymerase chain reaction by which individual gene segments are amplified through sequential cycles of polymerization, heat denaturation, and reannealing.

Phenotype: Individual traits or characters.

Physical mapping: Gene order based on actual physical measurements in terms of chromosome bands or DNA base pairs.

Pleiotropy: Multiple traits determined by a single cause, often a gene mutation.

Point mutations: Nucleotide substitutions.

Polymorphism: Multiple alleles at a locus, producing amino acid or DNA sequence variation.

Polypeptide chains: Proteins or, in the case of multiple subunits, components of proteins formed by peptide bonds between amino acids.

Polyploidy: Abnormal chromosome number that is a multiple of the haploid karyotype, e.g., 69,XXY or 92,XXXX.

Positional cloning: Isolation of gene segments based on chromosome location.

Primary relative: First degree relative, i.e. those sharing 50% of genes.

Primer: Oligonucleotide used to begin nucleic acid polymerization at a particular site on a DNA strand, e.g., with PCR or reverse transcriptase.

Proband: Individual bringing family to attention, indicated by arrow in pedigrees.

Prometaphase analysis: Karyotype prepared from synchronized cells arrested in early prophase; these studies require prior notice to the laboratory.

Propositus: Same as proband.

Protein polymorphism: Products of alternate alleles at a locus exemplified by the ABO or HLA systems.

Quantitative traits: Incremental phenotypes such as height or blood pressure.

Recombinant DNA: Chimeric DNA molecules produced by joining of segments from different species, often using the complementary "sticky ends" produced by restriction endonucleases.

Recombination: Breakage and reunion of DNA strands.

Repetitive DNA: DNA sequences that have multiple copies in a genome.

Restriction endonuclease: A bacterial enzyme designed for defense against bacteriophage that recognizes and cleaves at specific nucleotide sequences.

Reverse genetics: Genetic analysis proceding from chromosomal location to cloned gene; positional cloning is now the preferred term.

Robertsonian translocations: Joining of two acrocentric chromosomes at their short arms to produce a single translocation chromosome.

Sequence: A cascade of primary and secondary events that are consequences of a single primary malformation or a disruption.

Somatic mosaicism: Variation in DNA sequence or karyotype among different somatic cells of an organism.

Sporadic: Isolated case, often implying lack of inheritance or genetic causation.

Submicroscopic deletion: Small chromosome deletions that can be visualized only by DNA analysis.

Syndrome: Multiple anomalies thought to be pathogenetically related and not representing a sequence.

Syndrome variability: Differing phenotypic manifestations among individuals with the same syndrome.

Targeting sequences: Amino acid regions that direct proteins to particular cellular locations.

Teratology: The study of abnormal development, particularly with regard to the disruptive influence of drugs, chemicals, and physical agents.

Threshold: A theoretical barrier at which an individual's combination of genes and environmental exposure crosses from predisposition to actual defect.

Translocation breakpoint: The region of recombination between two chromosomes.

Translocation carriers: Individuals with "balanced" translocations that have no extra or missing chromosome material.

Triplet repeat amplification: Increased number of tandemly repeating 3-bp units that can alter gene expression, as in fragile X syndrome or myotonic dystrophy.

Trisomies/monosomies: Karyotypes with extra or missing entire chromosomes.

Uninformative: Genetic linkage study where parental alleles and therefore the risk for disease transmission cannot be distinguished.

Uniparental disomy: Two copies of a chromosome pair derived from one parent.

Variable expressivity: Variable symptoms among affected individuals in a family.

Zygotic expression: Synthesis of gene products from zygotic DNA rather than maternal RNA molecules.

Part I

Approach to the child with special needs

Children with special health care needs account for a substantial proportion of pediatric hospital and outpatient visits. While the individual disorders causing chronic disease may be rare, the aggregate impact of chronic care occupies a significant fraction of the health professional's time. From the perspective of health insurance, it is often cited that the sickest 1 percent of the population consumes 30 percent of the health care resources, and the sickest 5 percent consumes 50 percent. The impact of chronic illness is similarly exaggerated in pediatric practice, with disproportionate demands on practitioners. Preventive management offers an important opportunity to minimize complications in children with special health care needs, and the key to preventive management is a specific diagnosis and approach. This section summarizes different types of genetic disease and developmental disability, with emphasis on the assignment of disease categories.

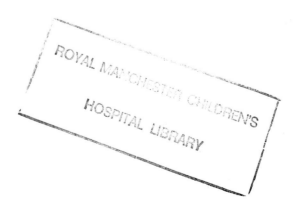

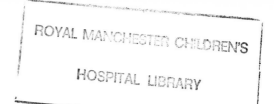
1

Approach to the child with genetic disease

Medical genetics is a harlequin specialty. One side is bright with the power of DNA diagnosis and genotyping; the other is darkened by ignorance of complex phenotypes. Fortunately, the molecular revolution is proceeding so rapidly that even complex syndromes are being drawn into the light of genetic analysis. For a growing number of developmental and/or metabolic disorders, proper recognition and referral can lead to definitive diagnostic testing. It is thus extremely important for practitioners to be familiar with common presentations of genetic and developmental diseases, allowing affected children and their families to receive the benefits of informed management and genetic counseling.

A correct diagnosis is the gateway to anticipatory guidance and case management. Although the primary care physician may not be the first practitioner to establish the correct diagnosis, it is essential that he or she be able to incorporate specialty opinions and laboratory data into a comprehensive care plan. It is not necessary for practitioners to know long lists of eponymic disorders, but it is necessary that they recognize the possibility of genetic or congenital disease so that appropriate referrals and information can be obtained. Textbooks (and computerized databases) such as *Mendelian Inheritance in Man* (McKusick, 1994), *Medical Genetics* (Jorde et al., 1994), *Recognizable Patterns of Human Malformation* (Jones, 1997), *Syndromes of the Head and Neck* (Gorlin et al., 1990), and *The Metabolic and Molecular Bases of Inherited Disease* (Scriver et al., 1995a) are available to provide details on particular diseases. This chapter will review the clinical approach to children with morphologic and/or metabolic alterations, focusing on the needs of those who are not genetic specialists. Italicized terms are defined in the glossary after the foreword in this book.

Categories of genetic disease

Hereditary factors are involved in more than 5000 diseases. The hereditary contribution may be partial, as with *multifactorial inheritance* of cleft palate, or major, as with *Mendelian inheritance* of sickle cell anemia. Because they are congenital disorders, malformation syndromes are included within the specialty of pediatric

Table 1.1 Number, frequency, mortality, and morbidity of genetic disease

Category	Number	Frequency (percent)	Mortality (percent)	Morbidity (percent)
Mendelian				
Autosomal dominant	2557	0.7	34	61
Autosomal recessive	1477	0.25	74	87
X-linked	310	0.5	62	85
Multifactorial	>100	3–5	>50	>50
Chromosomal	>100	0.5	95	98
Syndromal	>1000	0.8	>90	98

Source: McKusick (1994); Wilson (1992); Costa et al. (1985).

genetics even though many, including fetal alcohol syndrome, are caused by environmental factors. Table 1.1 summarizes the number, frequency, morbidity, and mortality of genetic diseases and syndromes classified according to their mode of inheritance (Wilson, 1990, 1992). Several studies have suggested that genetic disorders are estimated to account for 17 to 27 percent of admissions in a general pediatric hospital (Emery & Rimoin, 1990, pp. 1–3). Recently, Yoon et al. (1997) estimated that 12 percent of hospital admissions in the states of California and South Carolina were related to birth defects and genetic diseases, generating about twice the charges per patient compared to other diseases.

Table 1.2 indicates that patients with genetic diseases come to attention in three ways: those requiring genetic counseling, those with congenital anomalies, and those with metabolic disorders. Each patient category is associated with particular inheritance mechanisms and laboratory evaluations (Table 1.2). Individuals requiring genetic counseling represent the largest category, since genetic diseases can affect any organ system. The patient with cystic fibrosis or the patient with sickle cell anemia is usually not managed by geneticists, but these patients share a need for genetic counseling. Because genetic counseling is frequently a complex process, it will often involve individuals with specialized training. Nevertheless, the key role of practitioners in bringing families to attention mandates that they be aware of risk factors such as the multiple miscarriages, consanguinity, or advanced parental age listed in Table 1.2.

A second category of patients referred for genetic evaluation is the child with congenital anomalies (*dysmorphology*). This category includes children with single anomalies, multiple anomaly syndromes, or chromosomal disorders and accounts for 3–5 percent of all births. The third category of referral consists of inborn errors of metabolism, which affect an estimated 1 in 600 births (Waber, 1990; Berry &

Table 1.2 Categories of pediatric genetic disease

Category	Characteristics	Laboratory evaluations
Genetic counseling	Relative with genetic disorder	DNA testing
	Parental consanguinity	Parental chromosomal studies
	Advanced maternal age (>35 years)	
	Advanced paternal age (>40 years)	
	Multiple miscarriages	
Dysmorphology	Breech presentation	Routine karyotype
	Intrauterine growth retardation	FISH studies
	Major and minor anomalies	Skeletal radiographs
	Microcephaly, macrocephaly	DNA testing
	Skeletal disproportion	
	Developmental and/or growth delay	
	Growth acceleration	
Acute metabolic disease	Lethargy, coma	Blood glucose, ammonia
	Developmental delay, seizures	Blood pH, lactate
	Hypoglycemia, particularly when no ketosis	Blood amino acids
		Blood carnitine
	Acidosis with increased anion gap	Blood acylcarnitine profile
	Lactic acidosis	Urinary ketones
	Neutropenia, thrombocytopenia	Urinary reducing substances
	Unusual odors	Urinary organic acids
Chronic metabolic disease	Hypotonia, seizures	Skin, liver, or muscle biopsy
	Developmental delay, regression	Leukocyte preparations
	Retinal or corneal changes	Enzyme assays
	Visceromegaly	Skeletal radiographs
	Skeletal changes	DNA diagnosis

Note:
FISH, fluorescent in situ hybridization.
Source: Wilson (1990), Friedman (1990), Waber (1990).

Bennett, 1998). Metabolic disorders may present in the neonatal period, but often become evident in later infancy or childhood when symptoms of episodic illness, visceromegaly, and/or neurodegeneration become evident.

The categories of morphologic and metabolic disease present with different signs and symptoms, and their diagnosis requires different laboratory measurements (Table 1.2). Intrauterine growth retardation and breech presentation frequently accompany congenital malformations and syndromes, as do altered head size, delayed or accelerated growth, and skeletal disproportion. Subtle (minor) anomalies such as epicanthal folds or single palmar creases raise questions of a syndrome pattern, particularly when several are detected. Observation of a surgically or cosmetically significant (major) anomaly should always initiate a search for other anomalies, so the different prognoses for children with isolated versus multiple anomalies are correctly assigned. Since the nervous system is affected in at least 55 percent of hereditary syndromes (Wilson, 1992), developmental delay is also an indication for syndrome evaluation. Chromosomal and skeletal radiographic studies are important laboratory considerations in a child with growth and/or developmental delay.

Inborn errors of metabolism may occasionally present with congenital malformations, but maternal metabolic compensation will usually protect fetal morphogenesis. A common scenario is the normal newborn who becomes irritable, lethargic, and comatose after feeding, often with accelerated physiologic jaundice or unusual odors. Hypoglycemia and acidosis are also frequent accompaniments of metabolic disease, particularly when the hypoglycemia is not combined with the appropriate ketotic response. Other presentations for metabolic disease include visceromegaly, bone marrow suppression, developmental delay or regression, and episodic vomiting or hypoglycemia.

Approach to genetic counseling

Genetic counseling is an educational process that provides individuals with information about a genetic disease and their recurrence risks. A definition of genetic counseling has been formulated by the American Society of Human Genetics. Its essence is that genetic counseling is a communication process which deals with the occurrence, or the risk of occurrence, of a genetic disorder in a family. During this communication process, appropriately trained individuals assist the family to understand (1) the diagnosis and management options for the disorder; (2) the contribution of heredity to the disorder and how this translates to recurrence risks among family members; and (3) the alternatives (i.e., prenatal diagnosis) for dealing with these recurrence risks. The counseling process should also assist the family choose a course of action based on their particular family goals or ethical/religious background and to make the best possible adjustment to the presence and future implications of a genetic disorder.

The need for genetic counseling often arises from a family history, which should be part of every medical evaluation. Depending on the reason for clinical presentation, a family history may consist of a few questions about primary relatives (e.g., parents, siblings of the patient) or require the drawing of a pedigree. A pedigree is simply a codified family history, with generations, individuals, and the presenting patient (*proband* or *propositus*) diagrammed in a standard format (Fig 1.1).

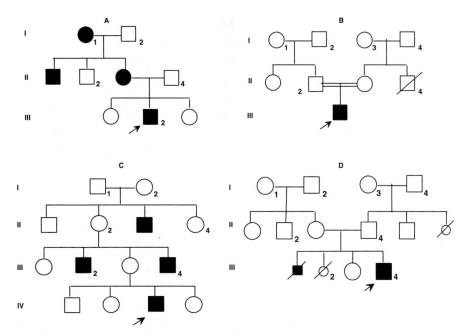

Fig. 1.1   Pedigrees typical of A, autosomal dominant; B, autosomal recessive; C, X-linked recessive; and D, chromosomal inheritance displaying symbols for males (squares), females (circles), affected individuals (filled symbols), consanguinity or inbreeding (double line), abortions (small symbols), death (diagonal line), and individuals coming to medical attention (arrows).

Numbering of the generations (Roman numerals) and individuals (Arabic numerals) facilitates documentation beneath the pedigree. If preliminary questioning or the reason for presentation mandates a detailed pedigree, then it is helpful to construct a readable diagram that other health professionals can refer to.

The person who prompts medical attention (proband, propositus or proposita) is highlighted by an arrow to establish the reference point of the pedigree. The scope of the pedigree will be determined by screening questions to determine how many (if any) relatives have relevant disease manifestations; it is usual to represent at least patient siblings, parental siblings, and grandparents if the pedigree is drawn, but additional information will depend on the indication. After the presence of genetic disease is documented by a preliminary family history, a genetic specialist may be called upon to construct a complete and accurate pedigree diagram.

Once a pedigree is constructed, inheritance mechanisms are often evident from the pattern of affected individuals. Autosomal dominant or X-linked inheritance often exhibits a vertical inheritance pattern, with male-to-male transmission ruling out the possibility of X-linked inheritance. Horizontal patterns of affected individuals (i.e., siblings) suggest the operation of autosomal recessive inheritance, and this mechanism is sometimes made more plausible by parental consanguinity (inbreeding).

In order to begin the process of genetic counseling, the physician must document the family history, inspect the pedigree for evidence of inherited diseases, and understand the genetic risks implied by particular inheritance mechanisms. The book *Mendelian Inheritance in Man* (McKusick, 1994), available for query on the World Wide Web (http//:www3.ncbi.nlm.nih.gov/omim), provides a useful reference for deciding which, if any, inheritance mechanism has been established for a pediatric disease. Since diseases may exhibit genetic heterogeneity with several possible inheritance mechanisms (e.g., Charcot–Marie–Tooth disease, retinitis pigmentosa, cleft palate), referral to a genetic specialist is often necessary for accurate genetic counseling. Practitioners can then review this specialty counseling with the family, utilizing their rapport and knowledge of the family to place the genetic information in context.

It is important to avoid a judgmental attitude towards reproductive options or disabilities, since overly negative portrayals of disorders such as Down syndrome can rupture the parent–physician relationship. In the case of prenatal diagnosis, anticipation, adoption or foster care should be mentioned as alternatives to abortion. Parent support groups are very useful in arranging contact with affected individuals so at-risk families can become familiar with disease manifestations.

For a growing number of diseases, genetic counseling can include the provision of DNA diagnosis for at-risk family members. Some understanding of the methods and requirements for DNA diagnosis are useful for practitioners, and these are summarized below. It is important that pediatricians be attuned to genetic risks in parents (or other relatives) that result from a child's diagnosis.

Diagnostic approach to the child with congenital anomalies

The term dysmorphology literally means painful or abnormal shape, and its presence orients the physician toward abnormalities of embryonic and fetal development. Until better laboratory measures of morphogenesis are available, the physical examination is paramount in the evaluation of children with congenital anomalies (Fig. 1.2). The recognition of subtle anomalies often guides the diagnostic and management plan.

Table 1.3 summarizes the categories of single and multiple anomaly disorders (Aase, 1992; Opitz & Wilson, 1996). As emphasized previously, isolated anomalies (cleft palate, spina bifida) affect a single body region and commonly are associated with multifactorial determination. When a child has multiple anomalies affecting different organ systems, the underlying cause is more likely to involve chromosomal or Mendelian disease. Genetic causation is particularly likely if the pattern of minor and major anomalies is associated with the recognizable facial appearance

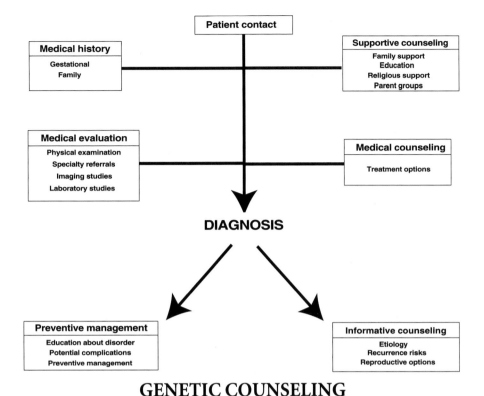

GENETIC COUNSELING

Fig. 1.2   Approach to the patient with a congenital disorder, demonstrating the parallel processes of medical evaluation (left side) and family counseling (right side).

that characterizes a *syndrome*. Although exceptions such as the fetal alcohol syndrome certainly occur, more than 75 percent of the syndromes listed in Jones (1996) are due to Mendelian or chromosomal disease.

The first principle of evaluation is then to ask whether a child has a single or multiple anomalies (Figs 1.3 and 1.4, color plates). Children with isolated anomalies will usually have normal mental development (unless the anomaly involves the brain), while the child with multiple congenital anomalies is at high risk for mental disability. Single anomalies such as cleft palate, pyloric stenosis, congenital heart disease, or congenital hip dislocation are usually amenable to surgical correction and imply a low (2–3 percent) recurrence risk for parents. When several anomalies occur together, concern about a syndrome will mandate consideration of a karyotype and/or skeletal radiologic survey; imaging studies to search for anomalies of the brain, heart, and kidneys; and a complex preventive management plan that includes the possibility of mental disability. Even when the family history is unremarkable, malformation syndromes often result from Mendelian or chromosomal inheritance that mandates referral for genetic evaluation and counseling.

Table 1.3 Types of congenital anomalies

Category	Subcategory	Definition	Example
Isolated defect			
Normal variant		Present in >4% of population, not abnormal	Mongolian spot
Anomaly		Deviation from expected or average type in structure, form and/or function which is interpreted as abnormal	
	Major anomaly	Anomaly of surgical or cosmetic consequence	Cleft palate
	Minor anomaly	Little impact on individual well-being	
	Malformation	Morphological defect resulting from an intrinsically abnormal developmental process	Radial aplasia
	Sequence	Pattern of anomalies derived from a single known or presumed prior anomaly or mechanical factor	Robin sequence
Multiple defects	Syndrome	Multiple anomalies thought to be patho-genetically related and not representing a sequence	Zellweger syndrome
	Association	Non-random occurrence in one or more individuals of several morphologic defects not identified as a sequence or syndrome	VACTERL association

Note:
VACTERL: vertebral, anorectal, cardiac, tracheo-esophageal, radial, renal.

Isolated congenital anomalies

Every health professional must learn to distinguish anomalies from family or racial characteristics that have no medical significance. *Normal variants*, such as the lumbar Mongolian spot or the aural (Darwinian) tubercle, are sometimes distinguished by their occurrence in more than 4 percent of the population (Table 1.3; Opitz & Wilson, 1996). *Major anomalies* are those with cosmetic or surgical consequences (e.g., cleft palate, atrial septal defect, malformed pinna; Stevenson et al., 1993). *Minor anomalies*, despite their diagnostic significance, occur in less than 4 percent of individuals and have little impact on well-being (e.g., epicanthal fold, single palmar crease, fifth finger clinodactyly, shawl scrotum). A scoresheet is available for > 90 common minor anomalies that may be recognized during the physical examination (Opitz & Wilson, 1996). The presence of three or more minor anomalies should arouse suspicion of a syndrome; multiple minor anomalies also confer increased risk for a major anomaly. In children with Down syndrome, minor anomalies of the face and hands (e.g., epicanthal folds, upslanting palpebral fissures, flattened facial profile, single palmar crease) often alert the physician before signs or symptoms of major anomalies (e.g., cardiac defects) become manifest. The detection of minor anomalies is thus an integral part of the genetic examination, allowing the child with a surgically correctable major anomaly to be distiguished from the child with a complex multiple anomaly syndrome.

Because the developing embryo has a dynamic anatomy, an isolated embryonic anomaly may lead to several abnormalities in the infant. A *sequence* represents a cascade of secondary events that derive from a primary anomaly (Spranger et al., 1982). Sequences, like isolated anomalies, are usually associated with sporadic occurrence or multifactorial determination. Examples include spina bifida sequence with lower limb hypoplasia and club feet; Pierre Robin sequence with small jaw, protruding tongue, and posterior cleft palate; or Potter sequence with facial changes, limb contractures, lung hypoplasia, and oligohydramnios due to renal agenesis. The key is to recognize that the several consequences of a sequence are related to a single cause; that, like isolated anomalies, they have a lower risk for mental disability or genetic etiology.

Congenital anomaly patterns

When several minor anomalies are recognized, the probability of major defects and of a syndrome is increased. Minor anomalies also help to distinguish syndromes from *associations*, which are groups of major defects thought to derive from a brief period of embryonic injury (Lubinsky, 1986). Associations, like sequences and isolated anomalies, will generally have lower genetic risks than syndromes.

Syndromes (literally, running together) are patterns of major and minor anomalies that relate to a single cause. In many cases, the cause is unknown. Malformation syndromes are exemplified by disorders such as Goldenhar syndrome, which involves multiple orofacial, cardiac, limb, and vertebral malformations. Note the involvement of several embryologically independent regions in a syndrome (eye, ear, heart, vertebrae, thumb) in contrast to the localized branchial arch error involving ear and jaw in hemifacial microsomia sequence.

Associations consist of major anomalies with similar embryologic timing (Lubinsky, 1986). The *VATER* association of Vertebral, Anorectal, Tracheo-Esophageal, Radial, and Renal defects involves mesodermal derivatives that begin differentiation at 20–25 days of embryogenesis (see Chapter 5). Associations usually lack minor anomalies, since there is no persistent influence like an extra chromosome to produce subtle alterations throughout gestation. As a result, individuals with associations do not have a characteristic facial appearance. For associations, identification of a characteristic anomaly stimulates a search for others; for syndromes, facial recognition often prompts evaluation for the characteristic anomaly pattern. In a child with a normal facial appearance, radial aplasia with tracheo-esophageal atresia should prompt concern for associated renal defects that occur in the VATER association. If the craniofacies is abnormal with a prominent occiput and malformed ears, the child should have chromosome studies to evaluate the possibility of trisomy 18 syndrome. Suspicion of the more devastating syndrome requires attention to minor anomalies of the face, ears, chest, hands, and feet; recognition of the trisomy 18 phenotype will then prompt imaging studies to search for major anomalies of the brain, heart, and kidneys.

Diagnostic approach to the child with metabolic disease

Despite the number and variety of metabolic disorders, consideration of the age of onset and the presenting manifestations (Table 1.4) allows a systematic approach to diagnosis. As with other categories of genetic disease, the complexity of laboratory tests and therapies will require the involvement of metabolic disease specialists. However, it is again the primary health care professional that must recognize the initial symptoms. For purposes of recognition, the metabolic disease category can be divided into acute disorders, involving smaller molecules with rapid turnover, and chronic disorders, involving larger molecules with slow turnover (e.g., *storage diseases*). This classification is of course oversimplified, and a more detailed summary of algorithms for metabolic disease can be found in Saudubray & Charpentier (1995). Since metabolic disorders almost always exhibit autosomal or X-linked recessive inheritance, the family history may be helpful in showing consanguinity or siblings with deaths in early childhood. Special laboratory evaluations are also implied for acute versus chronic metabolic diseases, and a definitive diagnosis has the added value of allowing prenatal diagnosis.

Acute metabolic disorders

The metabolic pathways responsible for the interconversion of small molecules are crucial as sources of energy and building blocks for the organism. Amino acids, sugars, fatty acids, and nucleotides are examples of small molecules that are interconverted by enzyme action to form intracellular networks that are much like a highway interchange; when an enzyme is missing due to a genetic mutation, the proximate molecules (substrates) accumulate and the distal molecules (products) are deficient. Diseases result from these accumulations and/or deficiencies, and from the diversion of substrates into alternative pathways.

Because of rapid interconversion and turnover, small-molecule diseases tend to be acute or episodic in presentation, with hypoglycemia, acidosis, anion gap, or unusual odors, as summarized in Table 1.4. These features contrast with large-molecule diseases, in which protein, carbohydrate, or lipid polymers cannot be cata-

Table 1.4 Presentations of metabolic disease

Presentation	Disease examples	Laboratory abnormalities
Small molecule diseases		
Lethargy, coma, alkalosis, tachypnea	Urea cycle disorders	Elevated ammonia, abnormal amino acid screen (e.g., elevated glutamine)
Hypoglycemia, lethargy, coma, acidosis	Organic acidemias	Anion gap, low pH, hypoglycemia, abnormal organic acid screen (e.g., methyl malonate)
Hypoglycemia, lethargy, coma, acidosis	Maple syrup urine disease	Abnormal amino acid screen (elevated leucine, isoleucine, valine), abnormal organic acid screen (elevated ketoacids)
Sepsis, hepatic disease, hepatomegaly	Galactosemia	Urine reducing substances
Hypoglycemia, hepatic disease, hepatomegaly	Tyrosinemia	Abnormal amino acid screen (tyrosine), elevated serum succinylacetone
Hypoglycemia ± hepatic disease, hepatomegaly	Fatty acid oxidation disorder	Decreased serum carnitine, abnormal organic acid screen (e.g., dicarboxylic acids), abnormal acylcarnitine profile (e.g., dicarboxyl carnitine)
Developmental delay, seizures	Phenylketonuria	Abnormal amino acid screen (phenylalanine)
Large molecule diseases		
Hypoglycemia, hepatic disease, hepatomegaly	Glycogenoses	Hyperuricemia, hyperlipidemia, glycogen on liver biopsy
Developmental regression, seizures ± hepatomegaly	Neurolipidoses	Storage substances in retina, brain, leukocytes, liver biopsy
Developmental regression, dysotosis, hepatomegaly	Mucopolysaccharidoses	Storage substances in brain, leukocytes

bolized and slowly accumulate in affected tissues. Acute metabolic diseases are not covered in this book because the frequency of specialist involvement and the need for dietary modifications are not easily summarized using the checklist approach. Several of these disorders allow true primary prevention, where disease is eliminated by avoidance of offending metabolites. Large-molecule (storage) disorders often have a chronic onset with symptoms such as neurodegeneration and/or hepatosplenomegaly. These more chronic and incurable disorders do require secondary or tertiary preventive management to minimize their complications. Chapter 19 deals with the management of chronic metabolic disorders.

When a child presents with catastrophic illness, the clinician should first consider toxic or infectious etiologies. Toxicants such as ethylene glycol or sepsis that causes cardiorespiratory failure can present with severe acidosis and an anion gap.

If toxicants are ruled out by history or urine screen, and if the symptoms seem out of proportion to the fever or possible infectious source, then a metabolic etiology should be considered. Routine evaluation of acutely ill children will usually provide a complete blood count together with serum glucose, electrolytes, pH, lactic acid, and hepatic transaminase values. Extending the testing to detect most metabolic diseases involving small molecules will require four additional tests: blood ammonia, blood amino acids, urine organic acids, and urine for reducing substances. If a fatty acid oxidation disorder is suspected, then a serum carnitine and acylcarnitine profile should be obtained.

Several categories of acute metabolic diseases will be evident from the initial panel of laboratory tests (Tables 1.2, 1.4). Marked elevations of blood ammonia in a child with lethargy, coma, and mild alkalosis/tachypnea suggest a urea cycle disorder, although transient hyperammonemia of the newborn can occur. A large anion gap with acidosis is suggestive of an organic acidemia. Examples include methylmalonic or propionic acidemia, which often manifest neutropenia due to bone marrow suppression. Because intermediary metabolism is a network of interconversions, urea cycle disorders will have elevations of certain amino acids (e.g., citrulline, ornithine, glutamine, lysine) and certain organic acidemias will have elevated blood ammonia. Hypoglycemia can also occur in methylmalonic or propionic acidemia, but often suggests a disorder of carbohydrate metabolism like galactosemia. Patients with galactosemia will have reducing substances in the urine. Certain disorders with hypoglycemia (e.g., galactosemia), aminoacidemia (e.g., tyrosinemia), or disorders of fatty acid oxidation (e.g., medium chain coenzyme A dehydrogenase deficiency) may present with hepatic disease.

Some children with accumulation of small molecules will not have acute presentations. Classical phenylketonuria is an example where symptoms are minimal until substantial neurologic damage occurs. Organellar diseases involving the peroxisomes or mitochrondria are also intermediate in this classification; they may be associated with lactic acidosis or hepatic disease, but usually have an indolent presentation (see Chapter 19). On the other hand, disorders involving large molecules like the glycogen storage diseases may have an acute presentation because of limited availability of substrate. The inability to degrade glycogen can produce hypoglycemia with seizures and acidosis (Table 1.4). These exceptions emphasize that categorization into small- and large-molecule disorders offers a simplistic approach that must be refined for actual patients.

The clinical goal for children with acute metabolic illness is to stabilize them by treating the acidosis, hypoglycemia, coagulopathies, and/or sepsis until the definitive results of blood amino acids and urine organic acids are available. Children with hyperammonemia or large elevations of organic acids may require peritoneal or hemodialysis for successful therapy, although pharmacologic treatment can reduce milder elevations of ammonia (Waber, 1990). Once stabilized, the definitive metabolic diagnosis can be made through enzyme assay of leukocytes, cultured fibroblasts, or biopsied liver. A few disorders can be diagnosed specifically by amino acid or organic acid profile (e.g., phenylketonuria), but most require confirmatory demonstration of an enzyme deficiency. Another general characteristic of small-molecule disorders is that they often can be treated by vitamin supplementation or dietary modifications. The diagnosis of disorders such as phenylketonuria or galactosemia not only allows the anticipation and prevention of neurosensory problems, but also dramatically alters the clinical course through dietary therapy.

Disorders involving large molecules

The prototypes for large-molecule disorders are enzyme deficiencies that cause accumulation of polymers in affected tissues. These "storage diseases" are usually more chronic in onset and less susceptible to dietary modification than disorders of small molecule metabolism. Examples include the glycogen storage diseases, neurolipidoses, and mucopolysaccharidoses (Table 1.4). Instead of acute alterations in amino acid or organic acid profiles, large-molecule disorders are categorized by examination of brain, retina, liver, leukocytes, bone marrow, and/or skeleton for evidence of storage. Recognition of the retinal cherry red spot in Tay–Sachs disease, bone marrow foam cells in Gaucher disease, or leukocyte granules in Hurler disease leads to confirmatory studies such as brain or skeletal imaging. The definitive diagnosis again rests on the demonstration of a specific enzyme deficiency using leukocytes, fibroblasts, or liver. Although dietary therapy is rarely available (continuous starch feedings for glycogenoses being an exception), diagnosis of a storage disease often leads to important preventive measures such as screening for hydrocephalus in the mucopolysaccharidoses (see Chapter 19).

The laboratory diagnosis of genetic/metabolic disease

The direct diagnosis of genetic disease using chromosomal, DNA, or enzyme analysis provides the most reliable information for genetic counseling. In thinking about genetic laboratory diagnosis, it is important to conceive of a typical cell with its large and small molecules in the cytoplasm and chromosomes in the nucleus. Chromosomal analysis (karyotyping) examines the chromosomes for numerical or structural alterations, while DNA analysis examines the structure of a specific gene on one of the 23 chromosome pairs. Metabolic testing examines the protein product of a specific gene by enzyme/antibody assay or, less precisely, by measuring altered metabolite levels that are created by enzyme deficiency. An advantage of DNA diagnosis is the ability to detect mutant alleles in all cell types, while assay of specific tissues may be required for the demonstration of protein or enzyme deficiency. If the diagnostic change in chromosomal, DNA, or enzyme analysis is detectable in amniotic or chorionic villus cells, then prenatal diagnosis can be offered to the at-risk couple.

For couples with multiple miscarriages, or children with a dysmorphic appearance and developmental delay, a chromosomal study or *karyotype* should be considered (Table 1.2). A routine karyotype demonstrates the number of chromosomes in peripheral blood leukocytes, and allows inspection of the paired metaphase chromosomes for rearrangements (Fig. 1.5, color plate). Standard *cytogenetic notation* describes the karyotype in terms of total chromosome number (typically 46), the type of sex chromosomes (typically XX or XY), and particular abnormalities relative to landmarks (light and dark *bands*). The chromosomal bands are designated by their location on the short (*p*) or long (*q*) chromosome arms and given consecutive numbers according to their distance from the centromere (e.g., band 15q11 on the chromosome 15 long arm or band 6p21 on the chromosome 6 short arm). Notation such as 47,XX+21 then describes altered chromosome number in a female with Down syndrome, and 46,XY,del(5)(5p14) describes a deletion of chromosome 5 extending to band p14 on the short arm in a male with cri-du-chat syndrome.

Although routine chromosomal analysis is an excellent screening test in children with dysmorphology or developmental delay, fluorescent in situ hybridization (FISH) technology allows the search of specific chromosome regions for subtle rearrangements. Small deletions in disorders such as Williams syndrome (chromosome 7q deletion), Prader–Willi syndrome (chromosome 15q deletion), or Shprintzen syndromes (chromosome 22q deletion) are diagnostic if the characteristic alteration is suspected and probed (see Chapter 9). FISH technology has largely replaced prometaphase analysis in which high resolution chromosome banding patterns were produced by arrest in early metaphase.

Because genes are segments of chromosomal DNA analogous to beads on a string, radioactive or fluorescent DNA probes can be designed to distinguish normal from abnormal alleles based on altered *DNA sequences*. DNA diagnostic testing is specific for the disorder in question (e.g., sickle cell anemia), since probes must be targeted to a particular genetic locus (e.g., the A or S β-globin gene alleles). Limitations of DNA diagnosis include disorders where every abnormal allele is different (e.g., Marfan syndrome), single gene disorders where the causative gene has not been identified or isolated (e.g., autosomal recessive Bardet–Biedl syndrome), or polygenic disorders involving environmental and genetic factors (e.g., diabetes mellitus). For many multifactorial diseases (e.g., diabetes mellitus, coronary artery disease, schizophrenia, Alzheimer disease) DNA analysis of family members allows the identification of predisposing alleles with risk modification.

The involvement of genetic specialists and DNA diagnostic laboratories is often required in the planning of DNA diagnostic studies, since the selection of at-risk family members and the interpretation of results may be quite complex.

The fragile X syndrome is an example of a disorder where DNA analysis is definitive, but complex to interpret. Like Huntington chorea, Friedreich ataxia, and Steinert myotonic dystrophy, fragile X syndrome is caused by the expansion of DNA regions composed of three nucleotide repeating units. The fragile X syndrome was first correlated with a site on the X chromosome that appeared broken or fragile in affected males. Although fragile X chromosomal analysis is often included in the initial chromosomal study of males with developmental delay, DNA analysis is much more sensitive. Fragile X syndrome is also unique in that female carriers may have altered behavioral and mental disability despite moderate expansion of triplet repeating units on one X chromosome. DNA analysis is thus required for female carriers, since their clinical severity and their risk for severely affected sons can be predicted by documenting the extent of triplet repeat expansion. Fragile X syndrome thus illustrates the power and complexity of DNA diagnosis, and emphasizes the need for genetic referral when single gene disorders are recognized.

While DNA testing is available for some inborn errors of metabolism, laboratory diagnosis usually involves products of the abnormal allele (e.g., enzyme assay) or metabolites that accumulate as a result of enzyme deficiency. Acute metabolic disorders often present with alterations of blood electrolyte, pH, glucose, ammonia, or lactate levels as listed in Table 1.2, while the more chronic storage diseases present with organ enlargement, progressive brain dysfunction, and the accumulation of polymers in affected tissues. The goal is to characterize the abnormal metabolites in plasma, urine, or affected tissues, which will in turn guide selection of the gene or enzyme to be tested. Participation of a metabolic disease specialist in the initial diagnostic evaluation is strongly recommended for interpretation of complex laboratory results (e.g., urine organic acid profiles). After recognition, referral, and diagnosis, the primary physician assumes an important role by ensuring dietary compliance or coordinating the preventive management program.

2

Approach to the child with a developmental disability

Primary health care providers are uniquely positioned to identify and initially evaluate developmental differences in young children. They are familiar with aspects of the family history and with psychosocial factors that may place a child at higher risk for developmental delay. Primary health care providers are aware of birth events and usually provide for the care of newborns. For those developmental disabilities that are identifiable prenatally or at birth or that result from perinatal complications, early detection is possible. Finally, and most important, the primary health care professional provides longitudinal anticipatory care during which alterations in developmental course can be recognized, followed, investigated, and managed. For most parents, the primary care physician is the first and most trusted respondent to their worries or concerns about their young child's development. It is important that all primary care physicians feel comfortable with this responsibility, confident in their skills at developmental screening, clear about the resources for intervention and further evaluation, and knowledgeable about management, coordination and advocacy.

This chapter provides an overview of the approach to the child with a developmental delay or disability from the perspective of primary care (Rubin & Crocker, 1989; Batshaw, 1994). Taking a generic approach that is intended to complement the specific guidelines of other chapters, we review the epidemiology of developmental disabilities. Developmental screening in primary care is discussed, with guidelines for referral to community-based agencies and for further medical evaluation. The adaptation of families to developmental difference in their children is discussed with reference to the facilitating role that primary health care providers may play in that adjustment. Finally, the concept of Chronic Condition Management (CCM) in primary care is introduced to clarify the important but often underemphasized ways in which primary health care providers complement specialists in the long-term health care of children with developmental disabilities.

Definitions and epidemiology

Estimates of the incidence of developmental disabilities, like those of chronic illnesses in children, vary depending on the definitions used and the method of ascertainment. Epidemiologic data can be derived from population surveys like the National Health Interview Survey conducted by the National Center for Health Statistics, in which a random selection of households are surveyed, providing information about over 17,000 children (Boyle et al., 1994). Case registries provide more categorical data, but are limited to the range of data sources used by the registry and the timing of registration. Registries that focus on birth and neonatal information may not detect developmental disabilities that become apparent later in the life cycle, and those that focus on identifiable conditions (e.g., birth defects registries) may not include children with developmental delays of unknown cause. Finally, administrative ascertainment data reflect the number of children receiving disability-related services such as special education, early intervention, or financial benefits (e.g., Supplemental Security Income, or SSI). Obviously, such data will include only those children who apply and are then found eligible for the service under study.

Estimates of the incidence of developmental disabilities in children range from 5 to 20 percent. When higher-prevalence, lower-severity conditions such as speech and language disorders and learning disabilities are included, estimates approach 20 percent, while a focus on conditions of higher severity shifts the rate toward 3–5 percent. The World Health Organization estimates the incidence world-wide at around 15–20 percent, while the National Health Interview Survey data based on parent interviews in the United States suggest a rate of 17 percent (Lipkin, 1991; Boyle et al., 1994). Figures for enrollment in special education services show wide variability from state to state, but provide a national average of about 10 percent (Ayers, 1994). Most special education services are for learning disabilities, speech, and attentional-behavioral disabilities.

When the focus shifts to specific conditions, each of the identifiable developmental disabilities (except for learning disabilities and attention deficit/hyperactivity disorder) is relatively rare. Though the "bell-shaped curve" for intelligence would predict a 2.5 percent incidence of mental retardation in the population, actual population data suggest a rate closer to 1 percent (Munro, 1986). Cerebral palsy occurs in 0.25–0.4 percent of children, while developmental language disorders affect up to 5 percent. Though most developmental disabilities have a similar incidence across ethnic groups and national boundaries, the rates for some vary inversely with income. Males significantly outnumber females for many developmental disabilities, including mental retardation, autism, and attentional disorders. This sex difference suggests sex-linked genetic mechanisms, ascertainment biases, or enhanced vulnerability of males to adverse developmental sequellae when exposed to biological or psychosocial risk factors.

Of major importance is the distinction of developmental disabilities from those that occur in adult life as a result of trauma, stroke, or aging. Developmental disability refers to a long-term impairment in the ability to perform or achieve age-appropriate skills in one or more areas that has its onset prenatally or during the developmental years. By definition, developmental disabilities involve families that require a wide range of supports, services, and professional disciplines, all with varied objectives and definitions of "developmental disability." These variable definitions, services, and outcome goals may cause confusion among families and professionals.

Another distinction in the definition of developmental disabilities has been between a categorical and a functional approach. The former fits within a traditional medical model and, for many years, was used to identify individuals eligible for a variety of services and supports. Categories such as mental retardation, cerebral palsy, sensory impairment, autism, learning disability, and language disorder are familiar chapter or section headings in pediatric textbooks and on benefit application forms. In the early 1980s, the federal government's Administration on Developmental Disabilities adopted a functional definition in which individuals must manifest impairments in at least three of seven functional categories with onset before age 22 in order to be developmentally disabled. This definition is used in many states to determine eligibility for some nonmedical benefits for people with developmental disabilities such as family support services. More recently, new SSI regulations for children require that the determination of eligibility of children for SSI benefits include an individual functional assessment if the child was not found eligible on a categorical basis. These changes reflect the fact that many children who experience obvious developmental disability do not have an identifiable cause or specific diagnosis.

What are the causes of developmental disabilities? Unlike the major chronic illnesses of adult life, the chronic disabling conditions affecting children are often rare. The more severe disorders such as Down syndrome, fragile X syndrome, or cerebral palsy are rare enough that an individual primary care physician may follow only one or two affected children at any time. More common conditions such as borderline cognitive disability or attention deficit disorder will be more familiar to practitioners, but are less likely to be associated with definitive diagnostic tests or etiologies. Given uncertainties of diagnosis and the bias of referral selection, the experience of a tertiary-based developmental evaluation clinic can be summarized as follows (Munro, 1986; Lipkin, 1991; Boyle, 1994):

- First, prenatal events are responsible for nearly half of developmental disabilities with genetic and teratogenic factors influencing up to one-third.

- Second, 20 percent of developmental disabilities were felt to have stemmed from environmental/behavioral influences in which the biologic effect on etiology was absent or of less apparent importance.
- Third, one-third of children with developmental disability referred for evaluation to a tertiary center remained without a specific diagnosis.

Recognizing developmental differences in a primary care setting

Responding to the newborn with a condition causing development disability

Some conditions associated with developmental disabilities are recognized at birth based on the presence of birth defects or physical features that characterize a specific syndrome or condition. Down syndrome, cleft lip/palate, and spina bifida, which are usually identified in the newborn period, are classic examples. In addition, children with adverse perinatal events (complications of prematurity or low birth weight, asphyxia, or infections) may have obvious early neurologic impairments or may be identified as being at "high risk" for later developmental delays. In these instances of very early identification of developmental concerns, the primary care physician has a series of responsibilities and opportunities to foster optimal outcomes for the child and the family.

Once a disabling condition is recognized (e.g., Down syndrome or evidence of neurologic impairment via seizures, abnormal tone, hydrocephalus), the primary health care provider may be responsible for conveying this news to the parents. Health care providers have learned a great deal in the past decade about how this news should be shared. Though nothing can turn bad news into good, it is possible for the process to help parents to a good start toward adaptation instead of prolonging their recovery from shock or grief. This process of breaking news should be regarded as an active one of empowering parents in the care of their new child in the face of events that have occurred beyond their control. Table 2.1 provides some guidelines about informing parents of diagnoses that were developed from surveys of parents regarding their satisfaction with the process.

In one study, when these simple steps were implemented, parental satisfaction with "how they were told" improved from about 25 percent to 100 percent (Cunningham et al., 1984). Informing parents of a diagnosis of disability in their child is not so much a single event as an ongoing process. Initial office visits may need to be more frequent to help support parents through this time and ensure their successful adaptation. They will need access to accurate, comprehensible information that addresses both the challenges ahead and the reasons for hope. The primary physician can aid optimism by listening, emphasizing positive aspects of the child (e.g., the child is a child first with assets as well as challenges), and prioritizing supports. Most parents indicate an interest in meeting other parents who have children

Table 2.1 Recommended techniques for informing parents of the diagnosis of Down syndrome in their child

---

Parents should be informed:

---

1. By someone with sufficient knowledge to inspire credibility
2. As soon as possible
3. With both parents together, if possible
4. With the baby present, if possible; refer to the baby by name
5. In a private, comfortable place, away from disturbances, with a minimal audience
6. In a straightforward manner, using understandable language; allow time for questions
7. With a balanced point of view, instead of a catalogue of problems; state something positive
8. With follow-up discussion arranged and provide a telephone number to call at any time for information
9. Followed by uninterrupted time in a private place for parents and child to be alone together

---

Source: Cunningham et al. (1984).

with the same or similar conditions. These parent-to-parent contacts can be arranged informally with other families in the same primary care practice or through parent advocacy or regional parent-to-parent organizations. Parents might also be encouraged to join regional and national organizations for families who have children with specific conditions. These organizations provide access to information, facilitate contact with other families, and often produce informative newsletters and conferences. Primary care practices should refer parents to appropriate organizations through the annual resource guide of Exceptional Parent magazine (P.O. Box 3000, Department EP, Denville NJ, 07834) or the Alliance of Genetic Support Groups (35 Wisconsin Circle, Suite 440, Chevy Chase, MD, 20815–7015). Many parent support groups now have home pages on the Internet that can be found through standard search engines. Parent support groups provide an enormous, if undistilled, source of information for both parents and professionals.

A recent scenario is the prenatal diagnosis of a birth defect or condition associated with developmental disability. Though the majority of prenatal tests for genetic conditions involve parents who plan to terminate the pregnancy in the event of an abnormal finding, some parents use such tests as information about the status of their child-to-be and plan to continue the pregnancy regardless of the result. When such parents are found to have a fetus affected by Down syndrome or spina bifida, they require the same attentive, careful "news breaking" as the parents of newborns. They may wish to meet other parents who have made the same decision to continue a pregnancy, and they usually will want the same access to information as the parents of an affected newborn. There may be further information about the fetus that will allow the anticipation of additional medical needs or assist planning for the delivery (e.g., looking for congenital heart disease or bowel anomalies in a fetus with Down syndrome or planning a Cesarean delivery for a child with spina bifida). Such parents may be able to prepare family and friends for the arrival of a child with challenges, allowing them to be more supportive and helpful at the time of birth.

All children who have a specific condition that is likely to cause developmental delay or disability (as well as all children simply found to be delayed, but without a diagnosis) should be referred to early intervention services (Majnemer, 1998). All states in the United States currently receive federal funding to provide early intervention services for children with established conditions causing developmental delays or with documented delays, but no specific diagnosis. Some states also provide these services for children who meet "at risk" criteria established by the state, but who are not yet experiencing delays. Many early intervention services are provided through regular home visits by early childhood professionals, though some programs offer "center-based" services in addition to or instead of home visits. Since the passage of the Individuals with Disabilities Education Act (IDEA) in 1986 and several revisions since, early intervention services have been an entitlement for eligible children. Early intervention services have used a family-centered model in which parents are actively involved in the planning and implementation of interventions. Though most early intervention programs include therapeutic services such as physical and speech therapy, they also provide "family support services" such as help with coordinating care, access to information, assistance with applications for benefits, transportation, and respite care. Physicians should not attempt to judge which children with disabling conditions or developmental delays in their practice should be referred, but should simply offer referral to all. The early intervention providers and parents will go through a process of evaluation and develop an Individual Family Service Plan (IFSP) once the referral is made. Involvement of the primary care physician and input into the IFSP process are usually welcome, though busy schedules and lack of reimbursement sometimes make such participation difficult.

In addition to making appropriate referrals, primary care physicians serve two important quality monitoring functions. First, they can make sure that the system is responsible to families with cerebral palsy, Down syndrome, spina bifida, epilepsy, failure to thrive, and technology dependence. Second, they can emphasize that developmental goals must emphasize a whole child perspective with learning through play, exploration, and quality social interaction as the key programmatic components.

Finally, primary health care providers need to be aware of and respond to the condition-specific health care needs associated with specific diagnoses. To a large measure, this book is intended to provide guidelines for the specific primary and specialty care needs of children with genetic and prenatally determined conditions. Generally, it is important for primary care providers to know that many genetic conditions place an affected child at risk for other medical complications, some of which are preventable and some of which will require specific interventions.

Screening for developmental differences as part of primary care

When prenatal or neonatal diagnosis of a genetic cause of developmental disability is not possible, suspicions usually emerge during the course of well-child care visits or when a change in health suggests an underlying condition that was not previously recognized. Such physical findings as alterations in muscle tone, movement, or reflexes, failure to grow, small or large head circumference, the presence or emergence of skin lesions, impairment of vision, or enlargement of liver and spleen may be clues to an underlying, identifiable syndrome or condition. When such findings are combined with developmental delays, the likelihood of a specific diagnosis increases.

In the majority of children with developmental disabilities, the first clues are delays in expected developmental progress. What constitutes the best approach to developmental screening in primary care is a subject of ongoing debate (Meisels, 1989). Nevertheless, every primary health care provider or agency should have a set of policies and practices aimed at the early identification of developmental delay and the initiation of appropriate interventions. Developmental screening is most effective when it is an ongoing process permeating various aspects of primary care. In this respect, the British experience with "developmental surveillance" is worth reviewing for its success in identifying children and its emphasis that every encounter is an opportunity to consider developmental issues (Dworkin, 1989).

Among the most reliable and least credited developmental screening tools is parental concern. When compared with a variety of more formal developmental screening tools, parental opinions or worries have a comparable degree of specificity and sensitivity (Glascoe & Dworkin, 1995). However, there is a temptation for clinicians to dismiss parents' concerns as the products of an anxious imagination or ignorance. Studies suggest that such an attitude is fraught with the risk of future recrimination for postponing the investigation of or intervention for a valid concern. Additional screening information is contained in the child and family's history in the form of "risk factors." Positive family history for developmental disabilities, exposure to risky events or behaviors during pregnancy, very low birth weight, or failure to thrive all are factors that tend to be associated with developmental delays. Furthermore, contributing social factors such as teenage parents, educational underachievement in parent or family members, a single parent with decreased social support, and a history of abuse or neglect increase the likelihood of developmental delay or disability.

Many primary care settings undertake periodic formal screening using a variety of standardized instruments. A review of the advantages and disadvantages of such tools is beyond the scope of this chapter, but a number of excellent reviews are available (Glascoe et al., 1990). Some of these tools require direct, hands-on-evaluation of the infant or child, but others are accomplished through information collected from parents. Some can be administered at any time or age, and others are standardized for use at specific ages or in association with specific well-child visits.

When clinicians encounter developmental delays in the course of well-child care, they should consider prompt referral for early intervention services. Such a referral provides (usually at no charge) further, more in-depth evaluation of all developmental domains by qualified professionals. If the child is found to be eligible for early intervention services, parents are supported in the feeling that "something is being done" in which they are able to play an important role. In addition, further family needs may be identified and addressed through the IFSP (discussed above). The referral for early intervention need not and should not be postponed until a cause for the developmental delays is identified. As we have seen, at least a third of children may never have a specific diagnosis, and for others, the diagnostic evaluation may take months or even years to complete.

The diagnostic evaluation selected by the primary care physician may vary depending upon the individual case. The primary care provider must constantly question the thoroughness of the undertaking and whether specialists consulted are focusing on narrow issues or broad possibilities. For example, if a child with delays is suspected of having seizures, did the pediatric neurologist simply "rule out" a seizure disorder or did he or she consider other neurologic or genetic conditions affecting development? Some children will benefit from a child development clinic diagnostic team evaluation, including a developmental pediatrician and other allied health professionals (physical therapist, occupational therapist, speech pathologist, psychologist, special educator). As genetic knowledge and technology continues its rapid growth, an increasing number of conditions can be identified through genetic testing and consultation. Most children with developmental delays, physical findings of note (e.g., microcephaly, unusual facial features), or positive family histories should be considered for a genetics or dysmorphology consultation. All older children with significant delays or mental retardation, whether they have other findings or not, should be considered for chromosome analysis and fragile X testing.

In addition to the identification of developmental delays in children, a primary care practice's collection of developmental information is necessary to recognize those children who are actually losing ground developmentally. Developmental regression as opposed to simple delay raises the more ominous possibilities of an ongoing metabolic disorder. Children showing regression require developmental monitoring and should be considered for prompt metabolic screening. In addition, infants and toddlers with seizures, intractable vomiting, failure to thrive, enlargement of liver and/or spleen, and unusual movements, muscle tone, or reflexes should prompt concerns about a metabolic disorder.

Many conditions causing developmental delays are associated with sensory impairments either on a direct neurologic basis or secondary to problems such as middle ear fluid. All children with significant developmental delays should undergo formal audiologic and, in most cases, pediatric ophthalmologic evaluations. These evaluations can be informative in infants and children of any age. They may provide clues about the diagnosis (e.g., the presence of optic atrophy or "cherry red" spots) as well as important secondary challenges that will need to be addressed to make developmental and educational interventions effective.

Parents of children with developmental disability but no clear diagnosis represent a group of families in need of particularly sensitive consideration. In their efforts to understand their child's challenges and to feel confident that nothing has been overlooked, they may require second opinions. Such parents may have difficulty coming to terms with the absence of a diagnosis and may need to revisit the process at intervals or, in particular, at significant transitions in the child's or family's life (e.g., a new pregnancy, transition into special education, the emergence of a new medical problem). Such reconsideration or reassessment may also be warranted from time to time on the grounds that new information and technology is constantly emerging and providing new approaches to diagnosis. Primary care providers should include questions about this issue at each health maintenance encounter.

Chronic Condition Management in primary care

Pediatric training and primary care practice has traditionally been structured around two basic activities: (1) health promotion and preventive health maintenance ("well-child care") and (2) the diagnosis and treatment of acute pediatric illnesses. Pediatric primary care providers have played less active roles in the long-term management of chronic conditions in children (Young et al., 1994). Primary care providers have been clear about the reasons for their lack of involvement in long-term care of chronic conditions. These reasons usually are related to issues of training and preparation, time and reimbursement, and poor communication about the roles and responsibilities of specialists and specialty clinics. Pediatric primary care providers have usually trained in settings where the model for care involves specialists. For example, the trainee is expected to learn about juvenile rheumatoid arthritis (JRA) from the rheumatologist and to experience long-term management of JRA in the rheumatology clinic. Seldom is a role for the primary care provider articulated or modeled. Needless to say, specialists play a crucial role in the diagnosis and management of chronic conditions in children, but primary care physicians should play an important co-management role. Primary care providers are well positioned for a coordinating role with schools and to help monitor such generic issues regarding chronic conditions as access to information, care coordination, instructions about self-care, and advocacy for needed services (Briskin & Liptak, 1995).

A further need is for the explicit definition of roles and services. Parents, school personnel, and health care providers are all subject to confusion about responsibility for various aspects of care (Liptak & Revell, 1989). Rarely do primary care physicians specify in their referral to a specialist the exact level of involvement that they would like the specialist to provide. Such involvement might range from a one-time opinion about a specific management issue to assuming complete responsibility for issues related to a child's chronic illness. Parents are usually left in the dark about whom to call when their child develops a symptom or problem that may be related to a chronic illness. School nurses or educators in need of information about the school implications of a chronic condition or wishing to report on a child's progress may be uncertain about whom to contact.

Unfortunately, most primary pediatric care offices and clinics are structured to provide acute and well-child care through a busy schedule of brief office encounters. The extra time needed by children with chronic conditions and their families is not easily incorporated into a typical office day. To be responsive to children with chronic conditions, primary care offices should consider offering a program of Chronic Condition Management (CCM) to children with developmental disabilities, in which the entire office system (appointments, record keeping, office visit, billing) and all personnel are geared to respond. Models for such Chronic Condition Management are being developed as generic primary care guidelines as the emergence of managed care places increased responsibilities in the hands of primary care providers (Cooley, 1994b). Formalizing such care may allow for the identification of children in need of broader primary care services and in turn allow for enhanced capitated or fee-for-service reimbursement to providers who offer CCM.

Supporting the families of children with disabilities

We have seen the importance of supportive informing about the diagnosis of a genetic or disabling condition to assist parents to the best possible adaptation to their child's needs. To continue to support this adaptation, primary care providers must view families in the light of recent research about coping strategies and resilience. Older theories and assumptions were based on models of either pathology (e.g., chronic sorrow) or grief resolution rather than efforts to evaluate family strengths and resilience (Summers et al., 1989; Singer, 1991). It is now clear from many studies that even when children are affected by the most severe handicaps, at least two-thirds of families cope well. Such families experience stress and periods of great difficulty, but do not have increased rates of divorce, serious mental illness, or other long-term dysfunction (Gath & Gumley, 1984). In fact, many such families frame their overall experience in terms of enrichment, empowerment, and spiritual growth. Much depends on the coping skills and strengths that families possessed prior to the identification of illness or disability in their child. However, it is also clear that families that cope well benefit from the presence of traditional social supports (extended family, friends, and community). Coping families also appear to develop a network of "reliable allies" among those supports. Primary care providers should strive to become and consider it a privilege to be one of those reliable allies (Cooley, 1994c).

Parents of children with disabilities and chronic conditions may be exquisitely sensitive to the words professionals use in characterizing their child. The use of dated or obsolete language not only damages the precarious hopes and self-esteem of parents but also may label the well-meaning professional as backward and out of date. Primary care providers should use care in their prognostic formulations, ensuring that they are speaking from knowledge and experience, not making baseless assumptions. Individuals with disabilities have shown a preference for "people first" language. This means referring to the child before the condition (e.g., the "child with Down syndrome," not the "Down syndrome child") and avoiding global references such as "the mentally retarded" instead of saying "people with mental retardation."

It is important for primary care providers to recognize the importance of the natural supports upon which all families depend, as described above. However, many families need additional formal supports, and these are available through state and community agencies (Cooley, 1994a). Such family support services often include assistance with access to information, contact with other families, and respite care. Some states provide family support in the form of a cash stipend to families to use at their own discretion, while others have discretionary funds for which families in need can apply. Family support services have been shown to make important contributions to the successful adjustment of families to the challenges of raising a child with a disability or other chronic condition. Primary care providers need to know how such services are organized in their communities, and need to consider referring all families of children who might benefit from family supports.

Parents of children with disabilities or other chronic conditions, like other parents, are experts about their child. Their expertise needs to be respected in the

Table 2.2 The key elements of family-centered care

1. Recognizing that the family is the constant in a child's life, while the service systems and personnel within those systems fluctuate
2. Facilitating family/professional collaboration at all levels of health care
3. Honoring the racial, ethnic, cultural, and socioeconomic diversity of families
4. Recognizing family strengths and individuality and respecting different methods of coping
5. Sharing with parents, on a continuing basis and in a supportive manner, complete and unbiased information
6. Encouraging and facilitating family-to-family support and networking
7. Understanding and incorporating the developmental needs of infants, children, and adolescents and their families into health care systems
8. Implementing comprehensive policies and programs that provide emotional and financial support to meet the needs of families
9. Designing accessible health care systems that are flexible, culturally competent, and responsive to family-identified needs

process of providing health care services at all levels. The development of a health care partnership between parents and professionals has been articulated as national public health policy. The Surgeon General of the United States has issued a directive that services for children with special health care needs be "family-centered, coordinated, community-based, and culturally competent" (U. S. Department of Health and Human Services, 1987). From this beginning, the characteristics of family-centered care have been further refined as standards against which health care settings, including clinics and physician offices, can measure their success or toward which they can aspire (Table 2.2).

In conclusion, developmental disabilities and chronic conditions affecting development are common in primary pediatric health care settings. This chapter provided an approach to the primary care of children with such conditions that promotes the best outcomes for health and independence as well as supporting family strengths in the process. When it is linked to the care guidelines for specific conditions described in the remainder of this book, sound and reliable primary health care may be achieved. The combination of the generic aspects of Chronic Condition Management in primary care, the elements of family-centered care, and the specific preventive health care needs of individual children provides a powerful enhancement of the role of pediatric primary care providers in community settings.

3

Approach to preventive management for children with disabilities

Preventive health care has received much attention in the past few decades, emphasized in the United States by a series of targeted health goals culminating in *Healthy People 2000* (U.S. Public Health Service, 1991). *Healthy People 2000* set forth three goals for American health care: (1) to increase the span of healthy life, (2) to reduce health disparities among individuals, and (3) to improve access to preventive services (McGinnis & Lee, 1995). Among the priority areas were family planning, mental health and mental disorders, maternal and infant health, and clinical preventive services, areas relevant to the care of children with congenital anomalies and syndromes. In their mid-decade assessment of progress toward the goals of *Healthy People 2000*, McGinnis & Lee (1995) cited reductions in childhood lead poisoning and accidents, with increases in childhood immunization rates. These results provide optimism that targeted health care goals can improve preventive care in the general pediatric population. This chapter will consider the rationale, justification, and practical approach to preventive care for a specialized pediatric population, those with congenital malformations. A major advantage of the preventive management approach to genetic disease is that it balances some of the negative consequences that may arise from genetic diagnosis (Holtzman, 1988, 1989).

General considerations in preventive medicine

Rose (1992) emphasized that few diseases are the inescapable lot of humanity, citing that 10 percent of eastern Indian children die before age 1 year while only 1 percent do here. This variability of disease offers opportunities for prevention if the causes and natural history of complications can be defined. Prevention is possible even for genetic diseases, where complications can be forestalled even if the disease cannot be treated. Phenylketonuria, sickle cell anemia, and cystic fibrosis are examples of genetic disorders where preventive management can greatly alter the natural history of disease.

Marge (1984), in the context of communication disorders, has discussed prevention as a primary, secondary, or tertiary process. Primary prevention would involve eliminating the onset of the disorder, as in the removal of an individual from a noisy workplace to prevent hearing loss. Secondary prevention would involve early detection of a problem that already has occurred, as in auditory screening of children at school. Tertiary prevention is reduction of the detected problem through rehabilitation, as in use of hearing aids for individuals with hearing loss (Marge, 1984). In the context of genetic diseases and congenital anomalies, primary prevention consists of genetic or medical counseling to prevent the occurrence of a disorder (e.g., avoidance of alcohol during pregnancy, folic acid supplementation to lower the incidence of neural tube defects). This book emphasizes secondary and tertiary prevention, exemplified by recognizing strabismus in a child with fetal alcohol syndrome and by providing optical or surgical treatment. Preventive management of genetic disorders can be defined as the avoidance or amelioration of complications in patients with genetic disease.

Justification of preventive strategies

Although the rationale for prevention as improving health is sound, the justification of particular preventive measures is often difficult. Table 3.1 lists several rationales for preventive strategies and juxtaposes them with conflicts that may arise. Health is a basic human right, but health, like beauty, is often in the eyes of the beholder. Doctors may define it as the absence of serious illness while the individual defines it as a sense of "well-being." The very definition of "health" is complex, since diseases are often extremes along a continuum of measurement (e.g., hypertension, hypoglycemia) rather than binary well/ill states (Rose, 1992). Lead poisoning is an example where the threshold of "disease" has dramatic implications for the efforts made in primary prevention (Schaffer & Campbell, 1994). Progressive lowering of the tolerable childhood lead level to 10 micrograms per deciliter of blood dramatically affects the costs and implications of intervention.

The process of diagnosis itself may lead to a loss of well-being because the person is now aware of his or her differences and potential morbidity. Diagnoses may also become labels that cause family, employment, or insurance consequences (Holtzman, 1989). These problems emphasize that diagnostic screening for the purpose of prevention must lead to clear-cut medical benefits for the patient. Individual benefits may also conflict with societal benefits. A dramatic example is when maternal screening must be considered for the infant's health, as when routine HIV testing of pregnant women can lead to beneficial zidovudine therapy for their infant (Stiehm, 1995).

In estimating the medical benefits of early detection and screening, it is also a complex task to define the appropriate outcome measures (Wilkin et al., 1993). Justification of preventive measures for children with genetic disorders and/or disabilities may require degrees of functional and/or quality of life as outcomes, since

Table 3.1 Justifications for prevention

Rationale	Conflict
Ethics	
Health is a universal human right	Is health defined as the absence of disease or a feeling of well-being?
	Personal "well-being" versus personal knowledge of impending complications and labeling as "diseased"
Elimination of disease and disability from society	Individual freedom of choice versus benefits for society
	Is health defined as the absence of disease or a feeling of well-being?
Outcomes	
Preventive measure should improve patient outcomes	Mortality versus quality of life as outcomes
Epidemiologic	
Target diseases are sufficiently common to have important consequences for society	Large benefits to a community may offer little to each individual.
	Screening general population versus high-risk population
Cost-effectiveness	
Early detection of illness	Postponement rather than elimination of disease
	Screening general population versus high-risk population
Disease should be prevented or modified by early detection	Must be resources for counseling and follow-up care to realize benefits

overall morbidity or mortality may not be avoided (see below). Quality of life is often a difficult outcome measure (Hennessy et al., 1994).

Disease incidence is another general issue in prevention (Table 3.1): how many people are affected by a particular preventive strategy? Rose (1992) described a "prevention paradox" in which measures bringing large benefits to a community may offer little to each individual. People may avoid seat belts or helmets because the probability of self-injury is low, despite indisputable evidence of benefit to the general population. It is necessary to immunize several hundred children to prevent one death, and some parents seize on this fact to avoid the pain for their child.

These considerations point out the differences between general versus high-risk prevention strategies (Rose, 1992). In general or population strategies, all individuals undergo the intervention. General screening goes to the root of the problem and seeks to eliminate it from the entire population. All people undergo the same screening procedure, and there is no singling out of one group for specialized management until the screening results are obtained. From the viewpoint of genetic disease, diagnostic activities such as newborn screening would qualify as general population screening that leads to disease elimination by dietary therapy. False positive values can be a significant problem in general population screening, since large numbers of individuals may be identified as "abnormal" and require additional intervention.

The alternative strategy of focusing on a high-risk population allows the intervention to be more closely matched to needs of the individual (Rose, 1992). Furthermore, the screening can be more selective and cost-effective than mass screening (Table 3.1). A disadvantage of high-risk screening is that it labels the individual rather than initiating general measures for the entire population (e.g., cholesterol screening). This concern reiterates the need to have effective treatment as part of the rationale for preventive screening. A higher frequency of false positive values can be tolerated in high-risk screening, since fewer individuals will be affected. This rationale underlies the application of maternal serum α-fetoprotein screening to women over 35 rather than the entire population. However, as evidenced by the anxiety and additional testing that followed the adoption of maternal serum α-fetoprotein screening, any medical screening for complications must be weighed against the possibility of false positive or ambiguous results. High-risk screening is the major focus of this book, following the rationale that genetic or developmental diagnoses imply specific interventions and preventive measures.

Cost-effectiveness is a strong justification for prevention, and this has been accomplished effectively for measures such as the measles–mumps–rubella vaccine (White et al., 1985). However, prevention of heart attacks by decreasing cigarette smoking may be socially desirable but not cost-effective if the heart attacks are merely postponed to older ages (Rose, 1992). The eventual toll of age often requires humanitarian rather than strict economic arguments, returning again to quality-of-life outcomes rather than longevity. Cost and cost-effectiveness obviously depend on other characteristics of screening, such as incidence and severity of the target disease and its predictability in a selected population (Table 3.1).

In summary, the underlying themes of beneficence and health optimization offer powerful rationales for preventive medicine. Justification of specific preventive measures is difficult because of ambiguities in defining health, outcomes, and cost-effectiveness. The justification of any given preventive measure will usually involve several considerations (ethics, outcomes, costs) that may be difficult to assess in children with disabilities.

Problems with physician compliance and the value of preventive checklists

Despite their acceptance of preventive guidelines, physicians often are slow to implement them (Lewis, 1988; Scott et al., 1992). Several barriers for implementation have been cited, including (1) organizational rigidity of the health care system which can squelch new initiatives, (2) lack of compelling evidence for improved outcomes or lack of knowledge of these improvements, (3) a disease-oriented tradition that makes physicians reactive to symptoms rather than proactive towards prevention, (4) constraints that eliminate time required for additional history, examination and counseling, and (5) lack of resources (Thompson et al., 1995).

The rigidity of health care systems may reflect the growing input of non-physicians or a lack of education of older physician-managers. Chi-Lum (1995) commented on the inadequacy of education regarding preventive measures in medical school curricula. The difficulty of selecting and measuring outcomes has already been alluded to. Unfortunately, as cited in the foreword to *Bright Futures* (Greene, 1994), there are few studies demonstrating efficacy of biomedical preventive measures and virtually none demonstrating efficacy of psychosocial measures (Wilson, 1995). Funding is one of the most severe problems in implementing preventive care. Kottke et al. (1993) points out that funding and resources correlate well with the willingness of physicians to devote the extra time needed for preventive practices.

On the positive side, Thompson et al. (1995) reported the successes of a preventive care program operated within the Group Health Program of Puget Sound, a health maintenance organization. This program achieved an 89 percent completion rate for childhood immunizations, a change in bicycle helmet use from 4 to 48 percent, and a 67 percent decrease in bicycle head injuries. Thompson et al. (1995) concluded that several factors were responsible for these and other accomplishments: (1) a population-wide viewpoint to prioritize prevention objectives, (2) evidence-based criteria to demonstrate benefits of preventive measures, (3) involvement of practitioners in the formulation of the preventive guidelines, (4) provision of reminders and checklists to patients and physicians, and (5) feedback to practitioners on positive population trends.

To focus on a major strategy employed in this book, there have been several studies demonstrating benefits of checklists on the delivery of preventive care (Cheney & Ramsdel 1987; Maiman et al., 1988; Johns et al., 1992; Jackson, 1996). Regarding the use of a checklist for behavioral problems in pediatric practice, over half of the 556 pediatricians who responded to the survey felt that checklists were valuable but about 30 percent felt that they were overly time consuming (Cheng et al., 1996). Availability and ease of use are clearly important if the value of checklists is to be realized.

Defining the effectiveness of preventive measures

Types of outcomes in people with disabilities

A health outcome is a result or visible effect that occurs after a health care interven-tion. The circumstances of the intervention, such as the type of personnel, the dose of medication, the duration of therapy, are often called *inputs*. It is clear that health care objectives influence selection of outcome criteria (Wilkin et al., 1993), and that these objectives in turn reflect perceptions of health care needs. To speak of a need, such as inadequate immunization rates, is to imply a goal of health care; needs are subject to value judgments about what should be appropriate goals and what con-stitutes deficiency from these goals (Wilkin et al., 1993).

It follows that the outcomes selected for assessing the health care of children with congenital anomalies and syndromes are highly dependent on attitudes toward the disabled. When the goals of society were oriented towards primary prevention of mental retardation, as in the eugenics movement, then the outcome measure was existence and the ideal outcome elimination (Gould, 1981). When the purported benefits of natural settings led to enthusiasm for institutions, then the outcomes were proportions of individuals receiving these benefits. Now, when inclusive schooling and job training are encouraged to allow integration with society at large, degrees of independent function are more pertinent outcomes in assessing health care of persons with disabilities.

The shift from binary outcomes such as life or death to graded outcomes such as function has also occurred for chronic disease in general. Mortality outcomes can be useful endpoints, as shown by Blair et al. (1995) in demonstrating reduced mor-tality for males with greater physical fitness. However, in chronic diseases such as asthma, functional indicators such as school attendance, sports participation, etc., will be more appropriate for the endpoints of current interest: household smoking, newer bronchodilator medications, home nebulizers, etc. For chronic diseases, natural history becomes an important baseline against which outcomes can be measured (Wilkin et al., 1993). Because of the rarity of disorders and an emphasis on diagnosis, natural history is poorly defined for many genetic syndromes. Natural history comparisons also require long-term studies, while changes in levels of function can be measured year by year.

Functional outcomes in children with disabilities

In order to appreciate functional status as an endpoint of health care, definitions offered by the World Health Organization are helpful (Wilkin et al., 1993). As men-tioned previously, health can be defined as a state of complete physical, mental, and social well-being rather than merely the absence of disease or infirmity. In addition, the functional status of individuals can be categorized by the following definitions:

Impairment: Loss or abnormality of psychiatric, physiologic or anatomic structure and function (e.g., loss of limb).

Disability: restriction of ability to perform an activity in manner or range considered normal for age.

Handicap: Disadvantage to a person resulting from impairment or disability.

As a parallel to the usual sequence of disease leading to pathogenesis leading to manifestations, the following functional sequence can then be imagined: Disease (intrinsic situation) leads to an impairment (experience exteriorized), which leads to a disability (experience objectified), which leads to a handicap (experience socialized). Outcomes can be drawn from each level, with disease or impairment being measures of individual biology and disability or handicap being measures of individual and society. The modern perspective on children with special needs shifts emphasis from disease diagnosis and impairment to the ability of the child to lead a normal life (Wilkin et al., 1983).

The first instrument for measurement of functional status was the activities of daily living (ADL) scale developed by the staff at Benjamin Rose Hospital, Cleveland, in 1959. Their underlying concept was that disease caused loss of functional capacities in a particular order, and that rehabilitation restored these capacities in reverse order. Interventions could thus be evaluated by the level of function restored. While the ADL scale focuses on basic activities of daily living (mobility, dressing, toileting) appropriate for the severely disabled, other scales have evolved to evaluate more complex functions such as laundry, housework, managing money, or employment. Measures have thus become more inclusive, evaluating not only disease or impairment, but also disability and handicap as discussed above.

Despite the potential utility of functional scales in assessing preventive management interventions, there are virtually no studies combining such assessments with the natural history of particular genetic syndromes. Surprisingly, reliability and validity have not been well demonstrated even for the Cleveland ADL scale (Wilkin et al., 1993), which is not very sensitive to small changes in the patient's condition. Strict functional assessment is also rather limited, since mental health or social support will obviously influence function. Any overall quality-of-life measurement should also include some estimate of patient satisfaction or well-being. A positive sense of well-being correlates strongly with an individual's motivation for preventive health practices (Gill & Feinstein, 1994; Hennessy et al., 1994). Such estimates have obvious difficulties when applied to people with disabilities, but more emphasis on assessment of personal well-being would parallel the emphasis on self-advocacy in the disability movement.

Several types of measures will be needed for a meaningful assessment of quality of life for people with disabilities. Examples include nominal outcomes (e.g., male/female), ordinal outcomes (e.g., severe, moderate, mild), interval outcomes (e.g., temperature), or ratio outcomes (e.g., developmental quotients). Some of these measures are part of functional scales such as the Guttman (ordinal measure of ability to walk 5, 10 or 50 meters) and Likert scale (ordinal measures of "strongly agree" to "strongly disagree," "most important" to "least important"; Wilkin et al., 1993). The numerical approach facilitates statistical analysis for correlations with preventive measures and for inter-test reliability (i.e., Kappa analysis). Issues in the measurement of quality of life for individuals with disabilities include the definition of disease-specific norms against which the disabilities are measured and timing and validity of individual functional assessments.

Msall et al. (1994a, b) provided an instrument that assesses functional independence in children and correlates with their stage of development. The WeeFIM scale includes a broad range of activities plus some psychosocial factors such as parental circumstances (Msall, 1996). If combined with measures of self-satisfaction, the WeeFIM scale should be useful for assessing changes in outcome as a result of preventive interventions. Although there are few studies linking preventive measures with functional outcome in children with disabilities, some simple theoretical examples can illustrate the importance of anticipatory health care in improving quality of life. These examples provide rationales for the preventive checklists in this book, and are obvious avenues for future research.

Consider a child with Down syndrome who might be scored as full function (3 points), mildly impaired (2 points), moderately impaired (1 point), or severely impaired (0 points) for a variety of skills and activities enjoyed by the typical young adult (e.g., reading, sports, church attendance, cooking, biking, driving). For 50 activities evaluated on a typical daily living scale, an average adult would score 150 points, while an optimally functioning person with Down syndrome would score about 120 points (80 percent). The young adult with Down syndrome would have mild dysfunction in activities such as reading or writing, and severe dysfunction in activities such as driving a car or managing money.

If, on the other hand, the person with Down syndrome had unrecognized hypothyroidism or pulmonary hypertension due to inoperable cardiac disease, their estimated score would drop to 90 points (60 percent) or 70 points (46 percent), respectively. Prevention of these complications by early thyroid or cardiac screening as recommended on the Down syndrome checklist thus would have a dramatic improvement of the child's eventual quality of daily living. Outcome studies that build on this simple analysis should one day provide compelling justification for preventive measures in children with congenital anomalies and syndromes. The outcome analyses must take into account the average disability/handicap expected for a particular disorder, assess a full range of activities, avoid prejudice about capabilities, and include measures of self-satisfaction and well-being.

Cost and health efficiency issues: Influence of health care reform

Cost-effectiveness is also a complex issue when used to judge preventive management interventions for patients with disabilities. It is ideal when an intervention is cost-effective, as for measles–mumps–rubella immunization programs that save $14 for each dollar invested (White et al., 1985). Increased hospitalization or chronic care expenses will be substantial for disorders such as undetected pulmonary hypertension, but less dramatic for a child with undetected hypothyroidism. In fact, the costs of endocrinology referral and treatment/follow-up may increase costs compared to the individual that is never screened for hypothyroidism. In order to demonstrate cost-effectiveness for measures such as thyroid or audiology screening, the lost income and increased living costs resulting from the cognitive or hearing impairments must be calculated. These will obviously depend on the social context (handicap), since an adult living on the family farm may experience fewer economic consequences than an adult seeking employment and independent living in an urban setting.

While health care professionals must balance the importance of a preventive care measure against its cost, there is no simple formula that can take into account both cost and quality-of-life issues. The philosophy of this book is to include all preventive measures that can significantly impact the quality-of-life, consistent with the principles of screening mentioned above (e.g., screening where symptoms cannot be relied upon and where an abnormal result implies some type of beneficial intervention). An example would be the consideration of cranial MRI imaging for infants with craniosynostosis (Chapter 14) or mucopolysaccharidosis (Chapter 19) but not for children with neurofibromatosis (Chapter 13); the high frequency of asymptomatic hydrocephalus in the first two disorders, together with a discrete intervention (shunt surgery), provides the rationale. For interventions like MRI scanning, where children are subjected to inconvenience or risk (anesthesia), a footnote is always added to emphasize that clinical judgment is needed.

In the future, preventive care for children with disabilities is likely to be challenged by managed care and federal providers. Children with disabilities are part of a large fraction of children with chronic diseases – 25.2 percent between ages 6 and 11, 35.3 percent between ages 12 and 17 years (Jessop & Stein, 1995). Children with chronic disease are more costly for healthcare, and special "carve-outs" may be needed to protect families from loss of health insurance or exclusion from managed care organizations (Neff & Anderson, 1995). These considerations dramatize the need for outcomes analysis of preventive measures, but should not deter health care professionals from their responsibilities for good medical care.

Designing a preventive care plan for the child with disability

As summarized in previous sections, the overriding rationale for preventive care as presented in this book is improvement in quality-of-life. Although it is clear that more research is needed to prove the value and/or cost-effectiveness of many preventive measures, the prime determinants here are the frequency of a potential complication, its impact on quality of life, and the effectiveness of an intervention in avoiding the complication. Our concept of using a table of complications to design a preventive management checklist is drawn from the idea of a "burden of suffering" inflicted by an illness or medical complication. The "burden of suffering" combines the prevalence with the severity of illness, and has been used frequently in justifying prevention programs (U.S. Public Health Service, 1994). For a child with a congenital anomaly or syndrome, the frequency of a complication combined with its impact on quality of life would constitute the "burden of suffering" that justifies prevention.

General pediatric preventive measures

Some preventive measures are assumed rather than explicitly mentioned in this book. Ensuring that a patient has a health care funding source and an identified physician or clinic is extremely important. Insurance coverage resulted in a twofold probability of having regular medical care and a twofold increase in preventive measures (breast examination, digital rectal examination) as demonstrated a survey of 102,263 Americans (Centers for Disease Control, 1995). Regular pediatric health care is obviously a crucial prerequisite to prevention, and a major goal of this book is to give primary physicians confidence in providing their extensive expertise to children with developmental and genetic disorders.

In infants with severely disabling disorders, the first pediatric decision may be whether treatment is justified at all. The Baby Doe infant with Down syndrome and duodenal atresia prompted much discussion of treatment options and was a factor in the development of hospital ethics committees (Bucciarelli & Eitzman, 1988). It is now accepted that all infants should receive basic life support including feeding and fluids. Extraordinary surgical or resuscitative measures may be withheld after discussion with the parents and ethics committee (Raffin, 1991), but it is essential that accurate prognostic information be available. Parent group information can be very helpful in these decisions, and the *Exceptional Parent* magazine provides a directory of parent groups that is used frequently in this book.

Most infants with congenital anomalies and syndromes will survive the infantile period and require long-term pediatric management. Important sources of recommendations for preventive well-child care include the books *Bright Futures* (Greene, 1994) and *The Canadian Guide to Clinical Preventive Health Care* (Canadian Task Force on the Periodic Health Examination, 1994). The checklists in this book are based on the recommendations in *Bright Futures* (Greene, 1994), which include recommendations for adolescent care (Jenkins & Saxena, 1995).

Part of pediatric management is to monitor development, growth, and behavior, since abnormalities in these areas were estimated to occur in 27.3 percent of children in the average pediatric practice (Horwitz et al., 1992). However, in Australia, only 82 percent of pediatricians indicated that they did developmental screening (Rossiter, 1993). Specialized growth and developmental charts are available for some genetic disorders, and these are referenced in the appropriate chapters.

Anticipatory guidance is another aspect of pediatric practice which is not specifically listed in the preventive management checklists. Many of these recommendations must be modified or extended for the child with disabilities, as exemplified by the ages needing child-proofing of the house for medicines or toxins. The whole approach of preventive management is an aspect of anticipatory guidance, and the information on specific disorders should be useful in guiding the expectations and modifications adopted by families.

Preventive measures for children with disabilities

Children in general pediatric practices have a high risk for psychosocial and developmental problems, and these two factors often coincide (Horwitz et al., 1992). Knowledge about developmental disabilities is thus important, and extends beyond their association with many isolated anomalies and most syndromes discussed in this book. Prediction of developmental disability may arise from a syndrome diagnosis, or result from functional assessment during the first few years of life. While Chapter 2 reviews the management of children with developmental disabilities, the condensed recommendations mandated by a standard checklist format require some discussion here.

When a disorder confers a high risk of genetic recurrence, seizures, or chronic care/learning problems, then specific referral to the respective genetics, neurology, or developmental pediatric clinic is suggested on the checklist. Even when referral is not mandated by specific circumstances, evaluation by these three specialties should be considered in any child with developmental disability. The combined referrals should lead to a consensus diagnosis, discussion of prenatal diagnostic options, and (in the case of developmental pediatrics) give valuable insight into psychosocial problems and cognitive testing. Which of these specialties becomes more involved will then depend on the primary diagnosis and the specialty center. Many genetics clinics are oriented towards diagnosis rather than ongoing care, while disorders such as cerebral palsy or spina bifida are traditionally managed by developmental pediatricians. Knowledge of various neuropsychologic testing instruments and specific learning disorders is usually much greater in developmental pediatric or neurology clinics.

Coincident with appropriate specialty referral should be enrollment in an early intervention (ages 0–3 years) or special preschool (4–6 years) program. Early intervention is listed on the checklists, and this should be extended to include the appropriate preschool or special education programs when the disability is recognized after infancy. Also important during infancy is appreciation that the child with neurologic problems usually has feeding problems. These can result from hypo- or hypertonia and include a poor suck, dysphagia, chronic aspiration, gastroesophageal reflux, or textural aversions. A team approach is often effective (Couriel et al., 1993). Attention to feeding is indicated under the "evaluate" column of preventive management checklists.

One of the important roles of the primary physician is to provide information about various services and life decisions applicable to patients with disabilities and their families. Parents should know their rights for education under the Individuals with Disabilities Education Act (I.D.E.A.). This act mandates that an individualized educational plan (I.E.P.) be established for each child with disabilities, gives rights for parents to participate in their child's I.E.P., and provides due process as a recourse if the parents are unhappy with the plan for their child. In other words, the I.D.E.A. provides ammunition for inclusion of the child in at least some regular classrooms. Attention to school issues is indicated by "school progress" under the "evaluate" column of the preventive management checklists, and by "school options" under the "refer/counsel" column. Children require specific attention during transitions between school levels, particularly if they are required to change agencies as in the transition between early intervention and preschool programs.

Parents should also begin to learn about insurance and financial issues as soon as a disability is suspected in their child. In 1935, Title V of the social security act provided federal funds for care of "crippled" children, later designated as children with special health care needs (Biehl, 1996). In 1965, the medicaid program was created in Title XIX of the social security law, and eligibility will provide coverage for many costs of outpatient preventive care.

Financial counselors or social workers are available at most hospitals for consultation on these issues. Parents should also recognize that their child will become independent at age 18 and, together with exposure to possible abuse or fraud, will lose medicaid benefits if he or she has assets above certain limits. There are tax considerations in establishing guardianship to safeguard the child, and special needs trusts are available to avert loss of federal benefits after the parent is deceased. Most health care professionals are not expert in these issues, but should become familiar with community resources such as the ARC (Association for Retarded Citizens) and specialized legal services. Financial and insurance issues are included in the "family support" reminder under the "refer/counsel" column of the checklists (see the Preface for further discussion of the "family support" reminder).

Because many genetic and developmental disorders have increased risk for behavioral problems, screening for abnormalities in the child or family is an important aspect of health assessment. Behavioral screening instruments are available (Herman-Staab, 1994), and referral to psychologic or psychiatric specialists should be made early rather than later when adverse consequences have occurred. Counseling strategies can be effective, as shown by the 44 percent reduction in drug use achieved by annual workshops in a high school setting (Botvin et al., 1995).

Specific medical guidelines for congenital malformations and syndromes

As discussed previously, the rationales for improved quality of life (realization of functional potential) and for screening a high-risk population (defined by the anomaly or syndrome) provide a solid foundation for using preventive medical checklists in children with genetic and/or developmental disorders. Our standard checklist format uses separate columns for general pediatric, screening, examination (history or physical), and special counseling or referral needs. Checklists have been developed for two anomalies (cerebral palsy, spina bifida), two associations, and 26 syndromes (Table 3.2). Syndromes with an incidence above 1 in 25,000 were selected for consideration based on the likelihood that an average pediatric practice would include at least one affected individual. Less extensive discussion of preventive management recommendations is provided for an additional 120 disorders.

The preventive guidelines used here for Down syndrome, fragile X syndrome, achondroplasia, neurofibromatosis-1, and Marfan syndrome are essentially those of the American Academy of Pediatrics (Committee on Genetics, 1994, 1995a, b, 1996a, b). Even for these consensus recommendations, justification by outcomes analysis or cost-effectiveness has not been performed (see above discussion). In many cases, complications encountered in other disorders could be related to the consensus guidelines from the American Academy of Pediatrics. For example, the incidence of chronic otitis in Williams syndrome (43 percent) is comparable to that in Down syndrome (40–60 percent), allowing consensus recommendations for audiology screening in Down syndrome to be extrapolated to patients with Williams syndrome. Particular caution was exerted in recommending imaging studies or other interventions that would require anesthesia in young children; these recommendations are usually qualified by a footnote that emphasizes the need for clinical judgment.

An overview of the resulting guidelines for 30 disorders (assuming diagnosis in the neonatal period) shows that a total of 3140 preventive measures were derived for 20 pediatric visits from birth to age 18 years (104 recommendations per disorder). Nine types of preventive measures were specified including imaging studies (3.2 percent of recommendations), laboratory tests (6.7 percent), functional screening (3.6 percent), screening by examination (22 percent), screening by

Table 3.2 The more common pediatric syndromes and metabolic dysplasias

Syndrome (Incidence in live births)	Impairment or disability (Chapter)
Down syndrome (1 in 600–1000)	Mental, heart, thyroid, hearing, vision, spine (7)
VATER association (1 in 620)	Heart, kidney, lumbar spine (5)
Fetal alcohol syndrome (1 in 670)	Mental, heart, hearing, vision, skeleton (6)
Fragile X syndrome (1 in 800)	Mental, vision (8)
47,XXY (Klinefelter) syndrome (1 in 1000)	Hearing, vision (8)
Fetal hydantoin syndrome (1 in 2000)	Feeding, hearing, vision (6)
Noonan syndrome (1 in 1000–2500)	Mental, heart, hearing, vision (10)
Diabetic embryopathy (1 in 3000)	Heart, vision, spine (6)
Neurofibromatosis type I (1 in 3000)	Mental, brain, nerves, spine, skeleton (13)
Turner syndrome (1 in 5000)	Heart, hearing, kidney (8)
Goldenhar syndrome (1 in 5600)	Mental, heart, hearing, vision, kidney, lungs (15)
Trisomy 13/18 (1 in 8000)	Mental, hearing, vision, heart, kidney, skeleton (7)
Marfan syndrome (1 in 10,000)	Heart, vision, skeleton, joints (16)
Arthrogryposis, amyoplasia (1 in 10,000)	Feeding, lungs, joints, muscles (19)
Cornelia de Lange (1 in 10,000)	Mental, feeding, heart, hearing, vision (10)
Ehlers–Danlos syndromes (1 in 10–20,000)	Heart, vision, skin, joints (16)
Beckwith–Wiedemann (1 in 17,000)	Abdomen, liver, kidney, tumors (12)
Osteogenesis imperfectas (1 in 20,000)	Hearing, skeleton, joints (11)
Prader–Willi syndrome (1 in 16–25,000)	Mental, feeding, vision, skin (9)
Achondroplasia (1 in 16–25,000)	Skeletal, spine, foramen magnum, joints (11)
Glycogen storage diseases (1 in 20–25,000)	Liver, kidney, skeleton (20)
Saethre–Chotzen syndrome (1 in 25,000)	Cranial, spine, vision, hearing (14)
Tuberous sclerosis (1 in 25,000)	Mental, heart, kidney, skeleton (13)
Shprintzen/del (22) syndrome (1 in 25,000)	Mental, heart, hearing, vision (9)
CHARGE association (1 in 20–50,000)	Mental, heart, hearing, vision, skeleton (6)
Williams syndrome (1 in 20–50,000)	Mental, heart, hearing, vision (9)
Mucopolysaccharidoses (1 in 25,000)	Mental, brain, vision, hearing, skeleton (19)
Peroxisomal disorders (1 in 10–50,000)	Mental, hearing, vision, liver, kidney, skeleton (19)

history (29 percent), examination for key findings (10.5 percent), specialty referral (14 percent), referral for special services (7 percent), and counseling (4 percent). Timing of the preventive measures includes 35 percent for 7 visits during infancy, 33 percent for 6 visits between ages 15 months and 6 years, and 32 percent for 7 visits between ages 8 and 18.

The additional costs of these guidelines can be estimated relative to the baseline cost of routine pediatric care. These cost estimates are very general, since the costs of a well-child visit ($36.19 to $49.94) or standard immunizations ($9.95 to $25.51 for diphtheria-tetanus-pertussis and $11.25 to $28.00 for hemophilus influenza) are quite variable (Freed et al., 1996). The baseline cost for routine pediatric care was estimated to be $1500 (1995 dollars) with a range from $1320 to $1670 per healthy individual. Additional costs imposed by the preventive care recommendations (estimated from birth to age 18) was highest for children with Down syndrome or CHARGE association (3.2 times baseline) and lowest for children with Saethre–Chotzen syndrome (1.8 times baseline). Costs are heavily dependent on the need for specialty referral, reaching 5.5 times baseline in children with CHARGE or VATER association with long-term survival and multiple anomalies. Costs would also be higher if additional physician time (mean of 3 extra history/physical items per visit) is considered.

Because of the increased costs and time demanded by preventive care, physicians must decide about the utility of individual recommendations based on their patient, family, and experience. It is again emphasized that use of a preventive checklist improved compliance in several controlled studies (Cheney & Ramsdel, 1987; Maiman et al., 1988; Johns et al., 1992), and that the development of clinical practice guidelines has been endorsed by the Agency for Health Care Policy and Research (1993) and by the Division of Health Care Services at the Institute of Medicine (Field, 1994). Indeed, many managed care programs have emphasized preventive services and even designed their own clinical practice guidelines. These trends offer hope that measures to improve the quality of life of patients with congenital anomalies and syndromes will become an integral component of pediatric care.

Part II

The management of selected single congenital anomalies and associations

4

Congenital anomalies associated with developmental disability

Cerebral palsy and congenital brain defects

Terminology

Cerebral palsy embraces a range of conditions characterized by disordered movement or posture resulting from a nonprogressive brain lesion or injury occurring prenatally or in early childhood (Palmer & Hoon, 1995). Cerebral palsy may be further defined by its topography (quadraplegia, hemiplegia, diplegia) or by its pathophysiology (pyramidal or extrapyramidal). Pyramidal lesions are associated with spastic types of cerebral palsy, while extrapyramidal insults are associated with hypotonic, choreoathetoid, and ataxic cerebral palsy. Overlap among the forms of cerebral palsy is common.

Cerebral dysgenesis refers to alterations in the formation of the central nervous system (e.g., abnormal cellular migration or proliferation) resulting in congenital defects in the size, structure, and function of the brain. Most of these defects result in significant neurologic impairment, including cerebral palsy and mental retardation (Gabriel & McComb, 1985; Rosenbloom, 1995). For example, lissencephaly (smooth brain) or agyria is a disorder of neuronal migration associated with severe developmental consequences (Dobyns, 1987). Absence of the corpus callosum includes a spectrum of alterations in the formation of midline cortical structures with diverse etiologies and a wide range of developmental outcomes (Jeret et al., 1987). Porencephalic cysts result from a specific, destructive event such as a vascular accident *in utero*.

Historical diagnosis and management

Taxonomy and classification were of great interest to early clinicians resulting in much of the terminology still in use (Ingram, 1984). William Little, an orthopedic surgeon, is often credited with the earliest efforts at classification (Little, 1862) and cerebral palsy was once called Little's disease. Sigmund Freud advanced the notion of predisposing factors to expand upon the more narrow assumptions of Little that cerebral palsy resulted from obstetric trauma and anoxia. Freud was also critical of

49

early efforts to classify cerebral palsy on the basis of etiology or pathology rather than clinical findings until direct causal relationships could be established. With notable exceptions, such as the relationship between kernicterus and choreoathetoid cerebral palsy, the issue of causality remains unresolved one hundred years later (Freud, 1897).

Interventions for cerebral palsy have mostly been grounded in notions of massage, bracing, and orthopedic surgery (Cruickshank, 1976; Carlson et al., 1997; Scrutton and Baird, 1997); they have also aimed at the limitation of disability and enhancement of function. Neurosurgical and orthopedic surgical techniques attempted in the early 1900s provided the basis for the use of tendon release and relocation and dorsal rhizotomy in the present. Following the establishment of federal funding for "crippled children's services" in the United States in 1935, multidisciplinary clinics have emerged as the state-of-the-art approach to cerebral palsy.

Incidence, etiology, and differential diagnosis

As discussed in Chapter 2, incidence figures are subject to variability as the result of methodologic factors including definitions of cerebral palsy, exclusions by severity or other criteria, and ascertainment. The overall prevalence of significant cerebral palsy ranges from 1.5 to 2.5 per 1000 live births (Kuban & Leviton, 1994; Pharoah et al., 1998). Tables 4.1 and 4.2 portray the distribution of cerebral palsy according to various subtypes.

The largest prospective samplings of prevalence, causal associations, and risk factors for cerebral palsy have used data from the Collaborative Perinatal Study of the National Institute of Neurological and Communicative Disorders and Stroke. The outcomes for 43,437 *full-term* children were reviewed by Naeye et al. (1989). Among the 150 children with CP in this population, only 9 cases (6 percent) appeared attributable to birth asphyxia. Of the 34 children with quadriplegic cerebral palsy, possible causes were apparent in 71 percent with 53 percent appearing attributable to congenital disorders, 14 percent to birth asphyxia, and 8 percent to CNS infections. Among the children with nonquadriplegic CP, congenital disorders appeared to account for about one third of the cases and congenital infections for about 5 percent. Birth asphyxia was not significantly associated with nonquadraplegic CP, and no cause could be identified in 60 percent of these patients. In another analysis of the Collaborative Perinatal Project data for both term and preterm births, Nelson & Ellenberg (1986) found a "defect" (congenital malformation, low birth weight, microcephaly) in 91 percent of the children who developed cerebral palsy.

Table 4.3 summarizes data from many studies of risk factors associated with cerebral palsy according to the timing with respect to gestation and birth. Additional

Table 4.1 Distribution of types of cerebral palsy

Diagnosis	Number	Percentage of total number	Percentage of those of known type
Dyskinetic	52	9.8	12.5
Spastic	270	51.2	64.7
Ataxic	39	7.4	9.4
Dyskinetic spastic	40	7.6	9.6
Dyskinetic ataxic	3	0.5	0.7
Ataxic spastic	13	2.5	3.1
Other types and type not known[a]	110	21.0	
Total	527	100	100

Note:

[a] The dyskinetic group includes choreoathetosis and dystonia: six cases were described only as hypotonic, but these are included under other types as it was not clear how many had true hypotonic cerebral palsy.

Table 4.2. Distribution of subgroups described as spastic

	Number	Percentage
Hemiplegia	97	36
Diplegia	74	28
Quadriplegia	71	26
Monoplegia	6	2
Paraplegia	5	2
Other	17	6
Total	270	100

risk factors of interest include maternal use of thyroid or estrogen hormones during pregnancy, nonvertex and face presentations at birth, and family history of cerebral palsy. Birth asphyxia or related factors have proven to be weak predictors of later cerebral palsy. Newborn encephalopathy and recurrent neonatal seizures are more strongly linked with cerebral palsy, though this may be an associative rather than causal relationship (Kuban & Leviton, 1994).

In contrast to the weak associations of prenatal and birth events in term infants, a birth weight below 1500 grams confers a 25–30 times increased risk of cerebral palsy (Kuban & Leviton, 1994). One-third of all babies who later develop cerebral palsy weighed less than 2500 grams at birth: by far the strongest factors associated with low birth weight and the later development of cerebral palsy are the presence

Table 4.3 Factors identified in epidemiologic studies as associated with cerebral palsy

Before pregnancy
History of fetal wastage
Long menstrual cycles

During pregnancy
Low social class
Congenital malformation
Fetal growth retardation
Twin gestation
Abnormal fetal presentation

During labor and delivery
Premature separation of the placenta

During the early postnatal period
Newborn encephalopathy

of periventricular leukomalacia or other parenchymal brain injury. Whether periventricular leukomalacia causes cerebral palsy or simply shares a common origin remains uncertain. These factors provide strong justification for brain imaging in children at risk.

Though the differential diagnosis of cerebral palsy is rarely complicated, other causes for delayed motor development, altered movement and reflexes, and altered muscle tone deserve consideration. Spinal cord tumors or other lesions are usually notable for sparing involvement of muscle groups above the lesion, while even spastic diplegia may show some upper-extremity involvement. Spina bifida is not likely to be mistaken for cerebral palsy, but consideration of a tethered cord in a child with apparent diplegia or monoplegia is important. Lower motor neuron and myopathic conditions also deserve consideration in a child with hypotonia and motor delays.

Diagnostic evaluation and medical counseling

The diagnosis of cerebral palsy is made through neurologic and developmental observation. The process is complicated by its pattern of emergence and change over time. Spasticity is nearly always preceded by hypotonia, which, while delaying motor milestones, may be less obvious to parents and clinicians. On the other hand, early alterations in movement and tone may subsequently attenuate or disappear. Efforts to standardize or formalize such observations are helpful in infants at high risk or who have suspicious findings from developmental screening during well-child care. Clues during well-child visits include the persistence of infantile reflexes, delayed appearance of postural and protective reflexes, asymmetrical movements or reflexes, variations in muscle tone, and delays in the sequence of motor milestones. Primary care physicians can enhance their assessment through the use of a more rigorous neuromotor examination, such as that of Milani–Comparetti & Gidoni. (1976). Standardized instruments such as the Bayley Scales of Infant Development or the Movement Assessment of Infants (MAI) provide scores that may be predictive of long-term motor impairment (Harris, 1984). The average child with cerebral palsy is not diagnosed until about 12 months of age (Palfrey et al., 1987), and some have suggested that a definitive diagnosis should be deferred until 2 years of age (Kuban & Leviton, 1994). Referral to a pediatric neurologist, developmental pediatrics (child development) clinic, or neuromotor disorders clinic may be helpful in establishing the diagnosis, and are essential in long-term preventive management. Such specialists will assist the primary care physician and family in the development of an initial treatment and care plan.

The consideration of specific underlying causes for the motor delays and impairments found on neurologic examination may be important. Conditions for which an intervention might prove crucial, such as a treatable metabolic disorder or findings that suggest child abuse ("shaken baby syndrome"), must not be overlooked. Other identifiable syndromes and conditions may have prognostic significance, associated complications, or recurrence risks (e.g., Aicardi syndrome or familial forms of cerebral palsy). A dysmorphology or genetics consultation may be useful to rule out specific conditions in which cerebral palsy is one of the characteristics. Brain imaging, usually by MRI, should be carried out in nearly all cases.

When the primary care physician becomes suspicious of cerebral palsy, it is important that he or she shares those concerns with the parents. Parents will be more able to understand and cope with the eventual diagnosis of cerebral palsy if they have been partners in the diagnostic process. Furthermore, the symptoms and signs themselves, before they are sufficient for a diagnosis, may already be worrisome to parents and may justify a referral for early intervention services. These delays alone may also make some children eligible for Supplemental Security Income (SSI), which may in turn (in most states) provide eligibility for Medicaid.

When it becomes clear that a fixed pattern of altered movement, muscle tone, and reflexes is associated with delayed motor milestones, then a diagnosis of cerebral palsy is warranted. As with other developmental disabilities, care should be taken in the process of informing parents (see Chapter 2 and the section of Chapter 7 on Down syndrome). The diagnosis might be framed in provisional terms for a mildly involved child less than 2 years of age because of the possibility of improvement. The term "cerebral palsy" must be presented and discussed carefully with parents to avoid misunderstandings. The prognosis is uncertain in nearly all children at the time of diagnosis, particularly with respect to specific characteristics such as independent ambulation, language, and cognitive ability. Children with the most severe motor involvement (not rolling over or persistent infantile reflexes at 12 months or not sitting by 24 months) are less likely to walk independently though this may vary with the type of cerebral palsy (Molnar, 1979; Lepage et al., 1998). Plans need to be made with the family for a definitive diagnostic evaluation. Most children and families will benefit from a referral to a multidisciplinary neuromotor clinic or team. This team usually includes a pediatric orthopedist, developmental pediatrician or neurologist, nurse coordinator, pediatric physical therapist, and orthoticist.

Family and psychosocial counseling

Cerebral palsy usually occurs episodically. However, it is important to inquire about any family history of cerebral palsy, motor disability, other developmental disability (e.g., mental retardation), seizures, or known genetic conditions. Such information may provide clues to diagnoses other than or in addition to cerebral palsy. Furthermore, there are a number of uncommon, but well-described forms of familial cerebral palsy (Cooley et al., 1990).

Parents should be referred to a local or state parent-to-parent organization (a parent support group), which will facilitate specific, one-to-one connections with an experienced parent who has been trained to be a resource to parents of newly diagnosed children. Most parents would benefit from contact with national, state, or local organizations as listed in *Exceptional Parent* magazine. Generic support groups for families of children with various disabilities are available, or they may be specific for cerebral palsy as listed (checklist, part 1). Reading materials for parents are also helpful (Geralis, 1991; Miller & Bachrach, 1995).

The diagnosis of cerebral palsy may be the first of a series of "bad news" experiences for parents. Later conclusions that a child will not walk, will need orthopedic surgery, will require augmentative help with communication, or will have cognitive limitations constitute diagnostic events for which parents may need extra support. Many parents and, later, children with cerebral palsy are led to a perspective of "fixing" the cerebral palsy rather than coping, preventing secondary disability, and accommodating. Sometimes this leads children to the impression that they are "broken," that therapy is aimed at "fixing" them, and, to the degree that a "fix" does not occur, they – parents or child – have failed. This is damaging to self-esteem, morale, and family strengths. Clinicians should use care in how they frame the goals of intervention and ensure that parents and, eventually, the child have clear roles in articulating those goals. Siblings and other family members may require attention and support as well.

Most children with cerebral palsy will be eligible for early intervention services (from birth to age 3 years) and special education services (after age 3). The goals of these services are optimal functioning, safety, inclusion in school and community, and self-determination to the degree possible. It should be assumed that most children with cerebral palsy can receive and will benefit from school services provided in regular settings. Often the classroom or curriculum will require modifications to include the student with cerebral palsy. Some school districts have maintained that children with cerebral palsy who appear to have no cognitive impairment do not experience an educational handicap and are, therefore, not eligible for a special education program. While some parents and children may prefer this, primary care physicians should be prepared to advocate for children who have been inappropriately denied school services.

Older children and adolescents with cerebral palsy who do not have mental retardation remain at risk for specific learning disabilities and attention deficits that may not become apparent until elementary school begins. More significant issues of self-esteem and anger may emerge during these years. Innovative efforts including peer-to-peer supports and active programs promoting self-determination should be implemented by the middle school years (Olson & Cooley, 1996). Concerns about dating, sexuality, and other social relationships need to be addressed openly and thoughtfully.

Natural history and complications

Outcomes of cerebral palsy vary from profound, multi-domain disability to mild, almost inapparent involvement. By definition it is assumed that all individuals have a permanent, non-progressive motor impairment. The nature of this impairment (spastic or athetoid, diplegia or quadriplegia) may emerge gradually in the early months and years. All children pass through an initial hypotonic phase, so if spasticity is present at birth, then the initial insult followed by hypotonicity occurred during intrauterine life (Capute & Accardo, 1996). Twenty-five percent of people with cerebral palsy are non-ambulatory, though there is considerable variation among types of cerebral palsy (Table 4.4; Molnar, 1979).

Cerebral palsy can "worsen" through failure to address the orthopedic complications. All children with cerebral palsy should be evaluated and followed, if necessary, by a pediatric orthopedist. This is often best accomplished through a neuromotor team. This approach allows the institution of a comprehensive plan of physical therapy, noninvasive orthopedic techniques (e.g., serial casting), and orthotics to maintain the flexibility and mobility of joints. Therapy may also reduce wasting and weakness as a consequence of disuse. Secondary complications such as scoliosis and hip subluxation can be identified, monitored, and treated. Orthopedic surgery, stereotactic spinal cord surgery (dorsal rhizotomy), and medications affecting movement and tone may be considered for selected individuals.

Table 4.4 Ambulatory status and onset of walking in prenatal and perinatal cerebral palsy

Clinical type	Number[a]	Age at Onset of Walking					Ambulatory	
		1–2 yr	2–3 yr	4–5 yr	5–8 yr	Never	Yes (%)	No (%)
Hemiplegia	107	98	9				100	0
Diplegia	81	31	20	5	5	12	85	15
Quadriparesis	144	12	14	22	19	46	68	32
Athetosis	96	20	19	14	12	23	77	23
Spastic-athetoid	38	3	5	2	2	20	47	53
Ataxic	12	0	2	4	2	0	100	0
Rigid	21					21	0	100
Atonic	14					14	0	100
Total	513	164	69	47	40	136	73	27

Note:
[a] Includes some children walking later than 8 yr.

Cerebral palsy may also "worsen" or appear to progress when there is a failure to address nutritional issues, seizures, or an additional medical illness. In addition, on occasion cerebral palsy is not the correct diagnosis but is temporarily mimicked by another, possibly progressive neurologic condition (Table 4.5).

Epilepsy occurs in about one-third of people with cerebral palsy, with a prevalence of 50 percent in those with hemiplegia (checklist, part 1). At least 30 percent have mental retardation, with a greater percentage among those with spastic quadraplegia (Kuban & Leviton, 1994). On the other hand, cognition may be underestimated in individuals with choreoathetoid cerebral palsy due to the severity of the expressive language disorder (Palmer & Hoon, 1995). Even those without mental retardation may have learning disabilities. People with cerebral palsy are at increased risk for impairment of vision or hearing. Oral motor involvement is common in most forms of cerebral palsy, and this may complicate feeding. Some individuals have significant problems with drooling. Alterations in esophageal motility may result in reflux and aspiration hazards. In severe cases, feeding or gastrostomy tubes may be necessary. Inadequate caloric intake may be complicated by increased caloric consumption by spastic muscles and excess movements contributing to failure to thrive. Delays in the acquisition of bowel and bladder control are common. Urologic evaluation may be helpful to determine the nature of the bladder dysfunction and the best treatment (McNeal et al., 1983). Constipation may result from decreased overall mobility and spastic involvement of the anal sphincter (checklist, part 1).

Table 4.5 Neurodegenerative disorders that
may be mistaken for cerebral palsy

Disorder	Inheritance
Spasticity	
Leukodystrophy	
Krabbe	AR
Metachromatic	AR
Adrenoleukodystrophy	XLR
Syndromes	
Zellweger	AR
Cockayne	AR
Small molecule disorders	
Arginase deficiency	AR
Abetalipoproteinemia	AR
Movement disorders	
Wilson's disease	AR
Ataxia-telangiectasia	AR
Lesch–Nyhan syndrome	XLR

Note:
AR, autosomal recessive; XLR, X-linked recessive.

Cerebral palsy preventive medical checklist

Because children with cerebral palsy have such diverse manifestations, the preventive medical checklist is an outline that must be modified according to individual needs. Timely, comprehensive care in early childhood can prevent chronic secondary disability, emphasizing the importance of obtaining early consultation from a neuromotor multidisciplinary team. Early assessment of feeding (Reilly et al., 1996), neuromotor (Capute & Accardo, 1996; DeLuca, 1996), and orthopedic (Ebara et al., 1996; Wilmshurst et al., 1996; Carlson et al., 1997; Scrutton & Baird, 1997) problems is particularly important, with consideration of new therapies such as intrathecal baclofen (Gerszten et al., 1998), botulinum toxin (Gooch & Sandell, 1996), or glycopyrrolate (Bachrach et al., 1998; Blasco & Stansbury, 1996). It is also essential to involve all children with early intervention or preschool special education. The careful evaluation and monitoring of hearing and vision by qualified specialists should become a regular aspect of preventive care for the child with cerebral palsy. Thorough initial consideration of possible neuropathologic, metabolic, genetic, or familial diagnoses should always be undertaken. The issue of causation and specific diagnosis should be revisited periodically as new knowledge and developments in fields such as genetics or brain imaging may offer fresh diagnostic opportunities.

Though the majority of families of children with moderate to severe cerebral palsy are not permanently disrupted by this challenge, about one-third of such families sustain serious consequences (e.g., divorce, abuse, mental health problems; Singer & Irvin, 1991). The families who cope successfully are more likely to have social and other supports and to have regained a sense of mastery of their situation. Primary care physicians can contribute to positive coping by families by facilitating connections with formal (programs, entitlements, information) and natural sources of support (friends, neighbors, churches, etc.). Even such minor actions as asking about and advocating for a "handicap" license plate may significantly relieve daily stresses for some families. Primary care physicians should strive toward a collaborative partnership with family caregivers rather than a prescriptive, paternalistic approach to care.

Hydrocephalus

Terminology

Hydrocephalus is a condition with diverse etiologies characterized by unbalanced formation and absorption of cerebrospinal fluid resulting usually in the enlargement of the cerebral ventricles and often in increased CSF pressure (Gabriel & McComb, 1985). Non-communicating hydrocephalus involves obstruction of the flow of CSF at or before the outlet of the fourth ventricle, while communicating hydrocephalus refers to a more distal obstruction that may also interfere with the reabsorption of CSF (Kinsman, 1996). Arrested and compensated hydrocephalus are terms implying a balance between production and the reabsorption of CSF. There is disagreement among experts regarding the usefulness and validity of this notion. A distinction is sometimes made between congenital and acquired hydrocephalus, depending on the timing of the etiologic event with respect to birth.

Arnold Chiari malformations, which are regarded as neural tube defects account for 40 percent of cases of hydrocephalus (Gabriel & McComb, 1985). Hydrocephalus results from the herniation of abnormal cerebellar or brain stem structures through the foramen magnum. In the Dandy Walker syndrome, which accounts for 5 percent of cases, the fourth ventricle dilates and herniates caudally due to the lack of an opening in its roof (Table 4.6).

Incidence, etiology, and differential diagnosis

Congenital hydrocephalus occurs in 2 per 1000 live births, with 25–50 percent of these cases associated with spina bifida (Jackson, 1990). "Acquired" hydrocephalus usually occurs as the result of infection, neoplasm, abnormal vascularity, or trauma

Table 4.6 Potential complications and consequences of hydrocephalus

General	
Life cycle	Increased mortality associated with cause[a]
	Increased mortality (50%), if untreated,
	20% of untreated children reach adulthood
Learning	Cognitive disability (verbal IQ scores exceed performance IQ scores)[b]
	Impaired "executive functions," learning differences
	Hyperverbal syndrome, handwriting and reading problems
	Problems with mathematics, problems with visual scanning
Facial	
Face	Altered cranial growth, prominent forehead, broad nasal root
Eyes	Strabismus, "sun-setting"
Skeletal	
Cranial	Macrocephaly, bulging fontanelle, split sutures
Limbs	"Cortical" thumbs
Internal	
Digestive	Vomiting as symptom
Neural	
CNS	Accumulation of cerebrospinal fluid, elevated intracranial pressure
Sensory	Vision deficits, visuomotor, visuospatial problems

Note:
[a] e.g., neoplasm, CNS infection; [b] frequent shunt infections lower IQ scores.

that results in bleeding. Kinsman (1996) suggested classifying hydrocephalus according to etiology as follows: malformation (e.g., Arnold Chiari), genetic process (e.g., X-linked or autosomal recessive), inflammation (e.g., meningitis), chemical irritation (e.g., bleeding), and neoplasm.

In newborns and infants, an enlarging head circumference is often accompanied by a bulging fontanel and splitting of sutures. Downward deviation of the eyes ("sunset sign") may occur. Symptoms such as irritability, vomiting, lethargy, poor feeding, apnea, and changes in respiratory pattern may also ensue (Nitahara et al., 1996; Marcus, 1996; Taylor & Madsen, 1996). In older children (after age 3), head enlargement is unlikely and symptoms will depend on the rapidity of onset of the hydrocephalus and associated changes in CSF pressure. Headaches are usually present, particularly in the morning, along with vomiting, abnormal eye movements, and altered level of consciousness. Papilledema may be evident.

The differential diagnosis includes conditions that either cause head enlargement or the symptoms associated with increased intracranial pressure. The former include subdural hematoma due to trauma, familial or genetic forms of macrocephaly (e.g., Sotos syndrome), certain metabolic storage diseases, and brain tumors. The latter include central nervous system infections, pseudotumor cerebri with its variety of causes, and ingestions such as lead poisoning. When imaging studies demonstrate enlarged ventricles, conditions in which this has resulted from cerebral atrophy rather than the accumulation of CSF under excess pressure must be considered.

Diagnostic evaluation and medical counseling

The diagnosis of hydrocephalus depends on some form of brain imaging to identify the presence of ventriculomegaly (Kinsman, 1996). Ultrasonography may be performed in infants with patent fontanelles, providing a quick, often crib-side assessment without sedation. In most instances, more complete imaging will be necessary using CT or MRI scans. Since sedation or anesthesia will be necessary in infants and young children for either study, the more informative MRI scan is usually preferable. This provides better detail of some structures and regions (James, 1992). In some individuals, serial studies will be necessary to differentiate static ventriculomegaly from true hydrocephalus.

When a clinician strongly suspects hydrocephalus, confirmation and treatment are urgent matters. Referral to an experienced pediatric neurosurgeon for further evaluation and surgical management is mandatory. However, it is also important to consider a variety of underlying etiologies which might be facilitated through consultations from a geneticist or a pediatric neurologist. Treatment is first directed at the underlying cause (for example, removal of a tumor). In some cases, particularly in neonates, decompression is accomplished through intermittent lumbar or ventricular punctures or through an external drainage system. When long-term decompression is needed, the installation of a ventriculoperitoneal (VP) shunt is the treatment of choice in most situations. The child with hydrocephalus is at high risk for both obvious and subtle developmental disabilities which may warrant monitoring through a developmental pediatrics consultation and referral to early intervention or special education programs. The nature and severity of the disability will depend in part on the etiology of the hydrocephalus and any associated alterations in CNS structures. However, there are a number of learning disabilities associated specifically with hydrocephalus (Wills, 1993; Fletcher et al., 1996).

Family and psychosocial counseling

As with other serious chronic conditions in children, the clinician should convey the news of the diagnosis of hydrocephalus with warmth, empathy, and clarity in the manner described in Chapter 2 and for Down syndrome in Chapter 7. If trauma is a possible etiology, consideration of child abuse is important. A number of familial forms of hydrocephalus exist, so a careful family history should be elicited.

While parents need reassurance about the prognosis of this condition, they will want to understand the developmental consequences that may occur. Hydrocephalus may have a direct impact on development or may be associated with other brain anomalies (e.g., absence of the corpus callosum) that affect brain function (Fletcher et al., 1992). While all families benefit from accurate, understandable information, the families of children who have severe impairments may require access to family support services, financing sources, and parent-to-parent linkages. Education about the monitoring of intracranial shunt functioning must be balanced with encouragement of normal childhood activities to avoid an overly protective "vulnerable child" scenario. National organizations may provide helpful information and support:

Hydrocephalus Opens People's Eyes (HOPE), 104–47 120th Street, Richmond Hill NY 11419; Guardians of Hydrocephalus Research Foundation, 2618 Ave. Z, Brooklyn NY 11235, (800) 458–8655; Hydrocephalus Association, 870 Market St. Suite 955, San Francisco CA 94102, (415) 732–7040, hydroassoc@aol.com, www.neurosurgery.mgh.harvard; Hydrocephalus Support Group, Inc., P. O. Box 4236, Chesterfield MO, 63006–4236, (202)-944–3285(314)532–8228; hydro@inlink.com; National Hydrocephalus Foundation, 12413 Centralia Rd., Lakewood CA, 90715–1623, (562) 402–3523; hydrobrat@earthlink.net; www.geocities.com/HOTSPRINGS/villa/2300.

Natural history and complications

In the past, untreated hydrocephalus was associated with a mortality of 50 percent, with severe mental retardation and disability occurring in 50 percent of survivors (Gabriel & McComb, 1985). Two-thirds of patients with untreated "spontaneously arrested" hydrocephalus experience disabling neurologic impairments. Assuming that hydrocephalus is promptly diagnosed and treated, the complications involve those associated with malfunction or infection of the intracranial shunt, those of the conditions causing or associated with the hydrocephalus, and the specific neuropsychologic consequences that have been associated with hydrocephalus (Table 4.6).

Hydrocephalus preventive medical needs

A number of articles, aimed at primary and allied health care professionals, describe principles of management in narrative form (Jackson, 1990; James, 1992). Special preventive medical measures for children with hydrocephalus relate primarily to the monitoring of shunt status (Iskandar et al., 1998), of developmental/educational progress and programming, and of family support needs. In other respects, their preventive health care is similar to that of other children. Children in whom hydrocephalus is associated with spina bifida are discussed in the next section of this chapter.

Linear growth of children with hydrocephalus may be delayed during childhood followed by acceleration during precocious puberty (Lopponen et al., 1995). Head circumference monitoring is important, particularly in the first three years, and the measurements should be plotted on head circumference charts extending from birth to age 18 (Nellhaus, 1986). Such charts also allow plotting of the head sizes of parents and other family members to rule out familial macrocephaly. Regular vision assessment (Gaston, 1996) and monitoring for signs of early puberty (Lopponen et al., 1996) should also be considered.

Spina bifida

Terminology

Spina bifida or rachischisis refers to a bony defect of the spine in which enclosure of the spinal cord is incomplete. This defect may be covered by normal skin (spina bifida occulta) or there may be a protruding sac (spina bifida cystica). When such a sac contains only meninges and cerebrospinal fluid, it is called a meningocele. The combination of spina bifida and meningomyelocele is sometimes referred to as myelodysplasia (Golden, 1979; Shurtleff et al., 1986).

Neural tube defects include central nervous system malformations that arise during the first 28–30 days of gestation as the result of incomplete formation, folding, or closure of the neural tube. Neural tube defects range from the most severe with holoanencephaly (complete absence of the brain) and craniorachischisis (absence of the covering skull) to the most distal sacral meningomyelocele in which spinal cord disruption may be minimal. Encephalocele and skin covered spinal cord lesions are sometimes included as neural tube defects though they occur after formation of the neural tube and neuronal disruption may be minimal or absent.

Historical diagnosis and management

Skeletal remains dating back over 10,000 years have revealed evidence of spina bifida (Feremback, 1963). Medical descriptions of spina bifida did not occur until the seventeenth century, and the association with hydrocephalus was first reported in 1769. Efforts to remove, close, or protect the herniated sac began in the nineteenth century with recognition by the early twentieth century that infection and hydrocephalus were the two most common lethal complications (Shurtleff, 1986). By the 1930s, early closure of the sac to prevent infection was advised, but debate remained about whether sac excision exacerbated hydrocephalus. Gradually the contemporary practice of skin closure over the sac and prompt shunting has emerged as the standard of care. The issue of "selection" of infants for aggressive management based on the severity of the lesion remains a topic of controversy. Few, if any, centers impose rigid selection criteria; most favor initial closure followed by a process of empowering parents as decision-making partners.

Incidence, etiology, and differential diagnosis

The prevalence at birth of neural tube defects has a distinct variability with geography and ethnicity as well as over time. For example, prior to 1980, the eastern United States experienced a rate of 3 to 3.5 per 1000 births while in the West the rate was 1 to 1.5 per 1000 births (Seller, 1994). However, over time this geographical distinction in the United States has been lost with a general decline in prevalence while in the United Kingdom, the birth prevalence has fallen from 4.5 per 1000 births in 1970 to 0.18 per 1000 in 1991. In the United States, the rate of neural tube defects has declined from 1.3 per 1000 births in 1970 to 0.6 per 1000 in 1989 (Yen et al., 1992).

Most reviews of causative factors for neural tube defects support etiologic heterogeneity. Neural tube defects are associated with chromosomal alterations (e.g., trisomies 13 and 18), prenatal exposures such as alcohol, rubella, or valproic acid, maternal diabetes, prenatal folic acid deficiency, and, rarely, Mendelian inheritance patterns (Shurtleff et al., 1986). Clear ethnic differences have been noted with increased prevalence among those of Celtic, Hispanic, and northern Native American origins and lower prevalence among Blacks, Asians, and Pacific Islanders (Centers for Disease Control, 1992). The recurrence risk in siblings which historically approached 5 percent in the United Kingdom, is now around 2 percent (Shurtleff et al., 1986).

Neural tube defects are usually readily suspected at birth based on the visible sac. However, care and expertise are required to determine the severity of the lesion and to identify associated complications or malformations. Careful tertiary level, multidisciplinary evaluation is essential to this process which is likely to involve intensive neonatal care with neurosurgical, pediatric neurologic, genetics, pediatric urologic, and pediatric orthopedics consultations as well as brain and spinal cord imaging. Rarely, apparent neural tube defects will prove to be more simple meningoceles with minimal neurologic impairment or involve lipomas of the spinal cord. Lipomas of the cord may occur in association with meningomyelocele, duplication of the spinal cord (diplomyelia), or tethering of the cord (Shurtleff et al., 1986).

Diagnostic evaluation and medical counseling

All women having relatives with neural tube defects should receive preconceptional supplementation of folic acid in amounts similar to those in standard multivitamins (Mulinare et al., 1988). Prenatal screening and diagnostic techniques have increased the frequency with which neural tube defects are identified during pregnancy. Maternal serum alpha-fetoprotein (MSAFP) levels are used for general population

Table 4.7 Degree of paralysis and functional implications

Paralysis	Hydrocephalus (%)	Ambulation	Bowel/bladder incontinence (%)
Thoracic or high lumbar (L1, L2)	90	May walk with extensive braces and crutches	>90
Mid lumbar (L3)	85	Can walk with either extensive, moderate, or minimal braces, and usually with crutches	>90
Low lumbar (L4, L5)	70	Will walk with moderate, minimal, or no bracing with or without crutches	>90
Sacral (S1 to S4)	60	Will walk with minimal or no braces and usually without crutches	>90

Source: Charney (1990).

screening with an accuracy of 75–80 percent in detecting an affected fetus (Johnson et al., 1990). The measurement of AFP in amniotic fluid has an accuracy of close to 95 percent, but fails to identify 5 percent of the defects in which there is a covering of epithelial tissue. AFP levels are also elevated in other malformations that disrupt the integrity of the fetal epithelium or that result in the loss of fetal (or placental) blood into the amniotic fluid. Ultrasonography can identify all but the smallest lesions including those with coverings of skin (Nadel et al., 1990).

Prenatal diagnosis allows for the provision of counseling, information, and support to parents. When the diagnosis is made within allowable legal gestational limits for abortion, some parents may elect to terminate the pregnancy. However, all parents should be provided access to balanced information about outcomes including the same information provided to parents of newborns with spina bifida and, upon request, contact with parents of older affected children. Prenatal diagnosis permits planning for the safest delivery (often by Cesarean) in a medical center that can provide an immediate response to the newborn's medical needs. In some instances, prenatal diagnosis may also allow ameliorative prenatal surgery, for example, to remove cerebrospinal fluid.

Whether the diagnosis has occurred prenatally or following birth, early, thorough evaluation of the newborn and implementation of appropriate care may substantially improve the outcome. To prevent the occurrence of infection, the meningomyelocele defect is usually closed in the first few days after birth. At this time, the level of the lesion may be clarified (Table 4.7). Lesions in the thoracic or high lumbar areas (L1 or L2) are regarded as "high level" and likely to result in complete paralysis of the lower extremities. Mid-level lesions around L3 may allow hip flexion and knee extension, while low lumber lesions at L4 or L5 allow flexion at hips, knees, and ankles with extension at knees and ankles. Hip extension and ankle flexion may remain weak. Sacral lesions result in mild weakness at the ankles, and toes. The higher the lesion the greater the ambulatory limitation and the need for assistive devices and equipment. Lesions at all levels are likely to affect bowel and bladder function (checklist, part 1).

   All newborns with spina bifida require brain imaging for the associated presence of CNS malformations, especially Arnold–Chiari malformation type II in which the brain stem and portions of the cerebellum are herniated downward into the foramen magnum. This malformation occurs in the majority of children with spina bifida, resulting in obstruction of cerebrospinal fluid movement and hydrocephalus (Griebel et al., 1991). In most cases, hydrocephalus will require surgical treatment as early as possible. This usually involves the placement of a ventriculo-peritoneal (VP) shunt to drain CSF from the enlarged cerebral ventricles to the peritoneal cavity (see the hydrocephalus section of this chapter for additional information).

Family and psychosocial counseling

When a neural tube defect is not suspected prenatally and is diagnosed at birth, care and attention is needed to counsel and inform parents. Immediate information about severity and complications may not be readily available. However, it is crucial that the informant be knowledgeable about the range of prognoses for newborns with spina bifida as well as appropriate interventions. Principles used to inform parents of a diagnosis like Down syndrome (see Chapter 7) apply in this instance as well. The informing interview should begin an active process of re-empowerment and support as parents cope with and adapt to the news. Parents should be supported by being together in the case of two parents or by the presence of another family member or close friend in the case of a single parent. The baby should be present, if possible, referred to by name, and held or otherwise acknowledged as a baby first and affected by a diagnosis second. Ample time for questions according to the parents' agenda of needs and concerns should be provided with frequent follow-up and ready access for parents to sources of information. Some parents may welcome contact with an experienced family of a child with spina bifida (Cerniglia, 1997). Rarely, parents may be interested in the availability of specialized foster care or adoption for babies with spina bifida.

   A history of the pregnancy including prenatal care and nutrition, ultrasound and other tests, and exposure to potential teratogens should be reviewed. This may not only identify etiologic factors, but more likely eliminate sources of parental fear or guilt about unrelated occurrences. The family history should be reviewed for other cases of neural tube and related defects as well as notation of the family's ethnic and geographic background.

As with other developmental disabilities, parents of children with spina bifida require ongoing information, advocacy, and support from primary care providers as well as members of a multidisciplinary specialty team (Liptak et al., 1988; Sarwark, 1996). Early referral to such a team located at the nearest tertiary care medical center, at an outreach location for such a medical center, or through the state's program for children with special health care needs is very important. Ideally, this referral connection will be made during the initial hospitalization as a newborn. In addition to the needed medical and surgical specialists working collaboratively, most spina bifida teams have a specialty nurse coordinator who provides the family with an accessible source of information, support, parent-to-parent contact, and care coordination. Such nurse coordinators can often provide community-based professionals (primary care physicians, early intervention professionals, teachers, etc.) with consultation, technical assistance, in-service training, and reading about spina bifida.

Depending on factors such as family income, many children with spina bifida are eligible for benefits such as Medicaid insurance, Supplemental Security Income (SSI) from the Social Security Administration, and possible financial and other supports from the state's program for children with special health care needs. Some states provide special "family support services" for families of children with developmental disabilities that may include respite care, discretionary funds, stipends or loan programs, advocacy and care coordination, and parent-to-parent contacts. Primary care physicians should ask about and confirm that families have access to these programs. Nearly all young children with spina bifida are eligible for state early intervention services from birth to age 3 years and preschool special education services from age 3 to age 5 or 6. Prompt connection with these services will benefit most families.

Parents will require specific information to help them maintain and monitor their child's status and well-being. Spina bifida team nurse coordinators often provide parents with training and information about clean intermittent catheterization techniques (Bomalaski et al., 1995; Johnston & Borzyskowski, 1998) and about the signs of ventriculoperitoneal shunt malfunction or infection. Additional information about home physical therapy and the encouragement of ambulation and other developmental tasks will come both from the nurse coordinator and from community-based therapists and early interventionists. The encouragement of parents to provide their children a normal range of regular experiences with siblings and other children their age will help to avoid creating a "vulnerable child" situation.

The specific issue of mobility will be an important one for parents and for the

child. Depending on the level of the lesion, a goal of independent bipedal ambulation may require a range of training, therapy, orthotics, orthopedic interventions,
and assistive devices. However, this goal should be supported in most individuals
with spina bifida even in situations where the eventual primary mode of community mobility is likely to be a wheelchair. Restricted mobility may be associated with
skin lesions and slow healing (Srivastava, 1995).

Older children should be gradually incorporated into discussions and treatment
planning activities while they are given increasing responsibility for their own self-
care. Information about spina bifida and its specific manifestations in the individual child should be provided in age appropriate language as early as possible.
Children should be taught to perform their own self-catheterization during the
early school age years according to the child's readiness and interest. Careful counseling about sexuality and reproductive health is important beginning in the grade
school years. The spina bifida team coordinator should have helpful information
in this regard. Many children might benefit from periodic meetings with an older
peer mentor who has spina bifida (Olson & Cooley, 1996).

Additional information of benefit to individuals with spina bifida, their families,
and their caregivers can be obtained from the Spina Bifida Association of America
(checklist, part 1). The SBAA publishes a well-written newsletter entitled *Spina
Bifida Spotlight* on specific topics of interest.

Natural history and complications

The natural history and complications of neural tube defects are highly dependent
on the severity of the primary defect and on the nature of any associated birth
defects (checklist, part 1). Neural tube defects may be uniformly lethal (anen-
cephaly) or associated with lethal combinations of other defects (e.g., trisomy 13).
On the other hand, they may be so mild as to have limited impact. Assuming the
presence of a spinal cord lesion (as opposed to a cranial lesion), over 90 percent of
babies who receive early surgical treatment survive into adulthood (Shurtleff,
1986). Early handling and management is aimed at avoiding infection of the CSF,
spinal cord, or brain before, during, and after closure of the back. As soon as surgical closure is achieved, plans for installation of a VP shunt under uninfected conditions should be carried out since the majority (up to 90 percent) of babies will
have hydrocephalus. There is growing evidence that shunting should be considered
in nearly all neonates with spina bifida even in the absence of an enlarging head
circumference. Intellectual outcomes seemed improved by such an aggressive
approach. Shunt malfunction or infection remain complications for the child with
spina bifida which require prompt diagnosis and management.

Nearly all children will have bowel and bladder incontinence (Bomalaski et al.,
1995; Johnston & Borzyskowski, 1998). While bowel function can usually be

managed with a combination of behavioral and dietary plans, urinary retention can lead to a series of complications including urinary tract infection, reflux, and hydronephrosis. Depending on the initial cystometric evaluation, a child's program may involve anticholinergic medication, clean intermittent catheterization, and antibiotics. Urinary diversions such as vesicostomy are rarely indicated. Some children (about 10–20 percent) who have repeated infections despite adequate bladder regimens and prophylaxis may require anti-reflux surgery (Bauer, 1994).

A tethered cord may develop in up to 10 percent of individuals as the result of scarring and adhesions at the surgical site or due to small cysts or lipomas of the cord. Newer surgical methods have been aimed at reducing the incidence of tethered cord. Unfortunately, the highest risk occurs among children with the lowest lesions who may experience the most relative loss of function due to tethered cord (Humphreys, 1986). Early diagnosis is important. Back and radiating leg pain, worsening of gait, scoliosis, bladder or bowel control, or long track neurologic findings are important signs and symptoms that suggest a tethered cord.

The presence of partial or complete lower extremity paralysis results in an increased risk for secondary orthopedic deformity. Many infants have club foot deformities when the lesion is at the L3 level or higher. Milder ankle and foot deformities may also require orthopedic attention. The hips are vulnerable to imbalanced musculature which may lead to contractures or hip dislocation (Frawley et al., 1996). Scoliosis occurs in a large number of children particularly those with thoracic or high-lumbar levels of involvement (in whom the incidence of scoliosis approaches 90 percent; Mayfield, 1991).

An increased risk of allergic hypersensitivity to latex-containing products is now well-recognized in people with spina bifida (Leger & Meeropol, 1992; Kwittken et al., 1995). Prevention from exposure is not only crucial for those with established sensitivity in whom severe reactions can occur, but also among all others beginning as newborns to reduce the likelihood of acquiring sensitivity. Many products used by infants contain latex (e.g., bottle nipples, pacifiers, teething toys, changing pads and mattress covers, and some diapers). Medical equipment must also be checked (bandages, tape, catheters, gloves, crutch arm pads, brace linings). Common childhood toys such as balloons, balls, racquet handles, water toys must be carefully evaluated. Household products such as rubber cement, erasers, sneakers, spandex products, condoms, and diaphragms (for birth control) contain latex. There may be some cross-reactivity with certain foods (bananas, kiwi, avocados).

Cognitive functioning and school performance are affected in the majority of children with spina bifida though usually in the context of a pattern of strengths and challenges (Wills et al., 1990; Dise & Lohr, 1998). It has become increasingly apparent that spina bifida is not associated with a universal reduction in overall intelligence, but some variation occurs depending on the level of the lesion and the priority given to careful management of hydrocephalus and shunt care. Shurtleff found that lesions below L3 were associated on the whole with average performance on IQ tests, while higher lesions tended to result in lower scores (Shurtleff, 1986). Children with VP shunts that have been carefully managed (prompt recognition and treatment of malfunction and infection) show verbal intelligence scores in the same range as controls without spina bifida (McClone et al., 1982).

More detailed profiling of cognitive abilities often reveals strengths in the verbal areas with better performance in reading and spelling compared to math. Visual perceptual skills affecting eye-hand coordination may also be impaired causing difficulty with handwriting and other fine motor tasks. There may also be an increased risk for more subtle neuropsychological challenges affecting attention, memory, sequencing, or reasoning (Cull & Wyke, 1984).

Spina bifida preventive medical checklist

Health promotion and preventive care for the child with spina bifida involves the coordination of important services from several medical and surgical subspecialties with attentive and accessible primary health care services. Children with spina bifida require all of the usual immunizations, health supervison, anticipatory guidance, and treatment of common acute health problems as their brothers and sisters (checklist, parts 2–4). In addition, primary care providers must be attentive to the extra child and family needs that may accompany a chronic condition. These needs include condition-specific areas of health supervision (e.g., avoidance of latex exposure in spina bifida) as well as generic issues such as the need for information, contact with other similar families, access to family support services and financial assistance, and school issues. Usually these needs are best addressed in an atmosphere of collaborative partnership between primary care providers and parents.

Growth with respect to weight and length/height requires monitoring in spina bifida. Obviously, careful attention to head circumference measurements is important prior to closure of cranial sutures. In some individuals, the measurement of arm span may be used as a substitute for height. Short stature and obesity have been reported with increased frequency in individuals with spina bifida. Careful evaluation for underlying contributing causes and, in the case of obesity, helpful life style guidance is important.

All children with spina bifida require the services of multiple medical and therapeutic specialists. These services are best provided through a multidisciplinary team which will develop and implement a care plan aimed at coordinating needed treatment and follow-up and communicating with community-based care-givers. The spina bifida medical checklists identify regular contact with the spina bifida team, but they do not attempt to specify the precise nature and timing of specific sub-specialty interventions that will vary from team to team and from child to child.

As with cerebral palsy, the spina bifida checklist presented here incorporates guidelines from a number of state programs or tertiary care centers that provide multidisciplinary services for children with spina bifida (Sarwark, 1996). Other authorities recognized by the checklist include the single page "Healthwatch for the person with myelodysplasia" (Crocker, 1989). The Spina Bifida Association of America's Professional Advisory Council has also published a well-referenced outline organized by age groups and by specialty areas including primary care roles (Rauen, 1990). Additional information of benefit to individuals with spina bifida, their families, and their care-givers can be obtained from the Spina Bifida Association of America (checklist, part 1; Spina Bifida Association of America, 1994).

Preventive Management of Cerebral Palsy

Clinical diagnosis: Clues during well-child visits include the persistence of infantile reflexes, delayed appearance of reflexes, asymmetrical movements or reflexes, variations in muscle tone, and delays in the sequence of motor milestones. Early alterations in movement and tone may subsequently attenuate or disappear. Often not diagnosed until age 1–2 years.

Diagnostic aids: Standardized instruments such as the Bayley Scales of Infant Development or the Movement Assessment of Infants (MAI) provide scores that may be predictive of long term motor impairment (Harris, 1984).

Incidence: 1.5–2.5 per 1000 births.

Genetics: Broad category of disease with most cases having a low recurrence risk. Many genetic disorders can be associated with spasticity, producing a 25 percent recurrence risk in some cases.

Key management issues: Early consultation from a neuromotor multidisciplinary team, involvement in early intervention and preschool special education, monitoring of hearing and vision, connections with formal (programs, entitlements, information) and natural sources of support (friends, neighbors, churches, etc.).

Growth charts: Arm/leg length or other segmental measurements may be substituted for height as a method of following long bone growth over time (Stevenson, 1995).

Parent groups: United Cerebral Palsy Association Inc., 1660 L. St. NW Suite 700, Washington DC, 20036-5602, (800) 872-5827, ucpainc@aol.com, http://www.ucpa.org; Ontario Federation for Cerebral Palsy, 1630 Lawrence Ave. W. Suite 104, Toronto ON, Canada M6L 1C5, (416) 244-8003, ofcp@ofcp.on.ca, http://www.ofcp.on.ca; Scope, 6 Market Road, London N7 9PW, (0171) 619-7100, http://www.scope.org.uk

Basis for management recommendations: "Healthwatch" table for cerebral palsy (Rubin and Crocker, 1989), other guidelines (Capute, 1998; Miller & Bachrach, 1995).

Summary of clinical concerns

General	Learning	Cognitive disability (30%), **learning differences** (40%), delayed motor skills, athetoid speech
	Behavior	Attention deficit hyperactivity disorder, autism
	Growth	Prematurity, low birth weight, dysphagia, failure to thrive, muscle wasting
Facial	Eye	Oculomotor dysfunction, **refractive errors** (50%), amblyopia (14%)
	Mouth	Oromotor dysfunction, dysphagia, feeding problems
Skeletal	Cranial	Decreased brain growth, later microcephaly
	Axial	Upper motor dysfunction, abnormal tone, scoliosis
	Limbs	Lower motor dysfunction, hip subluxation, contractures, deformities
Internal	Digestive	Oral hypotonia, autonomic dysfunction, vomiting, GE reflux, drooling, decreased bowel motility, altered sphincter tone, constipation, fecal incontinence
	Pulmonary	Aspiration, bacterial pneumonia
	Circulatory	Restrictive cardiopathy due to scoliosis
	Excretory	Altered sphincter tone, urinary incontinence
Neural	CNS	**Spasticity** (65%), **hemiplegia** (50%), **seizures** (30%), hypotonia, ataxia (10%), dyskinesis (19%), choreoathetosis
	Motor	**Hypotonia, oromotor dysfunction, motor delays**
	Sensory	Optic nerve injury, **vision deficits** (50%), hemianopsia that is more frequent with hemiplegia, acoustic nerve injury, hearing deficits that are increased in kernicterus and infectious etiologies, altered somatosensation, **abnormal stereognosis** (50%)

bold: frequency > 20%

Key references

Capute, A. J. (1998). *Pediatrics* 102:233–4.

Harris, S. (1984). *Journal of Developmental and Behavioral Pediatrics* 5:336.

Miller, F. & Bachrach, S. J. (1995). *Cerebral Palsy: A Complete Guide to Caregiving.* Baltimore: Johns Hopkins University Press.

Rubin, I. L. & Crocker, A. C. (eds.), *Developmental Disabilities.* Philadelphia: Lea & Febiger.

Stevenson, R. D. 1995. *Archives of Pediatrics and Adolescent Medicine* 149:658–62.

Cerebral Palsy

Preventive medical checklist (0–1yr)

Patient **Birth Date** / / **Number**

Pediatric	Screen	Evaluate	Refer/Counsel
Neonatal / / *Newborn screen* ❑ *HB* ❑	Head sonogram ❑ MRI scan[3] ❑ Hearing, vision[2] ❑	Muscle tone ❑ Movement ❑ Feeding ❑	Developmental pediatrics ❑ Neurology ❑ Genetics ❑ Ophthalmology ❑
1 month / /	Growth ❑ Hearing, vision[2] ❑ Audiology ❑	Feeding, stooling ❑ Nutrition ❑ Neuromotor ❑	Family support[4] ❑ Feeding specialist[3] ❑ Cardiology ❑
2 months / / *HB[1]* ❑ *Hib* ❑ *DTaP, IPV* ❑ *RV* ❑	Growth ❑ Hearing, vision[2] ❑	Feeding, stooling ❑ Nutrition ❑ Neuromotor ❑	Early intervention[5] ❑
4 months / / *HB[1]* ❑ *Hib* ❑ *DTaP, IPV* ❑ *RV* ❑	Growth ❑ Hearing, vision[2] ❑	Feeding, stools ❑ Nutrition ❑ Neuromotor ❑	Early intervention[5] ❑ Neuromotor clinic ❑
6 months / / *Hib* ❑ *IPV[1]* ❑ *DTaP* ❑ *RV* ❑	Growth ❑ Hearing, vision[2] ❑	Feeding, stooling ❑ Nutrition ❑ Neuromotor ❑	Family support[4] ❑
9 months / / *IPV[1]* ❑	Growth ❑ Hearing, vision[2] ❑	Neuromotor[6] ❑	
1 year / / *HB* ❑ *Hib[1]* ❑ *IPV[1]* ❑ *MMR[1]* ❑ *Var[1]* ❑	Growth ❑ Hearing, vision[2] ❑ Urinalysis, BP ❑	Feeding, stools ❑ Nutrition ❑ Neuromotor[6] ❑ Communication ❑	Family support[4] ❑ Early intervention[5] ❑ Neuromotor clinic ❑

Clinical concerns for Cerebral Palsy, ages 0–1 year

Feeding problems	Vomiting	Developmental delay
Seizures	Gastroesophageal reflux	Failure to thrive
Spasticity	Drooling	Muscle wasting
Hearing, vision loss	Urinary tract infections	Aspiration pneumonia

Guidelines for the neonatal period should be undertaken *at whatever age* the diagnosis is made; DTaP, acellular DTP; IPV, inactivated poliovirus (oral polio also used); RV, rotavirus; MMR, measles–mumps–rubella; Var, varicella; [1]alternative timing; [2]by practitioner; [3]as dictated by clinical findings; [4]parent group, family/sib, financial, and behavioral issues as discussed in the preface; [5]including developmental monitoring and motor/speech therapy; [6]posture, drooling.

Cerebral Palsy

Preventive medical checklist (15m–6yrs)

Patient   **Birth Date**   /   /   **Number**

Pediatric	Screen	Evaluate	Refer/Counsel
15 months / / Hib[1] ❑ MMR[1] ❑ DTaP, IPV[1] ❑ Varicella[1] ❑	Growth ❑ Hearing, vision[2] ❑	Nutrition ❑	Family support[4] ❑ Early intervention[5] ❑
18 months / / DTaP, IPV[1] ❑ Varicella[1] ❑ Influenza[3] ❑	Growth ❑ Hearing, vision[2] ❑	Neuromotor[6] ❑	Assistive technology[7] ❑
2 years / / Influenza[3] ❑ Pneumovax[3] ❑ Dentist ❑	Growth ❑ Hearing, vision[2] ❑ Audiology ❑ Urinalysis, BP ❑	Nutrition ❑ Neuromotor[6] ❑	Family support[5] ❑ Assistive technology[7] ❑ Neuromotor clinic ❑ Ophthalmology ❑
3 years / / Influenza[3] ❑ Pneumovax[3] ❑ Dentist ❑	Growth ❑ Hearing, vision[2] ❑ Audiology ❑ Urinalysis, BP ❑	Nutrition ❑ Neuromotor[6] ❑ Communication ❑	Family support[4] ❑ Preschool transition[5] ❑ Assistive technology[7] ❑ Neuromotor clinic ❑ Ophthalmology ❑
4 years / / Influenza[3] ❑ Pneumovax[3] ❑ Dentist ❑	Growth ❑ Hearing, vision[2] ❑ Audiology[3] ❑ Urinalysis, BP ❑	Nutrition ❑ Neuromotor[6] ❑ Neurobehavioral[8] ❑	Family support[4] ❑ Preschool program[5] ❑ Neuromotor clinic ❑ Ophthalmology ❑
5 years / / DTaP, IPV[1] ❑ MMR[1] ❑	Growth ❑ Hearing, vision[2] ❑ Audiology ❑ Urinalysis, BP ❑	Nutrition ❑ Neuromotor[6] ❑ Neurobehavioral[8] ❑ Sleep apnea ❑	School transition[5] ❑ Neuromotor clinic ❑ Ophthalmology ❑ Assistive technology[7] ❑
6 years / / DTaP, IPV[1] ❑ MMR[1] ❑ Dentist ❑	Growth ❑ Hearing, vision[2] ❑ Audiology ❑ Urinalysis, BP ❑	School progress ❑ Nutrition ❑ Neuromotor[6] ❑ Neurobehavioral[8] ❑	Family support[4] ❑ Neuromotor clinic ❑ Assistive technology[7] ❑ Urology[3] ❑

Clinical concerns for Cerebral Palsy, ages 15m–6 years

Microcephaly	Amblyopia	Cognitive disability
Seizures	Refractive errors	Muscle wasting
Spasticity	Gastroesophageal reflux	Aspiration pneumonia
Hearing, vision loss	Urinary, fecal incontinence	Sleep apnea

Guidelines for prior ages should be undertaken *at the time of diagnosis*; DTaP, acellular DTP; IPV, inactivated poliovirus (oral polio also used); MMR, measles–mumps–rubella; Var, varicella; [1]alternative timing; [2]by practitioner; [3]as dictated by clinical findings; [4]parent group, family/sib, financial, and behavioral issues as discussed in the preface; [5]including developmental monitoring and motor/speech therapy; [6]continence, drooling; [7]position, ambulation, communication; [8]cognition, communication, psychosocial.

Cerebral Palsy

Preventive medical checklist (6+ yrs)

Patient   **Birth Date**   /   /   **Number**

Pediatric	Screen	Evaluate	Refer/Counsel
8 years / / *Dentist* ❑	Growth ❑ Hearing, vision[2] ❑ Audiology ❑	Nutrition ❑ Neuromotor[6] ❑ Neurobehavioral[8] ❑ Sleep apnea ❑	School options ❑ Neuromotor clinic ❑ Assistive technology[7] ❑ Ophthalmology ❑
10 years / /	Growth ❑ Hearing, vision[2] ❑ Audiology ❑	School progress ❑ Neuromotor[6] ❑ Neurobehavioral[8] ❑	Neuromotor clinic ❑ Assistive technology[7] ❑
12 years / / *Td[1], MMR, Var* ❑ *CBC* ❑ *Dentist* ❑ *Scoliosis* ❑ *Cholesterol* ❑	Growth ❑ Hearing, vision[2] ❑ Audiology ❑	Nutrition ❑ Neuromotor[6] ❑ Neurobehavioral[8] ❑ Puberty ❑	Family support[5] ❑ School options ❑ Neuromotor clinic ❑ Assistive technology[7] ❑ Ophthalmology ❑
14 years / / *CBC* ❑ *Dentist* ❑ *Cholesterol* ❑ *Breast CA* ❑ *Testicular CA* ❑	Growth ❑ Hearing, vision[2] ❑ Audiology ❑	School progress ❑ Neuromotor[6] ❑ Neurobehavioral[8] ❑ Puberty ❑	Neuromotor clinic ❑ Assistive technology[7] ❑ Urology ❑
16 years / / *Td[1]* ❑ *CBC* ❑ *Cholesterol* ❑ *Sexual[5]* ❑ *Dentist* ❑	Growth ❑ Hearing, vision[2] ❑ Audiology ❑	Nutrition ❑ Neuromotor[6] ❑ Neurobehavioral[8] ❑ Puberty ❑	Vocational planning ❑ Neuromotor clinic ❑ Assistive technology[7] ❑ Ophthalmology ❑
18 years / / *CBC* ❑ *Sexual[5]* ❑ *Cholesterol* ❑ *Scoliosis* ❑	Growth ❑ Hearing, vision[2] ❑ Audiology ❑	School progress ❑ Neuromotor[6] ❑ Neurobehavioral[8] ❑	Vocational planning ❑ Neuromotor clinic ❑ Assistive technology[7] ❑
20 years[9] / / *CBC* ❑ *Sexual[5]* ❑ *Cholesterol* ❑ *Dentist* ❑	Growth ❑ Hearing, vision[2] ❑ Audiology ❑	Nutrition ❑ Neuromotor[6] ❑ Neurobehavioral[8] ❑ Work, residence ❑	Family support[4] ❑ Neuromotor clinic ❑ Assistive technology[7] ❑ Ophthalmology ❑

Clinical concerns for Cerebral Palsy, ages 6+ years

Seizures   Refractive errors   Cognitive disability
Spasticity   Hearing, vision loss   Incontinence

Guidelines for prior ages should be undertaken *at the time of diagnosis*; Td, tetanus/diphtheria; MMR, measles–mumps–rubella; Var, varicella; [1]alternative timing; [2]by practitioner; [3]as dictated by clinical findings; [4]parent group, family/sib, financial, and behavioral issues as discussed in the preface; [5]birth control, STD screening if sexually active; [6]continence, drooling, [7]position, ambulation, communication; [8]cognition, communication, psychosocial; [9]repeat every decade.

Preventive Management of Spina Bifida

Clinical diagnosis: Although usually evident at birth, the level/severity of spina bifida and the presence of additional malformations must be determined. Rarely, apparent neural tube defects will prove to be more simple meningoceles with minimal neurologic impairment or involve lipomas of the spinal cord (Shurtleff et al., 1986). **Incidence:** 0.6–1.8 per 1000 births.

Genetics: Multifactorial determination with a 2–3 percent recurrence risk after one affected child. Preconceptional supplementation of folic acid in amounts similar to those in standard multivitamins significantly lowers the recurrence risk (Mulinare et al., 1988).

Key management issues: Intermittent catheterization techniques, signs of ventriculoperitoneal shunt malfunction or infection, control of bowel function, urological complications (urinary retention, urinary tract infection, reflux, and hydronephrosis), tethered cord (back or leg pain, worsening of gait, scoliosis, long-track neurologic findings), avoidance of latex-containing products, and early intervention/school monitoring for learning differences (Liptak et al., 1988).

Parent groups: Spina Bifida Association of America, 4590 MacArthur Boulevard NW, Suite 250 Washington DC, 20007–4226; (202) 944–3285, http://www.sbaa.org; Spina Bifida Association of Canada, 220–388 Donald St., Winnepeg, MB CAN R3B 2J4, (204) 925–3650; Association for Spina Bifida and Hydrocephalus, 42 Park Road, Peterborough PE1 2UQ, UK, postmaster@asbah.demon.co.uk, www.asbah.demon.co.uk/, 01-733-555-988

Growth charts: No specific charts are available.

Basis for management recommendations: Healthwatch for the person with myelodysplasia (Rubin & Crocker, 1989; Rauen, 1990).

Summary of clinical concerns

General	Learning	Cognitive disabilities (attention, memory, sequencing, reasoning) Learning differences (perceptual-motor problems, eye-hand coordination, language skills exceed math skills) Conversational ability may conceal problems with comprehension
	Behavior	School and behavioral problems; learning difficulties may compound adolescent adjustment to disability
	Growth	Feeding problems (hospitalization may delay feeding routines), dysphagia, early short stature, later obesity
Facial	Eye	Oculomotor dysfunction, **strabismus** (20%)
	Mouth	Oromotor dysfunction, dysphagia
Surface	Epidermal	Open skin wound, decreased mobility, decubital ulcers
Skeletal	Axial	Abnormal posture, **scoliosis** (up to 90%), orthotic and bracing needs
	Limbs	**Orthopedic problems** (hip dislocation, club foot deformity, osteoporosis), Muscle wasting (if non-ambulatory or following immobilization for orthopedic surgery), ambulation problems, appliance needs
Internal	Digestive	Bowel dysfunction, constipation, gastrointestinal and toileting problems
	RES	**Latex sensitivity** (20%)
	Excretory	**Bladder dysfunction** (100%), urinary incontinence, urologic problems (infection, urinary retention, reflux, hydronephrosis)
Neural	CNS	**Hydrocephalus** (90%), seizures (10%), anticonvulsant needs
	Motor	**Delayed motor skills,** lower extremity paralysis, impaired mobility, ambulation problems, appliance needs
	Sensory	Loss of sensation, impaired coordination

RES, reticuloendothelial system, **bold: frequency > 20%**

Key references

Rubin, I.L. & Crocker, A.C. (eds.) (1989). *Developmental Disabilities: Delivery of Medical Care for Children and Adults.* Philadelphia: Lea & Febiger.

Liptak, G., Bloss, J., Briskin, H., Campbell, J., Hebert, E. & Revell, G. (1988). *Journal of Child Neurology* 3:3–20.

Rauen, K. (ed.) (1990). *Guidelines for Spina Bifida Health Case Services throughout Life.* SBAA.

D. Shurtleff, ed. 1986, *Myelodysplasias and Exotrophies: Significance, Prevention, and Treatment.* Orlando, Florida: Grune and Stratton.

Spina Bifida

Preventive medical checklist (0–1yr)

Patient		Birth Date / /	Number

Pediatric	Screen	Evaluate	Refer/Counsel
Neonatal / / *Newborn screen* ❏ *HB* ❏	Hearing, vision[2] ❏ Renal function ❏ Head, spine MRI[3] ❏	Level of NTD ❏ Feeding, muscle tone ❏ Movement ❏ Hydrocephalus ❏ Bony deformities ❏	Family support[4] ❏ Early intervention[5] ❏ Spina bifida team[6] ❏ Spina bifida counsel[7] ❏ Avoid latex exposure ❏
1 month / /	Growth ❏ Hearing, vision[2] ❏ Shunt function ❏	Feeding, nutrition ❏ Bladder/bowel function ❏ Neuromotor status ❏	Developmental pediatrics ❏ Genetic evaluation ❏ Spina bifida team[6] ❏
2 months / / *HB[1]* ❏ *Hib* ❏ *DTaP, IPV* ❏ *RV* ❏	Growth ❏ Hearing, vision[2] ❏ Shunt function ❏	Feeding, nutrition ❏ Bladder/bowel function ❏ Neuromotor status ❏	Early intervention[5] ❏ Spina bifida team[6] ❏ Genetic counseling ❏
4 months / / *HB[1]* ❏ *Hib* ❏ *DTaP/IPV* ❏ *RV* ❏	Growth ❏ Hearing, vision[2] ❏ Shunt function ❏	Feeding, nutrition ❏ Bladder/bowel function ❏ Neuromotor status ❏	Early intervention[5] ❏ Spina bifida team[6] ❏ Spina bifida counsel[7] ❏
6 months / / *Hib* ❏ *IPV[1]* ❏ *DTaP* ❏ *RV* ❏	Growth ❏ Hearing, vision[2] ❏ Shunt function ❏	Feeding, nutrition ❏ Bladder/bowel function ❏ Neuromotor status ❏	Family support[4] ❏ Spina bifida team[6] ❏ Spina bifida counsel[7] ❏
9 months / / *IPV[1]* ❏	Growth ❏ Hearing, vision[2] ❏ Shunt function ❏	Neuromotor status ❏	
1 year / / *HB* ❏ *Hib[1]* ❏ *IPV[1]* ❏ *MMR[1]* ❏ *Var[1]* ❏	Growth ❏ Hearing, vision[2] ❏ Audiology ❏ Urinalysis, BP ❏ Shunt function ❏	Feeding, nutrition ❏ Bladder/bowel function ❏ Neuromotor status ❏ Prelanguage function ❏	Family support[4] ❏ Early intervention[5] ❏ Spina bifida team[6] ❏ Spina bifida counsel[7] ❏ Ophthalmology ❏

Clinical concerns for Spina Bifida, ages 0–1 year

Hydrocephalus, strabismus	Renal failure, hypertension	Incontinence, latex allergy
Shunt or urinary infection	Hip dislocation, scoliosis	Tethered cord

Guidelines for the neonatal period should be undertaken *at whatever age* the diagnosis is made; DTaP, acellular DTP; IPV, inactivated poliovirus (oral polio also used); RV, rotavirus; MMR, measles–mumps–rubella; Var, varicella; [1]alternative timing; [2]by practitioner; [3]as dictated by clinical findings; [4]parent group, family/sib, financial, and behavioral issues as discussed in the preface; [5]including developmental monitoring and motor/speech therapy; [6]including a nurse coordinator with specialists in pediatrics, neurosurgery, pediatric urology, and pediatric orthopedics – the timing of follow-up visits may vary from team to team and from patient to patient; [7]counsel avoidance of latex products, bowel management, signs of shunt malfunction.

Spina Bifida

Preventive medical checklist (15m–6yrs)

Patient   **Birth Date**   /   /   **Number**

Pediatric	Screen		Evaluate		Refer/Counsel	
15 months / / *Hib*[1] ❏ *MMR*[1] ❏ *DTaP, IPV*[1] ❏ *Varicella*[1] ❏	Growth	❏	Feeding, nutrition Bladder/bowel function Neuromotor status	❏ ❏ ❏	Family support[4] Early intervention[5] Spina bifida team[6]	❏ ❏ ❏
18 months / / *DTaP, IPV*[1] ❏ *Varicella*[1] ❏ *Influenza*[3] ❏	Growth Hearing, vision[2] Shunt function	❏ ❏ ❏	Feeding, nutrition Bladder/bowel function Neuromotor status	❏ ❏ ❏	Assistive technology[8] Seating/positioning Ambulation plans	❏ ❏ ❏
2 years / / *Influenza*[3] ❏ *Pneumovax*[3] ❏ *Dentist* ❏	Growth Hearing, vision[2] Audiology Urinalysis, BP Shunt function	❏ ❏ ❏ ❏ ❏	Feeding, nutrition Bladder/bowel function Neuromotor status	❏ ❏ ❏	Family support[4] Spina bifida team[6] Spina bifida counsel[7] Assistive technology[8]	❏ ❏ ❏ ❏
3 years / / *Influenza*[3] ❏ *Pneumovax*[3] ❏ *Dentist* ❏	Growth Hearing, vision[2] Audiology Urinalysis, BP Shunt function	❏ ❏ ❏ ❏ ❏	Feeding, nutrition Bladder/bowel function Neuromotor status	❏ ❏ ❏	Family support[4] Preschool transition[5] Spina bifida team[6] Spina bifida counsel[7] Assistive technology[8]	❏ ❏ ❏ ❏ ❏
4 years / / *Influenza*[3] ❏ *Pneumovax*[3] ❏ *Dentist* ❏	Growth Hearing, vision[2] Urinalysis, BP Shunt function	❏ ❏ ❏ ❏	Bladder/bowel function Neuromotor status Ambulation, nutrition Neurobehavioral[9]	❏ ❏ ❏ ❏	Family support[4] Preschool program[5] Spina bifida team[6] Spina bifida counsel[7]	❏ ❏ ❏ ❏
5 years / / *DTaP, OPV*[1] ❏ *MMR*[1] ❏	Growth Hearing, vision[2] Audiology Urinalysis, BP Shunt function	❏ ❏ ❏ ❏ ❏	Bladder/bowel function Neuromotor status Ambulation, nutrition Neurobehavioral[9]	❏ ❏ ❏ ❏	School transition[5] Spina bifida team[6] Spina bifida counsel[7] Ophthalmology	❏ ❏ ❏ ❏
6 years / / *DTaP, IPV*[1] ❏ *MMR*[1] ❏ *Dentist* ❏	Growth Hearing, vision[2] Shunt function	❏ ❏ ❏	School progress Bladder/bowel function Neuromotor status Nutrition	❏ ❏ ❏ ❏	Spina bifida team[6] Spina bifida counsel[7] Self-care planning Assistive technology[8]	❏ ❏ ❏ ❏

Clinical concerns for Spina Bifida, ages 1–6 years

Hydrocephalus, strabismus   Renal failure, hypertension   Incontinence, latex allergy
Shunt or urinary infection   Hip dislocation, scoliosis   Tethered cord

Guidelines for prior ages should be undertaken *at the time of diagnosis*; IPV, inactivated poliovirus (oral polio also used); MMR, measles–mumps–rubella; Var, varicella; [1]alternative timing; [2]by practitioner; [3]as dictated by clinical findings; [4]parent group, family/sib, financial, and behavioral issues as discussed in the preface; [5]including developmental monitoring and motor/speech therapy; [6]including a nurse coordinator with specialists in pediatrics, neurosurgery, pediatric urology, and pediatric orthopedics – the timing of follow-up visits may vary from team to team and from patient to patient; [7]counsel avoidance of latex products, bowel management, signs of shunt malfunction; [8]position, ambulation, communication.

Spina Bifida

Preventive medical checklist (6+ yrs)

Patient	Birth Date / /	Number

Pediatric	Screen	Evaluate	Refer/Counsel
8 years / / *Dentist* ❏	Growth ❏ Hearing, vision[2] ❏ Shunt function ❏	Bladder/bowel function ❏ Neuromotor status ❏ Ambulation, nutrition ❏ Neurobehavioral[9] ❏	School options ❏ Spina bifida team[6] ❏ Spina bifida counsel[7] ❏ Self-care planning ❏
10 years / /	Growth ❏ Hearing, vision[2] ❏ Shunt function ❏	School progress ❏ Bladder/bowel function ❏ Neuromotor status ❏ Self-care skills ❏	Spina bifida team[6] ❏ Spina bifida counsel[7] ❏ Self-care planning ❏ Assistive technology[8] ❏
12 years / / *Td[1], MMR, Var* ❏ *CBC* ❏ *Dentist* ❏ *Scoliosis* ❏ *Cholesterol* ❏	Growth ❏ Hearing, vision[2] ❏ Shunt function ❏	Puberty, nutrition ❏ Bladder/bowel function ❏ Neuromotor status ❏ Neurobehavioral[9] ❏	Family support[4] ❏ School options ❏ Spina bifida team[6] ❏ Spina bifida counsel[7] ❏ Self-care planning ❏
14 years / / *CBC* ❏ *Dentist* ❏ *Cholesterol* ❏ *Breast CA* ❏ *Testicular CA* ❏	Growth ❏ Hearing, vision[2] ❏ Audiology ❏ Urinalysis, BP ❏ Shunt function ❏	School progress ❏ Puberty, nutrition ❏ Bladder/bowel function ❏ Neuromotor status ❏	Spina bifida team[6] ❏ Spina bifida counsel[7] ❏ Assistive technology[8] ❏
16 years / / *Td[1]* ❏ *CBC* ❏ *Cholesterol* ❏ *Sexual[5]* ❏ *Dentist* ❏	Growth ❏ Hearing, vision[2] ❏ Shunt function ❏	Puberty, nutrition ❏ Bladder/bowel function ❏ Neuromotor status ❏ Self-care skills ❏ Neurobehavioral[9] ❏	Vocational planning ❏ Spina bifida team[6] ❏ Spina bifida counsel[7] ❏ Self-care planning ❏
18 years / / *CBC* ❏ *Sexual[5]* ❏ *Cholesterol* ❏ *Scoliosis* ❏	Hearing, vision[2] ❏ Shunt function ❏	School progress ❏ Bladder/bowel function ❏ Neuromotor status ❏ Neurobehavioral[9] ❏	Vocational planning ❏ Spina bifida team[6] ❏ Spina bifida counsel[7] ❏ Assistive technology[8] ❏
20 years[10] / / *CBC* ❏ *Sexual[5]* ❏ *Cholesterol* ❏ *Dentist* ❏	Hearing, vision[2] ❏ Urinalysis, BP ❏ Shunt function ❏	Bladder/bowel function ❏ Neuromotor status ❏ Self-care skills ❏ Work, residence ❏	Family support[4] ❏ Spina bifida team[6] ❏ Spina bifida counsel[7] ❏

Clinical concerns for Spina Bifida, ages 6+ years

Hydrocephalus
Shunt, urinary infections

Renal failure, hypertension
Scoliosis, tethered cord

Incontinence, latex allergy
Learning differences

Guidelines for prior ages should be undertaken *at the time of diagnosis*; Td, tetanus/diphtheria; MMR, measles–mumps–rubella; Var, varicella; [1]alternative timing; [2]by practitioner; [3]as dictated by clinical findings; [4]parent group, family/sib, financial, and behavioral issues as discussed in the preface; [5]birth control, STD screening if sexually active; [6]including a nurse coordinator with specialists in pediatrics, neurosurgery, pediatric urology, and pediatric orthopedics – the timing of follow-up visits may vary from team to team and from patient to patient; [7]counsel avoidance of latex products, bowel management, signs of shunt malfunction; [8]position, ambulation, communication; [9]including psychoeducational, emotional, cognition, communication, and self-esteem; [10]repeat every decade.

5

Single anomalies, sequences, and associations

Single anomalies are confined to one body region or organ system, while sequences and associations disrupt several systems. As discussed in Chapter 1, isolated anomalies and sequences usually have an excellent prognosis unless the brain is affected. Associations are clusters of major anomalies that tend to occur together; their difference from syndromes is discussed in Chapter 1 and in the section on associations below. Single anomalies, sequences, and associations usually have a low genetic recurrence risk in contrast to syndromes with likelihood of chromosomal or Mendelian inheritance. The single anomalies, sequences, and associations discussed in this chapter were selected because they are fairly common and have important implications for preventive management. They are listed in Table 5.1.

Single anomalies and sequences

Because the embryo is a dynamic structure, anomalies occurring at one stage in development may lead to consequences in later stages (see Chapter 1). Renal agenesis (an isolated anomaly) initiates a cascade of consequences including oligohydramnios, facial deformations, and club feet (Potter sequence). This cascade or "sequence" of events has the low recurrence risk expected of isolated anomalies rather than the likelihood of genetic or chromosomal etiology implied by syndromes. Preventive management can be lifesaving for disorders such as Pierre Robin sequence, or facilitate palliative care and postmortem counseling for disorders such as Potter sequence. In anomalies such as cleft palate, informed management prevents complications such as hearing loss and speech delay.

Amniotic band disruption sequence

The developing embryonic vascular system and the close apposition of embryo and extra-embryonic membranes provide numerous opportunities for morphologic catastrophe. Defects such as porencephaly (cystic lesion in the brain) or hemifacial microsomia (small ear and jaw on one side) have been related to vascular accidents in the fetal or embryonic period. Whether by vascular accidents or

Table 5.1 Single anomalies, sequences, and associations

Anomaly, sequence, or association	Incidence (live births)	Preventive measures
Isolated anomalies and sequences		
Amniotic disruption sequence	1 in 10,000	Orthopedic and/or craniofacial evaluation; hearing, vision, developmental assessment if craniofacial
Cleft lip/cleft palate	1 in 1000	Plastic surgery and craniofacial evaluation; hearing
Cleft palate	1 in 2500	assessment, evaluation for chronic otitis
Craniofacial deformations: plagiocephaly	~1 in 100	Evaluation for craniosynostosis, monitoring of head shape and growth, helmeting
Craniofacial deformations: torticollis	~1 in 500	Monitoring of head shape, neck extension
DiGeorge anomaly	~1 in 10,000	Cardiac, thymus, serum calcium evaluation; cellular immunity, hearing, ECI
Frontonasal malformation	~1 in 50,000	Craniofacial surgery, examination for frontal encephalocele, vision and hearing testing
Klippel–Feil anomaly, type I (severe)	1 in 6–10,000	Cervical spine flexion-extension radiographs, ophthalmology, audiology
Klippel–Feil anomaly, type II (mild)	1 in 100	None
Pierre Robin sequence	1 in 8500	Prone positioning, monitoring of growth, nasopharyngeal airway if obstruction
Associations		
VATER association	1 in 6000	See VATER checklist, parts 2–4
CHARGE association	1 in 20,000	See CHARGE checklist, parts 2–4

other mechanisms, the breakdown of the amnion may produce tissue remnants (bands) that encircle fetal parts and cause severe anomalies. As mentioned in Chapter 1, these mechanical or physiologic lesions are often called disruptions to separate them from true malformations; disruptions almost always occur sporadically, with no evidence for genetic transmission in patients with milder defects who survive to reproduce. A particularly high rate of disruptions occurs in monochorionic twins, where vascular connections in their common placenta can produce twin-to-twin shunting.

Amniotic bands have an incidence of about 1 in 10,000 live births, with a much higher incidence in abortuses (Levy, 1998). Amniotic bands may suggest facial clefts if other bands affecting the limbs are not noted (Kumar, 1996). Further inspection may reveal that the cleft has a geographic rather than embryonic distribution, more consistent with adhesion and tearing by a band than with a known embryonic cleavage. Depending on its timing and distribution, the amnion rupture sequence of anomalies includes limb, craniofacial, and/or lateral body wall defects

(Froster & Baird, 1993). Unfortunately, there are as yet no model systems that can distinguish among possible causes of the amnion rupture (i.e., amnion hypoplasia, inappropriate cell death, altered vascular supply, etc.). Genetic mechanisms may occasionally produce anomalies that resemble amniotic bands, as illustrated by certain mouse mutants (Elliot et al., 1995).

Preventive management begins with assessment of the distribution of anomalies and involvement of the appropriate surgical specialties. Most amniotic band disruptions involve the extremities and require the involvement of orthopedic surgery. More extensive craniofacial involvement should be managed by a craniofacial surgery team, with pediatric attention to early feeding, nutrition, growth, chronic otitis, hearing assessment, vision evaluations, and developmental assessment. Genetic counseling should be provided to ease parental guilt about contributing to the disruptions and to emphasize the usual low recurrence risk.

Cleft lip/cleft palate

Despite several centuries of observation, understanding of the pathogenesis of cleft palate is still rudimentary. The embryology is well documented, with failure of the primary palate involved in cleft lip/cleft palate and failure of the lateral palatine process fusion in cleft palate alone. Cleft lip with or without cleft palate occurs in about 1 in 1000 live births, and the incidence of cleft palate alone is 1 in 2500 live births (Milerad et al., 1997). If a parent has cleft palate, then there is an approximate 2–3 percent recurrence risk for primary relatives to have cleft palate; the same occurs with cleft lip/cleft palate. Both types of clefts "breed true" and are consistent with polygenic inheritance. Although there is considerable variation among studies, from 2–14 percent of patients with cleft lip and 13–64 percent of patients with cleft lip/cleft palate have associated anomalies (Milerad et al., 1997). Conversely, over 300 syndromes have cleft lip or cleft lip/cleft palate as a component defect. This large number of syndromes corroborates polygenic inheritance of the isolated anomalies and implicates many genetic loci in the causation of oral clefts.

Parent support groups for cleft lip/palate include the Cleft Palate Foundation (CPF), 104 South Estes Drive Suite 204, Chapel Hill NC, 27514 USA, (800) 242–5338 (800–24–CLEFT), cleftline@aol.com, http://www.cleft.com; Cleft Lip and Palate Association (CLAPA), 134 Buckingham Palace Road, London SW1A 9SA, telephone 0171–824–8110.

Preventive management of children with cleft lip consists of appropriate craniofacial and plastic surgery referral with later attention to dental care (Nguyen & Sullivan, 1993; Posnick & Thompson, 1995; Rohrich et al., 1996; Witt et al., 1997; Witt & Marsh, 1997). For children with cleft lip/palate, there are additional risks for chronic otitis and hearing loss, feeding problems, speech problems, sleep apnea

(Sheldon, 1998), and more severe dental anomalies (Robson et al., 1992). In general, the risk for missing or malpositioned teeth correlates with the severity of cleft and the degree of jaw hypoplasia (DeLuke et al., 1997). There is also a higher risk for growth delay in children with cleft lip/cleft palate, so growth, feeding, and nutrition should all be closely monitored (Lee et al., 1996; Cunningham & Jerome, 1997). Specialized nipples and prostheses are very helpful in the management of cleft lip/cleft palate, and referral to a specialized cleft palate team is ideal (Bardach et al., 1992). Complications after cleft palate surgery may include nocturnal enuresis due to airway obstruction (Nowak & Weider, 1998).

Management of isolated cleft palate is similar to that for patients with cleft lip/cleft palate, except that corrective surgery to improve appearance and parental acceptance is not as urgent. Submucous clefts may be subtle and require special diagnostic methods (Gosain et al., 1996a).

Craniofacial deformations – torticollis and plagiocephaly

Cranial deformations usually have an excellent prognosis once birth frees the baby from uterine constraints or compression during the delivery process. Congenital torticollis or wry neck is often accompanied by a mass (fibromatosis) of the sternocleidomastoid muscle, producing decreased extension and tilting of the head toward the affected side (Ackerman et al., 1996; Blythe et al., 1996). The anomaly is usually sporadic, rarely exhibiting multifactorial determination (Engin et al., 1997). Torticollis can occur secondary to gastroesophageal reflux (Sandifer syndrome) or ocular problems (Williams et al., 1996), necessitating treatment of the underlying cause. The primary anomaly usually resolves spontaneously, but sometimes requires bracing, range of motion exercises, or even botulinum toxin (Wheeler, 1997). Rarely, persistent torticollis may cause progressive craniofacial deformity, and surgery may be considered. Preventive management is limited to monitoring of feeding and craniofacial growth, with surgical referral for severe cases.

Plagiocephaly (cranial asymmetry) can occur because of uterine constraint, abnormal fetal presentation, or craniosynostosis (Roddi et al., 1995; Posnick, 1996; Huang et al., 1998). Breech presentation is a common cause of plagiocephaly and other deformities such as congenital hip dislocation, scoliosis, torticollis, and talipes equinovarus (Gorlin et al., 1990, p. 3). Recent recommendations for "baby on back" sleeping during infancy has increased the frequency of occipital plagiocephaly due to postnatal positioning (Argenta et al., 1996; Huang et al., 1996; Kane et al., 1996; Sadove, 1996; Jones et al., 1997; McAlister, 1998; Rekate, 1998). Preventive management of plagiocephaly consists of neonatal evaluation to assess severity, followed by close monitoring of head growth and head shape during the first month of life (Pollack et al., 1997; Belkengren & Sapala, 1998). In children with severe or progressive deformity, a cranial MRI scan is probably worthwhile to exclude brain anomalies, hydrocephaly, or craniosynostosis. If recognized during the childhood period when the cranium is flexible, plagiocephaly can be treated by remolding the head shape with plastic helmets. Children with significant plagiocephaly should be referred to a craniofacial surgery team for evaluation, including the exclusion of craniosynostosis through examination, skull films, or cranial MRI scan (Posnick, 1996).

DiGeorge anomaly

The DiGeorge anomaly involves malformation of the thymus, parathyroid, heart, and craniofacies, producing hypocalcemia, cardiac disease, and cellular immune deficiency. The craniofacial changes are suggestive of a branchial arch abnormality with micrognathia, middle ear anomalies, and down-turned corners of the mouth. The condition is most characteristically associated with a microdeletion of chromosome 22 (Lindsay et al., 1995; Cuneo et al., 1996, 1997), and it has considerable overlap with other chromosome 22 deletion phenotypes such as Shprintzen syndrome (see Chapter 9). Patients with DiGeorge anomaly may also have choanal atresia, laryngomalacia, or palatal defects, and similarities to the CHARGE association are discussed below (Markert et al., 1997). The DiGeorge anomaly is a component of many other chromosomal or teratogenic syndromes (including fetal alcohol syndrome) and has an incidence of about 1 in 10,000 births (Leitch & Winter, 1996).

Parent support groups for DiGeorge anomaly include the Velo-Cardio-Facial Syndrome Educational Foundation (VCFSEF), Jacobson Hall Room 707 University Hospital 750 East Adams Street, Syracuse NY, 13210 USA, (315) 464–6590, vcfsef@hscsyr.edu, http://www.hscsyr.edu/~vcfsef; The 22q and You Center, Clinical Genetics Center, The Children's Hospital of Philadelphia 34th & Civic Center Blvd, Philadelphia, PA 19104 USA, (215) 590–2920, mcginn@email.chop.edu, http://cbil.humgen.upenn.edu/VCFS/index.html; Primary Immunodeficiency Association, http://www.pia.org.uk, United Kingdom.

Preventive management is complex and can follow the deletion 22/Shprintzen checklist presented in Chapter 9. Correction of hypocalcemia and treatment of seizures may be required in the neonatal period, when chest radiographs, echocardiography, and examination of the palate and choanae are essential. Later management includes evaluation of cellular immunity (T-cell counts, phytohemagglutinen stimulation, candidal skin testing), avoidance of live viral vaccines until adequate immunity is demonstrated, and hearing assessments. Thyroid and gastrointestinal anomalies have been associated with the DiGeorge anomaly, and many who survive infancy have had mental deficiency (Gorlin et al., 1990, pp. 663–6; Jones, 1997, pp. 616–17). If a chromosome 22 deletion is found, testing of parents may be considered even though the likelihood of a positive finding and the recurrence risk are low.

Frontonasal malformation

This anomaly has been termed "frontonasal dysplasia" even though there is no evidence that tissue dysplasia is involved. There is striking hypertelorism with a broad nasal root, and it is important to realize that an encephalocele may be present in the midline. Associated problems may include epibulbar dermoids or colobomas of the eyes, optic disc anomalies (Hodgkins et al., 1998), malformed ears with conductive hearing loss, brain anomalies including hydrocephalus, and mental deficiency (Gorlin et al., 1990, pp. 785–89; Guion-Almeida et al., 1996; Qureshi & Khan, 1996; Jones, 1997, pp. 240–1). Preventive management should include referral to craniofacial surgery, monitoring of head circumference, hearing and vision testing, and cranial imaging to determine the presence of brain anomalies or frontal encephalocele. A specific syndrome involves frontonasal malformation with cranial and limb changes (Orr et al., 1997).

Klippel–Feil anomaly

Klippel–Feil anomaly involves fusion of the cervical vertebrae (Baba et al., 1995; Guille et al., 1995; Sarwark & Kramer, 1998). The fusion may be occult or, in more severe cases, associated with shortening of the neck, limitation of head movement, and pterygium colli (webbed neck). Some authors have called the occult form type II Klippel–Feil anomaly, while more severe fusions of the cervical and upper thoracic vertebrae have been called type I (Gorlin et al., 1990, pp. 886–8; Jones, 1997, pp. 618–19). The milder type II Klippel–Feil anomaly has an incidence of about 1 in 100 live births, while the more severe type I form has an incidence of 1 in 6–10,000 live births. As with other isolated anomalies, Klippel–Feil anomaly usually implies a low recurrence risk. The anomaly does occur as a component of several syndromes, including the Noonan, Wildervanck, and Goldenhar syndromes (Crockard & Stevens, 1995).

For patients with severe type I anomalies, the low hairline, short neck, and pterygium colli should alert the physician to obtain spinal radiographs to document the degree of fusion. Milder type II fusions will usually be detected on routine radiographs taken later in life; they require few precautions and do not pose a risk for military service (Gluck & Mawn, 1992). Eye anomalies (strabismus, nystagmus), hearing loss (25–50 percent), and cleft palate (17 percent) have been associated with severe cervical vertebral fusions, and congenital heart defects sometimes noted (Gorlin et al., 1990, 886–8).

Pizzutillo et al. (1994) reported two types of cervical spine mobility in type I Klippel–Feil patients that depend on the localization of fusion. Some have increased motion of the upper cervical segments with risk for neurological injury, while others have increased movement of the lower cervical segments with risk for degenerative arthritis. Neurologic complications, dysraphic lesions of the spinal cord (Steinbok, 1995; David et al., 1996), and even brain anomalies (Kennedy & McAuley, 1998) may be associated. Accordingly, preventive management of patients with extensive cervical fusions should include cervical spine flexion-extension radiographs to assess the pattern and mobility of cervical spine movements (Karasick et al., 1998; Rouvreau et al., 1998). All patients should be treated carefully during intubation or anesthesia, and monitoring by ophthalmology, audiology, and neurology is recommended. Patients with cleft palate should be watched for development of chronic otitis media and given speech therapy as appropriate.

Pierre Robin sequence

The variable definition of Pierre Robin sequence may account for incidence estimates that range from 1 in 2000 to 1 in 30,000 live births (Gorlin et al., 1990, pp. 700–5; Jones et al., 1997, 234–5). The classic description was by Pierre Robin in 1923, and the anomaly is a component of more than 20 syndromes (Gorlin et al., 1990, p. 701). The primary defect is thought to be mandibular hypoplasia, which interferes with tongue descent and produces a U-shaped cleft palate. All patients should be screened for associated anomalies, particularly the retinal detachment that may occur with Robin sequence in the Stickler syndrome (see Chapter 16). Preventive management includes prone positioning which may prevent respiratory complications (Shprintzen & Singer, 1992). Monitoring of growth and feeding is important since some patients have had growth and developmental delay that may reflect respiratory obstruction. The cleft may produce velopharyngeal immotility, requiring aggressive speech therapy (Witt et al., 1995). Monitoring of pulmonary functions and blood gases, together with sleep studies, should be considered in patients with poor growth. A nasopharyngeal airway should be inserted in patients with respiratory problems, since catch-up growth of the mandible can be anticipated. Most patients appear normal after a few years.

Associations

Although first promoted by Quan & Smith (1973), associations have long been emphasized in the surgical literature, where discovery was critical for operative outcome (e.g., Kirkpatrick et al., 1983). Associations describe anomalies that occur together more often than would be expected by chance and are like syndromes in defining a pattern of anomalies (Evans et al., 1993). Unlike syndromes, associations do not have an implied unique cause. Some view associations as statistical entities that will eventually disclose underlying syndromes or sequences (Spranger et al.,

1982). Others view associations as real biological entities that will highlight unique developmental mechanisms (Lubinsky, 1986; Evans et al., 1993; Opitz & Wilson, 1996). Progress with the CHARGE association (see below) suggests that both perspectives have merit.

How do associations differ from syndromes? A brief period of embryonic injury is hypothesized for associations, contrasting with the prolonged developmental impact of syndromes. In syndromes, the persistence of abnormal chromosomes or genes throughout the embryonic and fetal periods produces not only major malformations but also minor anomalies that reflect altered "fine-tuning" of structure (Lubinsky, 1986). Minor anomalies often produce a distinctive facies in syndromes that is lacking in associations. The major anomalies of associations usually share a critical embryonic period, illustrated by the embryonic day 20–25 period that characterizes abnormal vertebral, cardiac, and tracheo-esophageal development in VATER association. Lubinsky & Moeschler (1986) further supported this idea of a shared embryonic time period by demonstrating that defects of early cardiac morphogenesis (e.g., dextrocardia) occur together with early VATER anomalies (e.g., sacral defects, hydrocephaly), while later cardiac anomalies (e.g., septal defects) occur with tracheo-esophageal fistula. In contrast, syndromes include mixes of anomalies with very different critical periods, as shown by the septal defects, clinodactyly, and single palmar creases that occur in Down syndrome. One minor anomaly that does occur in VATER association is the single umbilical artery, present in 35 percent of cases.

An International Working Group (Spranger et al., 1982, p. 163) defined association as a "non-random occurrence in two or more individuals of multiple anomalies not known to be a polytopic field defect, sequence, or syndrome." Opitz (1993) emphasized the early embryonic timing by defining association as "idiopathic occurrence of multiple congenital anomalies during blastogenesis." In practice, the predominance of major anomalies and sporadic occurrence are the most important aspects of associations, for these guide the approach to diagnosis and counseling.

VATER association

Terminology

VATER association is an acronym that represents *V*ertebral defects, *A*nal atresia, *T*racheo–*E*sophageal fistula, *R*adial limb and *R*enal defects. Synonyms include VACTERL association, where the "C" and "L" are added to emphasize cardiac and limb defects (Rittler et al., 1996; Botto et al., 1997).

Historical diagnosis and management

Among many well-known associations of midline anomalies (e.g., Kirkpatrick et al., 1965), Say & Gerald (1968) drew attention to the frequent concurrence of polydactyly, imperforate anus, and vertebral anomalies. The grouping of anomalies was expanded and popularized by Quan & Smith (1973) as the VATER association, despite concerns by Say (1975) that the acronym would prove more confusing than helpful. Surgical advances have greatly improved the management of patients with VATER association, which even in recent studies has an infant mortality rate of 48 percent (Khoury et al., 1983).

Incidence, etiology, and differential diagnosis

More than 500 individuals with VATER association have been reported in the literature, and a 1968–79 population survey from metropolitan Atlanta yielded 400 patients with 2 VATER anomalies and 50 nonsyndromal patients with 3 or more VATER anomalies (Khoury et al., 1983). The survey included about 300,000 live births (11,366 individuals with birth defects), allowing the birth incidence for VATER association to be estimated at 1.6 per 1000. Based on the incidence of individual VATER defects in the population, only 29 rather than 400 persons with 2 VATER defects and 1 rather than 50 persons with three VATER defects would be expected by chance, demonstrating the strong tendency for these anomalies to cluster together.

The etiology of VATER association is unknown, although infants of diabetic mothers show an increased incidence. As currently defined, the diagnosis is excluded if a recognizable chromosomal or genetic syndrome is found. Risks for the full association to recur are minimal, but relatives with component defects of the association have been described in VATER families. For this reason, genetic contribution to VATER malformations is suspected and being pursued by several laboratories. The pathogenesis involves injury to developing mesoderm at 20–25 days postconception, resulting in abnormal development of vertebral, anorectal, cardiac, tracheo-esophageal, radial and renal derivatives. As discussed in the overview, dysmorphogenesis seems limited to major organ systems, with few minor anomalies of face, palate or limbs.

Differential diagnosis is large because many genetic and chromosomal syndromes include one or more components of the VATER association. Most dangerous is the misdiagnosis of patients with trisomy 18 as VATER association, since the management of their cardiac, radial ray, and renal defects may be inappropriately aggressive and fraught with the operative instability manifested by patients with chromosomal disease. Appreciation of minor anomalies such as malformed ears, aberrant palmar creases, prominent heels, or rocker-bottom feet allows suspicion of trisomy 18, with the use of bone marrow karyotype determination to make the diagnosis within 3–4 hours. Mendelian syndromes such as Holt–Oram (heart, limb defects), Fanconi anemia (heart, limb, vertebral defects), or Townes–Brock (heart, anal defects) may also resemble VATER association and lead to inappropriate

Table 5.2 Spectrum of anomalies in the VATER association contrasted with sacrococcygeal dysgenesis (caudal deficiency) and the Goldenhar complex

	VATER Association		Sacral dysgenesis	Goldenhar complex
	Weaver et al.	Duncan et al.	Duncan et al.	Rollnick et al.
Anomalies	(1986)	(1991)	(1991)	(1987)
Vertebral				
Cervical		10	3	22
Thoracic		18	22	
Lumbar		22	55	
Sacrococcygeal		50	35	
Percentage with vertebral anomaly	60	100[a]	100[a]	24
Anorectal	56	88	0	≤2
Cardiac	73	24	0	5
Tracheo-esophageal fistula	60	28	0	—
Renal	74	85	26	5[b]
Limb, upper	44	29	0	2
Limb, lower	43	30	73	3
Eye	—	4	0	20
Ear	39	10	0	99
Branchial arch/jaw	9	—	—	100[a]
Cleft lip +/− palate	13	3	0	22
Genital	44	55	3	5[b]
SUA[c]	33	10	0	—
CNS[d]	5	16	69	13

Notes:
[a] Ascertained by this anomaly; [b]both genital and urinary tract; [c]single umbilical artery; [d]central nervous system, including spina bifida, hydrocephalus and lower limb dysfunction. Percentages that distinguish the disorders are underlined.

genetic counseling (David et al., 1996; Rossbach et al., 1996; Lurie & Ferencz, 1997; Lomas et al., 1998). Radial ray defects can occur in VATER association as well as in association with the chromosome 22q11 deletion (Digilio et al., 1997).

Considerable overlap of the VATER spectrum of anomalies (Rittler et al., 1996; Botto et al., 1997) with those of the caudal regression and Goldenhar syndrome/hemifacial microsomia complexes is indicated by the terms "axial mesodermal dysplasia spectrum" (Russell et al., 1981) and "sacrococcygeal dysgenesis association" (Duncan et al., 1991) – see Table 5.2. The admonition of Say (1975) to go beyond the VATER acronym and consider a broad spectrum of anomalies should thus be heeded.

Table 5.2 compares the frequency of anomalies in the VATER association, sacrococcygeal dysgenesis association, or caudal regression sequence (Duncan et al., 1991), and the hemifacial microsomia/Goldenhar complex (Rollnick et al., 1987). The predominance of cardiac, tracheo-esophageal, renal, upper limb, and genital anomalies in VATER association is highlighted, but overlap occurs with anorectal, lower limb, eye, ear, palatal, and central nervous system anomalies. Vertebral anomalies are categorized according to their highest level of affliction (Duncan et al., 1991); the caudal positioning of VATER and sacral dysgenesis association defects contrasts with but is not exclusive of the cervical bias in Goldenhar syndrome. While different anomaly patterns are certainly evident in VATER association, the manifestations of sacral dysgenesis and Goldenhar/hemifacial microsomia complex must be considered in the management of VATER patients.

Diagnostic evaluation and medical counseling

Since there is no biological marker for VATER association, the diagnosis is made by documenting component anomalies. Severe anorectal, cardiac, tracheo-esophageal, and limb defects will present with obvious signs or symptoms, but milder anomalies of these systems plus vertebral or renal defects may require laboratory and imaging studies for diagnosis. VATER association should be considered after one cognate defect is recognized, but the degree of suspicion will depend on the presenting anomaly. For example, children with tracheo-esophageal fistula have a 37 percent frequency of cardiac defects, while those with cardiac defects have only a 1.4 percent chance to have tracheo-esophageal fistula. It is thus more important to investigate cardiac status in children with tracheo-esophageal fistula than vice versa.

A reasonable approach to the diagnostic evaluation is to screen for all of the cognate VATER anomalies once two of them have been documented. For example, in the absence of identified syndromes, children with limb and cardiac defects should have spinal x-rays, renal sonogram, and surveillance for feeding/respiratory problems. Finding of a third cognate anomaly makes the diagnosis secure. Patients with tracheo-esophageal fistula certainly deserve echocardiography and renal sonography, as do patients with imperforate anus (31 percent likelihood of renal defects once imperforate anus is documented; Khoury et al., 1983). Patients with renal defects or vertebral defects also deserve echocardiography (26 and 25 percent respective risks for cardiac defects according to Khoury et al., 1983). Patients with initial ascertainment of cardiac or limb anomalies have low risks for associated anomalies (Khoury et al., 1983).

Family and psychosocial counseling

Patients having 3 or more of the cognate VATER association defects and no obvious pattern of minor anomalies can be given a firm diagnosis with low recurrence risk (< 1 percent). Although patients with tracheo-esophageal fistula and/or severe cardiac defects have considerable mortality (as high as 48 percent in some studies), the good chance for normal mental development warrants health professionals taking an optimistic attitude toward these children. Psychosocial counseling, as for any child with a serious medical illness, may be useful for emotional and social stresses associated with prolonged and difficult hospitalization. Parent support groups for VATER association are available (see the VATER checklist, part 1).

Natural history and complications

Most complications of VATER association are direct consequences of congenital anomalies (checklist, part 1). Occasional patients will have growth failure during infancy or more subtle abnormalities like strabismus, myopia, torticollis, scoliosis, hip dislocation, urinary tract infections, neurogenic bladder, or altered gait (Weaver et al., 1986; Duncan et al., 1991; Chestnut et al., 1992; Lu & Ridker, 1994). Urinary tract problems may lead to urolithiasis (Unuvar et al., 1998). These potential complications require surveillance in early childhood. Major roles of the primary physician are to ensure thorough evaluation, to coordinate surgical care, and to provide optimistic case management with the realization that most patients have normal neurologic outcomes. While infancy and early childhood may be turbulent periods for patients with VATER association, specialized adolescent and adult care is required only for residual problems from infantile anomalies.

A documented complication of VATER association is spinal dysraphism (Chestnut et al., 1992). This abnormality consists of intraspinal lipomas or dermoids, tethering of the distal conus by a thickened filum terminale, diastematomyelia, etc. In 50 percent of patients, the dysraphism may be heralded by cutaneous surface markers such as lipomas, hemangiomas, sacral sinuses, sacral dimples, or asymmetric gluteal folds. If not detected in infancy, compression or traction of the spinal cord may lead to deterioration of walking, asymmetric leg musculature and strength, enuresis and poor bladder control. Myelomeningocele is a well-documented complication of VATER association, and spinal dysraphism represents the milder side of this spectrum. Although the frequency of spinal dysraphism in VATER association has yet to be established, Chestnut et al. (1992) reported six VATER patients with this problem and suggest routine spinal ultrasound in infants or spinal MRI in older children with VATER association.

VATER association preventive management checklist

The most critical period of management for children with VATER association is in the nursery, where documentation of the component anomalies has immediate medical and surgical consequences (checklist, part 1). Patients with tracheo-esophageal fistula or anorectal anomalies certainly warrant echocardiographic investigation as discussed above. Renal anomalies are sufficiently frequent in all VATER association groups that ultrasound study is also justified. Even without surface markers in the sacral area, ultrasound of the lower spine to evaluate spinal dysraphism is justified based on later consequences in several VATER patients. Once the patient is past the early childhood period, care is similar to that for the general population unless residual problems from congenital anomalies are present (see checklist, parts 3–4).

CHARGE association

Terminology

CHARGE is an acronym that was formulated by Pagon et al. (1981) for the association of Coloboma, Heart disease, Atresia choanae, Retarded growth and development, Genital anomalies, and Ear anomalies. Facial similarities in some patients (Fig. 5.1, color plate) and occasional familial occurrence has caused some to prefer the term "CHARGE syndrome."

Historical diagnosis and management

Multiple congenital anomalies associated with coloboma and choanal atresia were recognized for at least 20 years before their designation as CHARGE association (Angelman, 1961; Hall, 1979; Harvey et al., 1991). As with VATER association, surgical improvements have lengthened survival for CHARGE association patients.

Incidence, etiology, and differential diagnosis

CHARGE association is sufficiently frequent that more than 250 cases have been reported. Based on the incidence of bilateral choanal atresia (1 in 8000 live births) and its 50 percent risk for associated anomalies, an incidence of 1 in 20,000 live births for CHARGE association seems reasonable (Harris et al., 1997). Its prevalence in older children will be diminished by significant infant mortality. The choanae are formed between days 35 and 38 of gestation; cardiac septation begins on day 38 of gestation, and closure of the fetal choroid fissure (that fails in colobomata) occurs from 28 to 35 days of gestation, establishing a critical period for causation of CHARGE association (Opitz, 1993).

Differential diagnosis includes consideration of VATER association, where heart defects and esophageal atresia may occur. Craniofacial disorders such as the Crouzon or Treacher – Collins syndrome may include choanal atresia, while Kallman syndrome includes central nervous system and genital defects (Jones, 1988). As emphasized by Pagon et al. (1981), occurrence of colobomata and cardiac disease in patients with trisomy 13, dup(22q), or del(4p) syndromes mandates a

Table 5.3 Comparison of anomalies in CHARGE association, DiGeorge anomaly, and Shprintzen syndrome

| Anomaly | CHARGE Association | | | | | | DiGeorge | Shprintzen |
	A	B	C	D	(Total)	%	E, F (%)	G (%)
Colobomata	16/19	17/20	43/47	15/16	(91/102)	89	7	3
Heart defect	12/21	16/20	42/50	14/17	(84/108)	78	95	82
Atresia choanae	13/21	13/20	28/50	6/17	(60/108)	55	—(low)	—(low)
Retarded growth	20/21	17/20	39/43	7/7	(83/91)	92	—(high)	33
Devel. delay	20/21	12/20	26/34	2/7	(60/82)	73	—(low)	40
Genital defect (M)	11/15	14/14	28/29	—	(53/58)	92	3	10
Ear anomaly	17/21	20/20	50/50	17/17	(104/108)	97	46	70
Renal anomaly	—	6/20	12/50	6/11	(24/81)	30	11	—(low)
Death by 1 yr	6/21	1/20	10/50	9/17	(26/108)	24	54	—(low)
Cleft lip/palate	5/21	—	—	6/17	(11/38)	29	6	98
Deafness	—	19/20	34/50	8/9	(61/79)	77	2	—(low)
Facial palsy	11/18	12/20	16/50	9/9	(48/97)	50	7	—(low)

Notes:

M, male; Percentages that distinguish the disorders are underlined.

Source: A, Pagon et al. (1981); B, Oley et al. (1988); C, Blake et al. (1989); D, Harvey et al. (1991); E, Greenberg (1993); F, Wilson et al. (1993); G, Goldberg et al. (1993).

normal karyotype before rendering a diagnosis of CHARGE association. An interesting exception to this rule may be the finding of deletions of the proximal long arm of chromosome 22 – del(22q11); these deletions are very common in patients with DiGeorge anomaly or Shprintzen syndrome (Devriendt et al., 1998). Since DiGeorge anomaly occurs in both CHARGE association and Shprintzen syndrome (face and palatal anomalies with conotruncal heart defects), and since the three disorders have similar types of cardiac anomalies, the "CATCH 22" spectrum of disorders (Wilson et al., 1993) may yield insight into the etiology of CHARGE association.

Diagnostic evaluation and medical counseling

Diagnosis of CHARGE association is based purely on the pattern of anomalies, since no diagnostic test is yet available. Comparison of anomalies in CHARGE association to those of the DiGeorge anomaly and Shprintzen syndrome is made in Table 5.3. CHARGE association frequencies are totaled from the series of Pagon et al. (1981), Oley et al. (1988), Blake et al. (1990), and Harvey et al. (1991) – each requiring that 4 of the cognate anomalies be present. Table 5.3 illustrates that high frequencies of coloboma, choanal atresia, male genital defects, deafness, and facial palsy distinguish CHARGE association from DiGeorge or Shprintzen syndrome. High frequencies of cleft lip/palate including velopalatine incompetence are characteristic of Shprintzen syndrome, while patients with isolated DiGeorge anomaly will lack cleft lip/palate and the coloboma/choanal atresia/facial palsy characteristic of CHARGE association. Despite these differences, patients with CHARGE association who also have DiGeorge anomaly and/or the prominent nose and palatal defects suggestive of Shprintzen syndrome deserve FISH studies for del(22)(q11) as part of their chromosome study (see Chapter 9). The presence of laryngeal anomalies and/or severe swallowing problems in CHARGE patients may also warrant evaluation of del(22)(q11), since the Opitz syndrome of dysphagia, reflux, and genital anomalies also has been related to this deletion (McDonald-McGinn et al., 1995).

Family and psychosocial counseling

Most cases are sporadic and predict a low recurrence risk for parents. However, several reports of familial CHARGE association (Pagon et al., 1981; Mitchell et al., 1985), including concurrence in identical twins (Oley et al., 1988), indicate a higher risk for certain families. Genetic factors may also be suggested by an increased paternal age (Tellier et al., 1996). Many patients with CHARGE association have a better prognosis for growth and development than would be predicted based on their early feeding problems and developmental delay (Blake et al., 1990; Harvey et al., 1991). Cautious optimism is thus warranted, particularly for those patients with normal neuroimaging and chromosome studies who survive infancy. Most families will require supportive counseling and services appropriate for raising a child with cognitive and physical disabilities. Parent groups are available (checklist, part 1).

Natural history and complications

The spectrum of complications in CHARGE association (checklist, part 1) is derived from the studies cited in Table 5.3. Intrauterine growth retardation occurs in 16 percent of patients with 92 percent showing growth delay during infancy. Mortality is high (28 percent) with about half dying in the neonatal period and half during infancy. Most exhibited developmental delay (73 percent), with 8 of 47 patients (17 percent) described as severe (Admiraal & Huygen, 1997; Blake et al., 1998). Cardiac anomalies tend to be severe, with tetralogy of Fallot, atrioventricular septal defect, ventricular septal defects, and patent ductus arteriosus being common in CHARGE association, as opposed to the interrupted aortic arch that is common in patients with DiGeorge anomaly. Pulmonary anomalies are also common (Markert et al., 1997; Sporik et al., 1997). Colobomata are often found in the fundus only (59 percent), emphasizing the importance of an ophthalmologic evaluation (Hayashi et al., 1998; Shah et al., 1998). Deafness may occur because of central nervous system or middle ear anomalies, and 77 percent of patients will have hearing deficits (Dhooge et al., 1998). Other anomalies include tracheo-esophageal fistula/esophageal atresia, omphalocele, facial palsy, cleft lip/palate, renal anomalies, and genital defects in males (checklist, part 1).

CHARGE association preventive management checklist

The high rate of central nervous system, airway, and neurosensory complications in CHARGE syndrome requires more comprehensive preventive care than in VATER association (Kaplan, 1989; Morgan et al., 1993; Bowling & Chandna, 1994). Blake et al. (1990, 1998) emphasized the importance of multidisciplinary management in CHARGE association, estimating that the number of exposures to general anesthesia could have been reduced by at least 25 percent using a more unified approach. The pediatrician's role as case manager can be extremely beneficial to these patients (checklist, parts 2–4). Blake et al. (1990, 1998) also point out the frequency of complications from aspiration; monitoring of patients after operations and thorough review of feeding/swallowing histories is thus important.

Neonatal evaluation of eyes, nose (airway), palate, heart, brain, kidney, and genitalia are indicated in CHARGE patients, along with early functional assessment of hearing and vision. Most patients will require extensive follow-up by ophthalmology and ENT specialists, and the high rate of growth/developmental problems mandates attention to nutrition, growth, early intervention, and school programs. Because the DiGeorge anomaly may occur, early chest x-ray to look for the presence of a thymus as well as calcium and white blood cell count measurements are indicated. The chest x-ray also is useful to screen for vertebral anomalies, and subsequent examinations for scoliosis should be performed. Significant risks for urinary tract anomalies warrant early sonographic screening and monitoring of urinalysis and blood pressure.

Preventive Management of VATER Association

Clinical diagnosis: VATER association is an acronym that represents *V*ertebral defects, *A*nal atresia, *T*racheo-*E*sophageal fistula, *R*adial limb and *R*enal defects, sometimes expanded to VACTERL to denote *C*ardiac and *L*imb defects (Quan & Smith, 1973).

Laboratory diagnosis: None available.

Incidence: 1.6 per 1000 births.

Genetics: Sporadic with less than 1% recurrence risk unless underlying syndromes like trisomy 18 or X-linked VACTERL with hydrocephalus are present.

Key management issues: Detection and surgical treatment of cardiac, renal, or tracheo-esophageal anomalies; monitoring of growth; alertness for complications such as hydrocephalus, choanal atresia, strabismus, myopia, torticollis with cervical spine anomalies, lower spine anomalies with scoliosis, hip dislocation, urinary tract infections, urolithiasis, tethered cord with neurogenic bladder or altered gait.

Growth Charts: Mapstone et al. (1986) distinguished two patient groups with VATER association, one with low-normal and one with delayed growth; many but not all of the delayed group had cardiac disease.

Parent groups: TEF/VATER Support Network, c/o Greg and Terri Burke, 15301 Grey Fox Rd, Upper Marlboro, MD 20772; (301) 952–6837; TOFS (Tracheo-Oesophageal Fistula Support Group), St. George's Centre, 91 Victoria Road, Netherfield, Nottingham, UK NG4 2NN, (44) (0115) 961-3092; info@TOFS.org.uk; http://www.tofs.org.uk

Basis for management recommendations: Complications noted below as documented by Quan & Smith (1973), Rittler et al. (1996), Weaver et al. (1986). It should be noted that spinal dysraphism is a recently recognized complication, and that the sensitivity of spinal sonography in detecting this anomaly is not known.

Summary of clinical concerns

General	Life span	Stillbirth (12%), **increased infant mortality** (48%)
	Growth	Low birth weight, dysphagia, failure to thrive
Facial	Eye	Microphthalmia, strabismus, myopia
	Ear	Chronic otitis, preauricular tags, **malformed pinna** (10–39%)
	Nose	Choanal atresia, respiratory obstruction
	Mouth	Cleft lip/palate, oromotor dysfunction
Surface	Neck/trunk	Klippel–Feil anomaly, torticollis, **inguinal hernia** (23%), hernia incarceration
Skeletal	Cranial	Large fontanelles, plagiocephaly
	Axial	Vertebral anomaly (80%), rib anomaly (23%), scoliosis (32%)
	Limbs	**Upper limb defect (35%** – radial aplasia, preaxial polydactyly); **lower limb defect (36%** – club foot, dislocated hip, flexion contractures)
Internal	Digestive	**Anorectal anomaly** (70%), gastroesophageal reflux, intestinal obstruction, vomiting, constipation
	Pulmonary	**Tracheoesophageal fistula** (28–60%), horseshoe Lung
	Circulatory	**Cardiac anomaly** (50% – VSD, ASD, PDA, tetralogy of Fallot, coarctation)
	Excretory	**Renal anomaly** (24–85% – renal agenesis, renal cysts, small or horseshoe kidney); **urinary tract anomaly** (48% – patent urachus, hydronephrosis, hydroureter); obstructive uropathy, urinary tract infections
	Genital	**Genital anomaly** (44–55% – cryptorchidism, hypospadias, micropenis, vaginal atresia)
Neural	CNS	Spina bifida, hydrocephalus, spinal dysraphism (tethered cord), enuresis
	Motor	Ambulation problems

Bold: frequency > 20%

Key references

Chestnut, R., James, H.E. & Jones, K.L. (1992). *Pediatric Neurosurgery* 18:144–8.

Mapstone, C.L., Weaver, D.D. & Yu, P.-L. (1986). *American Journal of Diseases of Children* 140:386–90.

Quan, L. & Smith, D.W. 1973. *Journal of Pediatrics* 82:104–7.

Rittler, M., Paz, J. E. & Castilla, E. E. (1996). *American Journal of Medical Genetics* 63:529–36.

Weaver, D.D., Mapstone, C.L. & Yu, P.-L. (1986). *American Journal of Diseases of Children* 140:225–9.

VATER Association

Preventive medical checklist (0–1yr)

Patient		Birth Date / /		Number	
Pediatric	**Screen**	**Evaluate**		**Refer/Counsel**	
Neonatal / / Newborn screen ❏ HB ❏	Echocardiogram ❏ Renal sonogram ❏ Spinal x-rays ❏ Spinal sonogram[1] ❏	Feeding/stooling ❏ Sacral dimple ❏ Hip click ❏		Genetic evaluation ❏ Cardiology, nephrology[3] ❏ Orthopedics[3] ❏ Pediatric Surgery[3] ❏ Neurosurgery[3] ❏	
1 month / /	Head size ❏	Feeding/stooling ❏ Urine stream ❏ Inguinal hernia ❏		Family support[4] ❏ Feeding specialist[3] ❏	
2 months / / HB[1] ❏ Hib ❏ DTaP, IPV ❏ RV ❏	Head size ❏ Growth ❏	Feeding/stooling ❏ Hip click ❏ Nutrition ❏		Early intervention[3,5] ❏ Feeding specialist[3] ❏ Genetic counseling ❏	
4 months / / HB[1] ❏ Hib ❏ DTaP/IPV ❏ RV ❏	Head size ❏ Growth ❏	Feeding/stooling ❏ Urine stream ❏ Nutrition ❏		Early intervention[3,5] ❏ Feeding specialist[3] ❏	
6 months / / Hib ❏ IPV[1] ❏ DTaP ❏ RV ❏	Head size ❏ Growth ❏ Urinalysis, BP ❏	Inguinal hernia ❏ Hip click ❏ Nutrition ❏		Family support[4] ❏ Dietician[3] ❏	
9 months / / IPV[1] ❏		Strabismus ❏ Nutrition ❏		Ophthalmology[3] ❏ Dietician[3] ❏	
1 year / / HB ❏ Hib[1] ❏ IPV[1] ❏ MMR[1] ❏ Var[1] ❏	Head size ❏ Growth ❏ Urinalysis, BP ❏ Spinal sonogram[1] ❏	Inguinal hernia ❏ Nutrition ❏		Family support[4] ❏ Early intervention[3,5] ❏ Genetics ❏ Dietician[3] ❏	

Clinical concerns for VATER Association, ages 0–1 year

Hydrocephalus	T-E fistula	Growth deficiency
Choanal atresia	Cardiac anomaly	Urinary tract anomaly
Cleft lip/palate	Vertebral anomaly	Cryptorchidism
Torticollis	Spinal dysraphism	Club foot

Guidelines for the neonatal period should be undertaken *at whatever age* the diagnosis is made; DTaP, acellular DTP; IPV, inactivated poliovirus (oral polio also used); RV, rotavirus; MMR, measles–mumps–rubella; Var, varicella; BP, blood pressure; [1]alternative timing; [2]by practitioner; [3]as dictated by clinical findings; [4]parent group, family/sib, financial, and behavioral issues as discussed in the preface; [5]including developmental monitoring and motor/speech therapy.

VATER Association

Preventive medical checklist (15m–6yrs)

Patient		Birth Date / /	Number

Pediatric	Screen		Evaluate		Refer/Counsel	
15 months / / *Hib[1]* ❑ *MMR[1]* ❑ *DTaP, IPV[1]* ❑ *Varicella[1]* ❑	Growth	❑	Nutrition	❑	Family support[4] Early intervention[3,5] Dietician[3]	❑ ❑ ❑
18 months / / *DTaP, IPV[1]* ❑ *Varicella[1]* ❑ *Influenza[3]* ❑	Growth	❑	Nutrition	❑	Dietician[3]	❑
2 years / / *Influenza[3]* ❑ *Pneumovax[3]* ❑ *Dentist* ❑	Growth Hearing, vision[2] Urinalysis, BP	❑ ❑ ❑	Gait Strabismus Scoliosis	❑ ❑ ❑	Family support[4] Neurosurgery[3] Ophthalmology[3] Orthopedics[3]	❑ ❑ ❑ ❑
3 years / / *Influenza[3]* ❑ *Pneumovax[3]* ❑ *Dentist* ❑	Growth Hearing, vision[2] Urinalysis, BP	❑ ❑ ❑	Gait Strabismus Scoliosis Inguinal hernia	❑ ❑ ❑ ❑	Family support[4] Preschool transition[3,5] Dietician[3]	❑ ❑ ❑
4 years / / *Influenza[3]* ❑ *Pneumovax[3]* ❑ *Dentist* ❑	Hearing, vision[2] Urinalysis, BP	❑ ❑	Gait Strabismus Scoliosis	❑ ❑ ❑	Family support[4] Preschool program[3,5] Cardiology[3]	❑ ❑ ❑
5 years / / *DTaP, IPV[1]* ❑ *MMR[1]* ❑	Hearing, vision[2] Urinalysis, BP Tethered cord	❑ ❑ ❑	Gait Strabismus Scoliosis Inguinal hernia	❑ ❑ ❑ ❑	School transition Neurosurgery[3] Ophthalmology[3] Orthopedics[3]	❑ ❑ ❑ ❑
6 years / / *DTaP, IPV[1]* ❑ *MMR[1]* ❑ *Dentist* ❑	Growth Hearing, vision[2] Urinalysis, BP	❑ ❑ ❑	School progress Gait Genitalia	❑ ❑ ❑	Family support[4] Cardiology[3] Neurosurgery[3] Pediatric surgery[3]	❑ ❑ ❑ ❑

Clinical concerns for VATER Association, ages 1–6 years

Cleft lip/palate	Urinary tract anomaly	Growth deficiency
Vertebral anomaly	Cryptorchidism, micropenis	Spinal dysraphism

Guidelines for prior ages should be undertaken *at the time of diagnosis*; DTaP, acellular DTP; IPV, inactivated poliovirus (oral polio also used); MMR, measles–mumps–rubella; BP, blood pressure; [1]alternative timing; [2]by practitioner; [3]as dictated by clinical findings tethered cord may present with symptoms of altered gait, enuresis; [4]parent group, family/sib, financial, and behavioral issues as discussed in the preface; [5]including developmental monitoring and motor/speech therapy.

VATER Association

Preventive medical checklist (6+ yrs)

Patient		Birth Date / /	Number

Pediatric	Screen	Evaluate	Refer/Counsel
8 years / / *Dentist* ❑	Growth ❑ Tethered cord ❑		
10 years / /	Hearing, vision[2] ❑ Urinalysis, BP ❑	School progress ❑ Genitalia ❑ Gait ❑	
12 years / / *Td[1], MMR, Var* ❑ *CBC* ❑ *Dentist* ❑ *Scoliosis* ❑ *Cholesterol* ❑	Tethered cord ❑	Puberty ❑ Genitalia ❑	Family support[4] ❑ Ophthalmology[3] ❑ Cardiology[3] ❑ Neurosurgery[3] ❑ Pediatric surgery[3] ❑
14 years / / *CBC* ❑ *Dentist* ❑ *Cholesterol* ❑ *Breast CA* ❑ *Testicular CA* ❑	Hearing, vision[2] ❑ Urinalysis, BP ❑	School progress ❑ Puberty ❑ Genitalia ❑ Gait ❑	
16 years / / *Td[1]* ❑ *CBC* ❑ *Cholesterol* ❑ *Sexual[5]* ❑ *Dentist* ❑	Tethered cord ❑	Puberty ❑	
18 years / / *CBC* ❑ *Sexual[5]* ❑ *Cholesterol* ❑ *Scoliosis* ❑	Hearing, vision[2] ❑ Urinalysis, BP ❑	School progress ❑ Gait ❑	Ophthalmology[3] ❑ Cardiology[3] ❑ Neurosurgery[3] ❑ Pediatric surgery[3] ❑
20 years[6] / / *CBC* ❑ *Sexual[5]* ❑ *Cholesterol* ❑ *Dentist* ❑	Hearing, vision[2] ❑ Urinalysis, BP ❑	Gait ❑	Family support[4] ❑ Ophthalmology[3] ❑ Cardiology[3] ❑ Neurosurgery[3] ❑

Clinical concerns for VATER Association, ages 6+ years

Cleft lip/palate Torticollis	Cardiac anomaly Urinary tract anomaly Cryptorchidism	Growth deficiency Spinal dysraphism

Guidelines for prior ages should be undertaken *at the time of diagnosis*; Td, tetanus/diphtheria; MMR, measles–mumps–rubella; Var, varicella; [1]alternative timing; [2]by practitioner; [3]as dictated by clinical findings – tethered cord may present with symptoms of altered gait, enuresis; [4]parent group, family/sib, financial, and behavioral issues as discussed in the preface; [5]birth control, STD screening if sexually active; [6]repeat every decade.

Preventive Management of CHARGE Association

Clinical diagnosis: CHARGE is an acronym that was formulated by Pagon et al. (1981) for the association of Coloboma, Heart disease, Atresia choanae, Retarded growth and development, Genital anomalies, and Ear anomalies. Facial similarities among certain patients and occasional familial occurrence has caused some to prefer the term "CHARGE syndrome".

Laboratory diagnosis: None.

Incidence: 1 in 20,000.

Genetics: A karyotype is often necessary to rule out chromosomal disorders, with most cases of CHARGE association being sporadic with a low recurrence risk. Occasional familial examples (Pagon et al., 1981; Mitchell et al., 1985) indicate higher risks for certain families.

Key management issues: Neonatal evaluation for choanal atresia, feeding problems, and cardiac defects; ophthalmology evaluation for colobomata or strabismus, audiology for hearing deficits due to CNS or middle ear anomalies, monitoring of feeding with alertness for tracheoesophageal fistula/esophageal atresia, omphalocele, facial palsy, cleft lip/palate, and urogenital anomalies.

Growth charts: Blake et al. (1993) summarize growth data from 44 affected children.

Parent groups: CHARGE Syndrome Foundation, 20084 Parkade Boulevard, Columbia MO, 65202-3121,(800) 442-7604; http://www.chargesyndrome.org

Basis for management recommendations: Blake et al. (1990) published recommendations for the multidisciplinary management of CHARGE association. The head MRI scan recommended at age 6 months may be delayed or omitted in children without neurologic problems.

Summary of clinical concerns

General	Learning	**Cognitive and learning differences** (73%); severe delay (17%), speech problems
	Growth	Low birth weight (16%); failure to thrive (77%); short stature (92%)
	Life cycle	**Increased infant mortality** (24%)
Facial	Eye	Oculomotor dysfunction, eye anomalies (**colobomata**, 89%; **iris defects**, 30%, **fundus defects**, 59%); **nystagmus** (26%), **strabismus** (32%).
	Ear	**External ear anomaly** (97%), **middle ear anomaly** (38%)
	Nose	**Choanal atresia** (64%), respiratory obstruction
	Mouth	**Feeding problems** (75%), **cleft lip/palate** (29%), dysphagia
Surface	Neck/trunk	**Short neck** (20%)
	Epidermal	Dry skin, alopecia, skin rashes
Skeletal	Cranial	**Microcephaly** (25%)
	Axial	Hemivertebrae, scoliosis (16%)
	Limbs	Clinodactyly, syndactyly
Internal	Digestive	**Gastroesophageal reflux** (37%), gastrointestinal obstruction, TE fistula/atresia (10%), omphalocele, anal atresia
	Pulmonary	**Respiratory problems, laryngeal anomaly** (20%)
	Circulatory	**Cardiac anomalies** (84%)
	Endocrine	Hormonal deficiencies (hypothyroidism; growth hormone deficiency, flat luteinizing hormone releasing hormone response, low testosterone)
	RES	DiGeorge anomaly (14%), immune deficiency (14%), frequent infections
	Excretory	Renal **anomaly** (30%), hydronephrosis
	Genital	Male genital anomaly (92% – micropenis, cryptorchidism)
Neural	CNS	**Brain anomalies** (50% – arrhinencephaly, cerebellar dysplasia); seizures
	Motor	**Facial palsy** (50%), **facial asymmetry**
	Sensory	Acoustic nerve dysfunction, **nerve deafness** (38%), **mixed hearing loss** (30%), **hearing deficits** (77%)

RES, reticuloendothelial system, GI, gastrointestinal system; **bold: frequency > 20%**

Key references

Blake, K. D. et.al (1990). *Archives of Diseases of Children* 65:217–23.

Blake, K. et al. (1993). *Archives of Diseases of Children* 68:508–9.

Mitchell, J. A. et al. (1985). *Ophthalmology and Pediatric Genetics* 6:31–5.

Pagon, R.A. et al. (1981). *Journal of Pediatrics* 99:223–7.

Wyse, R.K.H. et al. (1993). *Pediatric Cardiology* 14:75–81.

CHARGE Association

Preventive medical checklist (0–1yr)

Patient   **Birth Date**   /   /   **Number**

Pediatric	Screen	Evaluate	Refer/Counsel
Neonatal / / *Newborn screen* ❑ HB ❑ [*Modify for DiGeorge*]	Echocardiogram ❑ Head sonogram ❑ Renal sonogram ❑ Urinalysis ❑ Thymus, WBC ❑ Calcium, P ❑	Airway ❑ Iris/fundus ❑ Feeds/stools ❑ Genitalia ❑ Facial muscles ❑	Genetic evaluation ❑ Feeding specialist ❑ Ophthalmology ❑ Cardiology, ENT ❑ Genetic evaluation ❑ Endocrinology[3] ❑
1 month / /	Head size ❑ Hearing/vision[2] ❑ Audiology ❑	Feeding, stooling ❑	Family support[4] ❑ Feeding specialist[3] ❑
2 months / / HB[1] ❑ Hib ❑ DTaP, IPV ❑ RV ❑	Growth ❑ Head size ❑ Hearing/vision[2] ❑	Feeding, stooling ❑ Nutrition ❑	Early intervention[5] ❑ Developmental pediatrics ❑ Genetic counseling ❑
4 months / / HB[1] ❑ Hib ❑ DTaP/IPV ❑ RV ❑	Growth ❑ Hearing, vision[2] ❑	Feeding, stooling ❑ Nutrition ❑	Early intervention[5] ❑
6 months / / Hib ❑ IPV[1] ❑ DTaP ❑ RV ❑	Growth ❑ Hearing/vision[2] ❑ Head MRI[3] ❑	Feeding/stooling ❑ Nutrition ❑	Family support[4] ❑ Development pediatrics ❑
9 months / / IPV[1] ❑	Audiology ❑	Strabismus ❑ Immunity ❑	Ophthalmology ❑ ENT ❑
1 year / / HB ❑ Hib[1] ❑ IPV[1] ❑ MMR[1] ❑ Var[1] ❑	Growth ❑ Hearing/vision[2] ❑ Urinalysis ❑	Nutrition ❑ Immunity ❑	Family support[4] ❑ Early intervention[5] ❑ Developmental pediatrics ❑ Genetics ❑

Clinical concerns for CHARGE Association, ages 0–1 year

Choanal atresia	Cleft lip/palate	Developmental disability
DiGeorge anomaly	TE fistula, omphalocele	Brain anomalies, seizures
Iris or fundus coloboma	Laryngeal anomaly	Facial palsies
Ear anomalies, hearing loss	Cardiac anomaly	Urogenital anomalies

Guidelines for the neonatal period should be undertaken *at whatever age* the diagnosis is made; if DiGeorge anomaly suspected, avoid live vaccines; DTaP, acellular DTP; IPV, inactivated poliovirus (oral polio also used); RV, rotavirus; MMR, measles–mumps–rubella; Var, varicella; P, phosphorus; TE, tracheo-esophageal; [1]alternative timing; [2]by practitioner; [3]as dictated by clinical findings; [4]parent group, family/sib, financial, and behavioral issues as discussed in the preface; [5]including developmental monitoring and motor/speech therapy.

CHARGE Association

Preventive medical checklist (15m–6yrs)

Patient　　　　　　　　**Birth Date** / /　　**Number**

Pediatric	Screen	Evaluate	Refer/Counsel
15 months / / Hib[1] ❑　MMR[1] ❑ DTaP, IPV[1] ❑ Varicella[1] ❑	Growth ❑	Nutrition ❑	Family support[4] ❑ Early intervention[5] ❑
18 months / / DTaP, IPV[1] ❑ Varicella[1] ❑ Influenza[3] ❑	Growth ❑	Nutrition ❑	
2 years / / Influenza[3] ❑ Pneumovax[3] ❑ Dentist ❑	Growth ❑ Urinalysis, BP ❑ Audiology ❑	Nutrition ❑ Immunity ❑	Family support[4] ❑ Developmental 　pediatrics ❑ Genetics ❑ Ophthalmology, ENT ❑
3 years / / Influenza[3] ❑ Pneumovax[3] ❑ Dentist ❑	Growth ❑ Urinalysis, BP ❑ Audiology ❑	Nutrition ❑ Scoliosis ❑	Family support[4] ❑ Preschool transition[5] ❑ Ophthalmology ❑ ENT ❑
4 years / / Influenza[3] ❑ Pneumovax[3] ❑ Dentist ❑	Growth ❑ Audiology ❑ Urinalysis, BP ❑	Nutrition ❑ Immunity ❑	Family support[4] ❑ Preschool program[5] ❑ Developmental 　pediatrics ❑ Genetics ❑ Ophthalmology, ENT[3] ❑
5 years / / DTaP, IPV[1] ❑ MMR[1] ❑	Growth ❑ Audiology ❑ Urinalysis, BP ❑	Nutrition ❑ Scoliosis ❑	School transition[5] ❑
6 years / / DTaP, IPV[1] ❑ MMR[1] ❑ Dentist ❑	Growth ❑ Hearing, vision[2] ❑ Urinalysis, BP ❑	School progress ❑ Nutrition ❑ Genitalia ❑ Scoliosis ❑	Developmental 　pediatrics ❑ Genetics ❑ Family support[4] ❑ Ophthalmology, ENT[3] ❑

Clinical concerns for CHARGE Association, ages 1–6 years

Nystagmus, strabismus	Laryngeal anomaly	Developmental disability
Ear anomalies, hearing loss	Cardiac anomaly	Brain anomalies, seizures
Cleft lip/palate	Respiratory problems	Facial palsies
GE reflux, failure to thrive	Urogenital anomalies	Scoliosis

Guidelines for prior ages should be undertaken *at the time of diagnosis*; IPV, inactivated poliovirus (oral polio also used); MMR, measles–mumps–rubella; BP, blood pressure; [1]alternative timing; [2]by practitioner; [3]as dictated by clinical findings; [4]parent group, family/sib, financial, and behavioral issues as discussed in the preface; [5]including developmental monitoring and motor/speech therapy.

CHARGE Association

Preventive medical checklist (6+ yrs)

Patient   **Birth Date** / /   **Number**

Pediatric	Screen		Evaluate		Refer/Counsel	
8 years / / *Dentist* ❑	Growth	❑	Nutrition Genitalia	❑ ❑	School options Developmental pediatrics Genetics Endocrinology[3]	❑ ❑ ❑ ❑
10 years / /	Growth Hearing, vision[2] Urinalysis, BP	❑ ❑ ❑	School progress Nutrition Genitalia	❑ ❑ ❑		
12 years / / *Td[1], MMR, Var* ❑ *CBC* ❑ *Dentist* ❑ *Scoliosis* ❑ *Cholesterol* ❑	Growth	❑	Puberty Genitalia	❑ ❑	Family support[4] School options Developmental pediatrics Genetics Ophthalmology, ENT[3]	❑ ❑ ❑ ❑ ❑
14 years / / *CBC* ❑ *Dentist* ❑ *Cholesterol* ❑ *Breast CA* ❑ *Testicular CA* ❑	Growth Hearing, vision[2] Urinalysis, BP	❑ ❑ ❑	School progress Puberty Genitalia Scoliosis	❑ ❑ ❑ ❑		
16 years / / *Td[1]* ❑ *CBC* ❑ *Cholesterol* ❑ *Sexual[5]* ❑ *Dentist* ❑			Puberty Scoliosis	❑ ❑	Vocational planning Developmental pediatrics Genetics[3]	❑ ❑ ❑
18 years / / *CBC* ❑ *Sexual[5]* ❑ *Cholesterol* ❑ *Scoliosis* ❑	Growth Hearing, vision[2] Urinalysis, BP School progress	❑ ❑ ❑ ❑	School progress	❑	Vocational planning Ophthalmology[3] ENT[3]	❑ ❑ ❑
20 years[6] / / *CBC* ❑ *Sexual[5]* ❑ *Cholesterol* ❑ *Dentist* ❑	Hearing, vision[2] Urinalysis, BP	❑ ❑	Work, residence	❑	Family support[4] Ophthalmology[3] ENT[3]	❑ ❑ ❑

Clinical concerns for CHARGE Association, ages 6+ years

Strabismus, nystagmus	Cardiac anomalies	Cognitive disability
Middle ear anomalies	Hypothyroidism	Immune deficiency
Hearing loss	Urogenital anomalies	Short stature
Failure to thrive	Scoliosis	Growth hormone deficiency

Guidelines for prior ages should be undertaken *at the time of diagnosis*; Td, tetanus/diphtheria; MMR, measles–mumps–rubella; Var, varicella; BP, blood pressure; [1]alternative timing; [2]by practitioner; [3]as dictated by clinical findings; [4]parent group, family/sib, financial, and behavioral issues as discussed in the preface; [5]birth control, STD screening if sexually active; [6]repeat every decade.

6

Teratogenic syndromes

It is quite remarkable that only about 20 of the more than 50,000 drugs and chemicals in common use are proven human teratogens (Schardein, 1985, p. 2). Considerably more – about 180 of 2800 tested – are teratogenic in two or more animal species (Schardein, 1985, p. 2). The example of Dr. Lenz, the pediatrician who identified thalidomide babies in 1961 (Kalter & Warkany, 1983), emphasizes the need for physicians to be alert and knowledgeable about potential teratogens. The references of Shardein (1985) and Shepard (1992) offer excellent guides to the teratogenic literature, and telephone hotlines are available through governmental or academic centers. Although teratology is a general term for the study of developmental anomalies, it is used here in the more limited sense to describe anomalies caused by environmental agents – physical, chemical, or infectious.

Less common syndromes

Parents are frequently concerned about environmental exposures to substances such as pesticides or industrial agents when their child has a congenital anomaly. It is again reassuring that only one environmental chemical – methyl mercury – is a proven human teratogen. The many lawsuits concerning agents such as dioxin or Bendectin are truly an American tragedy (Brent, 1988). These unscrupulous awards provide sad testimony to our inadequate science of congenital anomalies.

Brent (1995) reviewed the criteria required to prove that an agent is a human teratogen:

1 Human population studies associate an agent with a syndrome or specific type of congenital anomaly.
2 Human population studies demonstrate a correlation between the frequency of the anomaly and exposure to the agent.
3 Animal models yield the same types of anomalies at equivalent dosage/exposure ranges of the agent.
4 The frequency and/or severity of anomalies show correlation with dosage of the agent.

Table 6.1 Human teratogenic syndromes

Causal agent	Complications	Preventive measures, evaluations
Ethanol	IUGR, DD, growth, brain, eye, heart, joints	ECI, ophthalmology, ENT cardiology
Hydantoin	IUGR, DD, growth	ECI, limb x-rays
Maternal diabetes	IUGR or macrosomia, brain, heart, skeleton	ECI, cardiology, head imaging, vertebral x-rays
Maternal hyperthermia	DD, brain, limbs, eye, craniofacies, genitalia	ECI, ophthalmology, ENT, orthopedics, urology
Maternal PKU	IUGR, DD, brain, heart, joints	ECI, head imaging, cardiology
Methyl mercury	IUGR, DD, brain, vision, hearing	ECI, head imaging, ENT, ophthalmology
Retinoic acid	DD, craniofacies, brain, heart	ECI, head imaging, ENT, ophthalmology, cardiology
TORCH	IUGR, DD, brain, eye, hearing, liver, spleen, blood	ECI, head imaging, ENT ophthalmology, GI, hematology
Trimethadione	IUGR, heart	Cardiology
Valproic acid	Neural tube, DD, heart	ECI, cardiology
Varicella	IUGR, DD, eye, limbs, skin	ECI, ophthalmology, dermatology
Warfarin	IUGR, craniofacies, nose	ECI, head imaging

Notes:

IUGR, intrauterine growth retardation; DD, developmental disability; TORCH, toxoplasmosis, other (syphilis), rubella, cytomegalovirus, herpes; ECI, early childhood intervention; PKU, phenylketonuria.

5 A mechanism for teratogenesis is understood and/or the results make biological sense.

All of these criteria are fulfilled for agents such as thalidomide or alcohol, while none is fulfilled for Bendectin. Claims that an agent increases the frequency of all types of congenital anomalies, rather than a pattern of specific malformations, are particularly suspect. It is important for physicians to emphasize the 2–3 percent risk of congenital anomalies in an average pregnancy, to allay parental guilt about exposures when appropriate, and to avoid naive or deliberate support for unscientific claims.

Table 6.1 lists many of the agents that fulfill the criteria for human teratogenesis, including major complications and preventive measures (Jones, 1997). Important among these are congenital infectious agents, some remembered by the TORCH acronym (Epps et al., 1995). Less common conditions that affect the embryo (embryopathy) or fetus (fetal syndrome) are then summarized, followed by detailed recommendations for the management of children with fetal alcohol syndrome, fetal hydantoin syndrome, and diabetic embryopathy.

Cocaine – a fetal cocaine syndrome?

The 30 percent of adults in the United States who admit to at least one use of cocaine, coupled with the 9–30% rates of positive cocaine testing at delivery indicate a potentially common neonatal disorder. Detection of cocaine may reach 70–80 percent when meconium or hair is screened after delivery of women who have had no prenatal care. Although severe effects of fetal cocaine exposure have been reported by specialists seeing referral populations (Fries et al., 1993), blinded examination of exposed newborns has failed to demonstrate a characteristic appearance (Little et al., 1996). Higher frequencies of pregnancy loss; dysmorphology including large fontanel, short nose, shallow nasal bridge, and small toenails; and neurologic complications such as hypertonia, sleep disorders, autism, learning problems, and attention deficit hyperactivity have been suggested for infants exposed to cocaine, but a higher frequency of urogenital anomalies is the only consistent finding among multiple studies (Konkol, 1994). Based on the mechanism of drug action in adults, fetal vascular disruptions might be anticipated as supported by higher frequencies of abortion, placental abruption, and prematurity in pregnant women using cocaine. At present, the lack of a consistently documented fetal cocaine syndrome mandates only careful monitoring of exposed children, with no specific preventive measures beyond alertness for urologic problems.

Cytomegalovirus: Fetal cytomegalovirus syndrome

Congenital infection with cytomegalovirus is estimated to be present in 1–3 percent of newborns, producing variable consequences that range from no symptoms (80 percent) to mild or disseminated neonatal disease with hepatosplenomegaly, coagulopathy, jaundice, and anemia (Weller, 1971; Watt-Morse et al., 1995). Survivors of disseminated neonatal disease have high frequencies of developmental disability (60 percent), hyperactivity with seizures or spasticity (35 percent), and hearing loss (30 percent) (Hanshaw, 1994; Steinlin et al., 1996). Fetal infection may produce intrauterine growth retardation, microcephaly, and optic atrophy in addition to the complications of acute neonatal disease. As with rubella or toxoplasmosis, continuing infection in the infant may cause chorioretinitis, hematologic abnormalities, obstructive hydrocephalus, and intracranial calcifications (Garcia et al., 1998). Inguinal hernias also occur. Preventive management should be directed towards the nervous system, with neonatal eye, hearing, and head MRI evaluations to document baseline abnormalities. Subsequent early intervention and monitoring of hearing/vision, liver, and bone marrow function are needed during early childhood. Since neonatal outcome is better in mothers with recurrent rather than primary cytomegalovirus infection (Fowler et al., 1992), the development of an effective vaccine offers the best hope for true prevention of fetal cytomegalovirus syndrome (Hanshaw, 1994).

Herpes – congenital and neonatal herpes infection

Neonatal infection with herpes virus occurs in 1500–2000 infants each year in the United States (0.5–0.75 per 1000 births), usually transmitted from mothers with primary genital infection (Overall, 1994; Kohl, 1997; Jacobs, 1998; Witlin et al., 1998). Ninety percent of these infections are due to herpes simplex virus-2, and only 4 percent of herpes infections are truly congenital (acquired prenatally) as compared to 86 percent acquired natally and 10 percent postnatally (Overall, 1994). Preventive management of neonatal herpes infection mainly concerns Cesarean delivery to avoid exposure to genital lesions and subsequent treatment of exposed infants with vidarabine and acyclovir to lower mortality and neurologic sequellae. The diagnosis of neonatal infection is best made by viral culture from maternal genital lesions or fluids (establishing exposure) or from neonatal vesicles, eye swabs, mouth swabs, buffy coat, or cerebrospinal fluid (Elder et al., 1995). It is important to suspect the diagnosis in infants with pustular lesions (Wagner, 1997).

Even with antiviral treatment, infants with congenital or neonatally acquired infection have significant frequencies of neurologic sequellae. Among infants with congenital infection, 85 percent had low birth weight due to prematurity or intra-uterine growth retardation, 67 percent had microcephaly with seizures and intra-cranial calcifications, and 57 percent had microphthalmia and chorioretinitis (Overall, 1994). Neurologic sequellae were present in two-thirds of infant survivors with neonatal herpes encephalitis. Pediatric preventive management should therefore focus on neurological and neurosensory development, ensuring early intervention programs, family support services, and regular hearing/vision screening. Joint care with neonatal follow-up, ophthalmology, and neurology specialists would provide an ideal management team, with the pediatrician coordinating specialty and support services. Parental education and planning of future pregnancies with neonatal and obstetric specialists is also essential, since 5 to 7 percent of neonatal infections occur in offspring of women with recurrent or asymptomatic herpes virus shedding.

Human immunodeficiency virus – fetal and neonatal HIV infection

Over 1 million children worldwide acquire infection with human immuno-deficiency virus-1 (HIV-1), most due to congenital infection. Vertical transmission rates of 15–40 percent are documented by prospective studies, equally divided between transplacental or perinatal infection (including breast-feeding) from HIV-positive mothers (Luzuriaga & Sullivan, 1994). Prenatal treatment with antiviral agents can decrease the likelihood of HIV-1 transmission and improve the outcomes of infected infants; antiviral therapies including protease inhibitors are obviously indicated in HIV-positive infants. Nevertheless, the severity and frequency

(~0.3–0.5 per 1,000 births in the United States) of symptomatic congenital/neonatal HIV-1 infection is a considerable public health problem.

Although characteristic facial features such as frontal bossing, prominent eyes, hypertelorism, and thick lips have been described in infants with congenital HIV-1 infection, most complications seem due to postnatal rather than fetal alterations (Stevenson, 1993). As in adult HIV disease, the infantile immune system is impacted with susceptibility to frequent infections. Frequent upper respiratory infections may be muted with intravenous gammaglobulin, including specific immunoglobulin in children exposed to varicella (Luzuriago & Sullivan, 1994). Prophylaxis against *Pneumocystis* using trimethoprim sulfamethoxazole and against atypical mycobacteria using rifabutin should be considered in children with low CD4 T cell counts. Other complications include microcephaly, dermatitis, anemia, and growth failure, emphasizing the value of a multidisciplinary team devoted to HIV-positive children that is available in many large centers. Preventive management will involve nutrition, early intervention and developmental issues in addition to social and family supports needed for parents with chronic disease and/or orphaned children.

Retinoids: Retinoic acid embryopathy

The ingestion of large amounts of vitamin A (retinol) or smaller amounts of its potent derivatives (isotretinoin, retinoic acid) during pregnancy may be associated with a severe malformation syndrome (Lammer, 1985; Coberly et al., 1996). The pattern of malformations associated with retinoic acid embryopathy includes craniofacial anomalies with microcephaly, cerebellar anomalies, ocular anomalies (microphthalmia), cleft palate, micrognathia, and cardiac defects including septal defects or transposition. Similarity to the DiGeorge anomaly includes thymic aplasia, and there are a variety of less common but severe organ defects such as holoprosencephaly, liver, and renal disease.

Preventive management of children with retinoic embryopathy should begin with cranial MRI scan, echocardiography, renal ultrasonography, and a skeletal radiographic survey to define the extent of anomalies. Ophthalmology and otolaryngology evaluations should also be performed in early infancy, with subsequent monitoring of hearing, vision, growth, and development. Immune assessment should precede the administration of live viral vaccines, and monitoring of feeding is necessary because of the craniofacial anomalies and neurologic dysfunction. Mental deficiency is often severe, necessitating early intervention and parental counseling appropriate for children with severe mental disability.

Rubella — fetal rubella syndrome

Congenital rubella infection is now rare due to universal immunization programs. Occasional cases are encountered due to local outbreaks, usually among immigrants from countries without routine immunization (Centers for Disease Control, 1997b). The full-blown rubella syndrome includes deafness (96 percent), eye anomalies (52 percent), cardiac anomalies affecting the pulmonary artery (22 percent), and developmental disability (10 percent), with about half of affected children exhibiting growth delay (Stevenson, 1993; Webster, 1998). Deafness is usually sensorineural, and eye anomalies include cataract, glaucoma, microphthalmia, and myopia (Stevenson, 1993). Preventive management should therefore include neonatal auditory evoked response, ophthalmology, and echocardiography screening, followed by early intervention and monitoring of growth. Regular hearing and vision screening will then be indicated, with more intensive rehabilitation programs for those infants with growth delay since it correlates with neurodevelopmental problems. The best prevention is widespread immunization, since maternal antibodies to rubella virus prevent damage to the fetus.

Syphilis – fetal syphilis syndrome

Congenital syphilis, like other consequences of sexually transmitted diseases, has exhibited recent increases in frequency (Sison et al., 1997; Hollier & Cox, 1998). Although effective prevention and therapy is available through treatment of infected mothers, lack of prenatal care and unrecognized infection perpetuates the congenital syndrome. Diagnosis is available through the demonstration of IgM antibodies in the infant. Manifestations of congenital syphilis range from abortion or fetal hydrops to the well-known triad of eye keratitis, sensorineural deafness, and dental anomalies including notched teeth and tapering of the incisors (Stevenson, 1993). Fetal infection can cause intrauterine growth retardation and neurologic damage without the characteristic neonatal triad. For less severely affected neonates, early diagnosis through antibody testing allows treatment with penicillin or comparable antibiotics and produces an excellent prognosis (Finelli et al., 1998). Monitoring of development, growth, hearing, and vision is important, and formal audiology and ophthalmology evaluations may be useful to detect sensorineural hearing loss or chorioretinitis. Severely affected infants will need dental, neurologic, and orthopedic follow-up due to their bone and brain lesions. Mothers require treatment and counseling regarding future pregnancies (McFarlin & Bottoms, 1996).

Toluene – fetal toluene syndrome

Toluene sniffing during pregnancy may produce a fetal syndrome of microcephaly, micrognathia, renal anomalies, and growth failure (Hersch, 1989). The facies is subtle, so a maternal history is usually necessary to consider the diagnosis. Preventive management should consist of monitoring growth and development, with consideration of an abdominal ultrasound if renal anomalies are suspected through growth failure or urinary tract infection. Early intervention is needed because of developmental delay.

Toxoplasmosis – fetal toxoplasmosis syndrome

Congenital toxoplasmosis infection occurs at a rate of 0.1–2 per 1,000 births in the United States, with the overall rate of vertical transmission being 30–40 percent (Guerina, 1994; Beazley & Egerman, 1998; Dunn & Palmer, 1998; Phillips, 1998). Maternal infection during the first trimester is associated with more severe neonatal symptoms, with a transmission rate estimated at 15 percent. Maternal infection later in gestation is associated with higher transmission rates (~60 percent) but mild or asymptomatic neonatal disease. Prevention is best accomplished by maternal education to avoid contact with cat litter, undercooked meat, or soil through gardening or poorly washed vegetables. In France, where the incidence of toxoplasmosis and congenital infection is 2–3 fold higher than in the United States, spiramycin treatment of pregnant women with acute toxoplasmosis infection has been shown to lower fetal transmission and the severity of neonatal disease. A vaccine to lower the incidence of toxoplasmosis in cats and other hosts is under development.

Congenital toxoplasmosis infection may be asymptomatic or manifest during the neonatal or later infantile period. The acute presentation may include fever, respiratory illness, hepatosplenomegaly, anemia, and jaundice that mimics other congenital infections. Diagnosis by the detection of specific IgM antibody allows effective treatment using pyrimethamine, sulfadiazine, and folinic acid to ablate pyrimethamine toxicity (Guerina, 1994). Neonatal screening programs allowing early treatment have demonstrated effectiveness by lowering the frequency of subsequent neurologic and ophthalmologic complications. Initial clinical abnormalities in infants (Guerina, 1994) can include intracranial calcifications (25–71 percent), hydrocephalus (7–17 percent), seizures (6 percent), microcephaly (4–14 percent), retinal lesions (18–60 percent), and visual impairment (15–43 percent). After treatment, less than 4 percent of infants had motor deficits, none had cognitive or hearing deficits, and 8 percent acquired new retinal lesions with some visual impairment (unilateral only). Because of these complications, a specific preventive management program is recommended to accompany the treatment program (Guerina, 1994). An initial evaluation with cranial CT scan, lumbar puncture, ophthalmology examination, blood counts, liver function tests, urine culture (to exclude cytomegalovirus infection), and neurology examination is recommended. The initial evaluation is followed by biweekly blood counts during pyrimethamine therapy, monthly pediatric and neurodevelopmental assessment, ophthalmology examinations every 3 months with annual checks after age 18 months, and IgG/IgM antitoxoplasmosis antibody measurements every 3 months until age 18 months for monitoring of infection (Guerina, 1994).

Valproic acid – fetal valproate syndrome

In the two decades of experience with valproic acid therapy of epilepsy, a 2–4 fold increased frequency of spina bifida in exposed offspring has been demonstrated (Bantz, 1984; Hockey et al., 1996). Diverse reports of facial and organ defects suggest that there is a valproate syndrome, probably even an embryopathy (Gorlin et al., 1990, pp. 28–9). Facial features include metopic ridging with trigonocephaly and a narrow forehead. Organ anomalies include cardiac anomalies (ventricular septal defects, coarctation of the aorta), genital anomalies (hypospadias, cryptorchidism, Mullerian duct anomalies), and limb anomalies (digital anomalies, talipes equinovarus, nail hypoplasia). Preventive management would include recommendations for children with spina bifida in affected cases (Chapter 4), with monitoring for cardiac, genital, or limb defects in other exposed children. The extent and severity of the fetal valproate syndrome is not yet well defined, since most children have been exposed to a combination of anticonvulsant medications. Variability of effects between twins indicates the complexity of pathogenesis (Hockey et al., 1996).

Warfarin – fetal warfarin syndrome

Exposure of the fetus to coumarin anticoagulants during pregnancy may produce a syndrome of nasal hypoplasia and stippling of the epiphyses (chondrodysplasia punctata – Hanson & Smith, 1975b; Hall, 1976). The most characteristic anomaly is the "fleur-de-lys" nose with its shallow bridge and hypoplastic tip. Additional abnormalities include prenatal growth deficiency, failure to thrive, microcephaly, hydrocephaly, seizures, hearing loss, ocular anomalies (cataracts, strabismus), and choanal atresia. Preventive management should include an initial skeletal radiographic survey to assess the extent of skeletal involvement, monitoring of feeding and growth, monitoring of the head circumference, ophthalmology evaluation, and audiologic screening. The nasal hypoplasia and stippled epiphyses may occur in genetic disorders of vitamin K or peroxisomal metabolism (Pauli, 1988).

Fetal alcohol syndrome

Terminology

Fetal alcohol syndrome (FAS) denotes a pattern of physical and behavioral anomalies related to exposure to ethanol during pregnancy (Fig. 6.1, color plate; Jones & Smith, 1975; Duerbeck, 1997). Children with milder abnormalities from ethanol exposure, who lack the more severe and characteristic pattern of FAS, are described as having fetal alcohol effects (FAE).

Historical diagnosis and management

Dangers of drinking during pregnancy were mentioned in biblical times and were specifically emphasized during England's Gin Epidemic of 1720–1750 (Warner & Roset, 1975; Hill et al., 1989). Specific patterns of physical anomalies in offspring of alcoholic women were documented by Lemoine et al. (1968) and by Jones et al. (1973).

Incidence, etiology, and differential diagnosis

The incidence of fetal alcohol syndrome is heavily dependent on socioeconomic status and ethnic background. The overall incidence is now estimated at 0.97–1.9 cases per 1000 live births in the United States, reaching 43 per 1000 among "heavy" drinkers (Abel & Sokol, 1987; Abel, 1995; Centers for Disease Control 1995, 1997a, c). This general incidence is 10–20 times higher than in Europe and other countries (0.08 per 1000), representing higher rates in areas characterized by low socioeconomic status and African American or Native American background (2.29 cases per 1000; Abel, 1995). Because births with FAE are 3–4 times more common than those with FAS, 10–20 percent of all mental retardation may be related to pre-natal exposure to ethanol (Garro et al., 1992). Isolated communities with low socioeconomic status and high-risk ethnic backgrounds can have incidences reaching 1 in 5 (Robinson et al., 1987).

Brain anomalies and small eyes have been documented in several animal models of FAS, including rodents and nonhuman primates (Streissguth et al. 1991). Correlation of alcohol dosage and timing with teratogenesis establishes ethanol as the etiologic agent, but its mode of action has not been defined (Garro et al., 1992). Maternal nutrition seems to play a minor role, with acetaldehyde and prostaglan-dins implicated as mediators of teratogenesis (Garro et al., 1992). Intraperitoneal injection of mice with ethanol on gestational day 7 produced growth retardation, neural anomalies, and facial changes that were similar to human FAS (Sulik et al., 1981). Strain differences were observed in the patterns of anomalies produced, indicating that genetic background may influence human susceptibility to FAS and FAE.

Diagnosis of FAS is based on subjective recognition of minor anomalies com-bined with disproportionate microcephaly and failure to thrive. A quantitative cra-niofacial profile has been published (Astley & Clarren, 1995). Facial anomalies include small eyes, shallow nasal bridge, upturned nose, abnormal ears (posteriorly rotated or low-placed), thin upper lip, and absent philtrum. Burd & Martsolf (1989) presented a scoring system for the diagnosis of FAS or FAE that requires 12 points (10 points from major criteria and 2 points from minor criteria). Major cri-teria include mental retardation (1–3 points), growth retardation (1–3 points for height, weight, and head circumference), characteristic facial anomalies (1 point each), and documented gestational alcohol intake or infantile withdrawal (10 points each). Minor criteria include many of the complications of eyes, heart, skeleton, lungs, kidneys, and brain listed in the checklist, part 1, scoring 1 point for each anomaly. The scoring system is a useful checklist for FAS anomalies, but its specificity seems limited, since delayed growth and development with similar facial and somatic anomalies are found in many other disorders including Down syndrome.

Burd & Martsolf (1989) argued against the false dichotomy between FAS and FAE on the grounds that all teratogens exhibit a range of effects according to the severity of the exposure. Regardless of the terminology, it is important to realize that ethanol teratogenesis may not produce an obvious phenotype at birth. Little et al. (1990) used maternal toxicology data to show that most offspring with subsequent neurologic problems were not identified in the newborn period. Graham et al. (1988) reported that only half of children recognized as FAS by age 4 were identified at birth. Until a biochemical "footprint" of exposure to ethanol is defined that can be used for objective diagnosis, FAS has a very broad differential that includes many children with microcephaly and growth and developmental delay. Offspring of mothers with untreated phenylketonuria resemble those with FAS, as do children with a long list of genetic or chromosomal conditions with microcephaly and growth failure. Severely affected infants may have abnormal brains with heterotopias (abnormal cell migration), prompting consideration of other neurologic disorders. Milder effects of FAS include learning disabilities, poor impulse control, and hyperactivity that can be present in numerous other syndromes (Hanson et al., 1976). A broad differential diagnosis and high degree of suspicion are essential for FAS, since the definitive maternal history may require skill and experience to elicit (Hill et al., 1989; Centers for Disease Control, 1997a, c).

Diagnostic evaluation and medical counseling

A major aspect of diagnosis is a good parental history. As stressed by Hill et al. (1989), blunt or judgmental questions often meet with denial or underestimates of drinking that are classic for alcoholic persons. Questioning of both parents (social customs are often congruent), initial focus on non-threatening agents such as carbonated beverages, and specific mention of beer and wine (sometimes not considered "drinks") are important strategies (Hill et al., 1989). Smoking histories are important, since cigarette smoking is a common correlate of alcoholism that also contributes to fetal growth restriction.

Because of difficulties in neonatal diagnosis, follow-up is a key tool for diagnosis of FAS. Even with strong evidence of maternal alcoholism, the "hit" rate in offspring varies between 20 and 69 percent (Cooper, 1987; Graham et al., 1988). In the presence of a clearcut maternal history and the typical FAS appearance discussed above, cardiac, renal, and perhaps even head ultrasound are warranted in the newborn period. Examination for minor anomalies is warranted, with careful documentation of subsequent growth and development. When available, experienced dysmorphologists may assist in recognizing the diagnosis as confirmed by controlled studies (Graham et al., 1988). Since no medical test is diagnostic, counseling must emphasize abstinence in future pregnancies, but acknowledge uncertainty in relating specific infant problems to maternal drinking.

Recent debate concerns the reliability and specificity of a behavioral phenotype in FAE, vis-à-vis a report from the Institute of Medicine (Boschert, 1995). Of concern is the use of soft neurologic signs or behavioral symptoms as diagnostic criteria for FAE, particularly when objective changes in growth, craniofacial morphology, and organ development are not present. Heavy drinking does cause IQ deficits in offspring regardless of morphologic findings (Mattson et al., 1997).

Family and psychosocial counseling

Although most children with recognizable FAS are born to persons with chronic alcoholism, better awareness of the condition may identify moderate drinkers who have children with milder growth and behavioral problems (Hill et al., 1989). Intervention can be very successful in more moderate drinkers, and should be attempted with chronic alcoholic persons to prevent alcohol in breast milk or even in formula as an infant tranquilizer (Burd & Martsolf, 1989). Abel (1988) emphasized the familial nature of FAS by pointing out that 17 percent of older sibs and 77 percent of younger sibs had evidence of FAS after an index case was identified. The first goals of family counseling are to intervene in the cycle of alcohol abuse and to protect the newly diagnosed infant from the hazards of further alcohol exposure or neglect. Since the incidence of FAS is strongly correlated with low socioeconomic status, initial counseling and intervention will usually require the involvement of protective and social services.

Several parent groups and organizations for fetal alcohol syndrome are available as indicated on part 1 of the checklist.

Natural history and complications

Major complications of the fetal alcohol syndrome are listed in part 1 of the checklist. The impact of alcohol on the developing brain is evidenced by a high frequency of neurologic problems (Marcus, 1987) and learning deficits with a mean IQ of 41–65 (Hanson et al., 1976; Streissguth et al., 1991; Cooper, 1987; Hill et al., 1989; Mattson et al., 1997). Older children often have attention deficits with hyperactive, distractible, and impulsive behavior (Nanson & Hiscock, 1990). Children with fetal alcohol syndrome have different behaviors than controls with similar IQ (Streissguth et al., 1998), and are at risk for mental illness (Famy et al., 1998). Neurosensory damage is also common, with abnormal brain stem evoked response found in 79 percent of 29 FAS patients (Rossig et al., 1994), hearing loss in 13 of 14 FAS patients (Church & Gerkin, 1988), and diminished vision in as many as 50 percent of FAS patients due to optic nerve or eye anomalies (Miller et al., 1984; Strömland, 1987; Hellstrom et al., 1997). The cognitive and neurosensory problems produce a high incidence of speech delay that needs attention (Iosub et al., 1981; Church & Gerkin, 1988; Church & Kaltenbach, 1997).

Other organs affected in FAS include the cardiac, immune, and skeletal systems. The DiGeorge anomaly with hypoparathyroidism and immune defects has been described (Amman et al., 1982), and the incidence of many types of infections, including otitis media, is increased. Cardiac anomalies, found in 41 percent of 76 children in one series (Sardor et al., 1981), include atrial or ventricular septal defects, tetralogy of Fallot, peripheral pulmonary artery stenosis, and dextrocardia. Upper airway obstruction due to midface hypoplasia has produced apnea or chronic hypoxia in some patients, placing them at risk to develop pulmonary hypertension (Usowicz et al., 1986). Subclinical renal tubular defects with impaired acidification have been documented in FAS (Assadi, 1990), as have frank renal anomalies (Qazi et al., 1979). A variety of connective tissue defects occur, including Klippel–Feil anomaly, limb contractures, hip dislocation, scoliosis, chest deformities, and the radiographic finding of stippled epiphyses (Hanson et al., 1976; Burd & Martsolf, 1989; Leicher-Düber et al., 1990). An elevated cancer rate has been suggested for FAS, with examples of neuroblastoma, hepatoblastoma, sacrococcygeal teratoma, medulloblastoma, adrenal carcinoma, and acute lymphocytic leukemia being published (Zaunschirm & Munteau, 1984). Whether these tumors reflect carcinogenic effects of alcohol that have been documented in adults or increased scrutiny of FAS patients is unknown.

Fetal alcohol syndrome preventive medical checklist

Because of the relatively high incidence and economic impact of FAS and FAE, there is probably no condition in which preventive management can have greater importance. A major goal is family intervention before further damage is inflicted on the developing infant and sibs. Provision of alcohol in breast milk or as an infant sedative is well-recognized, and social/protective service intervention is mandated when the diagnosis of FAS is made (Burd & Martsolf, 1989). High rates of affected sibs (Abel, 1988) emphasize the need for family evaluation and a thorough parental history for children with suspect FAS or FAE.

In those cases where the diagnosis is recognized during infancy, imaging or x-ray studies for cardiac, vertebral, and renal anomalies are indicated. Physical examination for orthopedic defects, including congenital hip dislocation, is important. Sensorineural or conductive hearing loss and eye anomalies are as common as in Down syndrome, so similar recommendations for vision and hearing assessment are included in the checklist. The high frequency of failure to thrive (50–75 percent, checklist, part 1) and microcephaly (disproportionately small in 93 percent – Hanson et al., 1976; Cooper, 1987; Hill et al., 1989; Streissguth et al., 1991) mandates careful monitoring of growth and nutrition. Growth hormone secretion in children with FAS is lower than normal but comparable to that of other children with intrauterine growth retardation (Hellstrom et al., 1996).

Referral to early childhood intervention and assistance with social, school, and financial issues that affect children with special needs are appropriate. Challenging behaviors in most children with FAS or FAE should be emphasized in discussions with foster or adoptive parents, and avenues for behavioral therapy provided. Behavior problems are particularly difficult in the adolescent and adult, including poor judgment, distractibility, and difficulty perceiving social clues (Famy et al., 1998; Streissguth et al., 1991). Pregnancy counseling, school/job support, and violence prevention are thus of even greater importance in the care of adolescents with FAS.

Fetal hydantoin syndrome

Terminology

Fetal hydantoin syndrome refers to a pattern of growth deficiency, developmental delay, and malformations in children who were exposed to hydantoin during pregnancy (Lewis et al., 1998).

Historical diagnosis and management

Anticonvulsant therapy was initiated with the use of potassium bromide in 1853, with the first recognition of congenital anomalies in offspring of epileptic women occurring in 1963 (Schardein, 1985, pp. 142–89). The introduction of hydantoins in the 1930s was followed by a similar delay before Hanson & Smith (1975a) described a syndrome of craniofacial anomalies, nail and digital hypoplasia, intrauterine growth retardation, and mental deficiency in offspring of hydantoin-treated women. Management has emphasized minimal dosage of a single drug in epileptic mothers, and surgical and/or developmental intervention in affected children (Hanson, 1986).

Incidence, etiology, and differential diagnosis

It is estimated that 1 percent of all individuals have epilepsy, and that anticonvulsants account for about 0.5 percent of drug sales (Shardein, 1985, p. 143). These figures translate to at least 15,000 annual U.S. births to women on anticonvulsants. Since phenytoin-exposed fetuses have a 5–10 percent risk of developing the full-blown hydantoin syndrome (Adams et al., 1990), its incidence should be about 1 in 2000 live births, while those with more subtle effects may be 2–3 times more numerous.

The pathogenesis of major or minor anomalies caused by phenytoin is still unknown. General effects of maternal epilepsy on fetal development, and possible synergies of multiple anticonvulsant medications have not been adequately dissected from the effects of hydantoin itself. Animal studies offer the best evidence for primary hydantoin effects, including face/limb and behavioral abnormalities that are comparable to those produced in humans (Adams et al., 1990). Differences in response among mouse strains (Finnell & Chernoff, 1984) predicted genetic factors in human susceptibility. This prediction was validated by the study of Buehler et al. (1990), showing correlation between maternal oxidase levels and fetal abnormalities after hydantoin exposure. The results suggest a role for arene oxide metabolites of hydantoin in fetal teratogenesis.

Differential diagnosis includes conditions with hirsutism, nail or digital hypoplasia, and similar facial features. Fetal alcohol syndrome is associated with growth/developmental delays and nail hypoplasia, as are the genetic Coffin–Siris and Coffin–Lowry syndromes. The Noonan, Williams, and Aarskog syndromes also have some overlap, as do effects of other anticonvulsant drugs such as barbiturates, primidone, and valproic acid (Hanson, 1986). Maternal and family history together with the pattern of anomalies should differentiate these conditions from fetal hydantoin syndrome.

Diagnostic evaluation and medical counseling

When the positive maternal history, characteristic facial anomalies, and digital hypoplasia are present, few diagnostic tests are needed. Chromosomal and radiographic studies may be indicated when atypical anomalies or severe growth/developmental retardation are present. Counseling should focus on minimizing anticonvulsant dosage in subsequent pregnancies, with avoidance of multidrug therapy whenever possible (Hanson, 1986). Barbiturates, primidone, and valproic acid all have been implicated as teratogens, and maternal seizures may be damaging as well. Assessment of maternal oxidation status (Buehler et al., 1990) may allow titration of the hydantoin dosage to balance maternal-fetal risk, but these assays are still experimental.

Family and psychosocial counseling

New parents are confronted with risks for developmental and chronic medical problems in their child. Their shock may be heightened by guilt or blame attached to the maternal seizure disorder. Counseling regarding the common occurrence of congenital anomalies regardless of maternal status and an optimistic scheme for management may be helpful. Early childhood intervention should be encouraged and social and/or psychiatric services made available.

Natural history and complications

Major complications include pre- or postnatal growth delay, microcephaly with developmental delay, feeding problems due to gastrointestinal anomalies, and a variety of anomalies affecting the cardiovascular, skeletal, and urinary systems (checklist, part 1). The face may be distinctive, with hypertelorism, shallow and broad nasal bridge, short nose, and wide mouth. Eye anomalies include ptosis, colobomata, and strabismus. Cleft or high palate and broad alveolar ridges occur inside the mouth, and the neck is often short with webbing or redundant skin. Hypoplasia of the terminal digits and nails is the most distinctive skeletal anomaly, but congenital hip dislocation, club feet, rib anomalies, vertebral anomalies, and scoliosis can occur (Sabry & Farag, 1996; Trousdale, 1998). Cardiac septal defects, urinary outflow tract obstruction, micropenis or cryptorchidism in males, and occasional brain anomalies including holoprosencephaly have been reported (Hanson & Smith, 1975b; Hanson, 1986). A worrisome finding in mouse or rat models is the prominence of behavioral abnormalities, but their frequency in human patients is not defined (Adams et al., 1990). Tumors of neural crest origin occur at increased frequency in fetal hydantoin syndrome, and phenytoin is carcinogenic in adults (Hanson, 1986).

Preventive management is directed toward the treatment of neonatal anomalies and evaluation for abnormal growth, development, vision, skeletal, and urinary tract function. Neonatal evaluation for positional deformities such as club feet or congenital hip dislocation is important, since these have a cumulative frequency of 11 percent (Schardein, 1985, p. 160). Although developmental and behavioral problems are not as frequent or severe as with the fetal alcohol syndrome, early childhood intervention with occupational and speech therapy will be necessary for some patients. Eye problems such as strabismus and urinary tract infections due to anomalies of the outflow tract require appropriate screening and referral. Abdominal examination is important because of early risk for renal anomalies and later risk for neural crest tumors. The low frequency of these complications (less than 1 percent) probably does not justify routine abdominal ultrasound examinations. Also infrequent are cleft palate and dental anomalies due to high-arched palate, but occasional patients may require plastic surgery and/or dentistry referral.

Diabetic embryopathy

Terminology

Infants of diabetic mothers (IDM) have increased risk for congenital malformation that correlates with the degree of metabolic aberration during pregnancy. The malformation process and its resulting pattern of anomalies are referred to as diabetic embryopathy.

Historical diagnosis and management

As the complications of stillbirth, neonatal hypoglycemia, and respiratory distress syndrome were ameliorated through better maternal management, increased risk for malformation in IDM was recognized (Gabbe, 1977). Mills et al. (1979) pointed out that the common malformations in IDM all occur before 7 weeks of pregnancy, so that control of diabetes before conception must be emphasized to safeguard the embryo.

Incidence, etiology, and differential diagnosis

The prevalence of diabetes mellitus during pregnancy is about 3 percent, with about 0.3 percent being pre-existing diabetes. Of the 50 to 150,000 IDM that are born each year in the United States, those who experience problems with maternal diabetic control during gestation will have a 6–10 percent incidence of major congenital anomalies (Schardein, 1985, pp. 423–5; Reece et al., 1993). These anomalies account for 50 percent of all perinatal deaths (Reece et al., 1993).

The etiology of anomalies resulting from maternal diabetes is still unclear. Maternal vasculopathy was first implicated as a predisposing factor, with a 10–11 percent risk for anomalies in offspring of women with Class D or F diabetes, compared with 3–4.5 percent in Class B or C diabetes. More recent studies have not confirmed these trends, and experiments with *in vitro* embryo culture have emphasized the teratogenic effects of hypo- and hyperglycemia, ketonemia, and somatomedin inhibitors (Reece et al., 1993). Deficiencies of zinc and arachidonic acid, high levels of free oxygen radicals, and differences in genetic susceptibility have also received experimental support as factors in diabetic embryopathy. Of great interest is a paradoxical growth *retardation* in some severely affected IDM (Pedersen & Mølsted-Pedersen, 1979); delayed growth along with delayed maturation of lung and hematologic functions may be a unifying theme in the disorder (Wilson, 1988). Sadler et al. (1995) analyzed the pattern of malformations in diabetic embryopathy and suggest that somite mesoderm and cephalic neural crest cells may be prime targets in the embryo.

Diagnostic evaluation and medical counseling

Unless other disorders are suspected, neonates should be evaluated for major anomalies of the brain, heart, GI tract, urinary tract, and vertebrae – complications listed in the checklist, part 1. Since the frequency of any given anomaly is low, clinical examination rather than routine screening should guide the use of expensive imaging studies. Medical counseling should review the correlation of poor diabetic control with anomaly risk, particularly emphasizing the achievement of good control before attempting another pregnancy. Gestational diabetes is not associated with a higher risk for congenital anomalies, so these mothers can be reassured and their offspring evaluated for other causes of anomalies.

Family and psychosocial counseling

Diabetes mellitus is a multifactorial disorder with significant genetic predisposition. Parents with type I diabetes confer a 5–10 percent risk to their offspring for developing type I (insulin-dependent) diabetes. These offspring have an even higher risk for developing type II (adult-onset) diabetes. These risks increase slightly if additional family members are affected. As with other teratogens, maternal guilt and blame may be counseling issues that require specialty participation. For women who can achieve and maintain good control of their diabetes, an optimistic outlook for future pregnancies is appropriate. Many anomalies associated with diabetic embryopathy can be detected by prenatal ultrasound at or before 16–18 postmenstrual weeks.

Natural history and complications

The checklist, part 1 lists major anomalies affecting the eye, jaw, heart, gastrointestinal tract, urinary tract, and central nervous system that occur in IDM whose mothers had pre-existing diabetes mellitus (Cordero & Landon, 1993; Martínez-Frìas, 1994; Tyrala, 1996; Sperling & Menon, 1997; Suevo, 1997). All of the anomalies occur at fairly low frequencies (1–3 percent). Caudal regression, ranging from sirenomelia (mermaid anomaly) to sacral agenesis, is the most characteristic anomaly, being present in about 1 percent of patients (Adra et al., 1994). Some children may require orthopedic, urologic, and neurosurgical follow-up when severe caudal regression produces limb hypoplasia, bladder dysfunction, and/or tethered cord/diastematomyelia (Adra et al., 1994).

Diabetic embryopathy preventive management checklist

Preventive measures in diabetic embryopathy are oriented more toward physical examination than toward routine screening, since all of the characteristic anomalies occur at low frequency (checklist, parts 2–4). Neonatal evaluation for eye, ear, oral, cardiac, skeletal, urinary tract, and neurologic anomalies is important. Management during later childhood is focused on preventing obesity and detecting subtle neuro-developmental problems. For children with caudal regression, or the full VATER association of anomalies, more aggressive orthopedic, urologic, and neurosurgical management is required. In such children, the VATER association preventive check-list may be more appropriate as a guide for management.

Preventive Management of Fetal Alcohol Syndrome

Clinical diagnosis: Clinical pattern including low birth weight, microcephaly, growth failure, small eyes, shallow philtrum, thin upper lip, anomalous ears, ocular, orthopedic, and cardiac problems (Hanson et al., 1976; Streissguth et al., 1991).

Incidence: 1.5 to 1.9 per 1000, depending on socioeconomic status (Abel & Sokol, 1987).

Laboratory diagnosis: None.

Genetics: Sporadic disorder related to maternal alcohol use during pregnancy.

Key management issues: Monitoring of growth, vision, and hearing; surveillance for ocular, cardiac, and orthopedic problems, early intervention with alertness for behavior problems and school difficulties.

Growth Charts: None available; failure to thrive and microcephaly are characteristic.

Parent groups: National Organization on Fetal Alcohol Syndrome, 1815 H St. NW, Suite 1000, Washington DC, 20006; Fetal Alcohol Syndrome/Effects listserver, United Kingdom: http://SARGON.MMU.AC.UK/fetal.htm

Basis for management recommendations: Based on the complications listed below and the recommendations of Burd & Martsolf (1989), Hanson et al. (1976), Streissguth et al. (1991).

Summary of clinical concerns

General	Learning	Cognitive disability (60%), speech delay (93%), learning differences (89% – mean IQ 41–65)
	Behavior	Behavior problems (80%), hyperactivity, psychiatric problems
	Growth	Low birth weight (57–89%), short stature (84%), failure to thrive (50–75%)
	Cancer	Increased cancer risk (rhabdomyosarcoma, Wilms tumor, leukemias)
Facial	Eye	**Small eyes (92%), optic nerve defects (39%), myopia (88%), astigmatism (50%), strabismus (56%)**
	Ear	**Ear anomalies (22%), otitis media (93%), hearing loss (38%)**
	Nose	**Shallow nasal bridge (61%), chronic nasal discharge**
	Mouth	**Dysphagia (91%), high palate (30%)**, cleft palate (7%), dental anomalies
Surface	Neck/trunk	Pectus excavatum
Skeletal	Cranial	Microcephaly (93%)
	Limbs	Decreased fetal mobility, radioulnar fusion (14%), **hip dislocation (9–33%)**, limb contractures
Internal	Digestive	**Dysphagia, feeding problems (91%)**
	Pulmonary	Airway obstruction, apnea
	Circulatory	Cardiac defects (41–49% – septal defects, tetralogy of Fallot, transposition of great vessels)
	RES	DiGeorge anomaly, frequent infections
	Excretory	Renal defects (20–66% – pyelonephritis, hematuria, renal hypoplasia)
	Genital	Genital defects (46% – hypospadias, micropenis, cryptorchidism)
Neural	CNS	Brain anomalies, holoprosencephaly, neural tube defects (1–3%), seizures (10–50%), irritability
	Motor	**Hypertonia, oromotor dysfunction, motor delays**
	Sensory	**Vision and hearing deficits (20–30%)**

RES, reticuloendothelial system, **bold: frequency > 20%**

Key references

Abel, E. L. & Sokol, R. J. (1987). *Drug and Alcohol Dependence* 19:51–70.

Burd, L. & Martsolf, J. T. (1989). *Physiology and Behavior* 46:39–43.

Hanson, J. W. et al. (1976). *Journal of the American Medical Association* 235:1458–60.

Streissguth, A. P. et al. (1991). *Journal of the American Medical Association* 265:1961–7.

Fetal Alcohol syndrome

Preventive medical checklist (0–1yr)

Patient   **Birth Date** /   /   **Number**

Pediatric	Screen	Evaluate		Refer/Counsel	
Neonatal / / *Newborn screen* ❑ HB ❑	Renal sonogram[3] ❑	Feeding Hip dislocation Eye anomaly Genitalia	❑ ❑ ❑ ❑	Maternal counsel Foster care Social services Genetics evaluation	❑ ❑ ❑ ❑
1 month / /	Cardiac echo ❑	Torticollis Serous otitis Nutrition	❑ ❑ ❑	Family support[4] Cardiology	❑ ❑
2 months / / HB[1] ❑ Hib ❑ DTaP, IPV ❑ RV ❑	Growth ❑ Hearing, vision[2] ❑	Hip dislocation Eye anomaly Nutrition	❑ ❑ ❑	Early intervention[5] Social services Developmental pediatrics Genetic counseling	❑ ❑ ❑ ❑
4 months / / HB[1] ❑ Hib ❑ DTaP/IPV ❑ RV ❑	Hearing, vision[2] ❑	Hip dislocation Serous otitis	❑ ❑	Early intervention[5] ENT[3] Social services	❑ ❑ ❑
6 months / / Hib ❑ IPV[1] ❑ DTaP ❑ RV ❑	Growth ❑ Hearing, vision[2] ❑ Urinalysis, BP ❑	Strabismus Hip dislocation Serous otitis	❑ ❑ ❑	Family support[4] Social services	❑ ❑
9 months / / IPV[1] ❑	Audiology ❑	Strabismus Serous otitis	❑ ❑	Ophthalmology	❑
1 year / / HB ❑ Hib[1] ❑ IPV[1] ❑ MMR[1] ❑ Var[1] ❑	Growth ❑ Hearing, vision[2] ❑ Urinalysis, BP ❑	Strabismus Serous otitis Nutrition	❑ ❑ ❑	Family support[4] Early intervention[5] Social services Developmental pediatrics Genetic counseling	❑ ❑ ❑ ❑ ❑

Clinical concerns for Fetal Alcohol syndrome, ages 0–1 year

Low birth weight
Thin upper lip, absent philtrum
Eye and ear anomalies
Otitis media, hearing loss

Cardiac anomalies
Renal anomalies
Genital anomalies
Hip dislocation

Feeding problems, growth delay
Microcephaly
Irritability, seizures
Hypertonia

Guidelines for the neonatal period should be undertaken *at whatever age* the diagnosis is made; DTaP, acellular DTP; IPV, inactivated poliovirus (oral polio also used); RV, rotavirus; MMR, measles–mumps–rubella; Var, varicella; BP, blood pressure; [1]alternative timing; [2]by practitioner; [3]as dictated by clinical findings; [4]parent group, family/sib, financial, and behavioral issues as discussed in the preface; [5]including developmental monitoring and motor/speech therapy.

Fetal Alcohol syndrome

Preventive medical checklist (15m–6yrs)

Patient **Birth Date** / / **Number**

Pediatric	Screen		Evaluate		Refer/Counsel	
15 months / / *Hib[1]* ☐ *MMR[1]* ☐ *DTaP, IPV[1]* ☐ *Varicella[1]* ☐					Family support[4] Early intervention[5]	☐ ☐
18 months / / *DTaP, IPV[1]* ☐ *Varicella[1]* ☐ *Influenza[3]* ☐	Growth	☐	Nutrition	☐		
2 years / / *Influenza[3]* ☐ *Pneumovax[3]* ☐ *Dentist* ☐	Growth Hearing, vision[2] Audiology Urinalysis, BP	☐ ☐ ☐ ☐	Strabismus Serous otitis Nutrition	☐ ☐ ☐	Developmental pediatrics Genetics ENT[3] Ophthalmology	 ☐ ☐ ☐ ☐
3 years / / *Influenza[3]* ☐ *Pneumovax[3]* ☐ *Dentist* ☐	Growth Hearing, vision[2] Audiology Urinalysis, BP	☐ ☐ ☐ ☐	Strabismus Serous otitis Behavior Nutrition	☐ ☐ ☐ ☐	Family support[4] Preschool transition[5] Social services Ophthalmology[3]	☐ ☐ ☐ ☐
4 years / / *Influenza[3]* ☐ *Pneumovax[3]* ☐ *Dentist* ☐	Growth Hearing, vision[2]	☐ ☐	Nutrition Behavior	☐ ☐	Family support[4] Preschool program[5] Developmental pediatrics Genetics Ophthalmology[3]	☐ ☐ ☐ ☐ ☐
5 years / / *DTaP, IPV[1]* ☐ *MMR[1]* ☐	Hearing, vision[2] Audiology Urinalysis, BP	☐ ☐ ☐	Nutrition Behavior	☐ ☐	School transition[5]	☐
6 years / / *DTaP, IPV[1]* ☐ *MMR[1]* ☐ *Dentist* ☐	Growth Hearing, vision[2]	☐ ☐	School progress Phallus size Nutrition Behavior	☐ ☐ ☐ ☐	Family support[4] Social services[3] Developmental pediatrics Genetics Ophthalmology, ENT[3]	☐ ☐ ☐ ☐ ☐

Clinical concerns for Fetal Alcohol syndrome, ages 1–6 years

Thin upper lip, absent philtrum
Eye and ear anomalies
Otitis media, hearing loss

Cardiac anomalies
Renal anomalies
Genital anomalies
Hip dislocation

Feeding problems
Microcephaly
Irritability, seizures

Guidelines for prior ages should be undertaken *at the time of diagnosis*; DTaP, acellular DTP; IPV, inactivated poliovirus (oral polio also used); MMR, measles–mumps–rubella; BP, blood pressure; [1]alternative timing; [2]by practitioner; [3]as dictated by clinical findings; [4]parent group, family/sib, financial, and behavioral issues as discussed in the preface; [5]including developmental monitoring and motor/speech therapy.

Fetal Alcohol syndrome

Preventive medical checklist (6+ yrs)

Patient   **Birth Date** / /   **Number**

Pediatric	Screen	Evaluate	Refer/Counsel
8 years / / *Dentist* ❑	Hearing, vision[2] ❑ Urinalysis, BP ❑	Nutrition ❑ Behavior ❑	School options ❑ Developmental pediatrics ❑ Genetics ❑
10 years / /	Growth ❑ Hearing, vision[2] ❑	School progress ❑ Nutrition ❑	Social services[3] ❑
12 years / / *Td[1], MMR, Var* ❑ *CBC* ❑ *Dentist* ❑ *Scoliosis* ❑ *Cholesterol* ❑	Hearing, vision[2] ❑ Urinalysis, BP ❑	Puberty ❑ Phallus size ❑ Nutrition ❑ Behavior ❑	Family support[5] ❑ School options ❑ Developmental pediatrics ❑ Genetics ❑ Ophthalmology, ENT[3] ❑
14 years / / *CBC* ❑ *Dentist* ❑ *Cholesterol* ❑ *Breast CA* ❑ *Testicular CA* ❑	Growth ❑	School progress ❑ Puberty ❑ Phallus size ❑ Nutrition ❑	Social services[3] ❑
16 years / / *Td[1]* ❑ *CBC* ❑ *Cholesterol* ❑ *Sexual[5]* ❑ *Dentist* ❑	Hearing, vision[2] ❑ Urinalysis, BP ❑ ❑	Puberty ❑ Nutrition ❑ Behavior ❑	Vocational planning ❑ Developmental pediatrics ❑ Genetics ❑
18 years / / *CBC* ❑ *Sexual[5]* ❑ *Cholesterol* ❑ *Scoliosis* ❑		School progress ❑ Nutrition ❑ Behavior ❑	Vocational planning ❑ Social services[3] ❑
20 years[6] / / *CBC* ❑ *Sexual[5]* ❑ *Cholesterol* ❑ *Dentist* ❑	Hearing, vision[2] ❑ Urinalysis, BP ❑	Nutrition ❑ Behavior ❑ Work, residence ❑	Family support[4] ❑ Social services[3] ❑

Clinical concerns for Fetal Alcohol syndrome, ages 6+ years

Dental problems	Cardiac anomalies	Learning differences
Irritability, seizures	Renal anomalies	Behavioral problems
Hearing loss	Scoliosis	Increased cancer risk

Guidelines for prior ages should be undertaken *at the time of diagnosis*; Td, tetanus/diphtheria; MMR, measles–mumps–rubella; Var, varicella; BP, blood pressure; [1]alternative timing; [2]by practitioner; [3]as dictated by clinical findings; [4]parent group, family/sib, financial, and behavioral issues as discussed in the preface; [5]birth control, STD screening if sexually active; [6]repeat every decade.

Preventive Management of Fetal Hydantoin syndrome

Clinical diagnosis: Clinical pattern including a distinctive face with hypertelorism, shallow and broad nasal bridge, short nose, and wide mouth; eye anomalies including colobomata and strabismus; cleft palate or broad alveolar ridges, small terminal digits and nails; orthopedic anomalies including club feet, dislocated hip, or scoliosis; cardiac and urinary outflow defects.

Laboratory diagnosis: None available.

Incidence: 1 in 2000 live births with subtle fetal effects being 2–3 times more common.

Genetics: Sporadic disorder due to maternal hydantoin intake; epoxide hydrolase levels may influence effects on fetus (Beuhler et al., 1990).

Key management issues: Detection and treatment of neonatal anomalies such as club feet or congenital hip dislocation followed by monitoring for abnormal growth, development, vision, skeletal anomalies, urinary tract function, and tumors (Murray et al., 1996).

Growth Charts: Hanson & Smith (1975) illustrate the growth delay and microcephaly that occurs in 25 percent of patients.

Parent groups: American Epilepsy Society, 638 Prospect Ave., Hartford CT, 06105-4240, (860) 586-7505, info@aesnet.org, http://www.aesnet.org; Epilepsy Canada, 1470 Peel St. Suite 745, Montreal PQ, Canada H3A 1T1, (514) 845-7855; epilepsy@epilepsy.ca; The National Society for Epilepsy, Chalfont St. Peter, Gerrards Cross, Buckinghamshire SL9 0RJ, UK, http://www.erg.ion.ucl.ac.uk

Basis for management recommendations: The complications listed below as detailed by Hanson & Smith (1975), Schardein (1985), and Hanson (1986).

Summary of clinical concerns

General	Learning	Mild cognitive disability, **learning differences** (25%)
	Growth	**Low birth weight** (36%), **growth delay** (52%), **short stature**
	Cancer	Cancer diathesis, neural crest tumors, lymphomas
Facial	Eye	**Hypertelorism** (21%), ptosis (5%), colobomata, strabismus
	Nose	**Shallow nasal bridge** (21%)
	Mouth	Broad alveolar ridges, high palate, cleft palate, cleft lip (3%)
Surface	Neck/trunk	Short neck, cystic hygroma, inguinal hernias (9%)
	Epidermal	Nail hypoplasia (11%), hirsutism (3%)
Skeletal	Cranial	**Microcephaly** (29%), wide anterior fontanel (10%), cranial asymmetry, metopic ridging (8%)
	Axial	Rib and vertebral anomalies (<1%), scoliosis
	Limbs	Hypoplastic distal digits, hip dislocation, club feet
Internal	Digestive	GI anomalies (pyloric stenosis, duodenal atresia, imperforate anus, diaphragmatic hernia)
	Circulatory	Cardiac anomalies (3%), mitral valve prolapse
	RES	Hyposplenism, thrombosis, coagulopathy
	Excretory	Renal hypoplasia, urinary tract anomalies
	Genital	Hypospadias, cryptorchidism, micropenis, shawl (bifid) scrotum
Neural	CNS	Holoprosencephaly, seizures
	Motor	Motor delays
	Sensory	Vision problems

RES, reticuloendothelial system, GI, gastrointestinal system, bold: frequency > 20%

Key references

Buehler, B.A. et al. (1990). *New England Journal of Medicine* 322:1567–72.

Hanson, J. W. (1986). *Teratology* 33:349–53.

Hanson, J. W. & Smith, D. W. (1975). *Journal of Pediatrics* 87:285–90.

Murray, J. C. et al. (1996). *Journal of Pediatric Hematology and Oncology* 18:241–3.

Schardein, J. L. 1985. *Chemically Induced Birth Defects*. New York: Marcel Dekker, Inc., p.142–89.

Fetal Hydantoin syndrome

Preventive medical checklist (0–1yr)

Pa___nt   Birth Date   /   /   Number

Pediatric	Screen		Evaluate		Refer/Counsel	
Neonatal / / *Newborn screen* ❑ *HB* ❑			Head shape Eye anomaly Heart Hip dislocation Genitalia	❑ ❑ ❑ ❑ ❑	Maternal counsel Genetic evaluation	❑ ❑
1 month / /			Heart	❑	Family support[4] Cardiology[3]	❑ ❑
2 months / / *HB[1]* ❑ *Hib* ❑ *DTaP, IPV* ❑ *RV* ❑	Growth Hearing, vision[2]	❑ ❑	Nutrition Hip dislocation Eye anomaly	❑ ❑ ❑	Early intervention[3,5] Developmental pediatrics Genetic counseling Craniofacial team[3]	❑ ❑ ❑ ❑
4 months / / *HB[1]* ❑ *Hib* ❑ *DTaP/IPV* *RV* ❑	Hearing, vision[2]	❑	Nutrition Hip dislocation	❑ ❑	Early intervention[3,5]	❑
6 months / / *Hib* ❑ *IPV[1]* ❑ *DTaP* ❑ *RV* ❑	Growth Hearing, vision[2]	❑ ❑	Nutrition Strabismus Hip dislocation	❑ ❑ ❑	Family support[4]	❑
9 months / / *IPV[1]* ❑			Nutrition Strabismus	❑ ❑	Ophthalmology	❑
1 year / / *HB* ❑ *Hib[1]* ❑ *IPV[1]* ❑ *MMR[1]* ❑ *Var[1]* ❑	Growth Hearing, vision[2] Audiology[3] Urinalysis, BP	❑ ❑ ❑ ❑	Nutrition Strabismus Palate	❑ ❑ ❑	Family support[4] Early intervention[3,5] Developmental pediatrics Genetics	❑ ❑ ❑ ❑

Clinical concerns for Fetal Hydantoin syndrome, ages 0–1 year

Cranial asymmetry	Cardiac septal defects	Failure to thrive
Wide anterior fontanelle	Pulmonic stenosis	Learning differences
Strabismus, ptosis	Urinary tract anomalies	Nail hypoplasia
High palate	Genital anomalies	

Guidelines for the neonatal period should be undertaken *at whatever age* the diagnosis is made; DTaP, acellular DTP; IPV, inactivated poliovirus (oral polio also used); RV, rotavirus; MMR, measles–mumps–rubella; Var, varicella; BP, blood pressure; [1]alternative timing; [2]by practitioner; [3]as dictated by clinical findings; [4]parent group, family/sib, financial, and behavioral issues as discussed in the preface; [5]including developmental monitoring and motor/speech therapy.

Fetal Hydantoin syndrome

Preventive medical checklist (15m–6yrs)

Patient		Birth Date / /	Number

Pediatric	Screen	Evaluate	Refer/Counsel
15 months / / *Hib[1]* ❑ *MMR[1]* ❑ *DTaP, IPV[1]* ❑ *Varicella[1]* ❑			Family support[4] ❑ Early intervention[3,5] ❑
18 months / / *DTaP, IPV[1]* ❑ *Varicella[1]* ❑ *Influenza[3]* ❑		Nutrition ❑	
2 years / / *Influenza[3]* ❑ *Pneumovax[3]* ❑ *Dentist* ❑	Growth ❑ Hearing, vision[2] ❑ Urinalysis, BP ❑	Nutrition ❑ Strabismus ❑ Palate ❑	Family support[4] ❑ Developmental pediatrics ❑ Genetics ❑ ENT[3] ❑ Ophthalmology ❑
3 years / / *Influenza[3]* ❑ *Pneumovax[3]* ❑ *Dentist* ❑	Growth ❑ Hearing, vision[2] ❑ Urinalysis, BP ❑	Nutrition ❑ Palate ❑	Family support[4] ❑ Preschool transition[5] ❑
4 years / / *Influenza[3]* ❑ *Pneumovax[3]* ❑ *Dentist* ❑	Hearing, vision[2] ❑ Urinalysis, BP ❑	Nutrition ❑ Palate ❑ Heart ❑	Family support[4] ❑ Preschool program[3,5] ❑ Developmental pediatrics ❑ Genetics ❑ Ophthalmology[3] ❑
5 years / / *DTaP, IPV[1]* ❑ *MMR[1]* ❑	Growth ❑ Hearing, vision[2] ❑ Urinalysis, BP ❑	Nutrition ❑ Palate ❑ Heart ❑	School transition ❑
6 years / / *DTaP, IPV[1]* ❑ *MMR[1]* ❑ *Dentist* ❑		School progress ❑	Family support[4] ❑ Developmental pediatrics ❑ Genetics ❑ Ophthalmology ❑

Clinical concerns for Fetal Hydantoin syndrome, ages 1–6 years

Strabismus, ptosis	Cardiac septal defects	Failure to thrive
High palate	Pulmonic stenosis	Learning differences
Genital anomalies	Urinary tract anomalies	Nail hypoplasia

Guidelines for prior ages should be undertaken *at the time of diagnosis*; DTaP, acellular DTP; IPV, inactivated poliovirus (oral polio also used); MMR, measles–mumps–rubella; BP, blood pressure; [1]alternative timing; [2]by practitioner; [3]as dictated by clinical findings; [4]parent group, family/sib, financial, and behavioral issues as discussed in the preface; [5]including developmental monitoring and motor/speech therapy.

Fetal Hydantoin syndrome

Preventive medical checklist (6+ yrs)

Patient		Birth Date / /	Number

Pediatric	Screen	Evaluate	Refer/Counsel
8 years / / *Dentist* ❏	Growth ❏ Hearing, vision[2] ❏ Urinalysis, BP ❏	Nutrition ❏ Phallus size ❏	School options ❏ Developmental pediatrics ❏ Genetics ❏
10 years / /		School progress ❏ Phallus size ❏ Scoliosis ❏	Ophthalmology[3] ❏
12 years / / *Td[1], MMR, Var* ❏ *CBC* ❏ *Dentist* ❏ *Scoliosis* ❏ *Cholesterol* ❏	Hearing, vision[2] ❏ Urinalysis, BP ❏	Nutrition ❏ Puberty ❏ Behavior ❏ Heart ❏	Family support[4] ❏ School options ❏ Developmental pediatrics ❏ Genetics ❏
14 years / / *CBC* ❏ *Dentist* ❏ *Cholesterol* ❏ *Breast CA* ❏ *Testicular CA* ❏	Hearing, vision[2] ❏ Urinalysis, BP ❏	Nutrition ❏ Puberty ❏ Behavior ❏ Heart ❏	Family support[4] ❏ School options ❏
16 years / / *Td[1]* ❏ *CBC* ❏ *Cholesterol* ❏ *Sexual[5]* ❏ *Dentist* ❏	Hearing, vision[2] ❏ Urinalysis, BP ❏	Nutrition ❏ Puberty ❏ Behavior ❏ Heart ❏	Vocational planning ❏ Developmental pediatrics ❏ Genetics ❏
18 years / / *CBC* ❏ *Sexual[5]* ❏ *Cholesterol* ❏ *Scoliosis* ❏		School progress ❏ Nutrition ❏ Behavior ❏	Vocational planning ❏
20 years[6] / / *CBC* ❏ *Sexual[5]* ❏ *Cholesterol* ❏ *Dentist* ❏	Hearing, vision[2] ❏ Urinalysis, BP ❏	Nutrition ❏ Behavior ❏ Heart ❏ Work, residence ❏	Family support[4] ❏

Clinical concerns for Fetal Hydantoin syndrome, ages 6+ years

Growth delay	Scoliosis	Cognitive disability
Strabismus, ptosis	Urinary tract anomalies	Frequent or severe infections
Cardiac anomalies	Genital anomalies	

Guidelines for prior ages should be undertaken *at the time of diagnosis*; Td, tetanus/diphtheria; MMR, measles–mumps–rubella; Var, varicella; BP blood pressure; [1]alternative timing; [2]by practitioner; [3]as dictated by clinical findings; [4]parent group, family/sib, financial, and behavioral issues as discussed in the preface; [5]birth control, STD screening if sexually active; [6]repeat every decade.

Preventive Management of Diabetic Embryopathy

Clinical diagnosis: In addition to fetal macrosomia and hypoglycemia, maternal diabetes mellitus can produce an embryopathy consisting of cranial, cardiac, and caudal anomalies (sacral agenesis, lower limb hypoplasia, urogenital anomalies).

Laboratory diagnosis: Suggested by neonatal hypoglycemia, hypocalcemia, hypomagnesemia, and polycythemia.

Genetics: Diabetes mellitus is a multifactorial disorder with a 5–10% risk for primary relatives (e.g., offspring of mothers with type I diabetes) to become affected with type I diabetes.

Key management issues: Neonatal metabolic alterations including low glucose, calcium, magnesium and high blood count; neonatal anomalies including facial (eye and ear anomalies, cleft palate), cardiac (transposition, septal defects), vertebral, limb, and urogenital defects; potential developmental problems with later obesity and propensity for diabetes mellitus.

Growth Charts: None available, but predisposition to obesity beginning in mid-childhood (Reece et al., 1993).

Parent groups: American Diabetes Association, National Service Center, 1660 Duke Street, Alexandria VA 22314, (800) 342-2383; www.diabetes.org; Canadian Diabetes Association, 15 Toronto St. Suite 1001, Toronto ON, Canada M5C 2E3, info@eda-nat.org, www.diabetes.ca; British Diabetic Association, 10 Queen Anne Street, London W1M 0BD, UK, (0171) 323-1531, bda@diabetes.org.uk, http://www.diabetes.org.uk

Basis for management recommendations: Complications documented below (Abra et al., 1994; Martinez-Frias, 1994; Sadler et al., 1995; Suevo, 1997; Tyrala, 1997).

Summary of clinical concerns

General	Learning	Developmental delay, learning differences
	Growth	Large birth weight, macrosomia
Facial	Eye	Anophthalmia, microphthalmia
	Ear	Ear anomaly (2%), ear atresia, hearing loss, chronic otitis media
	Mouth	Oromotor dysfunction, cleft lip/palate (5%)
Skeletal	Cranial	Hemifacial microsomia, cranial asymmetry
	Axial	Rib and vertebral anomalies (<1%), scoliosis, sacral agenesis (1–2%)
	Limbs	Small lower limbs (1%)
Internal	Digestive	Gastrointestinal anomalies (intestinal obstruction, omphalocele, imperforate anus, situs inversus, heterotaxy)
	Pulmonary	Immature lungs, respiratory distress
	Circulatory	Cardiac anomalies (3% – transposition, ventricular septal defect)
	Endocrine	Hypoglycemia, hypocalcemia, hypomagnesemia, cyanosis, irritability, tetany, seizures
	RES	Polycythemia, jaundice, clotting diathesis
	Excretory	Renal agenesis, ureteral duplication, urinary tract anomalies, obstructive uropathy, urinary tract infections
	Genital	Micropenis, cryptorchidism
Neural	CNS	Holoprosencephaly, neural tube defects, seizures, developmental disability
	Motor	Motor delays
	Sensory	Vision or hearing deficits

RES, reticuloendothelial system, GI, gastrointestinal system, **bold: frequency > 20%**

Key references

Adra, A., Cordero, D., Mejides, A. et al. (1994). *Obstetrical and Gynecological Survey* 49:508–16.

Martínez-Frías, M.L. (1994). *American Journal of Medical Genetics* 51:108–13.

Reece, E.A., Hmko, C.J., Wu, Y.-K. & Wiznitzer, A. (1993). *Clinics in Perinatology* 20:517–32.

Sadler, L.S., Robinson, L.K. & Msall, M.E. (1995). *American Journal of Medical Genetics*, 55:363–6.

Suevo, D. M. (1997). *Neonatal Network* 16:25–33.

Tyrala, E. E. (1996). *Obstetrics & Gynecology Clinics of North America* 23:221–41.

Offspring of Diabetic Mothers

Preventive medical checklist (0–1yr)

Patient **Birth Date** / / **Number**

Pediatric	Screen	Evaluate	Refer/Counsel
Neonatal / / *Newborn screen* ❑ HB ❑	Glucose ❑ Calcium ❑ CBC ❑ Skeletal x-rays[3] ❑	Eyes ❑ Heart ❑ Lower limbs ❑ Kidneys ❑ Genitalia ❑	Genetic evaluation ❑ Ophthalmology[3] ❑ Orthopedics[3] ❑ Neurosurgery[3] ❑ Cardiology ❑
1 month / /	Head growth ❑ Growth ❑ Head MRI[3] ❑	Heart ❑ Palate ❑ Spine ❑	Family support[4] ❑ Neurosurgery[3] ❑
2 months / / HB[1] ❑ Hib ❑ DTaP, IPV ❑ RV ❑	Hearing, vision[2] ❑	Palate ❑ Lower limbs ❑	Early intervention[3,5] ❑ Diabetic counseling ❑ Genetic counseling ❑ Orthopedics[3] ❑ Neurosurgery[3] ❑
4 months / / HB[1] ❑ Hib ❑ DTaP/IPV ❑ RV ❑	Head growth ❑ Growth ❑		Early intervention[3,5] ❑
6 months / / Hib ❑ OPV[1] ❑ DTaP ❑ RV ❑	Hearing, vision[2] ❑	Heart ❑ Palate ❑ Spine ❑	Family support[4] ❑
9 months / / IPV[1] ❑			
1 year / / HB ❑ Hib[1] ❑ IPV[1] ❑ MMR[1] ❑ Var[1] ❑	Head growth ❑ Growth ❑ Hearing, vision[2] ❑ Urinalysis, BP ❑	Nutrition ❑ Limbs, gait, Spine ❑	Family support[4] ❑ Early intervention[3,5] ❑ Developmental pediatrics ❑ Genetics ❑ Orthopedics[3] ❑ Neurosurgery[3] ❑

Clinical concerns for Diabetic Embryopathy, ages 0–1 year

Low glucose, Ca, Mg	Cardiac anomalies	Developmental delay
Polycythemia	Urogenital anomalies	Brain anomalies
Microphthalmia, cleft palate	Vertebral anomalies	Frequent or severe infections
Hemifacial microsomia	Limb anomalies	

Guidelines for the neonatal period should be undertaken *at whatever age* the diagnosis is made; DTaP, acellular DTP; IPV, inactivated poliovirus (oral polio also used); RV, rotavirus; MMR, measles–mumps–rubella; Var, varicella; BP, blood pressure; [1]alternative timing; [2]by practitioner; [3]as dictated by clinical findings; [4]parent group, family/sib, financial, and behavioral issues as discussed in the preface; [5]including developmental monitoring and motor/speech therapy.

Offspring of Diabetic Mothers

Preventive medical checklist (15m–6yrs)

Patient		Birth Date / /	Number

Pediatric	Screen	Evaluate	Refer/Counsel
15 months / / <small>Hib[1] ❑ MMR[1] ❑ DTaP, IPV[1] ❑ Varicella[1] ❑</small>			Family support[4] ❑ Early intervention[5] ❑
18 months / / <small>DTaP, IPV[1] ❑ Varicella[1] ❑ Influenza[3] ❑</small>	Growth ❑	Nutrition ❑	
2 years / / <small>Influenza[3] ❑ Pneumovax[3] ❑ Dentist ❑</small>	Hearing, vision[2] ❑ Urinalysis, BP ❑	Nutrition ❑ Limbs, gait ❑ Spine ❑	Family support[4] ❑ Developmental 　pediatrics[3] ❑ Genetics ❑ Orthopedics[3] ❑
3 years / / <small>Influenza[3] ❑ Pneumovax[3] ❑ Dentist ❑</small>	Urinalysis, BP ❑	Nutrition ❑	Family support[4] ❑ Preschool transition[3,5] ❑
4 years / / <small>Influenza[3] ❑ Pneumovax[3] ❑ Dentist ❑</small>	Urinalysis, BP ❑	Nutrition ❑	Family support[4] ❑ Preschool program[3,5] ❑ Urologist[4] ❑ Dietician[3] ❑
5 years / / <small>DTaP, IPV[1] ❑ MMR[1] ❑</small>	Growth ❑ Urinalysis, BP ❑	Nutrition ❑ Diabetes ❑	School transition[3,5] ❑ Developmental 　pediatrics[3] ❑ Genetics ❑
6 years / / <small>DTaP, IPV[1] ❑ MMR[1] ❑ Dentist ❑</small>	Growth ❑ Urinalysis, BP ❑	School progress ❑ Obesity ❑ Phallus size ❑ Gait ❑	Family support[4] ❑ Dietician[3] ❑ Urologist[3] ❑

Clinical concerns for Diabetic Embryopathy, ages 1–6 years

Microphthalmia	Urogenital anomalies	Developmental delay
Hemifacial microsomia	Vertebral anomalies	Brain anomalies
Cardiac anomalies	Limb anomalies	Frequent or severe infections

Guidelines for prior ages should be undertaken *at the time of diagnosis*; DTaP, acellular DTP; IPV, inactivated poliovirus (oral polio also used); MMR, measles–mumps–rubella; BP, blood pressure; [1]alternative timing; [2]by practitioner; [3]as dictated by clinical findings; [4]parent group, family/sib, financial, and behavioral issues as discussed in the preface; [5]including developmental monitoring and motor/speech therapy.

Offspring of Diabetic Mothers

Preventive medical checklist (6+ yrs)

Patient   **Birth Date** / /   **Number**

Pediatric	Screen		Evaluate		Refer/Counsel	
8 years / / *Dentist* ❑	Growth Urinalysis, BP	❑ ❑ ❑	Obesity Nutrition Phallus size	❑ ❑ ❑	School options Developmental pediatrics[3] Genetics Dietician[3] Urologist[3]	❑ ❑ ❑ ❑ ❑
10 years / /	Urinalysis, BP	❑	School progress Obesity Nutrition Scoliosis	❑ ❑ ❑ ❑		
12 years / / *Td[1], MMR, Var* ❑ *CBC* ❑ *Dentist* ❑ *Scoliosis* ❑ *Cholesterol* ❑	Urinalysis, BP	❑	Nutrition Gait Diabetes	❑ ❑ ❑	Family support[4] Developmental pediatrics[3] Genetics	❑ ❑ ❑
14 years / / *CBC* ❑ *Dentist* ❑ *Cholesterol* ❑ *Breast CA* ❑ *Testicular CA* ❑	Urinalysis, BP	❑	School progress Nutrition Gait	❑ ❑ ❑		
16 years / / *Td[1]* ❑ *CBC* ❑ *Cholesterol* ❑ *Sexual[5]* ❑ *Dentist* ❑	Urinalysis, BP	❑	Nutrition	❑	Vocational planning[3] Developmental pediatrics[3] Genetics	❑ ❑ ❑
18 years / / *CBC* ❑ *Sexual[5]* ❑ *Cholesterol* ❑ *Scoliosis* ❑	Urinalysis, BP	❑	School progress Nutrition	❑ ❑	Vocational planning[3]	❑
20 years[6] / / *CBC* ❑ *Sexual[5]* ❑ *Cholesterol* ❑ *Dentist* ❑	Urinalysis, BP	❑	Nutrition Diabetes Work, residence	❑ ❑ ❑	Family support[4]	❑

Clinical concerns for Diabetic Embryopathy, ages 6+ years

Tethered cord (gait problems, enuresis)
Urinary tract anomalies

Scoliosis
Cryptorchidism, micropenis
Overgrowth, obesity

Learning and school problems
Diabetes mellitus (5–10% risk)
Frequent or severe infections

Guidelines for prior ages should be undertaken *at the time of diagnosis*; Td, tetanus/diphtheria; MMR, measles–mumps–rubella; Var, varicella; BP blood pressure; [1]alternative timing; [2]by practitioner; [3]as dictated by clinical findings; [4]parent group, family/sib, financial, and behavioral issues as discussed in the preface; [5]birth control, STD screening if sexually active; [6]repeat every decade.

Part III

Chromosomal syndromes

7

Autosomal syndromes

Embryonic or fetal death is most likely when chomosomes 1–22 (autosomes) are deficient or duplicated (chromosomal aneuploidy). Fetuses that do survive to be born will usually have multiple medical problems, including growth failure, developmental delay, predisposition to infection, and multiple major or minor anomalies. Table 7.1 summarizes anomalies that occur commonly in chromosomal disorders. Chromosomal imbalance seems to alter homeostasis (Shapiro, 1983), rendering patients more fragile and susceptible to operative stress or environmental insults. Since accurate diagnosis is required for preventive management and genetic counseling, chromosome studies are mandated for all children with multiple anomalies, particularly those with growth and/or developmental problems. Children with isolated malformations are unlikely to have chromosomal disorders unless subtle anomalies have been missed (see Chapter 1).

Less common aneuploidies

Each chromosomal excess or deficiency is associated with its own particular syndrome. The length of the unbalanced region is one factor, illustrated by the severity of trisomy 13 (2 times longer than chromosome 21) or trisomy 18 (1.5 times longer than chromosome 21) compared to Down syndrome. In addition to length (quantity), the particular genes on a duplicated chromosomal segment (quality) must be important in determining phenotypic severity. Chromosomes 16 and 18 are of about equal length, but trisomy 16 almost always presents as early miscarriage. There is much to learn about the mechanisms by which chromosomal aneuploidy causes an abnormal phenotype. Why, for example, would triploidy, with its extra 23 chromosomes in each cell, be more compatible with fetal survival than trisomy 16?

More than 100 chromosomal disorders involving a duplication or deletion of autosomal material have been described. Although trisomy 13, 18, and 21 are sufficiently common to be familiar, the average practitioner will not encounter many of the rarer aneuploidies. Complications of rare chromosomal disorders can

Table 7.1 Malformations characteristic of chromosomal syndromes

Common malformations	Uncommon malformations
Agenesis of corpus callosum, spina bifida	Anencephaly
Esophageal duodenal, anal atresia	Jejunal, ileal atresia, gastroschisis
Tracheo-esophageal fistula, omphalocele	Gastroschisis
Renal and urinary tract malformations	Exstrophy of the bladder
Cardiac anomalies	Situs inversus, acardius
Radial aplasia, postaxial polydactyly	Conjoined twins, teratomas
Microphthalmia, ocular colobomata	Phocomelia, ectrodactyly (lobster claw)
	Ulnar and fibular anomalies

Source: Schinzel (1984, p. 41).

be found in specialized references (de Grouchy and Turleau, 1984; Schinzel, 1984; Gorlin et al., 1990) and are summarized in Tables 7.2 and 7.3. Health professionals encountering one of these rare disorders can consult the appropriate table, note the most likely health problems, and include appropriate preventive measures in their medical care plan. Detailed preventive management checklists are presented for the more common disorders – trisomy 13/18 and trisomy 21.

Table 7.1 contrasts anomalies that occur frequently in chromosomal disorders with those that occur infrequently (Schinzel, 1984, p. 41). The frequent central nervous system, eye, cardiac, gut, and renal anomalies, together with problems of growth, development, and immunity, provide a general foundation for preventive management. If imaging studies of the brain, heart, and kidney were not obtained during evaluation of the infant with a chromosomal disorder, then they should be considered after the abnormal karyotype is documented. Clinical judgment should always be used, particularly for imaging studies requiring anesthesia in a compromised child. Knowledge of brain anomalies may not contribute to management decisions in chromosomal disorders with an extremely poor prognosis (e.g., trisomy 13/18 or triploidy). Early monitoring of growth and feeding is important for all children, as nutrition is often a prime parental concern even in the neuro-devastated child. For children with a reasonable prognosis, early intervention with vision, hearing, speech, occupational therapy and physical therapy assessments is essential.

Specific complications of chromosomal disorders are listed in Tables 7.2 and 7.3. Table 7.2 lists the more severe chromosomal disorders that resemble trisomy 13/18 in mortality and morbidity. Complications of moderate to mild chromosomal disorders, comparable in severity to Down syndrome, are listed in Table 7.3. While this classification as severe versus moderate is useful in terms of parental expectations

Table 7.2 Frequent complications of more serious chromosomal syndromes

Disorder	Aneuploid region	# Patients	Complications
Del(1p)	pter→p36	<10	Microcephaly, cleft, pulmonic stenosis, blindness
Del(1q)	q21→q25, q25→q32, q42→qter	10–50	FTT, seizures, agenesis corpus callosum, osteoporosis, cleft palate, cardiac a., genital a., hypoplastic kidneys
Dup(1p)	q25→qter	10–50	Eye a., cleft, thymic hypoplasia
Dup(1p)	q32→qter	10–50	FTT, cataracts, cardiac a., GI stenoses, genital a.
Del(2q)	q21→q31	<10	FTT, brain a., cataracts, cleft, cardiac a.
Dup(2p)	pter→p23	10–50	FTT, microcephaly, seizures, strabismus, cardiac a., scoliosis, renal a.
Ring(3)		<10	FTT, microcephaly, renal a., genital a.
Dup(3p)	pter→p23	10–50	FTT, cleft, cardiac a., genital a., ureteral duplication
Dup(3p)	pter→p21	10–50	FTT, brain a., microphthalmia, cleft, choanal atresia, GI atresias, genital a.
Del(4p)	pter→p16.1/p13 Wolf–Hirschhorn syndrome	>50	FTT, polymicrogyria, hydrocephalus, coloboma, nystagmus, cleft, cardiac a., urinary tract a., skeletal a.
Del(4q)	q31→qter	10–50	FTT, Robin sequence, TE fistula, cardiac a., renal a., rib a.
Dup(4p)	pter→p13/p11	10–50	Obesity, short stature, microcephaly, absence corpus callosum, hydrocephalus, coloboma, cleft, cardiac a.
Dup(4q)	q22/q25 →q31q/34	<10	FTT, microcephaly, seizures, choanal stenosis, hip dislocation
Del(5p) Ring(5)	pter→p11/p15 Cri-du-chat syndrome	10–50	FTT, microcephaly, cleft, malocclusion, cardiac a., scoliosis, cryptorchidism, hypospadias, GI malrotation, thymic dysplasia
Dup(5p)	pter→p14/p11	10–50	FTT, hydrocephalus, coloboma, corneal opacities, cleft, intestinal a., anal atresia, cardiac a., renal a., club feet
Del(6q)	q25/q26→qter	<10	Tall stature, seizures, choanal atresia, cleft, cardiac a., hip dislocation, hydronephrosis, club feet
Dup(6q)	q21/q25→qter	10–50	FTT, hydrocephalus, absent corpus callosum, microphthalmia, cleft, renal a., club feet, genital a., inguinal hernia
Del(7p)	pter→p22/p15	<10	FTT, craniosynostosis, cleft, cardiac a., joint contractures
Del(7q)	q11→q21	<10	FTT, seizures, hypothyroidism, cardiac a.,
Del(7q)	q32/q34→qter	10–50	FTT, microcephaly, coloboma, cleft, cardiac a., hydronephrosis, hypospadias, sacral agenesis
Dup(7p)	pter→p21/p13	<10	FTT, hydrocephalus, choanal atresia, cleft, cardiac a., renal a.
Dup(7q)	q11→q22/q31	<10	Renal tubular acidosis, hypoplastic kidney, cryptorchidism
Dup(7q)	q22/q31→qter	10–50	FTT, hydrocephalus, coloboma, cleft, cardiac a.

Table 7.2 (*cont.*)

Disorder	Aneuploid region	# Patients	Complications
Dup(8p)	pter→p21/p11	10–50	FTT, cataract, cleft, cardiac a., scoliosis, micropenis
Dup(8p)	q11/q23→qter	10–50	FTT, choanal atresia, cleft, cardiac a., renal a., hypospadias
Dup(9p)	pter→cen pter→q21/q22	>50	FTT, seizures, hydrocephalus, coloboma, strabismus, cleft, cardiac a., urinary tract a., scoliosis, genital a.
Trip(9p)	pter→cen	10–50	FTT, hydrocephalus, cleft, cardiac a.
Dup(9q)	q11/q31/q33 →qter	10–50	FTT, cleft, cardiac a., renal a., joint contractures, renal cysts
Trisomy 9	full (milder if mosaic)	10–50	FTT, perinatal asphyxia, microcephaly, hydrocephalus, coloboma, cataracts, cardiac a., renal a., scoliosis
Del(10p)	pter→p14/13	10–50	FTT, seizures, eye a., cleft, heart a., renal a., club feet, hypothyroidism, genital a.
Del(10q)	q25→qter	<10	FTT, cleft, cardiac a., anal atresia, genital a.
Dup(10p)	pter→p14/p11	10–50	FTT, coloboma, cleft, cardiac a., biliary atresia, renal cysts,
Dup(10q)	q22/q24/q25→qter	10–50	FTT, cataract, cleft, cardiac a., scoliosis, renal a., genital a.
Del(11q)	q22/q23→qter	10–50	FTT, eye a., pyloric stenosis, cardiac a., urinary tract a.
Dup(11p)	pter→p14/p11	<10	FTT, eye a., cardiac a., urinary tract a., malrotation
Dup(11q)	q21/q23→qter	<10	Short stature, seizures, brain a., eye a., cardiac a., genital a.
Dup(12p)	pter→p11 or trip (12p)	10–50	FTT, aniridia, cleft, cardiac a., renal a.
Dup(12q)	q24→qter	10–50	FTT, cardiac a., anal a., renal a., malrotation, hypospadias
Del(13q)	q22/q31→qter	10–50	FTT, brain a., coloboma, eye a., thymic or thyroid hypoplasia, cardiac a., renal a., vertebral a., anal atresia
Dup(13q)	q14/q21/q22→qter	10–50	Brain a., coloboma, glaucoma, cleft, cardiac a., urinary tract a.
Dup(14q)	q22/q23→qter	<10	FTT, glaucoma, deafness, cardiac a., urinary tract a.
Trisomy 14	mosaic	<10	FTT, cleft, cardiac a., renal a., deafness, eczema, hip dysplasia
Dup(15q)	pter→q14/q22	<10	FTT, cleft, cardiac a., scoliosis, renal a., joint contractures
Dup(15q)	q21/q25→qter	<10	FTT, craniosynostosis, cataract, cardiac a., renal a., genital a.
Del(16q)	q13→q22	<10	FTT, microphthalmia, cardiac a., renal a., malrotation, anal a.
Dup(16p)	pter→q11	10–50	FTT, cleft, cardiac a., gut atresias, ovarian dysgenesis
Dup(16q)	q21/q22→qter	<10	FTT, seizures, cleft, cardiac a., anal atresia, genital a.
Trip(18p)	pter→p11/q11	10–50	Ataxia, seizures, cardiac a., renal a., scoliosis
Dup(18q)	q11/q12→qter	10–50	FTT, cardiac a., renal a., similar to trisomy 18
Dup(18q)	q21→qter	10–50	FTT, seizures, coloboma, choanal atresia, cardiac a., renal a., malrotation
Dup(19q)	q13→qter	<10	FTT, seizures, cleft, cardiac a., urinary tract a., vertebral a.

Table 7.2 (cont.)

Disorder	Aneuploid region	# Patients	Complications
Ring(22)		10–50	FTT, brain a., coloboma, cleft, cardiac a., renal a.
Dup(22q)	q11/q13→qter	<10	FTT, brain a., cleft. cardiac a., renal a., genital a.
Trisomy 22	Full, mosaic	<10	FTT, renal a., malrotation, anal atresia, limb a., genital a.
Triploidy	Full	>50	FTT, brain a., eye a., cleft, cardiac a., TE fistula, club feet

Notes:
Dup, duplication; del, deletion; ter, terminus; cen, centromere; del(3p)(pter→p13/p15), short arm deletion of chromosome 3 from the terminus to between bands 13 and 15; # Patients, number of patients reported in literature; FTT, failure to thrive; a., anomalies; cleft, cleft lip and/or palate; GI, gastrointestinal; TE, tracheo-esophageal.
Source: Schinzel (1984).

and medical management, it must be emphasized that individual patients are highly variable and may have a better prognosis than is average for their disorder. The lack of long-term studies or comprehensive patient registries may bias natural history toward the most severe or unusual patients.

With these reservations, the particular risks outlined in Tables 7.2 and 7.3 can be melded with the general risks in Table 7.1 to produce a management plan for patients with rare chromosomal anomalies. Recall that cytogenetic notation uses a "p" to designate the chromosome short arm, "q" the long arm, and band numbers to indicate the region of deficiency ("del") or duplication ("dup"). Band numbers increase as they go from the centromere to the short or long arm terminus ("ter"). Characteristic abnormalities in patients with duplication of the long arm of chromosome 7 can be found by locating "Dup(7q)" in the tables, then ascertaining which entry matches the patient in question. Note that there are two entries for dup(7q) in Table 7.2 and one in Table 7.3; patients with duplication of region 7q32→7qter are mildly or moderately affected (Table 7.3), while those with duplications of 7q11→7q22/q31 or of 7q22/q31→7qter are severely affected (Table 7.2). Thus, the extent of deletion or duplication, as indicated on the cytogenetic laboratory report, may be important for anticipating complications. Once the relevant entry is located, the table lists the approximate number of reported patients and their characteristic anomalies. A caveat to this approach applies to the child with complex chromosomal rearrangements, where combined duplication and deficiency may hinder the forecast of complications.

Chromosomal disorders for which only 1 or 2 patients have been described are not listed in the tables. Natural history information is obviously unreliable even for listed disorders where fewer than 10 patients have been described. When there is

Table 7.3 Frequent complications of milder chromosomal syndromes

Disorder	Aneuploid region	# Patients	Complications
Ring(1)		10–50	Cleft palate, cardiac defects, leukemia
Dup(1p)	p31→p22	<10	FTT, microcephaly, cryptorchidism
Dup(1q)	q25→q32	10–50	Macrocephaly, eye a., dental dysplasia, cardiac a.
Dup(1q)	q42→qter	<10	Cardiac, renal, genital anomalies
Del(2p)	pter→p23/p21	<10	FTT, microcephaly, seizures, skeletal anomalies
Ring(2)		10–50	FTT, microcephaly, retinal dystrophy, cardiac a., genital a., lymphedema of hands and feet
Dup(2q)	q31→qter	10–50	FTT, cleft, cardiac a., eczema, genital a.
Dup(2)	q32/q34→qter	10–50	FTT, glaucoma, coloboma, cardiac a., renal a., skeletal a., intestinal atresias
Del(3p)	pter→p25	10–50	FTT, optic atrophy, cleft, cardiac a., renal a., scoliosis
Dup(3q) Dup(3q)/ Del(3p)	q21/q25→qter, q13/q21→qter/ del(pter→p25)	>50	FTT, seizures, hypoplasia of cerebellum, brain a., cataracts, glaucoma, cardiac a., renal a., GI malrotation, absent or streak ovaries, cryptorchidism, hypospadias
Del(4p)	p15→p12	<10	Glaucoma, urinary outflow obstruction
Del(4q)	q21/q23→q27/q32	<10	FTT, craniosynostosis, microphthalmia, hypothyroidism, chronic otitis, cardiac a., renal a.
Del(4q)	q32→qter	<10	Short stature, microphthalmia, Robin sequence, genital a.
Ring(4)		10–50	FTT, microcephaly, seizures, cleft, cardiac a., limb a.
Dup(4q)	q25/q27→qter	10–50	FTT, microcephaly, cleft, hip dislocation, club feet, renal a.
Del(5q)	q15→q31	<10	Short stature, optic atrophy, cleft, cardiac a., renal a., club feet
Dup(5q)	q11/q13→q22	<10	Short stature, cardiac a.
Dup(5q)	q31/q33→qter	10–50	FTT, hydrocephalus, strabismus, cardiac a., delayed puberty
Ring(6)		10–50	FTT, microphthalmia, strabismus, hip dislocation, genital a.
Dup(6p)	pter→p22/p21	10–50	FTT, hydrocephalus, microphthalmia, cataract, strabismus, cardiac defects, renal a., hydronephrosis, genital a.
Del(7)	p21→p15/p13	<10	FTT, skull defect, cardiac a., renal a., anal atresia, limb a.
Del(7)	q21→q22/q34	10–50	FTT, glaucoma, cleft, pancreatic hypoplasia, cardiac a.
Ring(7)		<10	FTT, cataract, nystagmus, coloboma, hypospadias, micropenis
Dup(7)	q32→qter	10–50	FTT, cardiac a., scoliosis
Del(8p)	pter→p21	10–50	FTT, hydrocephalus, microcephaly, nystagmus, cardiac a., vertebral a., genital a.
Del(8q)	q13→q22	<10	FTT, microphthalmia, cardiac a., genital a., limb a.,
Del(8q)	q22→q24		Langer–Giedion syndrome, ptosis, limb a., skeletal exostoses

Table 7.3 (*cont.*)

Disorder	Aneuploid region	# Patients	Complications
Ring(8)		<10	FTT, hip dislocation, inguinal hernia, cryptorchidism
Trisomy 8	mosaic	>50	Absent corpus callosum, eye a., cardiac a., renal a., limb a.
Del(9p)	pter→p22/p21	10–50	Cleft, cryptorchidism, hydronephrosis, rib and vertebral a.
Ring(9)		10–50	FTT, microcephaly, cleft, cardiac a., genital a., vertebral a.
Dup(9p)	pter→p22/p21	10–50	FTT, microcephaly, disproportionate speech delay
Ring(10)		<10	Short stature, microcephaly, cardiac a., urogenital a.
Dup(10q)	q11→q21	<10	FTT, coloboma, microphthalmia, hypospadias
Del(11p)	p14→p12	10–50	FTT, aniridia, eye a., Wilms tumor, genital a., gonadoblastoma
Ring(11)		<10	FTT, cardiac anomalies
Del(12p)	pter→p12/p11	<10	Short stature, microcephaly, cardiac a.
Ring(12)		<10	Short stature, microcephaly
Del(13q)	q12/q14→q14/q31	10–50	FTT, retinoblastoma, scoliosis, inguinal hernias, genital a.
Del(13q)	q32/q33→qter	<10	Short stature, microcephaly, brain a., club feet, hemivertebrae
Ring(13)		10–50	FTT, cleft, depigmentation, alopecia areata
Dup(13p)	pter→q12/q21	10–50	FTT, strabismus, cardiac a., cryptorchidism, skull defects
Ring(14)		10–50	FTT, seizures, high palate, renal hypoplasia, cryptorchidism
Dup(14q)	pter→q11//q22	10–50	FTT, microphthalmia, cleft, cardiac a., joint contractures
Del(15q)	pter→q13/q22	<10	FTT, hydrocephalus, cleft, cardiac a., club feet, genital a.
Del(15q)	q11→q12/q13	10–50	Obesity, genital a., Prader–Willi, Angelman syndromes
Ring(15)	full, mosaic	10–50	FTT, cardiac a., renal a., ectopic anus, behavior problems
Dup(15q)	pter→q11/q13	>50	High palate, strabismus, nystagmus, hip dysplasia, club feet
Ring(17)		<10	Seizures, retinitis, genital a.
Dup(17p)	pter→p11/p13	10–50	FTT, microcornea, corneal clouding, glaucoma, cleft, cardiac a., urinary tract a., joint contractures
Dup(17q)	q21/q23→qter	<10	FTT, coloboma, cleft, cardiac a., renal a., vertebral a., genital a.
Del(18p)	pter→p11/q11	>50	FTT, brain a., choanal stenosis, eye a., cleft,
Ring(18)			craniosynostosis, malrotation, vertebral a., autoimmune disorders, alopecia
Del(18p)	q11/q21→q21/q23	<10	FTT, cataract, skull defects, cleft, cardiac a., IgA deficiency
Del(18q)	q21→qter	>50	FTT, brain a., strabismus, cleft, cardiac a., vertebral a., scoliosis, renal a., conductive deafness
Dup(18p)	pter→p11/q11	10–50	Branchial sinus, hemifacial microsomia
Dup(20p)	pter→p11/q11	10–50	Cataract, coloboma, cardiac a., renal a., vertebral a.
Del(21q)	pter→q11/q21	<10	FTT, cloudy cornea, cleft, cardiac a., anterior anus, genital a.
Ring(21)		10–50	FTT, eye a., craniosynostosis,, cleft, cardiac a., vertebral a.

Table 7.3 (*cont.*)

Disorder	Aneuploid region	# Patients	Complications
Del(22q)	pter→q11	10–50	Short stature, microcephaly, cardiac a., DiGeorge a.
Dup(22q)	pter→q11/q13; trip(22)	10–50	FTT, coloboma, cardiac a., renal a., malrotation, biliary atresia
Dup(22q)/ Dup(11p)	pter→q11 q23→qter	>50	FTT, brain a., cleft, cardiac a., renal a., anal atresia, hypoplasia of diaphragm, hip dislocation, micropenis, cryptorchidism
Triploidy	mosaic	<10	FTT, asymmetry, coloboma, genital a.
Tetraploidy	mosaic	<10	FTT, microcephaly, cataract, cardiac a., renal a., thymic hypoplasia, scoliosis, Arnold–Chiari malformation

Notes:
Dup, duplication; del, deletion; ter, terminus; cen, centromere; del(3p)(pter→p13/p15), short arm deletion of chromosome 3 from the terminus to between bands 13 and 15; # Patients, number of patients reported in · literature; FTT, failure to thrive; a., anomalies; cleft, cleft lip and/or palate; GI, gastrointestinal.
Source: Schinzel (1984).

little experience with a disorder, general complications listed in Tables 7.1 to 7.3 can be used as a guide to preventive management. Developmental delay, learning disability, failure to thrive, microcephaly, seizures, infections of the respiratory tract, eye anomalies, cleft lip/palate, cardiac anomalies and urogenital anomalies are common complications of chromosomal disorders. A checklist such as that for trisomy 13/18 emphasizes assessment and monitoring of these problems, allowing its use as a general guide to the health care of children with rare chromosomal syndromes.

There are a growing number of parent support groups for chromosome disorders, and these can be found through the directories of the Alliance of Genetic Support Groups (http://www.medhelp.org/geneticalliance/) or Exceptional Parent magazine (www.eparent.com) – i.e., The Chromosome 9p- Network, 675 North Round Table Drive, Las Vegas NV, 89110, (720) 453–0788, http://www.9pminus.org; or Disorders of Chromosome 16 Foundation, 331 Haddon Circle, Vernon Hills IL, 60061, (847) 816–0627, http://members.aol.com. Trisomy 13/18

Trisomy 13/18

Terminology

Children with extra chromosomal material representing an entire chromosome 13 or chromosome 18 are affected with the trisomy 13 or trisomy 18 syndrome (Figs

7.1, 7.2, color plates). The extra chromosomal material may arise by trisomy or translocation. Although each syndrome has a distinctive pattern of anomalies, trisomy 13 and trisomy 18 are discussed together because they have many overlapping features and a similar natural history. Patients with mosaicism for trisomy 13 or 18 have variable proportions of normal and trisomic cells among different tissues. Those with low percentages of mosaicism as judged from blood or fibroblast karyotyping will have a much milder phenotype than is typical for trisomy 13 or trisomy 18 syndrome (Delatycki & Gardner, 1997).

Historical diagnosis and management

The terms "Patau syndrome" and "Edwards syndrome" indicate the respective descriptions of trisomy 13 (Patau et al.) and trisomy 18 (Edwards et al.) in 1960. Taylor (1968) compared the two disorders, concluding that 42 of 45 observed abnormalities occurred in both conditions.

Incidence, etiology, and differential diagnosis

Trisomy 13 due to nondisjunction or translocation occurs in about 1 in 12,000 livebirths, with a frequency in miscarriages some 100-fold higher (Gorlin et al., 1990, p. 40). Trisomy 18 is slightly more common, with a frequency between 1 in 5000 and 1 in 7000 live births. Aneuploidy leads to the characteristic pattern of malformation, but the pathogenesis is poorly understood. Brain anomalies often bias the facial appearance in trisomy 13, with variable degrees of microphthalmia, nasal hypoplasia, and/or cleft lip caused by underlying holoprosencephaly. Isolated holoprosencephaly, Meckel syndrome with encephalocele and polydactyly, and the Pallister–Hall syndrome of brain anomalies and polydactyly may be confused with trisomy 13. Patients with trisomy 18 often have a characteristic "clenched fist" with overlapping fingers. Following the general rule that no one anomaly is pathognomonic for a syndrome, the clenched fist may occur in other disorders associated with decreased movement or innervation of the hands. Patients with the Pena–Shokeir syndrome of arthrogryposis and microcephaly, other disorders with decreased fetal movement, and trisomy 13 may resemble patients with trisomy 18.

Diagnostic evaluation and medical counseling

Rapid laboratory confirmation of trisomy 13 or trisomy 18 is available using fluorescent in situ hybridization (FISH) or bone marrow karyotyping when surgical decisions are pending. Patients with trisomy 13/18 are at risk for a variety of internal malformations that require evaluation in the newborn period. Initial management often will require imaging of the brain, heart, urinary tract, and abdomen along with careful observation of feeding and respiratory status. Hypertonia, seizures, and uncoordinated swallowing place these patients at high risk for aspiration, which may further increase their risks for apnea. Cardiac anomalies in trisomy 13 or 18 include septal defects, polyvalvular disease, patent ductus arteriosus, coarctation of the aorta, and, in trisomy 13, dextrocardia with or without aberrant venous return and/or aortic positioning (trisomy 13/18 checklist, part 1). Medical counseling should emphasize the risks for internal anomalies and be realistic but not hopeless concerning the developmental potential of patients with trisomy 13 and trisomy 18.

Crucial perinatal decisions involve the aggressiveness of medical and surgical management. Trisomy 13 and trisomy 18 patients are often recognized prenatally, offering the opportunity to counsel the parents concerning delivery and neonatal resuscitation options. Avoidance of Cesarean delivery or extreme resuscitation measures is often appropriate, especially in infants with major organ anomalies who may not survive the infantile period. Early neonatal diagnosis facilitates medical counseling regarding the management of anomalies such as hydrocephalus, meningomyelocele, cleft palate, tetralogy of Fallot, ventricular septal defect, or cryptorchidism/hypospadias; each of these anomalies, together with requirements for artificial ventilation or gastrostomy feedings, involves different levels of intervention and different consequences from withholding therapy. A reasonable strategy is to recommend simple surgeries and supportive care that alleviate suffering or ease management for parents; more elaborate surgery or prolonged intensive care is usually not recommended (Bos et al., 1992; Paris et al., 1992). This is partly because of anesthetic risks (Pollard & Beasley, 1996). Appropriate fluid and nutritional support are always indicated, and an overly negative and dehumanizing outlook by the health professional may provoke parental resistance and delay agreement on palliative care. It is important to recall that about 10 percent of patients will survive at least 1 year, and to emphasize the preventive management that can be provided for these children. As with any medical crisis, social and pastoral services should be included as part of the medical counseling.

Family and psychosocial counseling

For patients with free-standing trisomy of chromosome 13 or 18, the recurrence risk is about 1 percent, increasing in the usual way with maternal age (2–3 percent total risk by maternal age 40 years). Parental karyotyping is required if the infant has translocation 13 or 18, with risks in the 5–10 percent range if one parent is a balanced translocation carrier. If genetic counseling is not available during the neonatal period, then referral to a genetics clinic is essential. Prenatal diagnosis is an option for subsequent pregnancies, with chorionic villus biopsy or amniocentesis recommended rather than the less specific lowering of maternal serum α-fetoprotein (MSAFP).

The most crucial counseling issue concerns the high infant mortality and severe developmental disability faced by patients with trisomy 13/18. Survey of more than 100 families with trisomy 18 demonstrated some developmental progress in these children (Baty et al., 1994a, b), so initial counseling should be realistic but not overly bleak (see below). Options for palliative care, including the chance to ameliorate some of the disabilities, should be mentioned when the parents have had a chance to adjust to the diagnosis. Parent support groups are listed in part 1 of the trisomy13/18 checklist.

Natural history and complications

Root & Carey (1994) calculated a median survival of 4 days among 64 patients with trisomy 18, with survival to 1 month in 35 percent of patients and 1 year in 5 percent. Gorlin et al. (1990, pp. 41–4) reported survival rates in trisomy 18 of 70 percent for 1 month and less than 10 percent for 1 year. Patients without cardiac anomalies live longer, with a mean survival of 40 days (Gorlin et al., 1990, p. 44; Jones, 1997, p. 14). Survival in trisomy 13 is somewhat better, with 55 percent surviving 1 month and 14 percent surviving 1 year (Gorlin et al., 1990, p.40; Jones, 1997, p. 18). Mortality figures vary considerably among studies, influenced by occasional long-term survivors. Patients with full trisomy 13 or 18 have survived into their late teens.

Baty et al. (1994a, b) documented the natural history of 130 patients with trisomy 13/18 using parental questionnaires and medical record review. Brain anomalies with seizures are common in both syndromes, with holoprosencephaly being prevalent in trisomy 13. Each disorder may include early hypertonia with clenched fists, although this sign is more emphasized in trisomy 18. Eye, external ear, and inner ear anomalies are common, causing visual and/or hearing impairment in most patients who are properly assessed (e.g., Holmes & Coates, 1994). Severe feeding problems with failure to thrive and multiple internal anomalies can be expected (checklist, part 1). Urinary tract infections occurred in 11–19 percent of patients with trisomy 13/18 according to the survey of Baty et al. (1994a). Other complications include spinal dysraphism (Wainwright et al., 1995; Herman and Siegel, 1997), myeloid malignancy (Mehta et al., 1998), and pigmentary lesions (Pillay et al., 1998).

An important addition to the literature is the study of Baty et al. (1994b) that documents some psychomotor development in patients with trisomy 13/18. Developmental quotients (developmental age divided by chronologic age) averaged 0.18 in 50 trisomy 18 individuals (ages 1–232 months) and 0.25 in 12 trisomy 13 individuals (ages 1–130 months), according to assessments from the medical record (Baty et al., 1994b). Older children responded to words or phrases, communicated with simple words or signs, crawled, used a walker, interacted with others, and achieved some toileting skills. Woldorf & Johnson (1994) described a 7-year-old girl with trisomy 18 who can use a walker.

Trisomy 13/18 preventive management checklist

After initial evaluations for internal anomalies, agreement on the various surgical versus palliative care options should be reached with the parents. Neurologic dysfunction may superimpose poor feeding on underlying pre- and postnatal growth retardation, particularly in patients with trisomy 18. Careful monitoring of growth, feeding, and nutrition is thus necessary throughout life, and feeding specialists may be required to achieve adequate caloric intake in these hypertonic, irritable, and neurologically immature patients (checklist, parts 2–4). Malformations of the eye, external ear, and inner ear are frequent, emphasizing the need for frequent hearing and vision assessment to ensure maximal function. Urinary tract anomalies are frequent in both trisomies, and hepatoblastoma or Wilms tumor has been encountered in longer survivors with trisomy 18. These risks should be monitored by performing periodic urinalyses and abdominal palpation. The debilitated state of many patients requires vigilance for respiratory infections and attention to social or local services such as social work, clergy, occupational or physical therapy, respite, and hospice care. The medical interventions listed on the trisomy 13/18 checklist, parts 2–4 should obviously be tailored to prognosis, since palliative care is appropriate for patients with severe anomalies.

Down syndrome

Terminology

Patients with an entire extra copy of chromosome 21 have Down syndrome. The extra chromosome may arise by nondisjunction (trisomy 21) or translocation (translocation Down syndrome). Patients with mixtures of normal and trisomic cells (mosaic Down syndrome) often have milder phenotypes, but it should be realized that percentages of normal cells among peripheral lymphocytes used for karyotyping may differ from percentages in brain.

Historical diagnosis and management

Down syndrome was first described in 1866 by Dr. J. H. Langdon Down, a British physician. Diagnosis was clinical until 1959, when Lejeune reported the extra number 21 chromosome in patients with Down syndrome. Early in this century, patients with Down syndrome and those with congenital hypothyroidism ("cretinism") were mistaken for each other because each displayed mental retardation, hypotonia, thyroid dysfunction, and growth failure (Volpe, 1986). Patients with Down syndrome, like others with moderate mental retardation, were often institutionalized because of overly pessimistic views of their potential. Improvements in cardiac surgery, immunizations, and thyroid treatment have ameliorated the major complications of Down syndrome and provided the modern expectations of family living, inclusive schooling, and prolonged life span (Cooley & Graham, 1991).

Incidence, etiology, and differential diagnosis

The incidence of Down syndrome is 1 in 650 to 1 in 1000 live births and shows little variation by ethnic groups (Gorlin et al., 1990, p. 33; Staples et al., 1991). Increasing maternal age is a significant risk factor, rising from about 1 in 2000 at age 20 to 1 in 50 at age 40 (Hook & Lindsjö, 1978). The disorder is caused by duplicated material from the distal long arm of chromosome 21 through nondisjunction (trisomy 21) or translocation (translocation Down syndrome). Extensive mapping of genes on this "critical region" of chromosome 21 is under way as part of the human genome initiative. The mechanisms by which increased dosage of these genes leads to the Down syndrome phenotype are as yet unknown (Epstein, 1995).

The newborn with Down syndrome is often recognized because of an unusual facies (Fig. 7.3, color plate) and hypotonia. In some newborns, especially premature infants, facial recognition may be difficult. Characteristic minor anomalies may be needed for diagnosis, including a central hair whorl, brachycephaly, upslanting palpebral fissures, epicanthal folds, Brushfield spots, anteverted nares, redundant neck skin, single palmar creases, clinodactyly, broad space between the first and second toes, and a deep plantar crease. The tongue frequently protudes, more because of hypotonia than true enlargement. As with all syndromes, the pattern of minor and major defects in Down syndrome varies from individual to individual. None of the anomalies is pathognomonic.

Diagnostic evaluation and medical counseling

All patients with Down syndrome have duplicated chromosomal 21 material, but the origin of this duplicated material may vary. The most typical finding is trisomy 21 where the extra number 21 chromosome is free-standing. Translocation refers to joining or exchange of chromosome 21 material with another chromosome. Translocation of chromosome 21 usually involves an acrocentric chromosome (chromosomes 13–15, 21, 22) as an end-to-end "Robertsonian" translocation. When a translocation is found, the parents must be karyotyped to determine if they "carry" the translocation in a balanced form. Occasionally, patients with Down syndrome will be mosaic, having a mixture of normal and trisomy 21 cells. Trisomy 21 is the etiology for Down syndrome in 96 percent of cases, with translocation (3 percent) and mosaic Down syndrome (1 percent) being less common.

Initial disclosure that Down syndrome is suspected is best made during the neonatal period when both parents are present or when other family members are available for support (Cooley & Graham, 1991). Avoidance of pejorative terms such as "mongolism" or "simian" crease is desirable, and the use of people-first language (e.g., the infant with Down syndrome rather than the "Down's baby") is encouraged. Counseling should stress the improved prognosis for children with Down syndrome and emphasize the importance of anticipatory guidance. Genetic counseling can begin when the karyotype results are available, usually 1–2 weeks after birth. If counseling must be delayed for 1–2 months, karyotype results should be communicated as soon as possible, to minimize parental anxiety. The recurrence risk for trisomy 21 is 1 percent if the mother is under age 35 and increases with maternal age thereafter. Depending on the nature of the balanced translocation, carriers can have risks between 5 and 100 percent to have another child with Down syndrome. Prenatal diagnosis using chorionic villus biopsy or amniocentesis allows detection of fetuses with Down syndrome by documenting the fetal karyotype. Screening of maternal serum during pregnancy is also possible and is recommended as a standard of care for women over age 35 years (Frame et al., 1997).

Family and psychosocial counseling

Contact with representatives of a Down syndrome parent group is the best way for parents to begin learning about the many psychosocial issues involved in raising a child with disabilities. Such contacts can be facilitated through one of the national organizations listed below, with most urban areas having active Down syndrome guilds or parent groups (Down syndrome checklist, part 1).

Msall et al. (1991) discussed ways in which a partnership can be forged between families, health care professionals, and early intervention specialists. Natal psychosocial issues include the options for adoption or foster care for parents who cannot accept a child with a handicap or who have insufficient resources. Few parents will opt to place children for adoption if they receive supportive counseling from informed professionals and parent representatives. Institutionalization is no longer a realistic option and should be mentioned only as an example of negative and inaccurate information that may be found in the older literature on Down syndrome. Marital and sibling stress that occurs during the adjustment to a child with disabilities should be discussed and appropriate counseling resources provided. Sibling and parent workshops available through Down syndrome organizations are helpful with these adjustments.

Later issues include the challenges in obtaining educational resources faced by many parents. Local parent groups and chapters of the Association for Retarded Citizens are often helpful in preparing parents as advocates in the educational process. While there is controversy and some resistance surrounding inclusive education of children with moderate disabilities, much anecdotal evidence attests to positive experiences for both "normal" and disabled children. Key indicators will be the child's level of function and the availability of assistance for the teacher. Behavioral and psychiatric disorders are more prevalent in children with Down syndrome, ranging from attention deficit disorders to psychoses. Child psychologists and behavioral therapists may be needed, with the provision that observation for problems triggering the behavior should precede and accompany pharmacologic intervention.

Medical issues include educating the parents about the symptoms of atlantoaxial instability. Although 15 percent of individuals with Down syndrome have radiographic evidence of atlantoaxial instability, few are symptomatic (Committee on Sports Medicine and Fitness, 1995). It is symptomatic children who are at highest risk for spinal cord injury, and the Committee on Sports Medicine and Fitness (1995) suggested that counseling parents about the symptoms of atlantoaxial instability (easy fatiguability, abnormal gait, neck pain, limited neck mobility, head tilt, clumsiness, spasticity, hyperreflexia, extensor-plantar reflex, other upper motor neuron signs) is more important than the cervical spine radiographs. However, Pueschel (1998) has argued for continued cervical radiographic screening.

Issues for midchildhood and adulthood include sexuality, with education about appropriate personal boundaries and private behavior. Contraception is an important consideration in females. Job training is important to anticipate, beginning at ages 15–16 to prepare for the end of mandated education after age 21–22. Parents must also confront issues of guardianship and financial support of older dependent children. Resources to assist with legal and estate planning issues can be obtained through the Down syndrome organizations and the Association of Retarded Citizens. While parents are usually too overwhelmed to confront these later issues in the first counseling session, they should be addressed in early childhood so that the parents can begin investigation and planning. Books to aid parents include those by Pueschel (1978) and Stray-Gunderson (1986).

Natural history and complications

Cooley & Graham (1991) emphasized the improvements in the length and quality of life enjoyed by individuals with Down syndrome. They cite a 50 percent mortality by age 5 in 1965, compared with 80 percent survival to age 30 or beyond in 1991. Much of this improvement reflects advances in pediatric and cardiothoracic surgery, allowing the correction of the gastrointestinal and cardiac anomalies (Weinhouse et al., 1995) that are prominent among the complications listed on the checklist, part 1. If no congenital anomalies are manifest in the newborn period, then more subtle abnormalities of the ocular, otic, dental, immune, urinary, and skeletal systems must be suspected. Transient myeloid proliferation may occur, conferring an increased but still low (still less than 1 percent) risk for leukemia. Neonatal liver disease is also a rare complication (Yagihashi et al., 1995). Neonatal jaundice, feeding problems, anal stenosis are common problems that often respond to parental counseling and resolve spontaneously.

Respiratory infections are more frequent and severe in children with Down syndrome, including chronic otitis, sinusitis, and pneumonia. Tonsillectomy and adenoidectomy are often required, but these procedures may have postoperative complications (Jacobs et al., 1996; Goldstein et al., 1998). Correctable problems such as constipation, strabismus, hypothyroidism, dental anomalies, atlantoaxial instability, and cryptorchidism are important not to miss. Msall et al. (1990) reported consequences of not screening for atlantoaxial instability in 4 children. Developmental delays, learning differences, and speech problems are universal, and there is a 10 percent risk for psychiatric problems in older individuals with Down syndrome. Despite neuropathological changes typical of Alzheimer disease in 100 percent of individuals over 35, symptomatic dementia is fortunately much less frequent (Cooley & Graham, 1991; Epstein, 1995).

Down syndrome preventive management checklist

An early version of the preventive medical checklist was designed by Dr. Mary Coleman (Cohen, 1992). Rubin & Crocker (1989) have presented similar recommendations in their "Healthwatch" chart for Down syndrome (Cooley & Graham, 1991), as did Carey (1992) in his table for anticipatory guidance and health supervision. The guidelines in the checklist, parts 2–4 have been adapted from these sources and conform to the recommendations of the American Academy of Pediatrics (Committee on Genetics, 1994). Cooley & Graham (1991) provided a detailed, clinically oriented discussion of modern preventive management.

Neonatal evaluation of Down syndrome includes attention to feeding and bowel function, since cardiac and gastrointestinal anomalies may occur. All children need an echocardiogram in the first few weeks, since large septal defects may not be audible by auscultation and present later with inoperable pulmonary hypertension. Hypotonia often complicates breast feeding, so extra support and expertise should be provided to interested mothers. Blood for karyotyping should be obtained in all cases, with referral for genetic counseling, early intervention, and parent group support. These services are potentially coordinated by a Down syndrome clinic in areas where one is available. Preventive care in childhood includes annual thyroid testing, monitoring of hearing and vision, and referral to ophthalmology at age 8–10 months to prevent later amblyopia. A "high TSH" form of hypothyroidism is common, requiring repeat thyroid function tests and possible hormone therapy. X-rays of the cervical spine are recommended at age 3 years, and at 10-year intervals thereafter. Sleep apnea is common in children with hypotonia, obesity, and respiratory infections; a "GRIMES" acronym may be used as a screening tool. The acronym stands for Gasping respirations, Retractions, Inspiratory stridor, Mouth breathing, and Excessive Sweating in children with Down syndrome (Spahis, 1994). Because of their susceptibility to infection, children and adolescents with Down syndrome should receive all immunizations, including pneumococcal, varicella, and influenza vaccines in children with respiratory difficulties.

Pediatric visits should continue through adolescence with particular attention to moderating obesity, recognizing visual or auditory deficiencies, and early recognition of school and behavior problems. Nutritional monitoring, with encouragement of dieting and exercise, is important, and some children may be more susceptible to vitamin deficiencies (Cabana et al., 1997). There is a higher risk for several autoimmune disorders, including type I diabetes and celiac disease (Mehta et al., 1995). Pubertal males with micropenis may be subject to ridicule, and early testosterone treatment may be considered. Although males are rarely fertile, adolescents may be sexually active and need protection from sexually transmitted diseases and pregnancy. Many females with Down syndrome can schedule and manage birth control pills with supervision, and Norplant or depot hormone injections may be considered for individuals with lower function.

Simple preventive treatments may include eyewash scrubs for blepharitis and nasal saline drops for sinusitis. Blepharitis is evidenced by erythema and/or swelling of the eyelids and can result in unsightly deformities of the lid or even keratitis. Washing of the eyelids with baby shampoo (or saline, if shampoo is irritating) during baths is helpful. Nasal saline drops (2 in each nostril, morning and night) prevent drying of the mucosa and help with the rhinorrhea, nasal obstruction, and sinusitis that is so common in the first 3–4 years.

Several unproven therapies have been promoted for Down syndrome, including recent attention to the memory-enhancing drug Piracetam. This drug has been tried in European patients with Alzheimer disease, but has a minimal track record and no proven benefit in children with Down syndrome. Vitamin supplements have a long history of use in Down syndrome, despite a lack of scientific evidence for true vitamin deficiencies. Fortunately, neither Piracetam nor the common vitamin/nutrient mixtures seem to be harmful. Parents should be warned against costly biochemical analyses, "cellular" treatments by injection of animal cell mixtures, or "patterning" treatments that impose rigid schedules on families already dealing with the added stress of disability (Cooley & Graham, 1991). Plastic surgery to alter tongue size or to correct facial features is also controversial.

As discussed above, preventive medical checklists for Down syndrome have been used for more than 15 years and formally recommended by the American Academy of Pediatrics (Committee on Genetics, 1994). They are also used by more than 30 Down syndrome clinics across the United States. A major goal of the Down syndrome clinic directors is to establish a clinical database that can justify the checklist by outcome analysis. Areas of controversy include the frequency of thyroid studies, the value of cervical spine films in predicting risk of atlantoaxial instability, and the frequency of referrals to genetic or Down syndrome clinics. While yearly thyroid studies are often recommended, relaxation of this schedule in children with appropriate growth and development should be considered. As mentioned above, counseling for symptoms of atlantoaxial instability is considered more useful than cervical spine radiographs by the Committee on Sports Medicine and Fitness (1995). Pediatricians familiar with Down syndrome and its preventive health care recommendations are certainly capable of managing these families without involvement of a Down syndrome or genetics clinic. However, initial genetic referral for counseling and family support is essential, and referral to a multidisciplinary Down syndrome clinic is useful during transition stages (preschool, school, puberty, early adult).

Preventive Management of Trisomy 13/18

Clinical diagnosis: Clinical pattern known as Patau syndrome for trisomy 13 with scalp defect, microphthalmia, cleft lip and palate, polydactyly; pattern known as Edwards syndrome for trisomy 18 with small face and jaw, abnormal ears, clenched fists, convex soles, more frequent prenatal growth retardation. Both syndromes have high frequencies of major organ defects.

Incidence: Trisomy 13 occurs in 1 in 12,000 and trisomy 18 in 1 in 5,000–7,000 live births; they have a 50–100 fold higher frequency in miscarriages.

Laboratory diagnosis: Karyotype to demonstrate trisomy or translocation, occasional mosaicism.

Genetics: Approximate 1% recurrence for pure trisomy 13 or 18, 5–10% for translocation if a parent is a carrier.

Key management issues: Neonatal recognition of brain anomalies, seizures, apnea for trisomy 13; GI and cardiac anomalies for both trisomies; family support and palliative care options, hearing, vision, genitourinary anomalies.

Growth Charts: Baty et al. (1994) reported measurements from 76 individuals with trisomy 18 and 17 individuals with trisomy 13.

Parent groups: S.O.F.T, 2982 S. Union St. Rochester, NY 14624, (800) 716-7638, barbsoft@aol.com, www.trisomy.org; SOFT Canada, 769 Brant St. Suite 420, Burlington ON, Canada, L7R 4BB8; S.O.F.T. (UK), (0121) 351-3122, enquiries@soft.org.uk

Basis for management recommendations: Recommendations of Carey (1992) drawn from complications documented below (Baty et al., 1994; Taylor, 1968).

Summary of clinical concerns

General	Aging	**Infant mortality** (T13 – 45% at 1 month, 62–86% at 1 year; T18 – 30–65% at 1 month, 90–95% at 1 year)
	Learning	**Severe disability** (100%)
	Growth	**Failure to thrive** (T13 – 87%; T18 – 96%)
Facial	Eye	**Eye anomalies** (T13 – 74% – microphthalmia, 76%, iris coloboma, 33%; T18 – 27% – corneal clouding, cataracts, microphthalmia, glaucoma)
	Ear	**Malformed ears** (T18 – 88% ;T13 – 87%), inner ear defects
	Mouth	**Oromotor dysfunction**, cleft lip (T13 – 41–58%; T18 – 6%), **cleft palate** (T13 – 48–59%; T18 – 7%)
Surface	Neck/trunk	**Loose skin, nape,** short neck (T13 – 79%), **inguinal hernia** (T13 – 40%; T18 – 56%); umbilical hernia
	Epidermal	Scalp defect (T13 – 44–75%)
Skeletal	Cranial	**Microcephaly** (T13 – 86%; T18 – 70%)
	Limbs	**Polydactyly** (T13 – 52–76%), **overlap of fingers** (T13 – 68%;T18 – 89%), **clubfoot** (T13 – 15%;T18 – 89%)
Internal	Digestive	GI anomalies (T13 – omphalocele, 11%; T18 – omphalocele, 9%, esophageal atresia, anal atresia, meckel diverticulum)
	Circulatory	**Cardiac anomalies** (T13 – 59–94%, septal defects, 73–91, patent ductus arteriosus, 82%,dextrocardia, 14%; T18 – 85%, septal defects, 86%, patent ductus, 74%, coarctation of aorta, 20%)
	Endocrine	T13 – pancreatic dysplasia, exocrine insufficiency; T18 – ectopic pancreas, thyroglossal duct cyst, hypothyroidism
	Excretory	**Renal anomalies** (T13 – 70% – polycystic kidneys, urinary tract anomalies, 10–25%; T18 – 30%, cystic kidneys, horseshoe kidney, double ureter), urinary tract infections (T13 – 19%)
	Genital	**Cryptorchidism** (T13,T18 – 100%), **prominent clitoris** (T18 – 89%), bicornuate uterus (T13)
Neural	CNS	**Hypertonia** (T13, T18 – 60%), **seizures** (T13 – 37%; T18 – 45%), **apnea** (T13 – 58%), holoprosencephaly (T13 – 70%), spina bifida (T13 – 4%; T18 – 1%)
	Sensory	**Hearing deficits** (T13 – 50%), sensorineural deafness, blindness

RES, reticuloendothelial system, GI, gastrointestinal system, **bold: frequency > 20%**

Key references

Carey, J. (1992). *Pediatric Clinics of North America* 39:25–53.
Baty, B. J. et al. (1994). *American Journal of Medical Genetics* 49:175–188; 49:189–94.
Taylor, A. I. (1968). *Journal of Medical Genetics* 5:227–52.

Trisomy 13/18

Preventive medical checklist (0–1yr)

Patient   **Birth Date** / /   **Number**

Pediatric	Screen		Evaluate		Refer/Counsel	
Neonatal / / *Newborn screen* ❑ *HB* ❑	Newborn screen ❑ Karyotype ❑		Feeds/stools ❑ Eyes ❑ Apnea, seizures ❑		Genetic evaluation ❑ Ophthalmology[3] ❑ Feeding specialist[3] ❑	
1 month / /	Head MRI[3] ❑ Renal sonogram ❑ Cardiac echo ❑		Feeds/stools ❑ Respiratory ❑ Apnea, seizures ❑		Family support[4] ❑ Feeding specialist ❑ Cardiology ❑	
2 months / / *HB¹* ❑ *Hib* ❑ *DTaP, IPV* ❑ *RV* ❑	Growth ❑ Hearing, vision[2] ❑		Feeds/stools ❑ Eyes ❑ Respiratory ❑ Apnea, seizures ❑		Early intervention[5] ❑ Developmental pediatrics ❑ Genetic counseling ❑ Feeding specialist[3] ❑ Neurology[3] ❑ Hospice care[3] ❑	
4 months / / *HB¹* ❑ *Hib* ❑ *DTaP/IPV* ❑ *RV* ❑	Growth ❑ Hearing, vision[2] ❑		Feeds/stools ❑ Eyes ❑ Respiratory ❑ Apnea, seizures ❑		Genetics ❑ Early intervention[5] ❑ ENT[3] ❑ Feeding specialist[3] ❑	
6 months / / *Hib* ❑ *IPV¹* ❑ *DTaP* ❑ *RV* ❑	Growth ❑ Hearing, vision[2] ❑		Nutrition ❑ Respiratory ❑ Apnea, seizures ❑		Family support[4] ❑ Developmental pediatrics ❑ Feeding specialist ❑	
9 months / / *IPV¹* ❑	Audiology ❑		Strabismus ❑ Abdominal exam[6] ❑		Ophthalmology[3] ❑ Hospice care[3] ❑	
1 year / / *HB* ❑ *Hib¹* ❑ *IPV¹* ❑ *MMR¹* ❑ *Var¹* ❑	Growth ❑ Hearing, vision[2] ❑		Nutrition ❑ Feeds/stools ❑ Respiratory ❑ Apnea, seizures ❑		Family support[4] ❑ Early intervention[5] ❑ Feeding specialist[3] ❑ Developmental pediatrics ❑ Genetics ❑ Neurology[3] ❑	

Clinical concerns for Trisomy 13/18, ages 0–1 year

Microcephaly	Hearing loss, ear anomalies	Developmental disability
Holoprosencephaly	Cardiac anomalies	Failure to thrive
Seizures, apnea	GI anomalies	Frequent infections
Eye anomalies	Urinary tract anomalies	Wilms tumor[6]

Guidelines for the neonatal period should be undertaken *at whatever age* the diagnosis is made; DTaP, acellular DTP; IPV, inactivated poliovirus (oral polio also used); RV, rotavirus; MMR, measles–mumps–rubella; Var, varicella; [1]alternative timing; [2]by practitioner; [3]as dictated by clinical findings – abdominal examinations because of risk for Wilms tumor; [4]parent group, family/sib, financial, and behavioral issues as discussed in the preface; [5]including developmental monitoring and motor/speech therapy.

Trisomy 13/18

Preventive medical checklist (15m–6yrs)

Patient		Birth Date / /	Number
Pediatric	**Screen**	**Evaluate**	**Refer/Counsel**
15 months / / Hib[1] ☐ MMR[1] ☐ DTaP, IPV[1] ☐ Varicella[1] ☐	Renal sonogram[6] ☐	Nutrition ☐ Respiratory ☐ Abdominal exam[6] ☐	Family support[4] ☐ Early intervention[5] ☐
18 months / / DTaP, IPV[1] ☐ Varicella[1] ☐ Influenza[3] ☐	Growth ☐ Hearing, vision[2] ☐	Nutrition ☐ Respiratory ☐ Abdominal exam[6] ☐	Feeding specialist[4] ☐ Genetics ☐
2 years / / Influenza[3] ☐ Pneumovax[3] ☐ Dentist ☐	Growth ☐ Hearing, vision[2] ☐	Nutrition ☐ Respiratory ☐ Apnea, seizures ☐ Abdominal exam[6] ☐	Family support[4] ☐ Developmental pediatrics ☐ Genetics ☐ Feeding specialist[3] ☐ ENT, ophthalmology[3] ☐
3 years / / Influenza[3] ☐ Pneumovax[3] ☐ Dentist ☐	Growth ☐ Hearing, vision[2] ☐ Audiology ☐	Nutrition ☐ Respiratory ☐ Abdominal exam[6] ☐	Family support[4] ☐ Preschool transition[5] ☐ Feeding specialist[3] ☐
4 years / / Influenza[3] ☐ Pneumovax[3] ☐ Dentist ☐	Growth ☐ Hearing, vision[2] ☐	Nutrition ☐ Abdominal exam[6] ☐	Family support[5] ☐ Preschool program[5] ☐ Developmental pediatrics ☐ Genetics ☐ Ophthalmology[3] ☐
5 years / / DTaP, IPV[1] ☐ MMR[1] ☐	Hearing, vision[3] ☐ Audiology ☐	Nutrition ☐ Seizures ☐	School transition[6] ☐ Hospice care[4] ☐
6 years / / DTaP, IPV[1] ☐ MMR[1] ☐ Dentist ☐	Growth ☐ Hearing, vision[2] ☐	School program ☐ Nutrition ☐ Abdominal exam[6] ☐	Family support[4] ☐ Developmental pediatrics ☐ Genetics ☐ Ophthalmology ☐ ENT[3] ☐

Clinical concerns for Trisomy 13/18, ages 1–6 years

Microcephaly
Holoprosencephaly
Seizures, apnea
Eye anomalies

Hearing loss, ear anomalies
Cardiac anomalies
GI anomalies
Urinary tract anomalies

Developmental disability
Failure to thrive
Frequent infections
Wilms tumor[6]

Guidelines for prior ages should be undertaken *at the time of diagnosis*; DTaP, acellular DPT; IPV, inactivated poliovirus (oral polio also used); MMR, measles–mumps–rubella; [1]alternative timing; [2]by practitioner; [3]as dictated by clinical findings – abdominal examinations because of risk for Wilms tumor; [4]parent group, family/sib, financial, and behavioral issues as discussed in the preface; [5]including developmental monitoring and motor/speech therapy.

Trisomy 13/18

Preventive medical checklist (6+ yrs)

Patient   **Birth Date** / /   **Number**

Pediatric	Screen		Evaluate		Refer/Counsel	
8 years / / *Dentist* ❑	Growth Hearing, vision[2]	❑ ❑	Nutrition Abdominal exam[6] Scoliosis Seizures	❑ ❑ ❑ ❑	School options Developmental pediatrics Genetics	❑ ❑ ❑
10 years / /	Hearing, vision[2]	❑	School program Nutrition Abdominal exam[6] Scoliosis	❑ ❑ ❑ ❑	Ophthalmology[3] ENT[3] Hospice care[3]	❑ ❑ ❑
12 years / / *Td[1], MMR, Var* ❑ *CBC* ❑ *Dentist* ❑ *Scoliosis* ❑ *Cholesterol* ❑	Growth Hearing, vision[2]	❑ ❑	Nutrition Abdominal exam[6] Seizures	❑ ❑ ❑	Family support[4] School options Developmental pediatrics Genetics	❑ ❑ ❑ ❑
14 years / / *CBC* ❑ *Dentist* ❑ *Cholesterol* ❑ *Breast CA* ❑ *Testicular CA* ❑	Hearing, vision[2]	❑	School program Nutrition Abdominal exam[6] Scoliosis	❑ ❑ ❑ ❑		
16 years / / *Td[1]* ❑ *CBC* ❑ *Cholesterol* ❑ *Sexual[5]* ❑ *Dentist* ❑	Growth Hearing, vision[2]	❑ ❑	Nutrition Abdominal exam[6] Seizures	❑ ❑ ❑	Hospice care[3] Developmental pediatrics Genetics	❑ ❑ ❑
18 years / / *CBC* ❑ *Sexual[5]* ❑ *Cholesterol* ❑ *Scoliosis* ❑	Hearing, vision[2]	❑	School program Nutrition Scoliosis	❑ ❑ ❑		
20 years[7] / / *CBC* ❑ *Sexual[5]* ❑ *Cholesterol* ❑ *Dentist* ❑	Growth Hearing, vision[2]	❑ ❑	Nutrition Seizures Living situation	❑ ❑ ❑	Family support[4]	❑

Clinical concerns for Trisomy 13/18, ages 6+ years

Microcephaly	Cardiac anomalies	Cognitive disability
Seizures	Urinary tract anomalies	Failure to thrive
Eye anomalies	Cryptorchidism, micropenis	Frequent infections
Hearing loss, ear anomalies	Scoliosis	Wilms tumor[6]

Guidelines for prior ages should be undertaken *at the time of diagnosis*; Td, tetanus/diphtheria; MMR, measles–mumps–rubella; Var, varicella; [1]alternative timing; [2]by practitioner; [3]as dictated by clinical findings – abdominal examinations because of risk for Wilms tumor; [4]parent group, family/sib, financial, and behavioral issues as discussed in the preface; [5]birth control, STD screening if sexually active; [7]repeat every decade.

Preventive Management of Down syndrome

Clinical diagnosis: Syndrome with characteristic facial appearance, upslanting palpebral fissures, single palmar creases, 5th finger clinodactyly, large space between first and second toes, hypotonia.
Incidence: 1 in 800–1000 births.
Laboratory diagnosis: Karyotype showing extra chromosome 21 due to trisomy (96%), translocation (3%), mosaicism (1%).
Genetics: 1 in 200 risk at maternal age 35; 1% recurrence risk after child with trisomy 21; 10–95% risk if parental translocation.
Key management issues: Positive attitude with people-first language (child with Down syndrome); karyotype parents if translocation; neonatal feeding, vision, hearing, heart, thyroid, and behavioral problems.
Growth Charts: Cronk et al. (1988).
Parent groups: National Down Syndrome Congress, 1605 Chantilly Dr., Suite 250, Atlanta, GA, 30324, http://.members.carol.net/nsdc/, (800) 232-NDSC; National Down Syndrome Society, 666 Broadway, New York, NY, 10012; http://www.ndss.org, 800-221-4602; Down's Syndrome Association, 155 Mitcham Rd., London SW17 9PG UK, (0181)-682-4012, http://downs-syndrome.org.uk
Basis for management recommendations: Consensus guidelines from Cooley & Graham (1991), Cohen (1992), Committee on Genetics (1996), Pueschel & Pueschel (1992).

Summary of clinical concerns

General	Learning	Cognitive and learning differences, speech problems
	Behavior	Behavior problems (10%) – hyperactivity, oppositional, adjustment, adolescent mental health problems (depression, anxiety)
	Growth	Feeding problems, short stature, obesity
Facial	Eye	Myopia, **astigmatism** (70%), **strabismus**, (20–40%), blepharitis (2–46%)
	Ear	**Small ear canals** (53%), **chronic otitis** (40–60%), cholesteatoma
	Nose	**Shallow nasal bridge** (61%), chronic nasal discharge
	Mouth	**Tooth anomalies** (23–47%), **periodontal disease** (90%), **sleep apnea** (31%), protruding tongue
Surface	Neck/trunk	Lax connective tissue, inguinal hernias
	Epidermal	Dry skin, alopecia, skin rashes
Skeletal	Cranial	Microcephaly, brachycephaly
	Axial	Atlantoaxial or occipitoatlantal instability (2–5%)
	Limbs	Slipped femoral epiphysis, arthritis, joint dislocations
Internal	Digestive	**Neonatal jaundice** (60%), anal stenosis, **constipation** (30%), gastro-intestinal anomalies (10–18%), gastroesophageal reflux, celiac disease
	Pulmonary	Increased severity and frequency of respiratory infections
	Circulatory	**Cardiac anomalies** (40–50%), cardiac failure, pulmonary hypertension
	Endocrine	**Hypothyroidism** (22–40%), type I diabetes
	RES	Frequent infections (increased 12-fold), neonatal leukemoid reactions, leukemias (increased 10 to 20-fold)
	Excretory	Cystitis, renal anomalies
	Genital	**Cryptorchidism** (14–27%), micropenis, infertility
Neural	CNS	Early senescence, dementia, Alzheimer disease
	Motor	Hypotonia, oromotor dysfunction, motor delays
	Sensory	**Vision and hearing deficits** (50–70%)

RES, reticuloendothelial system; **bold: frequency > 20%**

Key references
Cohen, W. I. (1992). *Down Syndrome Papers and Abstracts for Professionals* 15:1–7.
Committee on Genetics, American Academy of Pediatrics (1994). *Pediatrics* 93:855–9.
Cooley WC, Graham JM Jr (1991): *Clinical Pediatrics* 30:233–53.
Cronk, C. et al. (1988): *Pediatrics* 81:102–10.
Pueschel, S. M. & Pueschel, J. K., ed., (1992): *Biomedical Concerns in Persons with Down Syndrome.* Baltimore: Paul H. Brookes.

Down syndrome

Preventive medical checklist (0–1yr)

| Patient | Birth Date / / | Number |

Pediatric	Screen	Evaluate	Refer/Counsel
Neonatal / / *Newborn screen* ❏ *HB* ❏	Karyotype ❏ CBC, differential ❏ ABR ❏	Feeding/stooling ❏ Cataracts ❏	Genetic evaluation ❏ Feeding specialist[3] ❏
1 month / /	Growth ❏ Echocardiogram ❏	Feeding/stooling ❏ Straining ❏ Constipation ❏	Family support[4] ❏ Feeding specialist[3] ❏ Cardiology ❏
2 months / / *HB[1]* ❏ *Hib* ❏ *DTaP, IPV* ❏ *RV* ❏	Growth ❏ Hearing, vision[2] ❏	Otitis ❏ Cataracts ❏ Blepharitis ❏	Early intervention[5] ❏ Genetic counseling ❏ Down syndrome clinic ❏ Anesthesia precautions ❏
4 months / / *HB[1]* ❏ *Hib* ❏ *DTaP/IPV* ❏ *RV* ❏	Growth ❏ Hearing, vision[2] ❏	Otitis ❏ Cataracts ❏ Nystagmus ❏	Early intervention[5] ❏ ENT[4] ❏ Ophthalmology[4] ❏
6 months / / *Hib* ❏ *IPV[1]* ❏ *DTaP* ❏ *RV* ❏	Growth ❏ Hearing, vision[2] ❏	Otitis, sinusitis ❏ Blepharitis ❏ Constipation ❏	Family support[4] ❏ Ophthalmology ❏ Developmental pediatrics ❏
9 months / / *IPV[1]* ❏	Audiology ❏	Otitis, sinusitis ❏ Strabismus ❏	
1 year / / *HB* ❏ *Hib[1]* ❏ *IPV[1]* ❏ *MMR[1]* ❏ *Var[1]* ❏	Growth ❏ Hearing, vision[2] ❏ T4, TSH ❏	Otitis, sinusitis ❏ Blepharitis ❏ Constipation ❏	Family support[4] ❏ Early intervention[5] ❏ Down syndrome clinic ❏

Clinical concerns for Down syndrome, ages 0–1 year

Feeding problems, jaundice	Cardiac anomalies	Hypotonia
Cataracts, nystagmus	Hypothyroidism	Developmental disability
Chronic otitis, hearing loss	Gastrointestinal anomalies	Motor and speech delay
Constipation, anal stenosis	Cryptorchidism, micropenis	Obstructive sleep apnea

Guidelines for the neonatal period should be undertaken *at whatever age* the diagnosis is made; DTaP, acellular DTP; IPV, inactivated poliovirus (oral polio also used); RV, rotavirus; MMR, measles–mumps–rubella; Var, varicella; [1]alternative timing; [2]by practitioner; [3]as dictated by clinical findings; [4]parent group, family/sib, financial, and behavioral issues as discussed in the preface; [5]including developmental monitoring and motor/speech therapy.

Down syndrome

Preventive medical checklist (15m–6yrs)

Patient		Birth Date / /	Number

Pediatric	**Screen**	**Evaluate**	**Refer/Counsel**
15 months / / *Hib¹* ❑ *MMR¹* ❑ *DTaP, IPV¹* ❑ *Varicella¹* ❑	Growth ❑ Hearing² ❑ Vision² ❑	Sleep apnea ❑ Otitis, sinusitis ❑ Strabismus ❑	Family support⁴ ❑ Early intervention⁵ ❑
18 months / / *DTaP, OPV¹* ❑ *Varicella¹* ❑ *Influenza³* ❑	Growth ❑ Hearing, vision² ❑		Anesthesia precautions ❑
2 years / / *Influenza³* ❑ *Pneumovax³* ❑ *Dentist* ❑	Growth ❑ Hearing, vision² ❑ Audiology ❑ T4, TSH ❑	Sleep apnea ❑ Otitis, sinusitis ❑ Strabismus ❑ OAI, AAI ❑	Family support⁴ ❑ Down syndrome clinic ❑ ENT³ ❑ Ophthalmology ❑
3 years / / *Influenza³* ❑ *Pneumovax³* ❑ *Dentist* ❑	Hearing, vision² ❑ Audiology ❑ C-spine x-rays¹ ❑ T4, TSH ❑	Sleep apnea ❑ Otitis, sinusitis ❑ Strabismus ❑ Blepharitis ❑	Family support⁴ ❑ Preschool transition⁵ ❑ Down syndrome clinic ❑ Ophthalmology ❑
4 years / / *Influenza³* ❑ *Pneumovax³* ❑ *Dentist* ❑	Growth ❑ Hearing, vision² ❑ T4, TSH ❑	Nutrition ❑ OAI, AAI ❑ Behavior ❑	Family support⁴ ❑ Preschool program⁵ ❑ Ophthalmology ❑
5 years / / *DTaP, IPV¹* ❑ *MMR¹* ❑	Hearing, vision² ❑ Audiology ❑ C-spine x-rays¹ ❑ T4, TSH ❑	Sleep apnea ❑ Nutrition ❑ Sinusitis ❑ Blepharitis ❑	Preschool program⁵ ❑ School transitional⁵ ❑ Development pediatrics ❑ Exercise, diet ❑
6 years / / *DTaP, IPV¹* ❑ *MMR¹* ❑ *Dentist* ❑	Growth ❑ Hearing, vision² ❑ T4, TSH ❑	School progress ❑ Diet, obesity ❑ Behavior ❑ OAI, AAI ❑	Family support⁴ ❑ Down syndrome clinic ❑ Ophthalmology, ENT³ ❑ Anesthesia precautions ❑

Clinical concerns for Down syndrome, ages 1–6 years

Strabismus, myopia	Hypothyroidism	Developmental disability
Chronic otitis, hearing loss	Atlantoaxial instability	Speech delay
Other respiratory infections	Obstructive sleep apnea	Behavior problems
Chronic sinusitis	Cryptorchidism, micropenis	Obesity, constipation

Guidelines for prior ages should be undertaken *at the time of diagnosis*; DTaP, acellular DTP; IPV, inactivated poliovirus (oral polio also used); MMR, measles–mumps–rubella; OAI, AAI occipito- or atlanto-axial instability; ¹alternative timing; ²by practitioner; ³as dictated by clinical findings; ⁴parent group, family/sib, financial, and behavioral issues as discussed in the preface; ⁵including developmental monitoring and motor/speech therapy.

Down syndrome

Preventive medical checklist (6+ yrs)

Patient		Birth Date / /	Number

Pediatric	Screen	Evaluate	Refer/Counsel
8 years / / _Dentist_ □	Growth □ Hearing[2] □ Vision[2] □	School progress □ Diet, obesity □ Phallus size □	Family support[4] □ School options □ Activities, exercise □ Endocrinology[4] □
10 years / /	Growth □ Hearing, vision[2] □	School progress □ Diet, obesity □ Sleep apnea □	Down syndrome clinic □ Ophthalmology[3] □ ENT[3] □ Cardiology[3] □
12 years / / _Td[1], MMR, Var_ □ _CBC_ □ _Dentist_ □ _Scoliosis_ □ _Cholesterol_ □	Growth □ Hearing, vision[2] □ T4, TSH □ C-spine x-rays □	Puberty □ Behavior □ OAI, AAI □ Blepharitis □	Family support[4] □ School options □ Activities, exercise □ Anesthesia precautions □
14 years / / _CBC_ □ _Dentist_ □ _Cholesterol_ □ _Breast CA_ □ _Testicular CA_ □	Hearing, vision[2] □ T4, TSH □	School progress □ Puberty □ Behavior □	Down syndrome clinic □ Activities, exercise □
16 years / / _Td[1]_ □ _CBC_ □ _Cholesterol_ □ _Sexual[5]_ □ _Dentist_ □	Hearing, vision[2] □ T4, TSH □	Diet, obesity □ Puberty □ Behavior □	Vocational planning □ Developmental pediatrics □ Cardiology[3] □ Ophthalmology[3] □
18 years / / _CBC_ □ _Sexual[5]_ □ _Cholesterol_ □ _Scoliosis_ □	Hearing, vision[2] □ T4, TSH □	Sleep apnea □ Nutrition □ Sinusitis □	Vocational planning □ Down syndrome clinic □ Exercise, diet □
20 years[6] / / _CBC_ □ _Sexual[5]_ □ _Cholesterol_ □ _Dentist_ □	Hearing, vision[2] □ T4, TSH □ C-spine x-rays □	Heart, joints □ Diet, obesity □ Behavior □ OAI, AAI □ Work, residence □	Down syndrome clinic □ Family support[4] □ Activities, exercise □ Cardiology[3] □ Ophthalmology[3] □

Clinical concerns for Down syndrome, ages 6+ years

Eye anomalies (myopia)	Hypothyroidism	Cognitive disability
Hearing loss	Atlantoaxial instability	Behavior problems
Chronic sinusitis	Obstructive sleep apnea	Obesity, constipation
Peridontal disease	Cryptorchidism, micropenis	Memory loss, regression

Guidelines for prior ages should be undertaken *at the time of diagnosis*; Td, tetanus/diphtheria; MMR, measles–mumps–rubella; Var, varicella; OAI, AAI occipito- or atlanto-axial instability; [1]alternative timing; [2]by practitioner; [3]as dictated by clinical findings; [4]parent group, family/sib, financial, and behavioral issues as discussed in the preface; [5]birth control, STD screening if sexually active; [6]repeat every decade.

8

Sex chromosome aneuploidy and X-linked mental retardation syndromes

Genes on the X chromosome have important roles in cognitive function, as illustrated by the excess of males with severe mental retardation. Remarkable also are the cognitive and behavioral abnormalities in sex chromosome aneuploidies such as the Klinefelter or XYY syndrome. The striking cognitive disability and psychiatric problems that are shared by many sex chromosome aneuploidy and X-linked mental retardation syndromes provide the rationale for their joint treatment in this chapter. The Turner, Klinefelter, and fragile X syndromes will be discussed in detail.

Sex chromosome aneuploidy

Sex chromosome imbalance usually has a milder phenotype than autosomal aneuploidy. Tables 8.1 and 8.2 summarize common sex chromosome aneuploidies in females and males. Mild cognitive disabilities, behavioral disorders, and reproductive problems predominate as complications of sex chromosome aneuploidy. Not listed in the tables are rare mosaic or chimeric individuals (e.g., individuals with mixtures of normal and aneuploid cells) that may cause pseudohermaphroditism or ambiguous genitalia. The presence of Y chromosome-containing cell lines in individuals without testes should trigger surveillance for intra-abdominal germinal tumors; these occur occasionally in X chromosome deletions (Table 8.1). Multidisciplinary management by urology, gynecology, and endocrinology is recommended in such cases.

Turner syndrome

Terminology

Females with short stature, immature sexual development, and webbed neck exhibit features first described by Bonnevie and Ullrich, later popularized by Turner (Fig. 8.1, color plate; Hall & Gilchrist, 1990). Bonnevie–Ullrich and Ullrich–Turner syndromes may be encountered as synonyms, but Turner syndrome is widely accepted. After the usual 45,X karyotype was defined in 1959, the

Table 8.1 Sex chromosome aneuploidy in females

Disorder	Karyotype	Incidence	Complications
Turner syndrome	45,X; 45,Xr(X)	1 in 5000	See Table 8.3; normal mental development
Del(Xp)	Xpter→p22/p21 Xpter→p12/p11 46,Xi(Xq)	10–50	Variable, mild features of Turner syndrome with short stature, menstrual irregularities, ovarian failure
Del(Xq)	Xq11/q12→qter Xq22/q24→qter	10–50	Variable features of Turner syndrome, gonadoblastoma
Trisomy X (Triple X)	47,XXX	1 in 2500	DD (25 percent), variable menstrual irregularity
Tetrasomy X	48,XXXX	>50	DD (IQ 30–80), menstrual irregularity, radioulnar synostosis, genital a., ovarian dysgenesis
Pentasomy X	49,XXXXX	10–50	DD, FTT, cleft, cardiac a., radioulnar synostosis, club feet, renal hypoplasia, genital a., ovarian dysgenesis

Notes:

p, short arm; q, long arm; r, ring, i, isochromosome; incidence – number per live births or reported cases; DD, developmental disability; FTT, failure to thrive; a., anomalies.

Source: Schinzel (1984, pp. 763–841), Gorlin et al. (1990, pp. 54–67), Staley et al. (1993).

minimal criterion for Turner syndrome became the deficiency of all or part of one X chromosome (Gorlin et al., 1990, p. 54; Jones, 1997, pp. 99. 81–2). The majority of patients have a 45,X karyotype or mosaicism with 45,X and 46,XX cell lines. Others have mosaicism involving unusual cell lines – isochromosome Xp or Xq, ring X, Xp or Xq deletion, and even male (46,XY) karyotypes. Rarely, Turner syndrome will involve smaller deletions of the X chromosome (Table 8.1). The term "male Turner syndrome" has been used imprecisely for Noonan syndrome, but the latter condition has a different, unknown etiology that does not involve obvious chromosomal changes (see below).

Historical diagnosis and management

Henry Turner described the Turner syndrome phenotype in 1938, and its chromosomal basis was recognized 21 years later (Hall & Gilchrist, 1990). Literature predating the use of hormone replacement therapy in Turner syndrome may exaggerate the severity of growth delay and sexual immaturity.

Incidence, etiology, and differential diagnosis

Turner syndrome is very common at conception, with 98–99 percent of affected pregnancies aborting spontaneously (Hall et al., 1982b). The birth incidence is 1 in

Table 8.2 Sex chromosome aneuploidy in males

Disorder	Karyotype	Incidence	Complications
Klinefelter syndrome	47,XXY	1 in 1000	See Table 8.4
XX males	46,XX	1 in 50,000	Similar to Klinefelter syndrome with lesser stature
Klinefelter variant	48,XXYY	1 in 50,000	DD, hypogonadism, aggression
Klinefelter variant	48,XXXY	>50	DD (IQ ~ 50), gynecomastia, radioulnar synostosis, kyphosis, hypogonadism
Klinefelter variant	49,XXXXY	>50	DD (IQ 20–60), FTT, cardiac a., radioulnar synostosis, scoliosis, micropenis, cryptorchidism
XYY syndrome	47,XYY	1 in 2000	Rare anomalies – urinary tract a., inguinal hernias, micropenis, hypospadias, cryptorchidism; behavioral a.
XYYY syndrome	48,XYYY	<10	DD, strabismus, pulmonic stenosis, genital a.
XYYYY syndrome	49,XYYYY	<10	DD, trigonocephaly, scoliosis, hydronephrosis
Del(Yq)	Yq11→qter	10–50	None; rare X-Y translocations may have severe DD, microcephaly, cardiac a., genital a. (Lahn et al., 1994).
Ring(Y)	46,Xr(Y)	<10	Short stature, cryptorchidism, hypospadias

Notes:
r, ring; incidence: number per live births or reported cases; DD, developmental disability; FTT, failure to thrive; a., anomalies.
Source: Schinzel (1984, pp. 763–841), Gorlin et al. (1990, pp. 54–67), Staley et al. (1993).

2500 female births, with one-third having demonstrable mosaicism (Schinzel, 1984, p. 768). Comparison of patients with X chromosome deletions indicates that deletion of the X short arm produces a more severe Turner phenotype than deletion of the X long arm; haplo-insufficiency of genes on the X short arm are thus responsible for the phenotype. Pathogenesis is still unknown. The characteristic webbed neck (pterygium colli) is a manifestation of the jugular lymphatic obstruction sequence that occurs in several conditions (Jones, 1997, pp. 620–1). Most similar is the Noonan syndrome of short stature, pterygium colli, broad chest, cardiac anomalies (usually of the pulmonary artery rather than aorta), and genital defects. In contrast, Noonan syndrome affects both sexes, has frequent mental disability, and often exhibits autosomal dominant rather than chromosomal inheritance.

Diagnostic evaluation and medical counseling

A karyotype is definitive for diagnosis, with about one-third of patients presenting in the newborn period, one-third during childhood, and one-third during adolescence because of delayed puberty (Hall et al., 1982b). A buccal smear to show the absence of a Barr body is not sufficient for diagnosis; older patients diagnosed on this basis should have a karyotype to rule out the presence of a Y chromosome. The ability to perform rapid screening for 45,X/46,XX or 45,X/46,XY mosaicism using fluorescent *in situ* hybridization (FISH) technology offers the opportunity for non-invasive karyotyping of buccal mucosa, urinary sediment, and peripheral blood in Turner females. Examination of several tissues in patients with Turner syndrome has indicated that mosaicism may be as frequent as 80% (Committee on Genetics, 1995c). Extensive search for X/XX mosaicism may be most helpful in older patients regrading their fertility, since growth and developmental outcomes in mosaic patients are not consistently better (Sybert, 1990). Search for X/XY mosaicism might be justified, since significant numbers of XY cells would indicate higher risks (15–25 percent) for developing gonadoblastoma or dysgerminoma in the abnormal gonads.

Initial counseling should emphasize the normal intellectual prognosis and life span expected for women with Turner syndrome. Gonadal dysgenesis causes infertility in 95 percent of 45,X females and 75 percent of mosaic 45,X/46,XX females (Turner syndrome checklist, part 1 – Hall & Gilchrist, 1990). Despite normal or above-average intelligence in many, learning differences regarding numerical abilities, spatial visualization, and fine motor execution have been described. The potential learning disabilities, together with the risk of early problems with feeding (Mazzocco, 1998), hearing and vision, warrant referral for early intervention services. An echocardiogram and abdominal sonogram to visualize cardiac or urinary tract anomalies (Turner syndrome checklist, part 2) are warranted as soon as the diagnosis of Turner syndrome is confirmed.

Family and psychosocial counseling

Having one child with monosomy X does not confer an increased risk of having subsequent children with chromosomal anomalies (Hall & Gilchrist, 1990). However, fertile women with mosaicism for 45,X or other abnormal cell lines have an increased risk of chromosomal anomalies in their offspring and should be offered prenatal diagnosis. If there is a structural rearrangement of an X chromosome, then parental karyotyping should be performed. All families should be referred for genetic counseling. When the diagnosis is made during infancy or early childhood, families should be informed about the possibility of growth hormone therapy so they can begin considering the large financial demands of this treatment. Some children will be mosaic with potential for fertility, and reproductive assessment with pelvic ultrasound (Mazzanti et al., 1997) together with counseling regarding pregnancy risks (Garvey et al., 1998) is warranted for some adolescent women. Turner syndrome support groups are useful in giving parents and affected individuals information about medical decisions, as well as the chance to meet adults with the disorder. Parent groups are listed in part 1 of the Turner syndrome checklist.

Natural history and complications

With modern preventive and surgical therapy, the survival of Turner patients should be normal. They are slightly smaller at birth, with weight of 2500–2900 g and length of 45–47 cm. Statural growth continues along the third centile until puberty, when untreated women will fall 3–4 standard deviations below the mean for age due to growth deceleration and the lack of a pubertal growth spurt (Hall & Gilchrist, 1990).

Holl et al. (1994) reported a study of 25 women with untreated Turner syndrome who averaged 148.7 cm in height, 16 cm below a control group. This compares with the median height range of 142–46 cm cited by Hall & Gilchrist (1990), although this may be changing with early androgen and growth hormone therapy (see below). Complications of Turner syndrome include eye, ear, cardiovascular, lymphatic, urinary tract, genital, and autoimmune problems (checklist, parts 2–4). Mosaic patients will generally have a milder course, except that patients with a Y chromosome-containing cell line face a 25 percent risk of the development of a gonadoblastoma in their streak gonad (Gorlin et al., 1990, pp. 54–7; Hall & Gilchrist, 1990). Biochemical abnormalities may be respresented by an increased risk for osteoporosis (Rubin, 1998) and aberrant lipid profiles (Ross et al., 1995).

Cardiac anomalies such as coarctation of the aorta and bicuspid aortic valve are sufficiently common that an echocardiogram should be considered during infancy (Hall & Gilchrist, 1990). Although the coarctation may not be clinically significant, these anomalies predispose to aortic aneurysm and atherosclerosis; yearly cardiology follow-up as well as antibiotic prophylaxis is indicated for these patients (Hall & Gilchrist, 1990), particularly since many develop mitral valve prolapse. Mosaic children who are fertile may have cardiac risks during pregnancy (Garvey et al., 1998). The aortic defects may underlie a general predisposition to vascular anomalies and hemangiomas that in the gastrointestinal tract may cause bleeding or protein-losing enteropathy. Renal ultrasound, periodic blood pressure determination, and urinalysis should be performed, since hypertension occurs independently of aortic or renal disease. There is increased risk of autoimmune disorders, including hypothyroidism and diabetes mellitus (Gorlin et al., 1990, pp. 54–7; Hall & Gilchrist, 1990). Obesity can also be a problem, necessitating counsel regarding appropriate diet and exercise.

The Turner syndrome preventive medical checklist

Consensus recommendations for the health supervision of children with Turner syndrome have been proposed by the Committee on Genetics, American Academy of Pediatrics (1995c). These suggestions, together with reasonable modifications removing unnecessary echocardiography (Noonan, 1997; Rappo, 1997; Roge et al., 1997), are the basis for the guidelines in parts 2–4 of the Turner syndrome checklist. Although the diagnosis is often missed in the nursery, unless characterisic pedal edema is present, karyotyping and possible pelvic sonography (Mazzanti et al., 1997) are crucial for management once the diagnosis is recognized. Bilateral removal of streak gonads during early childhood is indicated in children with mosaicism for Y chromosome-containing cells. A second peak in the risk of gonadoblastoma occurs at puberty, so review of diagnostic results and consideration of novel tests to detect Y material should be made in adolescent females. Alertness for tumors should be maintained in all women with Turner syndrome, since at least 5 examples of gonadoblastoma arising in 45,X patients without detectable Y chromosome material have been reported (Pierga et al., 1994).

Other problems during infancy and early childhood may include cardiac anomalies, chronic otitis and developmental delay. Peripheral pulses should be checked on newborns and older children with Turner syndrome. Early intervention is appropriate for some children along with vision, urinalysis, and blood pressure screening for all. Short stature may be associated with low self-esteem and other behavioral problems in Turner syndrome, justifying early referral to endocrinology. Some children may also need plastic surgery evaluation if their pterygium colli, nevi, or keloids are disfiguring. Improved growth velocity has occurred using oxandrolone and/or growth hormone therapy (Attanasio et al., 1995; Haeusler et al., 1995). Early and prolonged treatment with growth hormone (Plotnick et al., 1998), together with low dose estradiol treatment (Rosenfield et al., 1998; Ross et al., 1998), may offer the best outcome. Growth hormone treatment does not remove all of the behavior differences (Siegel et al., 1998), but estrogen treatment is useful in promoting normal puberty and avoiding osteoporosis (Rubin, 1998).

A final issue concerns behavioral and learning differences in women with Turner syndrome. A recent controlled study (McCauley et al., 1995) found weaker social relationships, school performance and self-esteem in 97 girls with Turner syndrome (ages 7–14 years) than in their peers. Like cognitive defects in spatial reasoning, it was not clear that these differences were severe enough to be clinically significant. While measures of map reading, figure drawing, geometry, or arithmetic may yield lower-than-average scores in Turner syndrome, many adolescents seem to catch up and perform well academically (Hall et al., 1982b); 80 percent of the adult women in the latter study had completed 4 years of college. Ross et al. (1995) reported significant discrepancy between verbal and performance IQ after study of 56 girls with Turner syndrome. Lower scores on tests of visual-motor, visual-spatial, and freedom from distractibility were significant in these women. The nonverbal IQ is thus lower than the verbal IQ in Turner syndrome.

Pavlidis et al. (1995) surveyed 80 adult women with Turner syndrome and found more conservative sexual attitudes and a more negative body image by comparison to controls. The frequency of sexual intercourse was also lower but correlated with positive body image, and sexually active women reported moderate to high levels of satisfaction (Pavlidis et al., 1995). There is clearly excellent potential for cognitive and gender function in Turner syndrome, but health care providers should be alert for signs of school or psychosocial problems.

Klinefelter syndrome

Terminology

Klinefelter syndrome describes males of increased stature with gynecomastia, small testes, and a 47,XXY karyotype. Klinefelter syndrome "variants" include disorders with more severe clinical features and additional X or Y chromosomes as the karyotypes 48,XXXY, 48,XXYY, and 49,XXXXY (Gorlin et al., pp. 58–61; Jones, 1997, pp. 72–3).

Historical diagnosis and management

Klinefelter described the syndrome in 1942, and the 47,XXY karyotype was reported in 1959 (Gorlin et al., pp. 58–61; Jones, 1997, pp. 72–3; Smyth & Bremner, 1998). Increased frequency of males with 47,XXY and 47,XYY syndrome have been found in mental or penal institutions, but prospective studies to document such associations have been controversial (Schwartz & Root, 1991).

Incidence, etiology, and differential diagnosis

The classic Klinefelter phenotype has a prevalence of 1.18 per 1000, with 80 percent having karyotypes of 47,XXY, 10 percent being 46,XY/47,XXY mosaics, and the remainder having multiple X or Y chromosomes (Table 8.2). More than 10 percent of males presenting with sterility and 3 percent with breast cancer will have Klinefelter syndrome. The additional X interferes with Leydig cell development in the testis, but the pathogenesis is unknown. The immature body habitus, feminine features (like gynecomastia, high voice, or sparse hair), and sterility reflect androgen deficiency. Differential diagnosis includes males with gonadotropin deficiency and other conditions with a lean, eunuchoid habitus such as homocystinuria or Marfan syndrome.

Diagnostic evaluation and medical counseling

Only 18 percent of individuals with 47,XXY Klinefelter syndrome will have major congenital anomalies, and most are recognized after puberty. The karyotype is diagnostic, and serum testosterone levels should be considered in postpubertal patients. For parents of young children, medical counseling should address the probable sterility and the increased risk of school and behavior problems. Adolescents and adults with Klinefelter syndrome should know about the possible benefits of testosterone supplements and cosmetic surgery.

Family and psychosocial counseling

Klinefelter syndrome, like most results of nondisjunction, is associated with advanced maternal age (Gorlin et al., 1990, p. 58; Jones, 1997, pp. 72–3). Genetic referral is needed for affected individuals and their parents. The recurrence risk of parents will be 1 percent or less, and family studies are needed only if unusual X or Y chromosome rearrangements are found. Occasional nonmosaic 47,XXY patients have been confirmed as fathers by paternity analysis; such couples warrant the option of prenatal diagnosis because of the increased risk of aneuploid offspring. Parent support groups are available (checklist, part 1).

Natural history and complications

Clark & Zuha (1977) speculated that men with Klinefelter syndrome may have the female pattern of longevity, with many examples unrecognized in old age. Precocious puberty has been reported in association with a germ cell tumor (Bebb et al., 1998). Patients should have normal life expectancy except for a 6-fold increased risk of cerebrovascular disease and a 1.6 percent incidence of neoplasia (Schwartz & Root, 1991; Bebb et al., 1998; Smyth & Bremner, 1998;). As shown in part 1 of the Klinefelter checklist, delayed speech is found in 51 percent, motor delays in 27 percent, and school maladjustment in 44 percent (Gorlin et al., 1990, p. 58; Mandoki & Sumner, 1991; Bender et al., 1993). Antisocial behaviors including theft or arson, alcoholism, and aggressiveness are described in some reports (Sørenson, 1992; Sørenson & Nielsen, 1977); others describe XXY men as having similar employment and social status to their peers (Porter et al., 1988; Schwartz & Root, 1991). Psychiatric disorders such as manic-depressive illness, psychosis, depression, and anorexia nervosa may be increased (Gorlin et al., 1990, p. 58; Sørenson, 1992).

Other medical complications include eye anomalies such as coloboma, strabismus or choroidal atrophy (Wolkstein et al., 1983), cleft palate, aortic stenosis or mitral valve prolapse, inguinal hernia, and genital anomalies such as cryptorchidism, hypospadias, and micropenis (Gorlin et al., 1990, pp. 58–9; Jones, 1997, pp. 72–3). Sørensen (1992) found frequent hearing deficits that were attributed to frequent respiratory tract infections during childhood; chronic otitis and sinusitis are not commented on in other studies. Increased frequency of autoimmune diseases such as collagen vascular disease or diabetes mellitus (Schwartz & Root, 1991), neurogenic amyotrophy (distal muscle weakness – Matsubara et al., 1994), and varicose veins have been reported.

Klinefelter syndrome preventive medical checklist

Patients with Klinefelter syndrome are rarely recognized in the newborn period unless identified through prenatal diagnosis. Mandoki & Sumner (1991) emphasize the advantages of early diagnosis so psychologic and/or pharmacologic therapy can be considered when school and behavior problems are recognized. Early care consists of screening for hearing or vision problems, plus physical and occupational therapy assessment for motor and speech delays (checklist, parts 2–4). Auditory evoked-response testing should be performed to rule out nerve deafness. If assessment reveals developmental delays, or if an early intervention program is the best way to obtain assessment, then the child should be referred. Eye and genital anomalies are sometimes found, so these regions should be carefully examined.

Many Klinefelter patients present because of behavior problems, abnormal pubertal development, or infertility. Puberty should be monitored carefully, since both delays and precocious puberty have been reported (Schwartz & Root, 1991). Gynecomastia, micropenis, or small testes can be a source of ridicule for teenagers and detract from self-image; Mandoki & Sumner (1991) described a patient for whom breast liposuction and orchiectomy followed by testicular implants improved self-image and behavior. Testosterone therapy is most beneficial if started at age 11–12 years. Nielsen et al. (1988) found that 77 percent of 30 adult males benefited from testosterone treatment (average 3.6 years) by showing better mood, less irritability, and more energy, endurance, and concentration. Depot injection or oral testosterone therapy may be tried, but side effects include priapism, salt and water retention, polycythemia, diabetes mellitus, and, in older patients, prostatic hypertrophy with sudden bladder obstruction (Schwartz & Root, 1991). Gynecomastia is not benefited by androgen therapy, although one study obtained benefit from dihydrotestosterone (Schwartz & Root, 1991). Priming of external genital development using testosterone may be indicated in males with a small phallus. For all of these reasons, endocrinology referral is strongly recommended.

Less common sex chromosome aneuploidies

47, XXX syndrome

Women with a 47,XXX or "triple X" karyotype typically have a normal appearance without congenital anomalies (Linden et al., 1995). Their main problems are with speech and developmental delay, mandating early intervention with speech therapy when the diagnosis is made during early childhood (usually by prenatal diagnosis).

One patient had a dysgerminoma of the ovary (Kemp et al., 1995). A higher frequency of behavioral problems ranges from immaturity to psychoses, but their frequencies are difficult to estimate because of ascertainment bias (Gorlin, 1990, pp. 63–4; Jones, 1997, pp. 78–80; Linden et al., 1995). When the diagnosis is made in older females, screening for behavioral difficulties with provision of counseling resources may be helpful. Some 47,XXX females have had decreased fertility, so reproductive evaluation and counseling is appropriate for adolescents.

Women with higher degrees of sex chromosome aneuploidy have more severe mental disability (average IQ of 55 in 48,XXX and 30–50 in 49,XXXX aneuploidy). Dental, cardiac, renal, and skeletal (club feet, joint laxity, radioulnar synostosis) occur at higher frequencies in these women, meriting attention to these problems during pediatric care (Table 8.1). Short stature and delayed puberty may occur, particularly in 49,XXXXX women, so endocrinology referral and growth hormone treatment might be considered in those with milder disabilities.

47, XYY syndrome

This disorder is often recognized incidentally in normal males or as an unexpected finding during evaluation of learning disabilities (Linden et al., 1995). The incidence is 1 in 1000 male live births, which is a small fraction of abundant 47,XYY sperm (1 percent) in the testis of normal males (Gorlin et al., p. 61). Congenital anomalies are infrequent, with a slightly higher incidence of genitourinary malformations and radioulnar synostosis that becomes frequent in the 48,XYYY or 49, XYYYY syndromes. The most striking complications are developmental and behavioral differences, including early clumsiness and fine motor problems, muscle weakness and incoordination, borderline mental disability (IQ 70 to 90) in 38 percent, impulsive behavior, and temper tantrums (Gorlin, 1990, pp. 61–2; Jones, 1997, pp.70–1). Several studies have demonstrated an increased frequency of 47,XYY men in penal institutions, but the causes are still debated (Linden et al., 1995).

Preventive management for 47,XYY males can begin with early intervention when the diagnosis is made prenatally. For older children, eliciting a behavioral history with provision of evaluation and counseling resources may help families; often parents have gone through considerable frustration that is clarified by the diagnosis. Occasionally, cryptorchidism, hypospadias, or small testes have occurred with decreased fertility. Genital examination and reproductive counseling are therefore indicated in the adolescent with 47,XYY syndrome.

Higher degrees of Y chromosome aneuploidy (48,XYYY, 49,XYYYY) are much more rare and severe disorders. Each has a high incidence of congenital anomalies and more severe disability, so they typically present in early childhood. Eye, cardiac, limb, and other skeletal anomalies are common in these syndromes, mandating early and periodic cardiac, ophthalmologic, and orthopedic assessments.

Table 8.3 X-linked mental retardation syndromes

Syndrome	Locus	Complications other than MR
Opitz GBBB	Xp22	Hypertelorism, hypospadias
Coffin–Lowry	Xp22	Coarse facies, broad fingers, joint laxity
Aarskog–Scott	Xp11	Short stature, hypertelorism, shawl scrotum, joint laxity
Norrie	Xp11	Blindness, hearing loss
Allan–Herndon–Dudley	Xp11–Xq21	Hypotonia, joint contractures
Opitz FG	Xp11–Xq22	Macrocephaly, brain a., gastrointestinal a., deafness
Renpenning	Xp21–Xq22	Short stature, microcephaly
α-thalassemia with MR	Xq13	Microcephaly, genital a., skeletal a., α-thalassemia
Simpson–Golabi–Behmel	Xq24–Xq28	Macrosomia, coarse facies, cardiac a., polydactyly, extra nipples
Borjeson–Forssman–Lehman	Xq26–Xq27	Short stature, obesity, microcephaly, hypogonadism
Fragile X	Xq27	Macrocephaly, long face, large ears, macro-orchidism
Otopalatodigital	Xq27–Xq28	Short stature, prominent brow, skeletal a., deafness
MASA, X-linked hydrocephalus	Xq28	Aphasia, shuffling gait, ataxia, spasticity

Note:

MR, mental retardation; a., anomalies.

Source: Lubs et al. (1996).

X-linked mental retardation syndromes

Aarskog syndrome

This condition was formally described in 1970 (Table 8.3), but had been recognized previously (Gorlin et al., 1990, p. 295; Jones, 1997, pp. 128–9). Aarskog syndrome exhibits X-linked inheritance, with affected males having short stature, hypertelorism, short fingers with other skeletal anomalies, and a characteristic "shawl" scrotum with cryptorchidism (Fryns, 1992; Teebi et al., 1993). Other characteristics include mild mental disability, odontoid hypoplasia with C1/C2 vertebral subluxation, pectus excavatum, inguinal hernia, cardiac defects, dental enamel hypoplasia, and the ability to position the fingers in a "swan's neck deformity" position (Gorlin et al., 1990, p. 295; Jones, 1997, pp. 128–9). Perinatal vascular accidents with resulting hemiplegia have been reported (Fryns & Descheemaeker, 1995). Female carriers often have some phenotypic features, and the causative gene has been isolated but is not routinely available for carrier screening (Pasteris et al., 1997).

Preventive measures for Aarskog syndrome should include careful growth measurements with the consideration that one patient had growth hormone deficiency. The fact that cervical vertebral anomalies occur in 50 percent of patients justifies lateral cervical spine radiographs at age 3–5 years as recommended for children with Down syndrome (Gorlin et al., 1990, p. 295). Early and consistent dental care, early childhood intervention, and careful examination for cryptorchidism or inguinal hernias should also be arranged. Ophthalmologic anomalies such as ptosis, strabismus, or tortuous retinal vessels are sufficiently common to make early referral to ophthalmology worthwhile (Pizio et al., 1994); cardiac anomalies, while reported, appear sufficiently infrequent that symptomatic evaluation without routine echocardiography should be adequate. The gene responsible for Aarskog syndrome has been localized to band Xp11.12 (Glover et al., 1993), so DNA diagnosis and reliable identification of female carriers can be anticipated in the near future.

Coffin–Lowry syndrome

Coffin–Lowry syndrome has a recognizable phenotype that includes a characteristic facies, soft and flexible hands, and short fingers. The locus has been mapped to the Xp22 chromosome region (Bird et al., 1995) and the causative gene identified (Trivier et al., 1997). Once the clinician is familiar with the condition, the facial appearance with down-slanting palpebral fissures and the characteristic handshake allows a rapid diagnosis. Many patients have been evaluated for hypothyroidism or mucopolysaccharidosis because of their clinical findings in infancy. There seems to be a general disorder of connective tissue, since inguinal hernias, pectus excavatum, and flat feet often occur (Gorlin et al., 1990, pp. 827–9; Jones, 1997, pp. 274–5). Speech is severely delayed, with average male IQ measured at 5–50 (Young, 1988). Other neurologic symptoms including cataplexy or drop attacks have been reported (Crow et al, 1998; Fryns & Smeets, 1998). Female carriers may exhibit mild manifestations of the condition (Plomp et al., 1995). Sensorineural hearing loss and premature tooth loss may be early manifestations of the disorder (Hartsfield et al., 1993; Higashi and Matsuki, 1994). Additional complications include dental malocclusion, cardiac anomalies, hydrocephalus, seizures (40 percent of patients), and agenesis of the corpus callosum (Soekarman & Fryns, 1994).

Preventive management for patients with Coffin–Lowry syndrome should include early intervention referral with emphasis on occupational, physical, and speech therapy. Monitoring of the head circumference to rule out hydrocephalus and alertness for manifestations of seizures are important. Early dental referral and alertness for cardiac or orthopedic anomalies are also recommended. As with all XLMR disorders, referral for genetic counseling is essential so that DNA diagnosis can be explored and carrier females identified.

FG syndrome

The FG syndrome of mental disability, absent corpus callosum, unusual facies with a frontal hair whorl, and intestinal anomalies was described in 1974 by Opitz and

Kaveggia (Opitz et al., 1988). The FG syndrome is somewhat intermediate between XLMR disorders with obvious distinguishing features (e.g., Lesch–Nyhan or Coffin–Lowry syndromes) and the nonspecific disorders that present only as developmental delay. Anomalies can be subtle in these nonspecific disorders, and it is important to remember the possibility of X-linked inheritance when evaluating male children with developmental delay. The term "FG" represents the initials of the first affected individual (Opitz et al., 1988).

Genetic mapping and gene characterization are increasingly helpful in sorting out different forms of XLMR, and make possible carrier detection and prenatal diagnosis once a genetic locus is defined. A disorder mapping to the region surrounding the X chromosome centromere is probably FG syndrome (Wilson et al., 1993), and confirmatory linkage to the Xq12 region was reported (Briault et al., 1997). Clinical manifestations include severe neonatal hypotonia in 90 percent, with consequent feeding problems and susceptibility to pneumonia. Ptosis, strabismus, ear anomalies, sensorineural hearing loss (30 percent), highly arched or cleft palate, and drooling are common problems. Joint contractures with flat feet and genu recurvatum can occur, with intestinal anomalies such as imperforate anus and malrotation (Gorlin et al., 1990, pp. 882–3; Jones, 1997, pp. 280–1). Inguinal and umbilical hernias, cryptorchidism, and hypospadias are frequent, and broad thumbs, keloids, and gingival hyperplasia occasional (Elia et al., 1995). Rare patients present with a fragile X-like phenotype (Piussan et al., 1996). Mental disability is severe to moderate, with brain anomalies ranging from partial to complete absence of the corpus callosum and defects of neuronal migration (Opitz et al., 1988). Some patients may have a severe and lethal course (Sorge et al., 1996).

Preventive management of FG syndrome should include an initial cranial MRI scan, ophthalmologic examination, and an electroencephalogram. Early monitoring of feeding and constipation is important, with gastroenterologic referral for severe reflux and aspiration. Milk of magnesia or other laxatives may be required for constipation. Regular pediatric evaluations for growth, development, orthopedic problems, and genital anomalies are important. Referral for early intervention and speech therapy, followed by evaluations for school placement and psychosocial support for the family, is essential. A thorough family history and genetic counseling are needed, since female carriers have no manifestations of the disease.

MASA syndrome and X-linked hydrocephalus

MASA is an acronym for mental retardation, aphasia, shuffling gait, and adducted thumbs. Study of over 100 patients has demonstrated that spasticity is an important part of the phenotype, with males having an average IQ of 50–75 (Macias et al., 1992). Several large families allowed genetic linkage of the MASA syndrome to the Xq28 chromosomal region (Macias et al., 1992; Schrander-Stumpel et al.,

1995). Families with X-linked hydrocephalus and clasped thumbs also showed linkage to Xq28, and it was subsequently recognized that both disorders result from mutations in a neural cell adhesion molecule called L1CAM (Vits et al., 1994; Schrander-Stumpel et al., 1995). DNA and prenatal diagnosis is now available for these families, and genetic counseling is an essential part of initial management.

Preventive management for patients with MASA syndrome will include early intervention with physical, occupational, and speech therapy. Hearing is not impacted in the disorder, and there have been few visceral anomalies. Rare patients have had brain anomalies and seizures, so MRI scan should be considered in severely affected individuals. Even though the syndrome is allelic with X-linked hydrocephalus, MASA individuals do not seem to develop hydrocephalus. Children with X-linked hydrocephalus usually have a severe course with prenatal onset, and many will receive palliative care appropriate for a lethal disease. Less severely affected patients can be managed as described for those with hydrocephalus in Chapter 4.

The fragile X syndrome

Terminology

Fragile X syndrome refers to a combination of mental and physical abnormalities exhibited by males and females with a fragile site at chromosome band Xq27. "Transmitting males" are asymptomatic males who transmit an X chromosome with the fragile site to their daughters. Female carriers have one normal X chromosome and one X chromosome with the Xq27 fragile site. "Triplet or trinucleotide repeats" refer to 3-base pair repeating units that occur in DNA at the fragile site. Males or carrier females with large numbers of triplet repeats (i.e., expanded length of the repeat region) exhibit the phenotype of fragile X syndrome.

Historical diagnosis and management

Fragile X syndrome was first described as an XLMR syndrome by Martin and Bell (1943), who recognized that affected males had a distinctive appearance with behavioral problems (Fig. 8.2, color plate). In the 1960s and 1970s, a specific marker or "fragile" X chromosome was visualized in Martin–Bell patients and shown to depend on culture of lymphocytes in tissue culture medium containing low amounts of folic acid. The ability to confirm clinical suspicion with chromosomal or DNA diagnosis has confirmed the fragile X phenotype of elongated body habitus, prominent jaw, large ears, lax connective tissue and large testes that Martin & Bell (1943) first observed (Giangreco et al., 1996; Tsuchiya et al., 1998).

Incidence, etiology, and differential diagnosis

The incidence of fragile X syndrome is about 1 in 1500 males and 1 in 2500 females, accounting for 30–40 percent of males with XLMR (Reiss et al., 1988; Warren & Nelson, 1994; Turk, 1995). After the fragile site focused attention on band Xq27 of the X chromosome, several laboratories isolated a gene from that region called "fragile X mental retardation-1" or "FMR-1" this gene was expressed in brain and testes and provided a good candidate for the cause of fragile X syndrome. Characterization of DNA near the FMR-1 gene demonstrated a cluster of trinucleotide repeating units that varied in normal individuals but were amplified dramatically in individuals with fragile X syndrome. Males or females with more than 200 triplet repeats exhibited symptoms of Martin–Bell syndrome due to inactivation of the FMR-1 gene. A DNA test based on the enumeration of triplet repeats became available to supplement chromosomal analysis for the diagnosis of fragile X syndrome (Turk, 1995; Hagerman, 1997).

Differential diagnosis includes other types of XLMR where there is a family history suggestive of X-linked inheritance. Older patients with the Klinefelter or XYY syndromes may prompt fragile X testing, since the males may be tall and have speech or behavior problems. Cerebral gigantism, with its accelerated early growth and hypotonia, may also be confused with fragile X syndrome (Gorlin et al., 1990, p. 67).

Diagnostic evaluation and medical counseling

All males with significant, unexplained developmental delay should have chromosomal studies including fragile X testing (Barnicoat, 1997; Turner et al., 1997). The cytogenetics laboratory must be alerted to test for fragile X syndrome, since the peripheral blood leucocytes must be cultured in low-folate medium. DNA testing for expanded repeats near the FMR-1 gene is more sensitive and precise; however, it will not screen for other chromosomal disorders in a child with developmental delay. Fragile X DNA testing is best used in a child with disability who has already had a normal karyotype, in potential carrier females assessed because of symptoms or family history, and in family studies to assign recurrence risks based on the identification of asymptomatic "transmitting" males or female carriers. Medical counseling is concerned with planning and services for a child with significant developmental disability.

Family and psychosocial counseling

The genetics of fragile X syndrome are quite complex because standard ratios for X-linked transmission must be modified according to gender and the number of amplified triplet repeats. All affected families must be referred for genetic counseling.

Normal individuals have 6–52 triplet repeats, individuals with unstable or "premutations" have 60–200, and individuals with Martin–Bell phenotype have 200–2000. Genesis of the premutation is not understood. Once a premutation of 60–200 repeats is present, further amplification occurs only during female meiosis. The risk of females with premutations depends on their number of triplet repeats – those with 60–80 will have lower risks for an affected male (200–2000 repeats) than those with 150–200 repeats. DNA testing is thus necessary for precise genetic counseling, since recurrence risk and phenotype often depend on the average number of triplet repeats (Hagerman, 1997). Prenatal diagnosis by chorionic villus biopsy or amniocentesis is now routine, and blastomere analysis before implantation (BABI) is under development at some centers. BABI and related technologies avoid the dilemma of abortion by selecting blastocysts for implantation that are female or lack high numbers of triplet repeats.

As with other conditions that cause severe to moderate developmental disability, initial psychosocial counseling is important for aiding parental adjustment to the child with fragile X syndrome. Complicating adjustment in some families are the subtle or manifest psychiatric problems in female carriers (Reiss et al., 1988; Freund et al., 1993; Baumgardner et al., 1995; Mostofsky et al., 1998). Females with less than 200 amplified triplet repeats at the fragile X locus ("premutation") exhibit no behavioral differences from control females having children with disabilities (Reiss et al., 1993). Females with more than 200 amplified repeats ("full mutation") have a greater frequency of avoidance and mood disorders, and the severity of both behavioral and cognitive problems was correlated with the size of DNA amplification. Hagerman et al. (1992) compared females with fragile X full or premutations to their normal sisters, and documented significant attentional difficulties in addition to cognitive and behavioral problems. Although these studies offer slightly differing views of the fragile X phenotype in females, it is clear that female carriers require evaluation for school and behavioral difficulties.

For males and females with fragile X syndrome, discussion of early intervention, speech, child behavior, social, and psychology/psychiatry services should be emphasized, and access to these services facilitated as needed. Parent support groups for fragile X syndrome are listed on the checklist, part 1.

Natural history and complications

Life span should be normal in fragile X syndrome, and large numbers of older individuals have been described (Saul et al., 1983). The fragile X checklist, part 1 indicates that there are few medical complications, with most problems caused by the mental disability. Gorlin et al. (1990, p. 66) reported an IQ range of 25 to 69, with

75 percent having IQs below 39. Saul et al. (1983) reported 4/21 patients with IQ above 55 and 11/21 with IQ below 39. Many patients are described as "autistic," with 7–15 percent of males with autism being positive for fragile X testing (Chudley & Hagerman, 1987; Jones, 1997, p. 126). Characteristics such as hand flapping, echolalia, aggressiveness, self-mutilation, and emotional instability are described in males and severely affected female carriers with fragile X syndrome. However, controlled studies have disputed the attribution of specific behavioral phenotypes to individuals with fragile X syndrome (Fisch, 1993). Seizures occur in 15 percent of affected males.

Although most children exhibit rapid growth, those with failure to thrive have received attention (Goldson & Hagerman, 1993). Predisposing factors may include gastroesophageal reflux, tactile defensiveness or food refusal with inadequate intake, and maternal psychiatric disease (Goldson & Hagerman, 1993). Physical abnormalities include large testes, which usually occur after puberty but can occur even in fetuses. Laxity of connective tissue may produce pectus excavatum, inguinal hernias, flat feet, and mitral valve prolapse. The frequency of mitral valve prolapse ranges from 6 percent in children to 80 percent in adults (Crabbe et al., 1993). The palate is high, and overbite or crossbite is common (Gorlin et al., 1990, p. 67). Both males and females are fertile, although few affected males have children.

Preventive medical checklist for fragile X syndrome

Preventive care is directed toward complications of mental disability, joint laxity, and dentistry (checklist, parts 2–4). Early medical concerns include chronic otitis and myopia or strabismus with the need for neurosensory screening. Mitral valve prolapse can be observed during childhood, and orthopedic problems such as flat feet or scoliosis can occur. Large testes may be noted, and the parents should be reassured that they are not signs of early puberty or sexual dysfunction. Supportive services such as early intervention, occupational therapy, physical therapy, behavioral assessment, and financial/school planning are particularly needed by fragile X families. Because of its association with fragile X expression in cultured cells, oral folic acid (10 to 50 mg per day) has been given to affected males without proven benefit (Hagerman, 1997). More important may be early recognition of seizures, hyperactivity, or psychiatric disorders that may be amenable to pharmacologic therapy. Carbamezapine has been effective for the treatment of epilepsy, and there is evidence that the incidence and treatment of hyperactivity or psychiatric disorders in fragile X syndrome are similar to those of the general population (Fisch, 1993). It is important to recognize female carriers with fragile X syndrome so that they receive adequate early intervention, school options, social services, and genetic counseling as appropriate. Female heterozygotes may have learning disabilities (15 percent) or frank mental retardation (35 percent) in addition to their risk of behavioral problems (Jones, 1997, pp. 150–1). These risks correlate with the number of repeats demonstrated by DNA analysis (Taylor et al., 1994).

Preventive Management of Turner syndrome

Clinical diagnosis: Malformation syndrome in females with neonatal pedal edema, webbed neck, heart anomalies and later short stature with immature sexual development.

Incidence: 1 in 2500 female births with 10–fold higher incidence at conception.

Laboratory diagnosis: 45,X karyotype in the majority with rarer deletions of Xp or Xq; 1/3 of patients are mosaic.

Genetics: Minimal recurrence risk for parents except in rare cases of translocation; mosaic females who are fertile have an increased risk for chromosomal anomalies in their offspring.

Key management issues: Karyotyping and possible pelvic ultrasound to define mosaicism and tumor risks; monitoring and therapy for growth and pubertal failure with growth hormone and estrogen; monitoring for eye, ear, thyroid, cardiovascular, lymphatic, urinary tract, genital, and autoimmune problems; alertness for GI bleeding, protein-losing enteropathy, or gonadoblastoma in the streak gonad.

Growth Charts: Lyon et al. (1985).

Parent groups: National Turner Syndrome Society of the United States, 15500 Wayzata Blvd., Minnetonka MN, 55391; Turner Syndrome Society of Canada York University, 768-214 Twelve Oaks, 4700 Keele Street, Toronto ON, Canada, M3J 1P3; The UK Turner Syndrome Society c/o The Child Growth Foundation, 2 Mayfield Ave., Chiswick, London, 44 (0181) 994-7625, cgflondon@aol.com

Basis for management recommendations: Consensus recommendations of the Committee on Genetics, American Academy of Pediatrics and the complications below as documented by Hall et al. (1982), Hall and Gilchrist (1990).

Summary of clinical concerns

General	Learning	Subtle differences (decreased fine motor execution, numerical abilities, spatial visualization)
	Behavior	Depression (10%), anorexia nervosa
	Growth	Short stature
	Tumors	Multiple nevi, hemangiomas, gonadoblastomas (25% if Y chromosome)
Facial	Eye	**Eye anomalies**, cataracts, strabismus (22%)
	Ear	**Chronic otitis** (80%)
	Nose	Choanal atresia (1%)
	Mouth	**Oromotor dysfunction**, **high palate** (36%), cleft lip/palate (2–3%)
Surface	Neck/trunk	**"Shield" chest** (53%), **pterygium colli** (46%), altered chest contour
	Epidermal	Cutaneous nevi, seborrhea, facial hirsutism, keloid formation
Skeletal	Cranial	Craniosynostosis
	Axial	Scoliosis, hypoplastic arch of atlas
	Limbs	**Cubitus valgus** (54%), **short metacarpals** 4/5 (48%), **osteoporosis** (50%), hip dislocation
Internal	Digestive	GI bleeding, GI lymphangiectasia, diarrhea, protein loss, malabsorption, enteropathy
	Circulatory	Cardiac anomalies (16% – coarctation of aorta, bicuspid aortic valve), **lymphedema** (63–80%), **hypertension** (20%)
	Endocrine	**Hypothyroidism** (20–30%), **delayed or absent puberty** (75–90%)
	RES	Autoimmune disorders – diabetes mellitus (adult onset, 5%), ulcerative colitis
	Excretory	Renal anomalies (anomalous ureters, horseshoe kidney, renal aplasia/hypoplasia)
	Genital	Gonadal dysgenesis, infertility (95%)
Neural	CNS	Rare cognitive disability, subtle learning differences
	Sensory	**Hearing deficits** (15–45%), **visual deficits** (22%)

RES, reticuloendothelial system, GI, gastrointestinal system; **bold: frequency > 20%**

Key references

Committee on Genetics (1995). *Pediatrics* 96:1166–73.

Hall, J. G. & Gilchrist, D. M.. (1990). *Pediatric Clinics of North America* 37:1421–40.

Hall, J.G., et al. (1982). *Western Journal of Medicine* 137:32–44.

Lyon, A. J. et al. (1985). *Archives of Diseases of Childhood* 60:932–6.

Turner syndrome

Preventive medical checklist (0–1yr)

Patient		Birth Date / /		Number	

Pediatric	Screen		Evaluate		Refer/Counsel	
Neonatal / / <small>Newborn screen ❑</small> <small>HB ❑</small>	Newborn screen ❑ Karyotype ❑		Feeding/stooling ❑ Cataracts ❑ Peripheral pulses ❑ Hips ❑		Genetic evaluation ❑ Feeding specialist[3] ❑	
1 month / /	Echocardiogram ❑ Renal sonogram ❑ BP ❑		Feeding/stooling ❑ Peripheral pulses ❑ Hips ❑		Family support[4] ❑ Cardiology ❑	
2 months / / <small>HB¹ ❑ Hib ❑</small> <small>DTaP, IPV ❑</small> <small>RV ❑</small>	Growth ❑ Hearing, vision[2] ❑		Feeding/stooling ❑ Otitis ❑		Early intervention[3,5] ❑ Genetic counseling ❑	
4 months / / <small>HB¹ ❑ Hib ❑</small> <small>DTaP/IPV ❑</small> <small>RV ❑</small>	Growth ❑ Hearing, vision[2] ❑		Feeding/stooling ❑ Otitis ❑		Early intervention[3,5] ❑ Genetics ❑ ENT[3] ❑	
6 months / / <small>Hib ❑ IPV¹ ❑</small> <small>DTaP ❑</small> <small>RV ❑</small>	Growth ❑ Hearing, vision[2] ❑ Urinalysis, BP ❑		Otitis ❑ Sinusitis ❑ Peripheral pulses ❑		Family support[4] ❑	
9 months / / <small>IPV¹ ❑</small>	Audiology ❑		Otitis, sinusitis ❑ Strabismus ❑			
1 year / / <small>HB ❑ Hib¹ ❑</small> <small>IPV¹ ❑</small> <small>MMR¹ ❑ Var¹ ❑</small>	Growth ❑ Hearing, vision[2] ❑ T4, TSH ❑		Otitis, sinusitis ❑ Peripheral pulses ❑ Cosmetic issues[3] ❑		Family support[4] ❑ Early intervention[5] ❑ Plastic surgery[3] ❑	

Clinical concerns for Turner syndrome, ages 0–1 year

Eye anomalies (strabismus)	Hypothyroidism	Learning differences
Chronic otitis	Coarctation of aorta	Keloid formation
Hearing loss	Bicuspid aortic valve	Seborrhea
Visual problems	Horseshoe kidney	Gonadoblastoma

Guidelines for the neonatal period should be undertaken *at whatever age* the diagnosis is made; DTaP, acellular DTP; IPV, inactivated poliovirus (oral polio also used); RV, rotavirus; MMR, measles–mumps–rubella; Var, varicella; [1]alternative timing; [2]by practitioner; [3]as dictated by clinical findings – cosmetic issues include webbing, nevi, keloids; [4]parent group, family/sib, financial, and behavioral issues as discussed in the preface; [5]including developmental monitoring and motor/speech therapy.

Turner syndrome

Preventive medical checklist (15m–6yrs)

Patient   **Birth Date** / /   **Number**

Pediatric	Screen		Evaluate		Refer/Counsel	
15 months / / *Hib[1]* ❏ *MMR[1]* ❏ *DTaP, IPV[1]* ❏ *Varicella[1]* ❏	Audiology Cardiac echo[3]	❏ ❏			Family support[4] Early intervention[5] Cardiology[3]	❏ ❏ ❏
18 months / / *DTaP, IPV[1]* ❏ *Varicella[1]* ❏ *Influenza[3]* ❏	Urinalysis, BP	❏	Strabismus	❏		
2 years / / *Influenza[3]* ❏ *Pneumovax[3]* ❏ *Dentist* ❏	Hearing, vision[2] Audiology T4, TSH Urinalysis, BP	❏ ❏ ❏ ❏	Otitis Sinusitis	❏ ❏	Family support[5] Genetics ENT[3] Ophthalmology	❏ ❏ ❏ ❏
3 years / / *Influenza[3]* ❏ *Pneumovax[3]* ❏ *Dentist* ❏	Hearing, vision[2] Audiology T4, TSH Urinalysis, BP Cardiac echo[3]	❏ ❏ ❏ ❏ ❏	Otitis Sinusitis	❏ ❏	Family support[5] Preschool transition[5] Genetics Cardiology[3]	❏ ❏ ❏ ❏
4 years / / *Influenza[3]* ❏ *Pneumovax[3]* ❏ *Dentist* ❏	Growth Hearing, vision[2] T4, TSH	❏ ❏ ❏	Nutrition	❏	Family support[5] Preschool program[3,5] Genetics Ophthalmology[3]	❏ ❏ ❏ ❏
5 years / / *DTaP, IPV[1]* ❏ *MMR[1]* ❏	Audiology T4, TSH Cardiac echo[3] Urinalysis, BP	❏ ❏ ❏ ❏	Sinusitis	❏	School transition[3,5] Cardiology[4] Endocrinology[1]	❏ ❏ ❏
6 years / / *DTaP, IPV[1]* ❏ *MMR[1]* ❏ *Dentist* ❏	Growth Hearing, vision[2] T4, TSH	❏ ❏ ❏	School progress Nutrition Scoliosis Cosmetic issues[3]	❏ ❏ ❏ ❏	Family support[5] Ophthalmology, ENT[3] Plastic surgery[3] Genetics Endocrinology[1]	❏ ❏ ❏ ❏ ❏

Clinical concerns for Turner syndrome, ages 1–6 years

Eye anomalies (strabismus)   Hypothyroidism   Learning differences
Chronic otitis   Coarctation of aorta   Keloid formation
Hearing loss   Bicuspid aortic valve   Seborrhea
Visual problems   Horseshoe kidney   Gonadoblastoma

Guidelines for prior ages should be undertaken *at the time of diagnosis*; DTaP, acellular DTP; IPV, inactivated poliovirus (oral polio also used); MMR, measles–mumps–rubella; [1]alternative timing; [2]by practitioner; [3]as dictated by clinical findings – cosmetic issues include webbing, nevi, keloids; [4]parent group, family/sib, financial, and behavioral issues as discussed in the preface; [5]including developmental monitoring and motor/speech therapy.

Turner syndrome

Preventive medical checklist (6+ yrs)

Patient _____ **Birth Date** / / **Number** _____

Pediatric	Screen		Evaluate		Refer/Counsel	
8 years / / *Dentist* ❏	Growth T4, TSH Cardiac echo[3] Urinalysis, BP	❏ ❏ ❏ ❏	Puberty Scoliosis Obesity	❏ ❏ ❏	School options Genetics Cardiology[3] Diet, exercise	❏ ❏ ❏ ❏
10 years / /	Hearing, vision[2] T4, TSH LH, FSH	❏ ❏ ❏	School progress Puberty Scoliosis	❏ ❏ ❏	Ophthalmology ENT[3] Endocrinology	❏ ❏ ❏
12 years / / *Td[1], MMR, Var* ❏ *CBC* ❏ *Dentist* ❏ *Scoliosis* ❏ *Cholesterol* ❏	T4, TSH LH, FSH Echocardiogram[3] Urinalysis, BP	❏ ❏ ❏ ❏	Puberty Behavior Obesity	❏ ❏ ❏	Family support[4] School options Genetics Cardiology[3]	❏ ❏ ❏ ❏
14 years / / *CBC* ❏ *Dentist* ❏ *Cholesterol* ❏ *Breast CA* ❏ *Testicular CA* ❏	Hearing, vision[2] T4, TSH LH, FSH	❏ ❏ ❏	School progress Puberty Behavior	❏ ❏ ❏	Genetics Endocrinology Diet, exercise	❏ ❏ ❏
16 years / / *Td[1]* ❏ *CBC* ❏ *Cholesterol* ❏ *Sexual[5]* ❏ *Dentist* ❏	T4, TSH Urinalysis, BP	❏ ❏	Puberty Behavior Obesity	❏ ❏ ❏	Vocational planning[3] Cardiology[3] Diet, exercise	❏ ❏ ❏
18 years / / *CBC* ❏ *Sexual[5]* ❏ *Cholesterol* ❏ *Scoliosis* ❏	Hearing, vision[2] T4, TSH	❏ ❏	School progress Puberty Behavior	❏ ❏ ❏	Vocational planning[3] Endocrinology[3]	❏ ❏
20 years[6] / / *CBC* ❏ *Sexual[5]* ❏ *Cholesterol* ❏ *Dentist* ❏	Hearing, vision[2] Cardiac sono[3] Urinalysis, BP	❏ ❏ ❏	Behavior Work, residence Obesity	❏ ❏ ❏	Family support[4] Dentistry Diet, exercise Cardiology[3]	❏ ❏ ❏ ❏

Clinical concerns for Turner syndrome, ages 6+ years

Hearing loss	Mitral valve prolapse	Learning differences
High palate, dental	Coarctation	Short stature
Hypothyroidism	Aortic aneurysm	Behavior problems
Diabetes mellitus	Scoliosis, osteoporosis	Delayed puberty
Hypertension	Gonadoblastoma	Keloid formation

Guidelines for prior ages should be undertaken *at the time of diagnosis*; Td, tetanus/diphtheria; MMR, measles–mumps–rubella; Var, varicella; FSH, follicle stimulating hormone; LH, luteinizing hormone; [1]alternative timing; [2]by practitioner; [3]as dictated by clinical findings – cosmetic issues include webbing, nevi, keloids; [4]parent group, family/sib, financial, and behavioral issues as discussed in the preface; [5]birth control, STD screening if sexually active; [6]repeat every decade.

Preventive Management of Klinefelter syndrome

Clinical diagnosis: Subtle pattern of manifestations including tall stature, asthenic habitus, small testes, gynecomastia, sexual immaturity.

Incidence: 1.18 per 1000 live births.

Laboratory diagnosis: 80 percent have karyotypes of 47,XXY, 10 percent of 46,XY/47,XXY, and the remainder multiple X or Y chromosomes.

Genetics: A recurrence risk of 1 percent or less, with family studies needed only for unusual X or Y chromosome rearrangements.

Key management issues: Monitoring for hearing or vision problems; physical and occupational therapy for motor and speech delays; endocrinology evaluation with possible testosterone therapy, monitoring for school and behavioral problems; higher aneuploidies (48,XXXY, 49,XXXXY) have more severe anomalies and cognitive deficits.

Growth charts: Regular charts can be used for the expected tall stature.

Parent groups: Klinefelter Syndrome and Associates, P.O. Box 119, Roseville, CA 95678-0119, (916) 773-2999 ksinfo@genetic.org, http://www.genetic.org/ks/; Klinefelter Syndrome United Kingdom (KSCUK), David Dennison, Co-ordinator, P. O. Box 60, Orpington BR6 8ZQ UK, http://hometown.aol.com/kscuk/kscinfo.htm

Basis for management recommendations: Derived from the complications below as documented by Schwartz & Root (1991), Smyth & Bremner (1998).

Summary of clinical concerns

General	Learning	Motor delays (27%), cognitive disability (mean IQ of 90 with 29% below 90)
	Behavior	Behavioral problems, antisocial behavior, poor self image, psychoses
	Growth	Tall stature
	Tumors	Cerebral germinoma, mediastinal teratoma, myeloproliferative diseases, breast cancer
Facial	Eye	Coloboma, choroidal atrophy, strabismus
	Ear	
	Nose	
	Mouth	Oromotor dysfunction, cleft palate, mandibular prognathism
Surface	Neck/trunk	Inguinal hernias, gynecomastia
	Epidermal	Sparse facial hair, varicose veins
Skeletal	Cranial	Microcephaly
	Axial	
	Limbs	Radioulnar synostosis (48,XXXY; 49,XXXXY)
Internal	Digestive	Omphalocele
	Circulatory	Cardiac anomalies (aortic stenosis)
	Endocrine	Growth hormone, testosterone deficiency; diabetes mellitus
	Genital	**Small testes**, **infertility**, cryptorchidism, micropenis
Neural	CNS	Cognitive deficits (especially 48,XXXY; 49,XXXXY)
	Motor	Neurogenic amyotrophy, decreased muscle mass
	Sensory	Neurosensory deafness

RES, reticuloendothelial system, GI, gastrointestinal system; **bold:** frequency > 20%

Key references

Hsueh, W. A., Hsu, T. H. & Federman, D. D. (1978). *Medicine* 57:447–61.

Schwartz, I. D. & Root, A. W. (1991). *Endocrinology and Metabolism Clinics of North America* 20:153–63.

Smyth, C. M. & Bremner W. J (1998*). Archives of Internal Medicine* 158:1309–14.

Klinefelter syndrome

Preventive medical checklist (0–1yr)

Patient　　　　　　　**Birth Date** / /　　**Number**

Pediatric	Screen	Evaluate	Refer/Counsel
Neonatal / / *Newborn screen* ❑ *HB* ❑	Karyotype ❑	Eyes ❑	Genetic evaluation ❑
1 month / /			Family support[4] ❑
2 months / / *HB[1]* ❑ *Hib* ❑ *DTaP, IPV* ❑ *RV* ❑	Hearing, vision[2] ❑		Early intervention[5] ❑ Genetic counseling ❑
4 months / / *HB[1]* ❑ *Hib* ❑ *DTaP/IPV* ❑ *RV* ❑	Hearing, vision[2] ❑		Early intervention[5] ❑
6 months / / *Hib* ❑ *IPV[1]* ❑ *DTaP* ❑ *RV* ❑	Hearing, vision[3] ❑	Strabismus ❑	Family support[4] ❑
9 months / / *IPV[1]* ❑	Hearing, vision[2] ❑ Audiology ❑ Urinalysis, BP ❑		
1 year / / *HB* ❑ *Hib[1]* ❑ *IPV[1]* ❑ *MMR[1]* ❑ *Var[1]* ❑	Hearing, vision[2] ❑	Strabismus ❑	Family support[4] ❑ Early intervention[5] ❑ Developmental pediatrics ❑ Genetics ❑

Clinical concerns for Klinefelter syndrome, ages 0–1 year

Eye anomalies (strabismus)　　Cryptorchidism　　　　Learning differences
Nerve deafness　　　　　　　Hypospadias　　　　　Motor and speech delay
Dental anomalies　　　　　　Micropenis

Guidelines for the neonatal period should be undertaken *at whatever age* the diagnosis is made; DTaP, acellular DTP; IPV, inactivated poliovirus (oral polio also used); RV, rotavirus; MMR, measles–mumps–rubella; Var, varicella; [1]alternative timing; [2]by practitioner; [3]as dictated by clinical findings; [4]parent group, family/sib, financial, and behavioral issues as discussed in the preface; [5]including developmental monitoring and motor/speech therapy.

Klinefelter syndrome

Preventive medical checklist (15m–6yrs)

Patient   **Birth Date**   /   /   **Number**

Pediatric	Screen	Evaluate		Refer/Counsel	
15 months / / *Hib[1]* ❑ *MMR[1]* ❑ *DTaP, IPV[1]* ❑ *Varicella[1]* ❑	Hearing, vision[2] ❑			Family support[4] Early intervention[5]	❑ ❑
18 months / / *DTaP, IPV[1]* ❑ *Varicella[1]* ❑ *Influenza[1]* ❑					
2 years / / *Influenza[3]* ❑ *Pneumovax[3]* ❑ *Dentist* ❑	Hearing, vision[2] ❑ Audiology ❑	Strabismus	❑	Family support[4] Developmental pediatrics Genetics	❑ ❑ ❑
3 years / / *Influenza[3]* ❑ *Pneumovax[3]* ❑ *Dentist* ❑	Hearing, vision[2] ❑ Audiology ❑	Strabismus	❑	Family support[4] Preschool transition[5]	❑ ❑
4 years / / *Influenza[3]* ❑ *Pneumovax[3]* ❑ *Dentist* ❑	Hearing, vision[2] ❑	Genitalia Behavior	❑ ❑	Family support[4] Preschool program[5] Developmental pediatrics Genetics	❑ ❑ ❑ ❑
5 years / / *DTaP, IPV[1]* ❑ *MMR[1]* ❑	Audiology ❑			School transition[5] Developmental pediatrics[3]	❑ ❑
6 years / / *DTaP, IPV[1]* ❑ *MMR[1]* ❑ *Dentist* ❑	Hearing, vision[2] ❑ Urinalysis, BP ❑	School progress	❑	Family support[4] Developmental pediatrics Genetics Endocrinology	❑ ❑ ❑ ❑

Clinical concerns for Klinefelter syndrome, ages 1–6 years

Eye anomalies (strabismus)	Cryptorchidism	Learning differences
Nerve deafness	Hypospadias	Motor and speech delay
Dental anomalies	Micropenis	

Guidelines for prior ages should be undertaken *at the time of diagnosis*; DTaP, acellular DTP; IPV, inactivated poliovirus (oral polio also used); MMR, measles–mumps–rubella; [1]alternative timing; [2]by practitioner; [3]as dictated by clinical findings; [4]parent group, family/sib, financial, and behavioral issues as discussed in the preface; [5]including developmental monitoring and motor/speech therapy.

Klinefelter syndrome

Preventive medical checklist (6+ yrs)

Patient   **Birth Date** / /   **Number**

Pediatric	Screen	Evaluate		Refer/Counsel	
8 years / / _Dentist_ ❑		Behavior	❑	School options Developmental pediatrics[3] Genetics Endocrinology	❑ ❑ ❑ ❑
10 years / /	Hearing, vision[3] ❑	School progress Heart Genitalia Behavior	❑ ❑ ❑ ❑	Endocrinology Cardiology	❑ ❑
12 years / / _Td[1], MMR, Var_ ❑ _CBC_ ❑ _Dentist_ ❑ _Scoliosis_ ❑ _Cholesterol_ ❑	Urinalysis, BP ❑	Puberty Phallus size Breast exam Behavior	❑ ❑ ❑ ❑	Family support[4] School options Developmental pediatrics Genetics Endocrinology	❑ ❑ ❑ ❑ ❑
14 years / / _CBC_ ❑ _Dentist_ ❑ _Cholesterol_ ❑ _Breast CA_ ❑ _Testicular CA_ ❑	Hearing, vision[2] ❑	School progress Puberty Genitalia Breast exam Behavior	❑ ❑ ❑ ❑ ❑	Endocrinology Self examination	❑ ❑
16 years / / _Td[1]_ ❑ _CBC_ ❑ _Cholesterol_ ❑ _Sexual[5]_ ❑ _Dentist_ ❑	Urinalysis, BP ❑	Puberty Phallus size Breast exam Behavior	❑ ❑ ❑ ❑	Vocational planning Developmental pediatrics Genetics Endocrinology Self examination	❑ ❑ ❑ ❑ ❑
18 years / / _CBC_ ❑ _Sexual[5]_ ❑ _Cholesterol_ ❑ _Scoliosis_ ❑	Hearing, vision[2] ❑	School progress Breast exam Genitalia Behavior	❑ ❑ ❑ ❑	Vocational planning Endocrinology	❑ ❑
20 years[6] / / _CBC_ ❑ _Sexual[5]_ ❑ _Cholesterol_ ❑ _Dentist_ ❑	Hearing, vision[2] ❑ Urinalysis, BP ❑	Breast exam Heart Behavior Work, residence	❑ ❑ ❑ ❑	Family support[5] Endocrinology Cardiology[3]	❑ ❑ ❑

Clinical concerns for Klinefelter syndrome, ages 6+ years

Delayed puberty	Aortic stenosis	Learning differences
Testosterone deficiency	Mitral valve prolapse	Behavioral problems
Gynecomastia	Pectus excavatum, scoliosis	Diabetes mellitus
Inguinal hernia	Breast carcinoma	Collagen vascular disease

Guidelines for prior ages should be undertaken _at the time of diagnosis_; Td, tetanus/diphtheria; MMR, measles–mumps–rubella; Var, varicella; [1]alternative timing; [2]by practitioner; [3]as dictated by clinical findings; [4]parent group, family/sib, financial, and behavioral issues as discussed in the preface; [5]birth control, STD screening if sexually active; [6]repeat every decade.

Preventive Management of Fragile X syndrome

Clinical diagnosis: Manifestations include elongated body habitus, prominent jaw, large ears, lax connective tissue, large testes, and behavioral differences.

Incidence: 1 in 1250–2500 males, 1 in 1600–5000 females.

Laboratory diagnosis: DNA testing reveals 50–200 trinucleotide repeats for asymptomatic males or females with "premutations," > 200 repeats for males or females with full mutations; 2/3 of females with full mutations have cognitive disability. The unstable trinucleotide repeats are near the fragile X gene at Xq27, where expansion leads to gene inactivation.

Genetics: Complex inheritance since the premutation expands only during female meiosis; individuals with full mutations simulate classical X-linked recessive inheritance (25% risk for affected or carrier females to have severely affected sons); premutations may be transmitted to asymptomatic children and become symptomatic in grandchildren (anticipation).

Key management issues: Early intervention and speech therapy for mental disability; monitoring for dental and connective tissue problems (pectus excavatum, mitral valve prolapse, inguinal hernias), family support with behavioral assessments and school planning.

Growth charts: Butler et al. (1992).

Parent groups: The National Fragile X Foundation, 1441 York St. Suite 303, Denver CO, 80206, (800) 688-8765, natfragx@ix.netcom.com; FRAXA Research Foundation Inc., P.O. Box 935, West Newbury, MA 01985-0935, (978) 462-1990, info@fraxa.org, http://www.qorxnet/fraxa; Fragile X Society, 53 Winchelsea Lane, Hastings, East Sussex TN35 4LG UK, (01424) 813-147.

Basis for management recommendations: Consensus guidelines from the Committee on Genetics, American Academy of Pediatrics (1996).

Summary of clinical concerns

General	Learning	**Cognitive disability** (100% – IQ range 25–69; 75% with IQ < 40), learning differences, speech problems (stuttering, repetitive phrases, dysfluencies, cluttered speech, rhythmic intonation)
	Behavior	**Aggressiveness** (50%); hyperactivity, emotional lability
	Growth	Early failure to thrive in some; later tall, asthenic habitus
Facial	Face	**Long and narrow face** (60%), prominent jaw
	Eye	**Strabismus** (40%), myopia, nystagmus
	Ear	Large, decreased cartilage
	Mouth	**High palate**, dental malocclusion
Surface	Neck/trunk	Pectus excavatum, inguinal hernia
Skeletal	Cranial	**Macrocephaly**, prominent occiput
	Axial	Scoliosis
	Limbs	**Flat feet** (40%), increased joint laxity
Internal	Digestive	Early feeding problems
	Circulatory	**Mitral valve prolapse** (80%), aortic dilatation (15%)
	Genital	**Macro-orchidism** (40–75%)
Neural	CNS	**Abnormal EEG** (50%), seizures (15%), irritability
	Motor	**Hypotonia**, hyper-reflexia

Bold: frequency > 20%

Key references

Butler, M. G., Brunschwig, A., Miller, L. K. & Hagerman, R. J. (1992). *Pediatrics* 89:1059–62.

Chudley, A. E. & Hagerman, R. J. (1987). *Journal of Pediatrics* 110:821–31.

Committee on Genetics, American Academy of Pediatrics (1996). *Pediatrics* 98:297–300.

Freund, L.S., Reiss, A. L. & Abrams, M. T. (1993). *Pediatrics* 91:321–9.

Hagerman, R. J. (1997). *Contemporary Pediatrics* 14:31–48.

Martin, J.P. & Bell, J. (1943). *Journal of Neurology and Psychiatry* 6:154–7.

Saul, R.A., Harden, K. J. Stevenson, R. E., et al. (1983). *Proc. Greenwood Genetics Center* 2:58–67.

Taylor, A. K., Safanda, J. F., Fall, M. Z. et al. (1994). *Journal of the American Medical Association* 271:507–14.

Fragile X syndrome

Preventive medical checklist (0–1yr)

Patient   **Birth Date** / /   **Number**

Pediatric	Screen	Evaluate	Refer/Counsel°
Neonatal / / *Newborn screen* ☐ *HB* ☐	DNA testing ☐	Feeding ☐ Strabismus ☐ Club feet ☐ Hip dislocation ☐	Genetic evaluation ☐ Feeding specialist[4] ☐
1 month / /		Feeding ☐ Maternal care ☐ Hip dislocation ☐	Family support[4] ☐ Gastroenterology[3] ☐ Feeding specialist[3] ☐
2 months / / *HB[1]* ☐ *Hib* ☐ *DTaP, IPV* ☐ *RV* ☐	Growth ☐ Hearing, vision[2] ☐	Feeding ☐ Strabismus ☐ Otitis ☐	Early intervention[5] ☐ Developmental pediatrics ☐ Genetic counseling ☐ Feeding specialist[3] ☐
4 months / / *HB[1]* ☐ *Hib* ☐ *DTaP/IPV* ☐ *RV* ☐	Growth ☐ Hearing, vision[2] ☐	Feeding ☐ Otitis ☐ Mitral valve ☐	Early intervention[5] ☐ Feeding specialist[3] ☐ Cardiologist[3] ☐
6 months / / *Hib* ☐ *IPV[1]* ☐ *DTaP* ☐ *RV* ☐	Growth ☐ Hearing, vision[2] ☐	Feeding ☐ Strabismus ☐ Otitis ☐ Hip dislocation ☐	Family support[4] ☐ Gastroenterology[3] ☐ Feeding specialist[3] ☐
9 months / / *IPV[1]* ☐	Audiology ☐	Feeding ☐ Strabismus ☐	Ophthalmology[3] ☐ ENT[4] ☐
1 year / / *HB* ☐ *Hib[1]* ☐ *IPV[1]* ☐ *MMR[1]* ☐ *Var[1]* ☐	Growth ☐ Hearing, vision[2] ☐	Feeding ☐ Strabismus ☐ Otitis ☐ Inguinal hernia ☐	Family support[4] ☐ Early intervention[5] ☐ Developmental pediatrics ☐ Genetics ☐

Clinical concerns for Fragile X syndrome, ages 0–1 year

Gastroesophageal reflux	Mitral valve prolapse	Developmental disability
Strabismus, nystagmus	Joint laxity	Hypotonia, seizures
High palate	Club foot, hip dislocation	Feeding problems
Serous otitis, hearing loss	Inguinal hernia	

Guidelines for the neonatal period should be undertaken *at whatever age* the diagnosis is made; DTaP, acellular DTP; IPV, inactivated poliovirus (oral polio also used); RV, rotavirus; MMR, measles–mumps–rubella; Var, varicella; [1]alternative timing; [2]by practitioner; [3]as dictated by clinical findings; [4]parent group, family/sib, financial, and behavioral issues as discussed in the preface; [5]including developmental monitoring and motor/speech therapy.

Fragile X syndrome

Preventive medical checklist (15m–6yrs)

Patient   **Birth Date** / /   **Number**

Pediatric	Screen	Evaluate	Refer/Counsel
15 months / / *Hib[1]* ☐ *MMR[1]* ☐ *DTaP, IPV[1]* ☐ *Varicella[1]* ☐	Growth ☐ Hearing, vision[2] ☐		Family support[4] ☐ Early intervention[5] ☐
18 months / / *DTaP, IPV[1]* ☐ *Varicella[1]* ☐ *Influenza[1]* ☐	Growth ☐	Feeding ☐ Strabismus ☐ Otitis ☐	
2 years / / *Influenza[3]* ☐ *Pneumovax[3]* ☐ *Dentist* ☐	Growth ☐ Hearing, vision[2] ☐	Feeding ☐ Strabismus ☐ Otitis ☐ Flat feet ☐	Family support[4] ☐ Developmental pediatrics ☐ Genetics ☐ Ophthalmology[3] ☐ ENT[3] ☐
3 years / / *Influenza[3]* ☐ *Pneumovax[3]* ☐ *Dentist* ☐	Growth ☐ Hearing, vision[2] ☐	Feeding ☐ Otitis ☐ Inguinal hernia ☐ Mitral prolapse ☐ Testes size ☐	Family support[4] ☐ Preschool transition[5] ☐ Cardiology[3] ☐ Ophthalmology[3] ☐ ENT[3] ☐
4 years / / *Influenza[3]* ☐ *Pneumovax[3]* ☐ *Dentist* ☐	Growth ☐ Hearing, vision[2] ☐	Nutrition ☐ Behavior ☐ Otitis ☐ Mitral prolapse ☐ Flat feet ☐ Staring spells ☐	Family support[4] ☐ Preschool program[5] ☐ Developmental pediatrics ☐ Genetics ☐ Cardiology, ENT[3] ☐ Neurology[3] ☐
5 years / / *DTaP, IPV[1]* ☐ *MMR[1]* ☐		Nutrition ☐ Behavior ☐ Strabismus ☐ Otitis ☐	School transition[5] ☐
6 years / / *DTaP, IPV[1]* ☐ *MMR[1]* ☐ *Dentist* ☐	Growth ☐ Hearing, vision[2] ☐ Testis size ☐	School progress ☐ Nutrition ☐ Behavior ☐ Mitral prolapse ☐	Family support[4] ☐ Developmental pediatrics ☐ Genetics ☐ Cardiology[3] ☐

Clinical concerns for Fragile X syndrome, ages 1–6 years

Feeding problems
Strabismus, nystagmus
High palate, dental problems
Serous otitis, hearing loss

Joint laxity, hip dislocation
Scoliosis
Club feet, flat feet
Inguinal hernia

Cognitive disability
Speech, behavioral problems
Tantrums, outbursts
Seizures

Guidelines for prior ages should be undertaken *at the time of diagnosis*; DTaP, acellular DTP; IPV, inactivated poliovirus (oral polio also used); MMR, measles–mumps–rubella; [1]alternative timing; [2]by practitioner; [3]as dictated by clinical findings – behavior problems can include hyperactive behavior, head banging, and hand biting; [4]parent group, family/sib, financial, and behavioral issues as discussed in the preface; [5]including developmental monitoring and motor/speech therapy.

Fragile X syndrome

Preventive medical checklist (6+ yrs)

Patient   **Birth Date** / /   **Number**

Pediatric	Screen	Evaluate	Refer/Counsel
8 years / / *Dentist* ❑	Growth ❑ Hearing, vision[3] ❑	Nutrition ❑ Behavior ❑ Pectus, scoliosis ❑ Flat feet ❑ Seizures ❑	School options ❑ Developmental pediatrics ❑ Genetics ❑ Orthopedics[3] ❑
10 years / /	Growth ❑ Hearing, vision[3] ❑	School progress ❑ Nutrition ❑ Behavior ❑ Testis size ❑	Neurology[3] ❑
12 years / / *Td[1], MMR, Var* ❑ *CBC* ❑ *Dentist* ❑ *Scoliosis* ❑ *Cholesterol* ❑	Growth ❑ Hearing, vision[3] ❑	Puberty ❑ Behavior ❑ Pectus, scoliosis ❑ Mitral prolapse ❑	Family support[4] ❑ School options ❑ Developmental pediatrics ❑ Genetics ❑ Cardiology[3] ❑
14 years / / *CBC* ❑ *Dentist* ❑ *Cholesterol* ❑ *Breast CA* ❑ *Testicular CA* ❑	Growth ❑ Hearing, vision[3] ❑	School progress ❑ Puberty ❑ Behavior ❑ Testis size ❑	
16 years / / *Td[1]* ❑ *CBC* ❑ *Cholesterol* ❑ *Sexual[5]* ❑ *Dentist* ❑	Hearing, vision[2] ❑	Puberty ❑ Behavior ❑ Pectus, scoliosis ❑ Flat feet ❑	Vocational planning ❑ Developmental pediatrics ❑ Genetics ❑ Orthopedics[3] ❑
18 years / / *CBC* ❑ *Sexual[5]* ❑ *Cholesterol* ❑ *Scoliosis* ❑		School progress ❑ Behavior ❑ Mitral prolapse ❑	Vocational planning ❑ Cardiology[3] ❑
20 years[6] / / *CBC* ❑ *Sexual[5]* ❑ *Cholesterol* ❑ *Dentist* ❑	Hearing, vision[2] ❑	Behavior ❑ Seizures ❑ Mitral prolapse ❑ Testis size ❑ Scoliosis ❑	Family support[4] ❑ Cardiology[3] ❑ Orthopedics[3] ❑ Neurology[3] ❑

Clinical concerns for Fragile X syndrome, ages 6+ years

Strabismus	Scoliosis	Cognitive disability
High palate	Club feet, flat feet	Behavioral problems
Dental anomalies	Inguinal hernia	Tantrums, outbursts
Joint laxity	Macro-orchidism	Seizures

Guidelines for prior ages should be undertaken *at the time of diagnosis*; Td, tetanus/diphtheria; MMR, measles–mumps–rubella; Var, varicella; [1]alternative timing; [2]by practitioner; [3]as dictated by clinical findings; [4]parent group, family/sib, financial, and behavioral issues as discussed in the preface; [5]birth control, STD screening if sexually active; [6]repeat every decade.

9

Chromosome microdeletion syndromes

Fluorescent in situ hybridization (FISH) technology allows the detection of subtle chromosome deletions by hybridizing fluorescent DNA probes to metaphase chromosomes. If targeted DNA segment is deleted, then the probe will not yield a fluorescent signal on that chromosome. Chromosome microdeletions may involve single genes or multiple genes, and their phenotypes can sometimes be explained according to the gene products that are missing.

Schmickel (1986) coined the term "contiguous gene deletion" to denote composite phenotypes that result when each deleted gene is associated with a standard Mendelian disease. One of the first examples was an X chromosome deletion that produced Duchenne muscular dystrophy, glycerol kinase, and adrenal hypoplasia in males (Francke et al., 1987). Each of these disorders had been described as a separate X-linked recessive disease, so their concurrence in one patient could be related to the deletion of contiguous genes. In other microdeletions exemplified by the Prader–Willi and Angelman syndromes, several mechanisms including genomic imprinting may act with the deficient gene products to produce the phenotype. Larger chromosomal deletions (e.g., the cri-du-chat deletion on chromosome 5) are never simple composites of Mendelian disorders since many different genes and intragenic regions are deleted.

Table 9.1 lists several chromosome microdeletion syndromes along with their major complications. The cytogenetics laboratory must be alerted when such disorders are suspected, since the FISH study must be performed with the appropriate DNA probe. In most of these disorders, understanding of the pathogenesis awaits better characterization of the genes and gene products within the deleted region. This chapter will provide brief discussion of the less common microdeletion syndromes, with more detailed review of the Williams, Prader–Willi, and Shprintzen/DiGeorge syndromes.

Rare contiguous gene deletion syndromes

Alagille syndrome

Five major features characterize Alagille syndrome, also known as arteriohepatic dysplasia (Alagille et al., 1987). These include unusual facies (95 percent), cholestasis (91

Table 9.1 Chromosome microdeletion syndromes

Deleted region	Disorder	Incidence	Complications
7q11	Williams syndrome	1 in 20,000–50,000	Short stature, cognitive disability, hypercalcemia, supravalvular aortic stenosis, hypertension
8q24	Trichorhinophalangeal syndromes I and II	> 100 cases	Short stature, microcephaly, sparse hair, bulbous nose, cardiac a., renal a., joint laxity
11p13	WAGR	> 50 cases	Wilms tumor–Aniridia–Genital anomalies–Retardation syndrome
13q14	Retinoblastoma, cognitive disability	> 50 cases	Retinoblastoma with or without cognitive disability
15q11q13(pat)	Prader–Willi syndrome	1 in 25,000	Short stature, obesity, cognitive disability, hypogonadism, hyperphagia, hypotonia
15q11q13(mat)	Angelman syndrome	> 50 cases	Growth failure, cognitive disability, prominent jaw, gelastic seizures, jerky movements
17p11.2	Smith–Magenis syndrome	> 50 cases	Growth failure, cognitive disability, self-mutilation, sleep disturbances
17p13.3	Miller–Dieker syndrome	> 50 cases	Lissencephaly, growth and developmental delay
20p11.2	Alagille syndrome	1 in 100,000	Unusual facies, cholestasis, vertebral anomalies, peripheral pulmonary stenosis, embryotoxon of eye
22q11	Shprintzen–DiGeorge	> 500 cases	Unusual facies, coloboma, conotruncal defects, hypoparathyroidism, immune deficiency
Xp21	Duchenne muscular dystrophy (DMD), other problems	> 10 cases	Combinations of DMD, chronic granulomatous disease, retinitis pigmentosa, glycerol kinase deficiency, adrenal hypoplasia
Xp22	Kallman syndrome, other problems	< 10 cases	Kallman syndrome, chondrodysplasia punctata, steroid sulfatase deficiency

percent), posterior embryotoxon of the eye (88 percent), vertebral defects (87 percent), and peripheral pulmonic stenosis (85 percent – Maródi et al., 1994). The incidence is about 1 in 100,000 births. Episodes of jaundice, pruritis, and xanthomas from hypercholesterolemia are frequent problems. In one series, growth retardation was present in 32 percent of the patients and mental retardation in 22 percent (Mueller et al., 1984). Deletion of the short arm of chromosome 20 has been found in several patients and offers a definitive diagnosis for some patients (Byrne et al., 1986). The deleted chromosome may be transmitted from parent to child, simulating autosomal dominant inheritance. Individuals with Alagille syndrome thus face a possible 50 percent recurrence risk.

The natural history indicates a shortened life span because of nutritional, infectious, cardiovascular, and hepatic diseases. The degree of lipid abnormality correlates with the severity of jaundice (Davit-Spraul et al., 1996), and children with early onset liver disease usually require transplantation. Over 25 percent of 80 patients reviewed by Alagille et al. (1987) had died by early adulthood. Preventive management should include cardiac imaging, radiographs to detect vertebral anomalies, and frequent monitoring of serum cholesterol and liver function. Alertness for renal problems is also needed, since some patients have had glomerular involvement (Maródi et al., 1994).

Angelman syndrome

First described by Dr. Harry Angelman in 1965, the pejorative but descriptive term "happy puppet syndrome" has been replaced by the eponymic term. Patients have severe mental disability with average IQ below 40 and no speech. There are jerky movements and gelastic (laughing) seizures that led to the "happy puppet" description. Dysmorphology is limited to microbrachycephaly, prognathism because of frequent jaw movements, and protrusion of the tongue with drooling (Williams & Frias, 1982). Knoll et al. (1989) demonstrated that patients with Angelman and Prader–Willi syndromes share a common chromosomal deletion at bands 15q11q13 but differ in the paternal origin of the deleted chromosome (Cassidy & Schwartz, 1998). Genes in the deleted region are subject to genomic imprinting, such that those derived from the mother are expressed differently from those derived from the father. As a result, deletion of maternally derived genes gives rise to the Angelman syndrome phenotype.

Preventive measures for Angelman syndrome will be focused on the severe neurologic disability, with the needs for rehabilitative, early intervention, and psychosocial services. In addition to seizures, self-mutilation, and frequent movements, children have a variety of ocular problems, including optic nerve atrophy, strabismus, and blindness (Massey & Roy, 1973). Visual assessment is thus important to encourage interactions and diminish autistic and self-mutilative tendencies.

Miller–Dieker syndrome

Lissencephaly is the major feature of Miller–Dieker syndrome, which was first reported in 1963 (Gorlin et al., 1990, p. 591). The syndrome is quite rare, with about 50 cases being reported. The lissencephaly and resulting hypotonia contribute to an abnormal face with bitemporal hollowing, high forehead, anteverted nares, and epicanthal folds. Patients also have abnormal palmar creases, clinodactyly, cryptorchidism, and occasional cardiac defects. Development is severely impaired, with over half of patients dying by age 6 months (Gorlin et al., 1990, p. 591.). A deletion at chromosomal band 17p13.3 has been demonstrated in 92 percent of patients with Miller–Dieker syndrome (Dobyns et al., 1993) – about two-thirds of these can be detected by cytogenetics and one-third by DNA analysis. The deletion led to the characterization of a gene called LIS-1 which also may be altered in patients with isolated lissencephaly (Dobyns et al., 1993). The LIS-1 gene product is absent in the brain of patients with Miller–Dieker syndrome (Mizuguchi et al., 1995). Preventive management should be concerned with the anticipation of pulmonary complications, rehabilitation services, and supportive care for the infant and family.

Smith–Magenis syndrome

A syndrome of microcephaly, craniofacial changes, digital anomalies, growth failure, and severe mental disability was described in 1982 (Greenberg et al., 1991, 1996). The patients have midface hypoplasia, severe speech delay, a hoarse, deep voice, and insensitivity to pain with mutilative behavior. Interesting in view of the associated 17p11.2 deletion are decreased deep tendon reflexes and muscle atrophy; a major locus for Charcot–Marie–Tooth disease has been mapped within the Smith–Magenis deletion region. Greenberg et al. (1991) suggested an incidence of 1 in 25,000 births, but the paucity of reported cases casts doubt on this figure. Under-ascertainment is probable because facial features may not stand out and DNA analysis is required for the recognition of the deletion in many patients. Besides rehabilitative and family supports for severe neurologic disease, preventive management should consider cardiac defects (31 percent), scoliosis (24 percent), flat feet (61 percent), and behavioral problems that occur at significant frequencies (Smith et al., 1998a; Greenberg et al., 1991). Sleep disturbance is a striking feature of Smith–Magenis syndrome (Smith et al., 1998b).

Trichorhinophalangeal syndromes

Smaller deletions in the chromosome 8q23q24 region produce the phenotype of trichorhinophalangeal (TRP) syndrome type I, while larger deletions produce the more severe phenotype of Langer–Giedion syndrome or TRP syndrome type II (Bühler & Malik, 1984). Both disorders have the cognate findings of sparse hair, prominent nose, and abnormally shaped fingers, and TRP II patients having microcephaly, mental disability, and multiple bony exostoses. Patients with type I TRP have normal intelligence with frequent upper respiratory tract infections, short stature, and joint laxity (Gorlin et al., 1990, pp. 806–11; Jones, 1987, pp. 290–3). Less frequent complications of type I TRP include cardiac anomalies (mitral valve prolapse), renal anomalies, dental anomalies (malocclusion, supernumerary teeth), and skeletal anomalies (scoliosis, flat feet, hip pain, and generalized arthritis; Dunbar et al., 1995). Preventive management should be directed to surveillance for otitis and upper respiratory infections, monitoring of growth, and alertness for cardiac, renal, and skeletal anomalies. Patients with TRP type II will need similar monitoring with the addition of early intervention and social support services because of mental disability. Chromosomal studies will be normal in some patients with TRP; these individuals may have submicroscopic deletions or mutations within putative TRP genes (Jones, 1997, p. 290–3).

Williams syndrome

Terminology

Williams et al. (1961) and Beuren et al. (1962) described children with supravalvular aortic stenosis, unusual facies, and other findings (Fig. 9.1, color plate). "Williams syndrome" or "Williams–Beuren" syndrome is the preferred terminology, since supravalvular aortic stenosis is not present in all patients. The "idiopathic hypercalcemia–supravalvular aortic stenosis syndrome" and "elfin facies syndrome" are equivalent terms (Gorlin et al., 1990, pp. 143–8; Jones, 1997, pp. 118–19).

Historical diagnosis and management

Numerous children with infantile hypercalcemia were described in Great Britain and Switzerland in the early 1950s (Jones, 1990). Many had feeding problems, constipation, and growth failure; a few developed azotemia and nephrocalcinosis. Concerns about a "milk-alkali" syndrome with excessive vitamin D intake led to changes in dietary recommendations for infants. Study of infantile hypercalcemia delineated a more severe group with persistent problems that probably corresponded to the Williams syndrome patients described by Williams et al. (1961) and Beuren et al. (1962).

Early reports of Williams syndrome focused on neonatal hypercalcemia and cardiac anomalies, and it was some time before the full syndrome of mental disability, unusual appearance, and multiple congenital anomalies would be appreciated (Jones & Smith, 1975; Jones, 1990). Supravalvular aortic stenosis was defined as a unique, autosomal dominant disorder before its recognition as part of Williams syndrome (Burn, 1986). Mapping of supravalvular aortic stenosis to a region of chromosome 7 containing the elastin gene led to the characterization of deletions in Williams syndrome (Ewart et al., 1993a, b; Wu et al., 1998).

Incidence, etiology, and differential diagnosis

The incidence depends on the accuracy of diagnosis, but is between 1 in 20,000–50,000 live births (Greenberg, 1990). Families containing some individuals with supravalvular stenosis and some with Williams syndrome have been reported, suggesting that milder patients may not be recognized (Gorlin et al., 1990, p.143). Deletion of one copy of the elastin gene presumably explains the supravalvular aortic stenosis and connective tissue alterations in Williams syndrome, with additional features caused by the deletion of contiguous genes (Ewalt et al., 1993b). The chief differential is between other syndromes with developmental disabilities and vascular problems; rubella embryopathy and Alagille syndrome can have pulmonary artery stenoses. Hypercalcemia occurs in hyperparathyroidism and vitamin D intoxication, but these disorders should be easily distinguished by history or physical examination (Gorlin et al., 1990, p. 147).

Diagnostic evaluation and medical counseling

Neonatal diagnosis of Williams syndrome is difficult unless hypercalcemia is detected. The characteristic face with stellate iris pattern, strabismus, periorbital fullness, thick lips, and long philtrum may not be obvious until early childhood. Once the diagnosis is suspected, chromosomal analysis can be performed using fluorescent in situ hybridization (FISH) to look for 7q11 microdeletions (Ewart et al., 1993b). Nickerson et al. (1995) report that over 90 percent of patients with classical Williams syndrome have a detectable 7q deletion; the diagnosis must be clinical in the remaining 10 percent. Medical counseling should emphasize the risks of ocular, cardiovascular, and renal anomalies, with mention of learning and behavioral problems (Williams syndrome checklist, part 1). The hypercalcemia is still not understood; it seems related to defective calcitonin release and diminished response to a calcium load (Jones, 1990). It may be the cause of acquired coarctation of the aorta that has been described (Dhillon et al., 1998).

Infancy is often difficult because of colic and feeding problems; parents may need considerable support during this period. Renal anomalies (Ichinose et al., 1996) and infantile spasms can occur (Tsao & Westman, 1997). During later childhood, subtle visual abnormalities (Olitsky et al., 1997) and learning differences are more problematic (Jarrold et al., 1998). The considerable verbal abilities and happy affect of children with Williams syndrome allow the health professional to be optimistic in describing the long-term outlook (Plissart et al., 1996).

Family and psychosocial counseling

Although Williams syndrome has exhibited rare parent–child transmission and concordance in identical twins, the recurrence risks for parents of affected children is less than 1 percent (Gorlin et al., 1990, p. 143; Jones, 1997, pp. 118–19). Rare families have demonstrated autosomal dominant inheritance, and referral for genetic counseling is important. Supportive counseling is required for the early feeding problems with colic, vomiting, or constipation; later difficulties with hyperactivity, distractibility, and learning differences will be stressful for most families and require psychosocial counseling and support. An article written by parents of a child with Williams syndrome provides useful insight for health professionals (Anonymous, 1985). Parent support groups are listed on the checklist, part 1.

Natural history and complications

The facial appearance of individuals with Williams syndrome changes considerably with age. Life span may be somewhat decreased because of cardiovascular or renal anomalies, but several studies described adults with excellent quality of life (Greenberg, 1990; Morris et al., 1990; Lopez-Rangel et al., 1992). The neonatal and infantile course may be turbulent, with feeding difficulties and hypercalcemia. Although supravalvular aortic or pulmonary stenosis, renal artery stenosis, and hypertension may cause problems, childhood is usually dominated more by behavioral than medical concerns. The loquacious, "cocktail-party" manner and happy affect are attractive, but the accompanying hyperactivity, emotional lability, and excessive anxiety may be taxing (Udwin & Yule, 1991). Hyperacusis is common, and extreme responses to doorbells or lawn-mowers may complicate behavioral management (Nigam & Samuel, 1994). Microcephaly and developmental delay are usual, with 59 percent of children having a global IQ under 70. Many children perform at age-appropriate levels in the areas of visual recognition, expressive language, and verbal recall (Udwin & Yule, 1991; Jarrold et al., 1998).

Later complications include mitral valve prolapse, peptic ulcer, cholelithiasis, obesity, urinary tract infections with bladder diverticular, and diabetes mellitus (Morris et al., 1990; Lopez-Rangel et al., 1992). Hypercalcuria persists in many adult patients, sometimes causing paradoxical release of parathormone. Nephrocalcinosis, renal artery, and other arterial stenoses cause hypertension to be a frequent complication, often with onset in the second or third decade. A few patients have had cerebral arterial stenosis with strokes at a young age (Kaplan et al., 1995; Soper et al., 1995). Urinary tract anomalies include bladder diverticula found in later life (Pober et al., 1993; Ichinose et al., 1996). Early graying of the hair, together with Alzheimer-like brain changes in one patient, suggests that aging may be accelerated (Golden et al., 1995).

Williams syndrome preventive medical checklist

Preventive management should begin at the time of diagnosis, with renal and cardiac sonography to document anomalies (checklist, parts 2–4). Hypertension may be associated with cardiovascular or renal disease, so frequent monitoring of blood pressure is important. Where possible, four-extremity blood pressures should be obtained so peripheral vascular stenoses can be recognized. Although feeding problems, colic, and constipation often complicate early growth, conservative management is indicated since gastrointestinal anomalies are rare. Chronic otitis is a frequent problem, necessitating frequent audiologic assessments and possible referral to otolaryngology. Dental anomalies are frequent, and dentistry with appropriate endocarditis prophylaxis should be an integral part of preventive care. Renal anomalies and urinary tract infections are sufficiently common that Pober et al. (1993) and Greenberg (1990) recommended frequent renal function tests. Renal sonography is recommended at least once in early childhood and once in later adolescence/adulthood (Greenberg, 1990).

In adolescence, blood pressure and urinary tract structure/function should be monitored, as indicated on the checklist, part 4. Williams syndrome is a "progressive, multisystem disorder" (Morris et al., 1990). Patients should be monitored for scoliosis and joint contractures. Those with mitral valve prolapse or other cardiovascular disease should be monitored by cardiology. Despite early feeding problems, obesity is a problem in 29 percent of patients (checklist, part 1) and nutritional counseling may be indicated. Performance and behavior in school should be followed, with referral to behavioral specialists as needed. Anxiety may cause peptic ulcer disease, and cholelithiasis should be borne in mind as a possible diagnosis in patients with abdominal pain. Community care networks are helpful if they can be established for adults with Williams syndrome (Udwin et al., 1998).

Prader–Willi syndrome

Terminology

The first report of Prader–Willi syndrome was by Prader et al. (1956), but several years elapsed before larger reviews established the full phenotype (Zellweger & Schneider, 1968). Occasionally the syndrome is referred to as Prader–Labhart–Willi syndrome to include all three original authors (Prader et al., 1956) or as the hypotonia–hypomentia–hypogenitalism–obesity (HHHO) syndrome (Zellweger & Schneider, 1968).

Historical diagnosis and management

The obese, sleepy boy immortalized in the Pickwick papers may have been the first reported case of Prader–Willi syndrome (Jones, 1997, p. 170). The condition remains "underdiagnosed and undertreated" (Cassidy, 1987), and consensus diagnostic criteria have been formulated (Holm et al., 1993). The disorder was one of the first examples of a contiguous gene deletion syndrome and, together with Angelman syndrome, is the prototypic clinical example of genomic imprinting in humans (Hall, 1990). Current interest includes the distinctive phases of natural history (see below), the unusual behaviors, and the disordered hypothalamic function exemplified by changes in appetite, temperature regulation, and sleep (Martin et al., 1998).

Incidence, etiology, and differential diagnosis

The incidence of Prader–Willi syndrome is 1 in 16,000–25,000 births (Zellweger & Soper, 1979; Burd et al., 1990). Occasional familial cases led to suspicion of a genetic etiology, and this was proven when approximately 70 percent of patients with a classical phenotype were shown to have a deletion on the paternally derived chromosome 15 between bands q13 and q15 (Holm et al., 1993). Many of the remaining 30 percent will have uniparental disomy for the maternally derived chromosome 15, thus being deficient in paternally derived genes from the 15q13q15 region. Rare patients have normal chromosome 15 structure and origin, but lack mechanisms for DNA methylation that are necessary for establishing the genomic imprint. Prader–Willi syndrome thus results from altered expression of genes within the 15q13q15 region, although the precise genes and mechanisms of dysmorphogenesis have not been defined.

The diagnosis is aided by facial changes including almond-shaped eyes, down-turned corners of the mouth, and bitemporal hollowing (Fig. 9.2, color plate). Karyotypic confirmation is especially needed in the infantile period before the development of hyperphagia. Differential diagnosis includes other disorders with neurologic dysfunction, severe hypotonia, and obesity. In the neonatal hypotonic phase, patients with the Prader–Willi syndrome may be confused with those of Down syndrome, Zellweger syndrome, or congenital neuropathies and myopathies. In the childhood obesity phase, disorders such as Cohen syndrome or Bardet–Biedl syndrome might be considered. Still unexplained is why rare patients with the fragile X syndrome have the obesity, hypogonadism, and growth failure of Prader–Willi syndrome (Schrander-Stumpel et al., 1994).

Diagnostic evaluation and medical counseling

Consensus diagnostic criteria have been formulated for Prader–Willi syndrome (Holm et al., 1993). Major criteria of neonatal/infantile hypotonia, infantile feeding problems, excessive weight gain between ages 1–6 years, compatible facial features, hypogonadism, global developmental delay/mental disability, hyperphagia and food obsession, and deletion/uniparental disomy for the chromosome 15q13q15 region. Minor criteria include decreased fetal movement; unstable, stubborn or oppositional behavior; sleep apnea; short stature; hypopigmentation; small hands and feet; strabismus; thick saliva; problems with speech articulation; and skin picking. Deletion or uniparental disomy of chromosome 15 is the keystone of diagnosis, provided the clinical features are compatible.

Most cytogenetic laboratories offer fluorescent in situ hybridization (FISH) analysis for the characteristic Prader–Willi deletion as a routine service. If a deletion is not detected in a patient with typical features, then DNA analysis for the origin of the number 15 chromosomes is available in some laboratories. If both chromosomes 15 contain polymorphic DNA segments indicating maternal origin, then a diagnosis of Prader–Willi syndrome owing to uniparental disomy is established. Further levels of testing are being developed for the 5–10 percent of patients who have Prader–Willi syndrome without deletion or uniparental disomy. Altered patterns of DNA methylation have been associated with parental imprinting of chromosomes. Prader–Willi syndrome can result when the chromosomes 15 have appropriate biparental origin but when the paternal 15 lacks its requisite pattern of DNA methylation. One can also anticipate that mutations in one or more of the contiguous genes in the 15q11q13 region will also cause Prader–Willi syndrome. At present, DNA methylation and future mutational analysis are experimental studies that are performed only by research laboratories.

Although early diagnosis of Prader–Willi syndrome confers the anticipation of improved muscle strength and function, the parents face considerable challenges in caring for a child with nutritional, motor, cognitive, and behavioral problems. The greatest emphasis of medical counseling will be weight management, since obesity is a large contributor to morbidity and early mortality (Greenswag, 1987). Later issues will include school arrangements, behavior management, and provision for adolescents and adults living in a controlled environment.

Family and psychosocial counseling

From data on more than 1500 families, Cassidy (1987) derived a parental recurrence risk of less than 1 in 1000. Most parents can be reassured about future reproduction without the need for prenatal diagnosis; however, fetal screening is possible when the index patient has a deletion or uniparental disomy. All families should be referred for genetic counseling. As for other disorders that inflict mental disability, supportive services such as psychology, social work, and grief counseling may be appropriate for some parents. Parent support groups are listed on the Prader–Willi syndrome checklist, part 1.

Natural history and complications

Few disorders exhibit the striking phenotypic changes observed in Prader–Willi syndrome. Prenatal hypotonia, decreased movement, and a propensity for breech positioning are followed by neonatal hypotonia that may be severe enough to mimic a congenital myopathy. Infantile hypotonia is associated with a weak suck and poor feeding that produces a "failure to thrive" picture until the change to hyperphagia occurs. Between ages 1 and 4 years, there is a transformation from growth failure to obesity caused by a voracious appetite. Abnormal eating behaviors include stealing food, nocturnal foraging for food, eating inappropriate foods, and binge eating. Morbid obesity may ensue that causes a shortened life span in Prader–Willi syndrome because of cardiopulmonary disease (Cassidy, 1987; Gorlin et al., 1990, pp. 345–7). Patients as old as 71 years have been reported (Carpenter, 1994), and it is interesting that all older reported patients have been females.

The most taxing complications of Prader–Willi syndrome are developmental and behavioral, but ocular, dental, cutaneous, and genital anomalies occur (checklist, part 1). Because oculocutaneous albinism occurs in 50 percent of patients with Prader–Willi syndrome, the misrouting of retinogeniculate-cortical projections as occurs in albinism has been invoked as a cause for strabismus (40–95 percent). However, Roy et al. (1992) did not find the asymmetric visual evoked response typical of nerve misrouting in 12 patients with Prader–Willi syndrome. Dental problems include increased caries and enamel hypoplasia, perhaps reflecting the high carbohydrate diet and decreased salivation in Prader–Willi syndrome (Cassidy, 1987). Rumination occurs in 10–17 percent of patients, and aspiration pneumonitis must be added to the cor pulmonale, temperature instability, and cardiac arrythmias that complicate anesthesia in patients with Prader–Willi syndrome (Hakonarson et al., 1995). Hypogonadotrophic hypogonadism, irregular menses, and infertility are common, joining with hyperphagia, disruption of the sleep cycle, and temperature instability as evidence of hypothalamic dysfunction. Rectal bleeding has been reported (Bhargava et al., 1996). Williams et al. (1994) did not find differences in thermoregulation between children with Prader–Willi syndrome and those with comparable developmental disabilities. Wilms tumor (Coppes et al., 1993) and three cases of leukemia (Gorlin et al., 1990, p. 347) have been reported, but an increased cancer risk is not yet documented.

Behavior problems dominate the management of Prader–Willi syndrome. Sleep disorders are common, with 50–90 percent of patients having daytime hypersomnolence. Although frequent snoring and a narrow upper airway occur in these patients, a central nervous system derangement of sleep is as common as obstructive sleep apnea (Kaplan et al., 1991). Violent outbursts, temper tantrums, obsessive-compulsive behavior, rigidity, manipulation, and stubbornness are common (Holm et al., 1993); older children and adults exhibit depression and a "refusal-lethargy syndrome" of hyperkinesis, refusal of food and drink, and soiling (Bartolucci & Younger, 1994). Skin-picking with cellulitis and scarring and recurrent nasal bleeding may reflect the obsessive-compulsive and oppositional aspects of the syndrome (Schepis et al., 1994). Spontaneous psychoses unrelated to other physical or behavioral problems have been reported in Prader–Willi syndrome, but their prevalence is not known (Clarke, 1993; Martin et al., 1998).

Developmental delay is most obvious in motor milestones, with sitting at an average age of 12–13 months, walking at 24–30 months, and riding a tricycle at 4.2 years (Cassidy, 1987). Cognitive functions that are independent of hypotonia are less severely delayed, with single words appearing at 21–23 months and sentences at a mean of 3.6 years (Cassidy, 1987). Articulation defects are common and the speech often has a nasal quality. Reading is a relative strength, with mathematics and social interactions being weaknesses (Cassidy, 1987; Curfs et al., 1991). Performance in solving mazes or codes was substantially above verbal performance that required auditory processing (Curfs et al., 1991); this profile may explain the clinical impression that many Prader–Willi patients enjoy puzzles. As noted on the checklist (part 1), 40 percent of patients have a global IQ that is above 70 and in the borderline or normal range. Poor performance in school often reflects specific learning disabilities, distractibility, or behavioral problems.

Preventive medical checklist for Prader–Willi syndrome

When the diagnosis is suspected based on infantile hypotonia, karyotyping and DNA analysis to establish chromosome 15 deletion or uniparental disomy are critical. Early diagnosis is useful, since the inculcation of needed dietary controls is more easily accomplished before the oppositional, stubborn, and obsessive behaviors of later childhood and adolescence are encountered. Close monitoring of feeding is necessary during infancy, since some children require enhanced-calorie formula or gavage feeding. Strabismus, sleep problems, dental anomalies, and early intervention for developmental problems are important aspects of management in early childhood.

Hyperphagia and morbid obesity are the major issues for later childhood and adolescence, but a wide variety of behavior problems require monitoring. Rumination can lead to gastric contents in the posterior pharynx during anesthesia, even after a 10-hour fast (Sloan & Kaye, 1991); reduction of acid secretion, decompression of the gastric contents, and body positioning to minimize reflux/aspiration are recommended for anesthesia. Pharmacologic treatment has been of benefit in skin-picking, using drugs such as fluoxetine (Prozac). Serotonergic drugs have also shown promise in controlling appetite, and have had beneficial results in ameliorating hyperphagia, obsessive-compulsive behavior, and self-mutilation in Prader–Willi syndrome (Stein et al., 1994). Haloperidol and thioridazine have also had anecdotal success for behavioral control, depression, and anxiety in Prader–Willi syndrome. Periodic evaluation of behavior is an important aspect of the checklist (parts 3–4), and involvement of school psychologists and/or behavioral therapists will often be required.

The most successful strategies for weight management involved close supervision to regulate intake and the encouragement of regular exercise (Cassidy, 1987). Patients with Prader–Willi syndrome do not experience satiety and have remarkable resistance to vomiting; unregulated caloric intake can approach 6000 kcal per day (Cassidy, 1987). Restriction of calories to 800–1100 per day in adolescents is usually necessary to achieve weight control. Education of parents and children is vital, and behavioral modification using rewards, restricted access to all food sources, and the promotion of exercise is necessary. Growth hormone therapy has been tried without remarkable benefits (Davies et al., 1998). Many adolescents and adults do best living in group homes restricted to Prader–Willi syndrome, so a uniform lifestyle can be designed. Despite these efforts, most patients become obese and require monitoring of cardiopulmonary status and blood pressure.

Shprintzen syndrome and the Del(22q) spectrum

Terminology

Shprintzen et al. (1978) described a syndrome with unusual facies, velopalatine insufficiency, and conotruncal anomalies, drawing together observations dating back to 1955 (Gorlin et al., 1990, p. 740; Jones, 1997, pp. 266–7; Olney & Kolodziej, 1998). The condition is also known as velocardiofacial syndrome. Some patients with Shprintzen syndrome have the absent thymus and parathyroid glands reported by DiGeorge (1965). Because a single error in branchial arch development is thought to be involved, the combination of thymic, parathyroid, and conotruncal cardiac anomalies is called DiGeorge sequence or DiGeorge anomaly (Conley et al., 1979). Monosomy 22 and then subtle deletions in chromosome band 22q11 were demonstrated in DiGeorge sequence. Soon it was demonstrated that some patients with isolated conotruncal cardiac anomalies had a 22q11 microdeletion, and the spectrum of Shprintzen syndrome, DiGeorge, and conotruncal anomaly was denoted as "CATCH 22" (Wilson et al., 1993; Johnson et al., 1995). The term serves as an acronym for cardiac defects, abnormal facies, thymic hypoplasia, cleft palate, and hypocalcemia that may result from chromosome 22 deletion, but its connotation of "can't win" is not flattering to patients and is replaced here by the Shprintzen syndrome/del(22) spectrum.

Recently, the del(22) spectrum has been further expanded by mapping of one form of Opitz syndrome – a condition with hypertelorism, severe dysphasia with laryngeal and/or esophageal clefts, and genital anomalies – to chromosome band 22q11 (Worthington et al., 1997). A patient with features of Opitz syndrome and del(22)(q11) presented with a vascular ring and pulmonary stridor (Zackai et al., 1996). Other terms for Opitz syndrome have included "G syndrome," "BBB syndrome," and "Opitz-Frias syndrome." The initials were derived from the surnames of affected children before the realization that the "G" and "BBB" patients exhibited different manifestations of the same disorder (Opitz, 1987).

Historical diagnosis and management

Because of subtle facial features in some patients, Shprintzen syndrome is probably underdiagnosed. Routine cytogenetic detection of the chromosome 22 deletion should allow earlier recognition of these patients and improve management of cardiac, orofacial, and immune problems. The spectrum of disorders united by the finding of chromosome 22 deletion, ranging from severe cardiac or orofacial anomalies to a normal appearance, is a significant example of how molecular advances can improve the understanding and management of clinical genetic disorders (Hall, 1993).

Incidence, etiology, and differential diagnosis

The incidence of the Shprintzen/del(22) spectrum is unknown, but is estimated to comprise about 8 percent of patients with syndromic cleft palate (Goldberg et al., 1993). Since as many as 44–64 percent of cleft lip/palate patients have associated anomalies (Gorlin et al., 1990, p. 698), and the incidence of cleft lip/palate is about 1 in 1000 live births (Gorlin et al., 1990, p. 695), overt cases of the Shprintzen/del(22) spectrum probably has a prevalence of about 1 in 25,000 births. Adding to this prevalence figure may be relatives of patients with Shprintzen syndrome who have behavioral and musculoskeletal features without oral or cardiac manifestations (Holder et al., 1993).

The frequency of chromosome 22 deletion is about 63 percent in patients with Shprintzen syndrome, 83 percent in patients with DiGeorge anomaly, and 29 percent of patients with nonsyndromic conotruncal anomalies (Hall, 1993). Haplo-insufficiency of genes in this deleted region is thus a prominent etiology for these conditions, and a candidate gene has recently been characterized (Fisher & Scambler, 1994). Differential diagnosis includes other conditions with orofacial and cardiac problems, including the orofacial digital syndromes. The DiGeorge sequence also occurs in CHARGE association (see Chapter 5), but the facial characteristics are different from those of Shprintzen syndrome.

Echocardiography, audiography, consideration of obstructive sleep apnea and close monitoring of feeding and palatal function are important in patients with suspected Shprintzen syndrome (Shprintzen checklist, part 1). In the presence of tetany or recurrent infections, chest x-rays, peripheral leukocyte counts, and serum calcium/phosphorus measurements should be obtained to evaluate the presence of DiGeorge sequence. Patients with the hypertelorism, genital anomalies, and dysphagia/aspiration that suggest a diagnosis of Opitz syndrome should have thorough investigation of their larynx, esophagus and swallowing function, since Nisen fundoplication and even upper esophageal ligation may be required to prevent irreversible pulmonary damage. Medical counseling should be optimistic for the entire del(22) spectrum, since ultimate cognitive function ranges from normal to mild mental retardation.

Family and psychosocial counseling

Before the discovery of the chromosome 22 deletion, Shprintzen syndrome was considered autosomal dominant and DiGeorge anomaly sporadic. Isolated conotruncal defects were usually multifactorial with a 2–3 percent recurrence risk, although occasional families would exhibit vertical transmission. If parents of affected children show any features of the Shprintzen/DiGeorge/del(22) spectrum, they should have FISH analysis for del(22)(q11). Parents without clinically sugges- tive physical or psychiatric features may also need del(22) analysis since the dele- tion has been found in apparently normal individuals. All families should be referred for genetic counseling. Individuals with the deletion or a presumptive clin- ical diagnosis of Shprintzen syndrome should be given a 50 percent recurrence risk, with the understanding that affected children will vary in their number and sever- ity of features. Psychosocial counseling may be quite important, since many affected children and occasional parents will have behavior problems ranging from poor social interaction to frank psychosis or phobic responses (Gorlin et al., 1990, pp. 740–2).

Parent support groups for the Shprintzen/DiGeorge deletion 22q11 spectrum are listed on the checklist, part 1.

Natural history and complications

Neonatal complications are particularly important to consider in Shprintzen/ del(22) syndrome, since their detection and management will have considerable influence on natural history. Cardiac anomalies and dysphagia may be severe and life-threatening, and failure to investigate the cardiovascular and gastrointestinal systems can lead to debilitating bronchiectasis or cardiopulmonary failure. The possibility of DiGeorge sequence must be considered from the perspective of early treatment and modification of the immunization schedule to omit live vaccines. The natural history of Shprintzen syndrome has three phases; a turbulent infantile course, with possible cardiac disease, severe dysphagia and reflux, obstructive sleep apnea and upper respiratory infections; a childhood compromised by hearing, speech, learning, and growth problems: and an adolescence/adulthood challenged by personality, school, and behavioral problems. The mental disability can relate to neuroanatomic changes such as cerebellar hypoplasia (Devriendt et al., 1996). Patients also have an increased risk of ocular, urinary tract, and genital anomalies, and increased connective tissue laxity confers risks of inguinal hernia in 30 percent of patients and scoloiosis in 13–15 percent (checklist, part 1). Aberrant arterial anatomy has been described, posing risks for otolaryngologic procedures (Ross et al., 1996; Olney & Kolodziej, 1998).

Although there is little information on adults with this recently described disease spectrum, life span in those surviving early complications is probably normal. Growth is slow early, but short stature was present in 2 of 5 adults studied by Goldberg et al. (1993); the short stature in 35 percent of children may thus repre- sent constitutional growth delay. Learning disabilities are almost universal in Shprintzen syndrome, and mental disability also occurs in the Opitz syndrome

(Opitz, 1987). Performance IQ is lower than verbal IQ in patients with Shprintzen syndrome, and hypernasal speech with articulation problems and language delay is common. A characteristic personality has been described (Goldberg et al., 1993), consisting of a bland affect, poor social interaction, and impulsive behavior (Gorlin et al., 1990, pp. 740–2). Psychosis and phobic reactions have been seen in some adults, including an apparently unaffected mother of 4 children with Shprintzen syndrome (Goldberg et al., 1993).

The presence of DiGeorge anomaly is essential to suspect and recognize so appropriate surveillance for infections and modification of the immunization schedule can be provided. Risks for upper respiratory infections are increased in most patients, necessitating aggressive treatment of chronic otitis and screening for hearing loss. In patients without overt cleft palate, submucous clefts may occur, with significant risks for otitis and speech problems. Many patients have feeding problems and failure to thrive, so feeding specialists may be needed to accomplish reasonable growth.

The care of older children and adolescents should focus on learning disabilities and potential school problems, which may be augmented by abnormal behaviors. Attention to speech, language, and hearing should continue, and awareness of the increased joint laxity may influence the recommendations for physical activity. Scoliosis and inguinal hernias occur at increased frequency, and the occurrence of genital anomalies in boys makes it important to monitor puberty.

Preventive Management of Williams syndrome

Clinical diagnosis: Characteristic pattern including neonatal hypercalcemia, characteristic facial appearance, periorbital fullness, prominent lips, stellate irides, early feeding problems and failure to thrive, happy personality in older children, hyperacusis, excellent musical and verbal skills (Udwin & Yule, 1991).

Laboratory diagnosis: Special chromosome (FISH) study demonstrating deletion on chromosome 7q including the elastin gene.

Genetics: Rarely inherited, recurrence risk < 1%.

Key management issues: Positive attitude, early intervention, feeding, vision, hearing, heart, renal, and behavioral problems.

Growth charts: Morris et al. (1988).

Parent groups: Williams Syndrome Association, PO Box 297, Clawson MI, 48107-0297, (241) 541-3630, members.aol.com/BobHazard/wsc.html; Canadian Association for Williams Syndrome PO Box 2115 Vancouver BC CAN, V6B 3T5, (604)852-2662 The Williams Syndrome Foundation (UK), 161 High Street, Tonbridge, Kent,TN9 1BX, England, (01732) 365-152, http://www. williams-syndrome.org.uk/

Basis for management recommendations: Complications cited by Greenberg (1990), Morris et al. (1988), Pober et al. (1993).

Summary of clinical concerns

General	Learning	**Cognitive and learning differences** (97%)
	Behavior	Behavior problems – hyperactivity, sensory integration problems
	Growth	**Feeding problems** (71%), **failure to thrive** (81%), **obesity** (21%)
Facial	Eye	**Oculomotor problems, esotropia** (50%), **hyperopia** (24%)
	Ear	**Hyperacusis** (95%), chronic otitis (43%)
	Mouth	**Dental malocclusion** (85%), **enamel hypoplasia** (48%), microdontia (55%)
Surface	Neck/trunk	**Pectus excavatum** (40%), **inguinal hernias** (38%), umbilical hernia
	Epidermal	Prematurely gray hair
Skeletal	Cranial	**Microcephaly,** brachycephaly
	Axial	**Kyphosis** (21%), scoliosis
	Limbs	**Contractures** (50%)
Internal	Digestive	**Early colic and vomiting** (40–67%), **constipation** (43%), peptic ulcer (18%), cholelithiasis (12%), rectal prolapse (12%)
	Circulatory	**Cardiac anomalies** (79%), **hypertension** (47–60%), arterial stenoses (18%)
	Endocrine	**Early hypercalcemia** (67%), diabetes mellitus (12%)
	Excretory	**Enuresis** (52%), **urinary tract infections** (29%), renal anomalies (18%)
	Genital	Micropenis
Neural	CNS	**Hypotonia, motor delays,** cerebral artery stenosis, strokes
	Sensory	**Hyperacusis** (95%), hearing loss, vision loss

Bold: frequency > 20%

Key references

Greenberg, F. (1990): *American Journal of Medical Genetics* suppl 6:85–8.

Jones, K. L. (1990): *American Journal of Medical Genetics* suppl 6:89–96.

Morris et al. (1988) in Saul et al. (1998): *Growth References: Third Trimester to Adulthood.* Greenville SC: Keys Printing, pp. 128–32.

Morris, C. A., Leonard, C. O., Dilts, C. & Demsey, S. A. (1990). *American Journal of Medical Genetics* 6:102–7.

Pober, B. R., Lacro, R. V., Rice, C., Mandell, V. & Teele, R. L. (1993): *American Journal of Medical Genetics* 46:271–4.

Udwin, O. & Yule, W. (1991): *Journal of Clinical and Experimental Neuropsychology* 13:232–44.

Williams syndrome

Preventive medical checklist (0–1yr)

Patient			Birth Date / /		Number	
Pediatric	**Screen**		**Evaluate**		**Refer/Counsel**	
Neonatal / / *Newborn screen* ❑ *HB* ❑	Total/ionized Ca ❑ FISH Del(7q) ❑		Feeding ❑ Inguinal hernias ❑		Genetic evaluation ❑ Feeding specialist[3] ❑	
1 month / /	Growth ❑ Cardiac echo ❑ Renal sonogram ❑		Feeding, colic ❑ GE reflux ❑		Family support[4] ❑ Cardiology ❑	
2 months / / *HB[1]* ❑ *Hib* ❑ *DTaP, IPV* ❑ *RV* ❑	Growth ❑ Hearing, vision[2] ❑		Feeding, colic ❑ GE reflux ❑ Otitis ❑		Early intervention[5] ❑ Developmental pediatrics ❑ Genetic counseling ❑ Gastroenterology[3] ❑	
4 months / / *HB[1]* ❑ *Hib* ❑ *DTaP/IPV* ❑ *RV* ❑	Growth ❑ Hearing, vision[2] ❑		Feeding, colic ❑ GE reflux ❑ Otitis ❑		Early intervention[5] ❑ ENT[3] ❑	
6 months / / *Hib* ❑ *IPV[1]* ❑ *DTaP* ❑ *RV* ❑	Growth ❑ Hearing, vision[2] ❑ Urinalysis, BP ❑		Feeding, colic ❑ GE reflux ❑ Otitis ❑ Constipation ❑		Family support[4] ❑ Feeding specialist[3] ❑ Ophthalmology ❑	
9 months / / *IPV[1]* ❑	Audiology ❑ Urinalysis, BP ❑		Otitis ❑ Strabismus ❑			
1 year / / *HB* ❑ *Hib[1]* ❑ *IPV[1]* ❑ *MMR[1]* ❑ *Var[1]* ❑	Hearing, vision[2] ❑ Total/ionized Ca ❑ BUN, creatinine ❑ Urinalysis, BP ❑		Feeding ❑ Otitis ❑ Strabismus ❑ Constipation ❑		Family support[4] ❑ Early intervention[5] ❑ Developmental pediatrics ❑ Genetics ❑ ENT[3] ❑	

Clinical concerns for Williams syndrome, ages 0–1 year

Feeding problems, colic	Cardiovascular anomalies	Hypotonia
Strabismus	Vascular stenoses	Developmental disability
Chronic otitis, hearing loss	Renal anomalies	Motor and speech delay
Constipation	Inguinal hernias	

Guidelines for the neonatal period should be undertaken *at whatever age* the diagnosis is made; DTaP, acellular DTP; IPV, inactivated poliovirus; RV, rotavirus; Var, varicella; GE, gastroesophageal; Ca, calcium; BP, blood pressure; [1]alternative timing; [2]by practitioner; [3]as dictated by clinical findings; [4]parent group, family/sib, financial, and behavioral issues as discussed in the preface; [5]including developmental monitoring and motor/speech therapy.

Williams syndrome

Preventive medical checklist (15m–6yrs)

Patient   **Birth Date** / /   **Number**

Pediatric	Screen		Evaluate		Refer/Counsel	
15 months / / Hib[1] ❑ MMR[1] ❑ DTaP, IPV[1] ❑ Varicella[1] ❑	Audiology Growth Hearing, vision[2]	❑ ❑ ❑	Feeding GE reflux Otitis Strabismus	❑ ❑ ❑ ❑	Family support[4] Early intervention[5] Cardiology	❑ ❑ ❑
18 months / / DTaP, IPV[1] ❑ Varicella[1] ❑ Influenza[3] ❑	Growth Hearing, vision[2]	❑ ❑	Strabismus	❑	Developmental pediatrics Genetics	 ❑ ❑
2 years / / Influenza[3] ❑ Pneumovax[3] ❑ Dentist ❑	Audiology Total/ionized Ca BUN, creatinine Urinalysis, BP	❑ ❑ ❑ ❑	Otitis Strabismus	❑ ❑	Family support[4] ENT[3] Ophthalmology[3] Cardiology	❑ ❑ ❑ ❑
3 years / / Influenza[3] ❑ Pneumovax[3] ❑ Dentist ❑	Audiology Total/ionized Ca BUN, creatinine Urinalysis, BP	❑ ❑ ❑ ❑	Otitis Strabismus	❑ ❑	Preschool transition[5] Developmental pediatrics Genetics ENT[3] Cardiology	❑ ❑ ❑ ❑ ❑
4 years / / Influenza[3] ❑ Pneumovax[3] ❑ Dentist ❑	Audiology Total/ionized Ca BUN, creatinine Urinalysis, BP	❑ ❑ ❑ ❑	Nutrition	❑	Family support[4] Preschool program[5] Ophthalmology[3]	❑ ❑ ❑ ❑
5 years / / DTaP, IPV[1] ❑ MMR[1] ❑	Audiology Total/ionized Ca BUN, creatinine Urinalysis, BP	❑ ❑ ❑ ❑	Nutrition	❑	School transition[5] Cardiology[3] Developmental pediatrics Genetics	❑ ❑ ❑ ❑
6 years / / DTaP, IPV[1] ❑ MMR[1] ❑ Dentist ❑	Hearing, vision[3] Total/ionized Ca BUN, creatinine Urinalysis, BP	❑ ❑ ❑ ❑	School progress Nutrition Scoliosis Behavior	❑ ❑ ❑ ❑	Family support[4] Ophthalmology[3] ENT[3]	❑ ❑ ❑

Clinical concerns for Williams syndrome, ages 1–6 years

Feeding problems	Aortic stenosis	Developmental disability
Growth failure	Dental anomalies	Speech delay
Eye anomalies (strabismus)	Renal arterial stenosis	Behavior problems
Chronic otitis, hearing loss	Urinary tract anomalies	Hyperactivity

Guidelines for prior ages should be undertaken *at the time of diagnosis*; Ca, calcium; BP, blood pressure; [1]alternative timing; [2]by practitioner; [3]as dictated by clinical findings; [4]parent group, family/sib, financial, and behavioral issues as discussed in the preface; [5]including developmental monitoring and motor/speech therapy.

Williams syndrome

Preventive medical checklist (6+ yrs)

Patient   **Birth Date**   /   /   **Number**

Pediatric	Screen	Evaluate	Refer/Counsel
8 years / / *Dentist* ☐	Total/ionized Ca ☐ BUN, creatinine ☐ Urinalysis, BP ☐	Scoliosis ☐ Behavior ☐	Family support[4] ☐ School options ☐ Cardiology[3] ☐ Endocrinology[3] ☐
10 years / /	Hearing, vision[2] ☐ Total/ionized Ca ☐ BUN, creatinine ☐ Urinalysis, BP ☐	School progress ☐ Scoliosis ☐ Behavior ☐	Ophthalmology ☐ ENT[3] ☐ Endocrinology[3] ☐
12 years / / *Td[1], MMR, Var* ☐ *CBC* ☐ *Dentist* ☐ *Scoliosis* ☐ *Cholesterol* ☐	Hearing, vision[2] ☐ Total/ionized Ca ☐ BUN, creatinine ☐ Urinalysis, BP ☐ Renal sonogram ☐	Puberty ☐ Behavior ☐	Family support[4] ☐ School options ☐ Developmental pediatrics ☐ Genetics ☐ Cardiology[3] ☐ Endocrinology[3] ☐
14 years / / *CBC* ☐ *Dentist* ☐ *Cholesterol* ☐ *Breast CA* ☐ *Testicular CA* ☐	Hearing, vision[2] ☐ Total/ionized Ca ☐ BUN, creatinine ☐ Urinalysis, BP ☐	School progress ☐ Puberty ☐ Scoliosis ☐ Behavior ☐	Endocrinology[3] ☐
16 years / / *Td[1]* ☐ *CBC* ☐ *Cholesterol* ☐ *Sexual[5]* ☐ *Dentist* ☐	Hearing, vision[2] ☐ Total/ionized Ca ☐ BUN, creatinine ☐ Urinalysis, BP ☐	Puberty ☐ Scoliosis ☐ Behavior ☐	Developmental pediatrics ☐ Genetics ☐ Vocational planning ☐ Cardiology[3] ☐
18 years / / *CBC* ☐ *Sexual[5]* ☐ *Cholesterol* ☐ *Scoliosis* ☐	Hearing, vision[2] ☐ Total/ionized Ca ☐ BUN, creatinine ☐ Urinalysis, BP ☐	School progress ☐ Behavior ☐	Vocational planning ☐
20 years[6] / / *CBC* ☐ *Sexual[5]* ☐ *Cholesterol* ☐ *Dentist* ☐	Hearing, vision[3] ☐ Total/ionized Ca ☐ BUN, creatinine ☐ Urinalysis, BP ☐	Behavior ☐ Work, residence ☐	Family support[4] ☐ Genetics clinic ☐ Cardiology[3] ☐

Clinical concerns for Williams syndrome, ages 6+ years

Peptic ulcer	Hypercalcemia	Cognitive disability
Cholelithiasis	Mitral valve prolapse	Short stature, obesity
Hypertension	Scoliosis	Behaviour problems
Renal failure	Urinary tract infections	Diabetes mellitus

Guidelines for prior ages should be undertaken *at the time of diagnosis*; Td, tetanus/diphtheria; Var, varicella; Ca, calcium; BP blood pressure; [1]alternative timing; [2]by practitioner; [3]as dictated by clinical findings; [4]parent group, family/sib, financial, and behavioral issues as discussed in the preface; [5]birth control, STD screening if sexually active; [6]repeat every decade.

Preventive Management of Prader–Willi syndrome

Clinical diagnosis: Pattern of manifestations including neonatal hypotonia and hypogonadism with later hyperphagia, obesity, and mental disability. A characteristic appearance may develop with almond-shaped palpebral fissures, down-turned corners of the mouth, small hands and feet.

Incidence: 1 in 16,000–25,000 live births.

Laboratory diagnosis: Chromosome and DNA diagnosis demonstrating microdeletion of band 15q13q15 (~60% of patients), maternal origin of both chromosomes 15 (uniparental disomy, ~25%), or defective DNA methylation (~5%). The latter test is positive for all three categories.

Genetics: Deletion, uniparental disomy, or defective DNA methylation are sporadic events with a low recurrence risk for parents of affected children.

Key management issues: Monitoring for eye, nutritional, motor, sleep apnea, cognitive, and behavioral problems. Emphasis on weight management is most important in order to avoid morbidity and early mortality from obesity.

Growth charts: Butler and Meaney (1991).

Parent groups: Prader–Willi Foundation, 223 Main Street, Port Washington NY, 11050, Prader–Willi Association, 2510 S. Brentwood Blvd.Suite 220, St. Louis MO,63144,Ontario Prader–Willi Syndrome Association,1910 Yonge St. 4th Floor,Toronto ON,Canada, M4S 3B2; Prader–Willi Syndrome Association (UK), 33 Leopold Street, Derby DE1 2HF, England, http://www.pwsa-uk.demon.co.uk/

Basis for management recommendations: Complications documented below as drawn from Cassidy (1987), Clarke (1993).

Summary of clinical concerns

General	Learning	**Cognitive disability** – normal/borderline (40%), mild (41%), moderate (12%); **learning and speech problems** (100%)
	Behavior	Behavior problems (hyperphagia, food foraging, manipulative behavior, tantrums, outbursts), psychoses, poor self image, poor social acceptance
	Growth	**Short stature**, **morbid obesity**, inactivity, decreased exercise
	Tumors	Leukemia (rare)
Facial	Eye	Myopia (25%), strabismus (40–95%)
	Mouth	**Decreased saliva**, **dental malocclusion** (40%), **increased caries** (44%)
Surface	Epidermal	Decreased pain sensitivity, **albinism** (50%), skin picking, cellulitis, scarring
Skeletal	Cranial	**Microcephaly**
	Limbs	Club foot (6%), hip dislocation (9%), osteoporosis
Internal	Pulmonary	Respiratory problems, sleep apnea, anesthesia precautions
	Circulatory	Congestive heart failure due to morbid obesity
	Endocrine	**Hypothalamic dysfunction**, diabetes mellitus (5–10%), **insulin requirement** (66%)
	Genital	Hypogonadism, cryptorchidism (80%), micropenis, labial hypoplasia, dysmenorrhea, male and female infertility
Neural	CNS	Sleep disorders – 50%, including daytime somnulence (50%), snoring (45%), restless sleep (40%), cataplexy (15%), sleep apnea; seizures (16–20%)
	Motor	Hypotonia, decreased muscle mass, weakness, inactivity
	Sensory	Misrouting of retinal-ganglion fibers, visual deficits

RES, reticuloendothelial system, GI, gastrointestinal system; **bold: frequency > 20%**

Key references

Butler, M.G. & Meaney, F.J. (1991). *Pediatrics* 88:853–60.
Cassidy, S. B. (1987). *Alabama Journal of Medical Sciences* 24:169–75.
Clarke, D. J. (1993). *British Journal of Psychiatry* 163:680–4.
Greenswag, L. R. (1987). *Developmental Medicine and Child Neurology* 29:145–52.
Zellweger, H. & Schneider H. J. (1968). *American Journal of Diseases of Children* 5:588–98.

Prader–Willi syndrome

Preventive medical checklist (0–1yr)

Patient   **Birth Date** / /   **Number**

Pediatric	Screen	Evaluate	Refer/Counsel
Neonatal / / *Newborn screen* ❑ *HB* ❑	Karyotype ❑	Feeding problem ❑ Constipation ❑	Feeding specialist[3] ❑ Genetic evaluation ❑
1 month / /		Feeding problem ❑ Constipation ❑	Family support[4] ❑ Feeding specialist[3] ❑
2 months / / *HB* ❑ *Hib* ❑ *DTaP, IPV* ❑ *RV* ❑	Growth ❑ Hearing, vision[2] ❑	Feeding problem ❑ Constipation ❑	Early intervention[5] ❑ Feeding specialist[3] ❑ Developmental pediatrician ❑ Genetic counseling ❑
4 months / / *HB[1]* ❑ *Hib* ❑ *DTaP/IPV* ❑ *RV* ❑	Growth ❑ Hearing, vision[2] ❑	Feeding problem ❑ Constipation ❑ Strabismus ❑	Early intervention[5] ❑
6 months / / *Hib* ❑ *IPV[1]* ❑ *DTaP* ❑ *RV* ❑	Growth ❑ Hearing, vision[2] ❑	Feeding problem ❑ Constipation ❑ Strabismus ❑	Family support[4] ❑
9 months / / *IPV[1]* ❑	Audiology ❑	Feeding problem ❑ Constipation ❑ Strabismus ❑	Ophthalmology ❑
1 year / / *HB* ❑ *Hib[1]* ❑ *IPV[1]* ❑ *MMR[1]* ❑ *Var[1]* ❑	Growth ❑ Hearing, vision[2] ❑	Feeding ❑ Salivation ❑ Strabismus ❑ Sleep apnea ❑	Family support[4] ❑ Early intervention[5] ❑ Dietician ❑ Developmental pediatrics ❑ Genetics ❑

Clinical concerns for Prader–Willi syndrome, ages 0–1 year

Poor feeding (infancy)   Hyperphagia (>2 years)   Developmental disability
Eye anomalies (strabismus)   Sleep apnea   Hypotonia
Decreased salivation   Cryptorchidism, micropenis   Speech delay
Dental anomalies   Behavioral problems

Guidelines for the neonatal period should be undertaken *at whatever age* the diagnosis is made; DTaP, acellular DTP; IPV, inactivated poliovirus (oral polio also used); RV, rotavirus; MMR, measles–mumps–rubella; Var, varicella; [1]alternative timing; [2]by practitioner; [3]as dictated by clinical findings; [4]parent group, family/sib, financial, and behavioral issues as discussed in the preface; [5]including developmental monitoring and motor/speech therapy.

Prader–Willi syndrome

Preventive medical checklist (15m–6yrs)

Patient _____ **Birth Date** / / **Number** _____

Pediatric	Screen		Evaluate		Refer/Counsel	
15 months / / *Hib[1]* ❏ *MMR[1]* ❏ *DTaP, IPV[1]* ❏ *Varicella[1]* ❏			Feeding Strabismus	❏ ❏	Family support[4] Early intervention[5]	❏ ❏
18 months / / *DTaP, IPV[1]* ❏ *Varicella[1]* ❏ *Influenza[3]* ❏	Growth Hearing, vision[2]	❏ ❏	Feeding Strabismus	❏ ❏	Ophthalmology	❏
2 years / / *Influenza[3]* ❏ *Pneumovax[3]* ❏ *Dentist* ❏	Growth Audiology	❏ ❏	Feeding Salivation Strabismus Sleep apnea	❏ ❏ ❏ ❏	Family support[4] Dietician Dentistry Genetics	❏ ❏ ❏ ❏
3 years / / *Influenza[3]* ❏ *Pneumovax[3]* ❏ *Dentist* ❏	Growth Audiology	❏ ❏	Feeding Salivation Strabismus Sleep apnea	❏ ❏ ❏ ❏	Family support[4] Preschool transition[5] Dietician Ophthalmology[3]	❏ ❏ ❏ ❏
4 years / / *Influenza[3]* ❏ *Pneumovax[3]* ❏ *Dentist* ❏	Growth Hearing, vision[2]	❏ ❏	Salivation Feeding Obesity	❏ ❏ ❏	Family support[4] Preschool program[5] Dietician Developmental pediatrics Genetics	❏ ❏ ❏ ❏ ❏
5 years / / *DTaP, IPV[1]* ❏ *MMR[1]* ❏	Growth	❏	Salivation Feeding Obesity	❏ ❏ ❏	School transition[5] Dietician Ophthalmology[3]	❏ ❏ ❏
6 years / / *DTaP, IPV[1]* ❏ *MMR[1]* ❏ *Dentist* ❏	Growth Hearing, vision[2]	❏ ❏	School progress Salivation Obesity Phallus size	❏ ❏ ❏ ❏	Family support[4] Dietician Developmental pediatrics Genetics	❏ ❏ ❏ ❏

Clinical concerns for Prader–Willi syndrome, ages 1–6 years

Poor feeding (infancy)	Hyperphagia (>2 years)	Developmental disability
Eye anomalies (strabismus)	Sleep apnea	Hypotonia
Decreased salivation	Cryptorchidism, micropenis	Speech delay
Dental anomalies		Behavioral problems

Guidelines for prior ages should be undertaken *at the time of diagnosis*; DtaP, acellular DTP; IPV, inactivated poliovirus (oral polio also used); MMR, measles–mumps–rubella; [1]alternative timing; [2]by practitioner; [3]as dictated by clinical findings; [4]parent group, family/sib, financial, and behavioral issues as discussed in the preface; [5]including developmental monitoring and motor/speech therapy.

Prader–Willi syndrome

Preventive medical checklist (6+ yrs)

Patient   **Birth Date** / / **Number**

Pediatric	Screen		Evaluate		Refer/Counsel	
8 years / / *Dentist* ☐	Growth	☐	Obesity Puberty Salivation Scoliosis	☐ ☐ ☐ ☐	School options Dietician Developmental pediatrics Genetics Endocrinology[6]	☐ ☐ ☐ ☐ ☐
10 years / /	Growth Hearing, vision[2]	☐ ☐	School progress Obesity Puberty Sleep apnea	☐ ☐ ☐ ☐	Dietician Activities, exercise Ophthalmology[3] Endocrinology[6]	☐ ☐ ☐ ☐
12 years / / *Td[1], MMR, Var* ☐ *CBC* ☐ *Dentist* ☐ *Scoliosis* ☐ *Cholesterol* ☐	Growth	☐	Puberty Phallus size Behavior	☐ ☐ ☐	Family support[4] School options Dietician Endocrinology[6] Developmental pediatrics Genetics	☐ ☐ ☐ ☐ ☐ ☐
14 years / / *CBC* ☐ *Dentist* ☐ *Cholesterol* ☐ *Breast CA* ☐ *Testicular CA* ☐	Growth Hearing, vision[2]	☐ ☐	School progress Puberty Phallus size Behavior	☐ ☐ ☐ ☐	Dietician Activities, exercise Endocrinology[6]	☐ ☐ ☐
16 years / / *Td[1]* ☐ *CBC* ☐ *Cholesterol* ☐ *Sexual[5]* ☐ *Dentist* ☐	Growth Hearing, vision[2]	☐ ☐	Behavior	☐	Vocational planning Dietician Developmental pediatrics Genetics Ophthalmology[3]	☐ ☐ ☐ ☐ ☐
18 years / / *CBC* ☐ *Sexual[5]* ☐ *Cholesterol* ☐ *Scoliosis* ☐	Growth Hearing, vision[2]	☐ ☐	Sleep apnea Behavior Cellulitis	☐ ☐ ☐	Vocational planning Dietician	☐ ☐
20 years[7] / / *CBC* ☐ *Sexual[5]* ☐ *Cholesterol* ☐ *Dentist* ☐	Growth Hearing, vision[3]	☐ ☐	Sleep apnea Behavior Cellulitis Work, residence	☐ ☐ ☐ ☐	Family support[4] Dietician Activities, exercise Endocrinology[6] Ophthalmology[3]	☐ ☐ ☐ ☐ ☐

Clinical concerns for Prader–Willi syndrome, ages 6+ years

Eye anomalies (myopia)	Short stature	Cognitive disability
Skin picking, cellulitis	Low testosterone, estradiol	Obesity
Scoliosis	Cryptorchidism, micropenis	Behavior problems
Osteoporosis	Clitorial, labial hypoplasia	Sleep apnea

Guidelines for prior ages should be undertaken *at the time of diagnosis*; Td, tetanus/diphtheria; MMR, measles–mumps–rubella; Var, varicella; [1]alternative timing; [2]by practitioner; [3]as dictated by clinical findings; [4]parent group, family/sib, financial, and behavioral issues as discussed in the preface; [5]birth control, STD screening if sexually active; [6]for consideration of growth hormone therapy, testosterone or estradiol supplementation; [7]repeat every decade.

Preventive Management of Shprintzen/Del(22q11) Spectrum

Clinical diagnosis: Pattern of manifestations including long face, narrow palpebral fissures, ear anomalies, velopalatine incompetence, cardiac anomalies, absent thymus and hypoparathyroidism due to DiGeorge anomaly, long and thin fingers, genital anomalies, speech and developmental disability. Adults may present with psychiatric disease.

Laboratory diagnosis: Deletion of band 22q11 demonstrated by FISH technology.

Incidence: Approximately 1 in 25,000 live births (some patients probably unrecognized).

Genetics: Sporadic inheritance with rare cases of parent–child transmission.

Key management issues: Neonatal feeding problems and cardiac anomalies, developmental disability with speech problems.

Growth charts: None available.

Parent groups: Velo-Cardio-Facial Syndrome Parent Support Group, 110-45 Queens Blvd., Forest Hills NY, 11375-5501, (718) 261-8049; Northeast VCFS Support Group, 2 Lansing Dr., Salem NH, 03079, (603) 898-6332, MLADJA@aol.com

Basis for management recommendations: Derived from the complications listed below as documented by Goldberg et al. (1993), Gorlin et al. (1990, pp. 740–42), Lipson et al. (1991).

Summary of clinical concerns

General	Learning	**Cognitive disability** (40% – verbal IQ 69–87, performance IQ 55–78), learning differences (99%), speech problems (nasality, articulation)
	Behavior	Behavior problems (bland affect, impulsive behavior, phobias, psychoses)
	Growth	Dysphagia, failure to thrive (25%), short stature (33–35%)
Facial	Eye	**Suborbital swelling** (35%), cataracts, colobomata (3%), blue sclerae, **tortuous retinal vessels** (35–50%)
	Ear	**Small auricles** (60%), **chronic otitis** (75%)
	Nose	Narrow choanae (75%)
	Mouth	**Cleft palate** (35%), submucous cleft palate, **velar paresis** (33%), **hypotonic pharynx** (90%), Robin sequence (17%), dental malocclusion
Surface	Neck/trunk	**Umbilical hernia** (23%), **inguinal hernia** (30%)
Skeletal	Cranial	**Microcephaly** (40%)
	Axial	Scoliosis (15%)
	Limbs	**Slender digits** (60%), increased joint laxity, club feet
Internal	Digestive	Gastroesophageal reflux, **aspiration** (90%), dysphagia
	Pulmonary	Stridor (vascular rings, laryngeal webs, laryngeal clefts)
	Circulatory	**Cardiac anomalies** (82% – ventricular septal defects, right-sided aortic arch, tetralogy of Fallot), Raynaud's phenomenon
	Endocrine	Hypocalcemia (10%)*, hypothyroidism
	RES	Thymic aplasia (10%)*, immune deficiency (10%)*
	Excretory	Ureteral reflux (10%)
	Genital	Hypospadias (10%), cryptorchidism
Neural	CNS	Seizures, cognitive disability
	Sensory	**Chronic otitis, conductive hearing loss** (75%), visual deficits

*particularly if DiGeorge present, RES, reticuloendothelial system; **bold**: frequency > 20%

Key references

Goldberg, R., Motzkin, B, Marion, R., et al. (1993). *American Journal of Medical Genetics* 45:313–19.

Gorlin, R. J., Cohen, M. M., Jr. & Levin, L. S. (1990). *Syndromes of the Head and Neck*, 3rd edn.

Lipson, A. H., Yuille, D., Angel, M., et al. (1991). *Journal of Medical Genetics* 28:596–604.

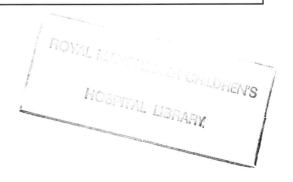

Shprintzen/Del(22q) Spectrum

Preventive medical checklist (0–1yr)

Patient		Birth Date / /	Number

Pediatric	Screen	Evaluate	Refer/Counsel
Neonatal / / *Newborn screen* ❑ HB ❑ [Modify for DiGeorge]	Chest x-ray ❑ Ca, P, WBC ❑ Karyotype ❑	Cataracts ❑ Dysphagia ❑ GE reflux ❑ Apnea, stridor ❑	Genetic evaluation ❑ Craniofacial team ❑ Feeding specialist[3] ❑
1 month / /	Cardiac echo ❑	Feeding ❑ Apnea, stridor ❑ Sleep apnea ❑	Family support[4] ❑ Cardiology ❑
2 months / / HB[1] ❑ Hib ❑ DTaP, IPV ❑ RV ❑	Growth ❑ Hearing, vision[2] ❑	Feeding ❑ Otitis ❑ Cataracts ❑	Early intervention[5] ❑ Developmental pediatrics ❑ Genetic counseling ❑ Gastroenterology[3] ❑ Dietician[3] ❑
4 months / / HB[1] ❑ Hib ❑ DTaP/IPV ❑ RV ❑	Growth ❑ Hearing, vision[2] ❑	Feeding ❑ Otitis ❑	Early intervention[5] ❑ ENT[3] ❑
6 months / / Hib ❑ IPV[1] ❑ DTaP ❑ RV ❑	Growth ❑ Hearing, vision[2] ❑	Feeding ❑ Otitis ❑ Sleep apnea ❑	Family support[4] ❑
9 months / / IPV[1] ❑	Growth ❑ Hearing, vision[2] ❑	Feeding ❑ Otitis ❑ Sleep apnea ❑	Family support[4] ❑
1 year / / HB ❑ Hib[1] ❑ IPV[1] ❑ MMR[1] ❑ Var[1] ❑	Growth ❑ Hearing, vision[2] ❑	Feeding ❑ Otitis ❑ Sleep apnea ❑ Immunity ❑	Family support[4] ❑ Early intervention[5] ❑ Developmental pediatrics ❑ Genetics ❑ Craniofacial team ❑

Clinical concerns for Shprintzen/Del(22q) Spectrum, ages 0–1 year

Dysphagia, failure to thrive	DiGeorge anomaly	Developmental disability
Eye anomalies (coloboma)	T-cell deficiency	Speech delay, nasal speech
Chronic otitis, hearing loss	Cardiac anomalies	Microcephaly, seizures
Dental anomalies	Obstructive sleep apnea	Ureteral reflux
Cleft palate, velar paresis	Laryngeal webs, clefts	Scoliosis

Guidelines for the neonatal period should be undertaken *at whatever age* the diagnosis is made; DTaP, acellular DTP; IPV, inactivated poliovirus (oral polio also used); RV, rotavirus; MMR, measles–mumps–rubella; Var, varicella; [1]alternative timing; [2]by practitioner; [3]as dictated by clinical findings; [4]parent group, family/sib, financial, and behavioral issues as discussed in the preface; [5]including developmental monitoring and motor/speech therapy.

Shprintzen/Del(22q) Spectrum

Preventive medical checklist (15m–6yrs)

Patient   **Birth Date** / /   **Number**

Pediatric	Screen	Evaluate		Refer/Counsel	
15 months / / Hib[1] ☐ MMR[1] ☐ DTaP, IPV[1] ☐ Varicella[1] ☐		Feeding Strabismus	☐ ☐	Family support[4] Early intervention[5]	☐ ☐
18 months / / DTaP, IPV[1] ☐ Varicella[1] ☐ Influenza[3] ☐		Feeding	☐	Nutritionist[3] ENT[3]	☐ ☐
2 years / / Influenza[3] ☐ Pneumovax[3] ☐ Dentist ☐	Growth ☐ Audiology ☐	Feeding Nutrition Sleep apnea Immunity	☐ ☐ ☐ ☐	Family support[4] Developmental pediatrics Genetics Craniofacial team Ophthalmology	☐ ☐ ☐ ☐ ☐
3 years / / Influenza[3] ☐ Pneumovax[3] ☐ Dentist ☐	Growth ☐ Audiology ☐ Urinalysis, BP ☐	Feeding Nutrition	☐ ☐	Family support[4] Preschool transition[5] Genetics Craniofacial team	☐ ☐ ☐ ☐
4 years / / Influenza[3] ☐ Pneumovax[3] ☐ Dentist ☐	Hearing, vision[2] ☐	Feeding Nutrition	☐ ☐	Family support[4] Preschool program[5] Ophthalmology	☐ ☐ ☐
5 years / / DTaP, IPV[1] ☐ MMR[1] ☐	Growth ☐ Audiology ☐ Urinalysis, BP ☐	Feeding Nutrition	☐ ☐	School transition[5] Genetics Craniofacial team	☐ ☐ ☐
6 years / / DTaP, IPV[1] ☐ MMR[1] ☐ Dentist ☐	Growth ☐ Hearing, vision[2] ☐	School progress Feeding Nutrition	☐ ☐ ☐	Family support[4] Ophthalmology ENT[3]	☐ ☐ ☐

Clinical concerns for Shprintzen/Del(22q) Spectrum, ages 1–6 years

Dysphagia, failure to thrive Chronic otitis, hearing loss Dental anomalies Cleft palate, velar paresis	T-cell deficiency Cardiac anomalies Obstructive sleep apnea Scoliosis	Developmental disability Speech delay, nasal speech Microcephaly, seizures Ureteral reflux

Guidelines for prior ages should be undertaken *at the time of diagnosis*; DTaP, acellular DTP; IPV, inactivated poliovirus (oral polio also used); MMR, measles–mumps–rubella; [1]alternative timing; [2]by practitioner; [3]as dictated by clinical findings; [4]parent group, family/sib, financial, and behavioral issues as discussed in the preface; [5]including developmental monitoring and motor/speech therapy.

Shprintzen/Del(22q) Spectrum

Preventive medical checklist (6+ yrs)

Patient   **Birth Date** / /   **Number**

Pediatric	Screen	Evaluate		Refer/Counsel	
8 years / / *Dentist* ❑	Growth ❑ Urinalysis, BP ❑			School options ❑ Developmental pediatrics ❑ Genetics ❑ Craniofacial team ❑	
10 years / /	Hearing, vision[2] ❑	School progress ❑ Scoliosis ❑		Ophthalmology ❑ ENT[3] ❑	
12 years / / *Td[1], MMR, Var* ❑ *CBC* ❑ *Dentist* ❑ *Scoliosis* ❑ *Cholesterol* ❑	Urinalysis, BP ❑	Puberty ❑ Behavior ❑		Family support[4] ❑ School options ❑ Developmental pediatrics ❑ Genetics ❑	
14 years / / *CBC* ❑ *Dentist* ❑ *Cholesterol* ❑ *Breast CA* ❑ *Testicular CA* ❑	Hearing, vision[2] ❑	School progress ❑ Puberty ❑ Behavior ❑ Scoliosis ❑		Craniofacial team ❑	
16 years / / *Td[1]* ❑ *CBC* ❑ *Cholesterol* ❑ *Sexual[5]* ❑ *Dentist* ❑	Hearing, vision[2] ❑ Urinalysis, BP ❑	Puberty ❑ Behavior ❑		Vocational planning ❑ Developmental pediatrics ❑ Genetics ❑	
18 years / / *CBC* ❑ *Sexual[5]* ❑ *Cholesterol* ❑ *Scoliosis* ❑	Hearing, vision[2] ❑	School progress ❑ Behavior ❑		Vocational planning ❑ Craniofacial team ❑ Psychiatry[3] ❑	
20 years[6] / / *CBC* ❑ *Sexual[5]* ❑ *Cholesterol* ❑ *Dentist* ❑	Hearing, vision[3] ❑ Urinalysis, BP ❑	Behavior ❑ Work, residence ❑		Family support[4] ❑ Psychiatry[3] ❑	

Clinical concerns for Shprintzen/Del(22q) Spectrum, ages 6+ years

Short stature	T-cell deficiency	Cognitive disability
Dental anomalies	Cardiac anomalies	Learning differences
Cleft palate, velar paresis	Ureteral reflux	Speech delay, nasal speech
Microcephaly, seizures	Scoliosis	Behavioral problems

Guidelines for prior ages should be undertaken *at the time of diagnosis*; Td, tetanus/diphtheria; MMR, measles–mumps–rubella; Var, varicella; [1]alternative timing; [2]by practitioner; [3]as dictated by clinical findings; [4]parent group, family/sib, financial, and behavioral issues as discussed in the preface; [5]birth control, STD screening if sexually active; [6]repeat every decade.

Part IV

Syndromes remarkable for altered growth

Syndromes with proportionate growth failure as a primary feature

Stature or length, limb segments, and head circumference are proportionate in symmetrical or harmonic growth failure, and disproportionate in asymmetrical or dysharmonic dwarfism. Disproportion of the head, thorax, or limbs often suggests a skeletal dysplasia as will be discussed in Chapter 11. Proportionate growth failure of stature and limbs may be accompanied by a slightly larger head circumference in nutritional deficiencies ("head sparing") or by a slightly smaller head circumference in some congenital syndromes. Table 10.1 summarizes various syndromes with proportionate growth failure, classifying them by time of onset (prenatal and/or postnatal) and by accompanying changes in head circumference (with or without microcephaly).

Syndromes with symmetrical intrauterine growth retardation include many chromosomal and teratogenic syndromes discussed in Chapters 5–7. Intrauterine growth retardation is a harbinger for congenital disease, and a thorough investigation of maternal health, gestational history, and the fetal karyotype is often indicated. Once disorders such as fetal alcohol syndrome, cri-du-chat syndrome, and trisomy 13/18 are excluded by physical and laboratory findings, the clinician should begin considering syndromes with primary growth failure. Since isolated fetal disease (e.g., cardiac anomaly, renal anomaly) rarely produces intrauterine growth failure, a more global process must be suspected. Table 10.1 lists the more common syndromes with growth failure that do not involve obvious karyotypic changes. These disorders will exhibit proportionately small birth measurements and/or symmetrical failure to thrive. Any clinician concerned about shortened limbs, small thorax, frontal bossing with a shallow nasal bridge, or certain skeletal anomalies should obtain a skeletal radiographic survey to evaluate the possibility of a skeletal dysplasia (dwarfism – see Chapter 11).

Follow-up may be necessary to recognize many of the primordial growth failure syndromes listed in Table 10.1. Children with the Russell–Silver, Donohue, Dubowitz, Niikawa, Seckel, or Williams syndrome may not exhibit obvious dysmorphology in the neonatal nursery. Many of the conditions have early feeding problems that may mask the underlying syndrome while gastrointestinal disorders

Table 10.1 Syndromes with growth failure

Syndrome	Incidence	Frequent abnormalities
Syndromes with prenatal growth retardation, normocephaly		
Russell–Silver	~150 cases	Facial, skeletal, renal, genital
Donohue (Leprechaunism)	~30 cases	Facial, epidermal, endocrine, genital
Syndromes with prenatal growth retardation, microcephaly		
Bloom	~130 cases	Facial, vascular, epidermal, skeletal, immune
Dubowitz	~30 cases	Facial, ocular, dental, skeletal, epidermal
Seckel	~30 cases	Ocular, dental, skeletal, genital
Smith–Lemli–Opitz	~50 cases	Facial, ocular, cardiac, GI, skeletal, genital
Syndromes with postnatal growth retardation, normocephaly		
Aarskog	~100 cases	Facial, skeletal, genital
Costello	~50 cases	Facial, cardiac, dental, epidermal
Noonan	1 in 2500 live births	Facial, ocular, dental, cardiac, skeletal, genital
Robinow	~50 cases	Facial, skeletal, genital
Syndromes with postnatal growth retardation, microcephaly		
Brachmann–de Lange	1 in 10,000 live births	Facial, ocular, cardiac, skeletal, GI, immune
Hallermann–Streiff	~150 cases	Facial, ocular, dental, skeletal, genital, epidermal
Niikawa–Kuroki	~150 cases	Facial, cardiac, skeletal, genitourinary
Rubinstein–Taybi	~600 cases	Facial, ocular, cardiac, skeletal, genital
Williams	1 in 25,000 live births	Facial, ocular, dental, cardiac, renal, genital

Note:
GI, gastrointestinal.

are evaluated. Some premature infants may be confused with small-for-gestational-age babies until catch-up growth is documented. Hand radiographs to evaluate the bone age may be helpful in evaluating older infants and toddlers with growth failure, since the bone age may be extremely delayed in endocrine problems such as hypothyroidism or growth hormone deficiency. By age 2–3 years, the evolution of dysmorphology, the presence of developmental delay, the accentuation of microcephaly, or the lack of catch-up growth should identify the child with a primary growth failure syndrome.

Rarer disorders

Of the disorders with growth failure listed in Table 10.1, most, like the Rubinstein–Taybi syndrome, are rare and will be discussed briefly. Brachmann–de Lange and Noonan syndromes are sufficiently common to warrant detailed preventive management (discussed later in this chapter). The Williams syndrome has been associated with a chromosome microdeletion, as was discussed in Chapter 9; Smith–Lemli–Opitz syndrome will be discussed in Chapter 19.

Bloom syndrome

Bloom syndrome was first described in 1954 as "congenital telangiectatic erythema resembling lupus erythematosus in dwarfs." This autosomal recessive syndrome involves pre- and postnatal growth retardation, mild microcephaly, immune deficiency, male hypogonadism, and sensitivity to sunlight producing erythematous malar and upper limb telangiectasia (Gorlin et al., 1990, pp. 297–8; German, 1993; Auerbach & Verlander, 1997; Jones, 1997, pp. 104–5). Chromosomal studies show a high rate of exchange between sister chromatids and breakage leading to unusual rearranged chromosomes. The chromosomal changes are diagnostic, and probably explain the predilection for neoplasia in patients with Bloom syndrome. Over 90 percent of neoplasms are malignant, with squamous and basal cell carcinomas, leukemias, lymphomas, adenocarcinomas of the gut or breast, and Wilms tumors being most frequent (German, 1993). Definition of the syndrome has been aided by the establishment of an international registry (German & Passarge, 1987). The syndrome exhibits autosomal recessive inheritance, with a 25 percent recurrence risk of parents of affected children. The causative BKM gene has been isolated and its product is located in the cell nucleus (Auerbach & Verlander, 1997).

Preventive management for Bloom syndrome will include monitoring of growth and stringent protection from the sun. Two patients had documented growth hormone deficiency and one responded to exogenous growth hormone (Gorlin et al., 1990, p. 299). Patients with frequent infections may have deficient immunoglobulins (IgA, IgG, or IgM) and may be candidates for gamma-globulin injections. Chronic upper respiratory infections often require otolaryngology involvement (Wong & Hashisaki, 1996). Occasional cardiac anomalies or skeletal anomalies such as unequal leg lengths, congenital hip dislocation, or club feet warrant surveillance during regular pediatric visits. Hypogonadism including small or undescended testes in males and menstrual irregularities in females may require evaluation during puberty, and diabetes mellitus has occurred in about 10 percent of adolescents and adults (German & Passarge, 1989). Most of the 61 cancers that appeared in 57 of 132 registered patients with Bloom syndrome had early onset, so prompt investigation of masses, ulcerated or pigmented skin lesions, anemias, bone or joint pain, asymmetric growth, or unusual gastrointestinal symptoms is essential. Mapping of the causative gene to chromosome band 15q26.1 (German et al., 1994) offers hope that a specific proto-oncogene may be characterized that will be useful for premalignant diagnosis.

Costello syndrome

Initially described in 1977 by Costello, the pattern of manifestations includes normal birth weight with subsequent short stature, normal or large head circumference, skin findings such as papillomas and acanthosis nigricans, curly hair, and joint laxity (Jones, 1997, pp. 124–5; Johnson et al., 1998; Sigaudy, 1998). The syndrome has similarities to Noonan syndrome in its facial appearance, short stature, and increased frequency of cardiomyopathies. Inheritance is autosomal dominant with most cases being sporadic (i.e., new mutations). Preventive management concerns will include early intervention for developmental delays (mean IQ 50–60) and feeding problems, assessments for congenital heart disease (pulmonic stenosis, ventricular septal defects) or arrythmias, and awareness of connective tissue laxity with monitoring for flat feet, joint dislocations, and mitral valve prolapse (Johnson et al., 1998).

Donohue syndrome (Leprechaunism)

Initially described in 1948, this autosomal recessive syndrome of pre- and postnatal growth, decreased subcutaneous tissue, hirsutism, nail hypoplasia, and genital hypertrophy has now been attributed to homozygous deletion of the insulin receptor gene (Wertheimer et al., 1993; Kosztolanyi, 1997; Ozbey et al., 1998). Subcutaneous atrophy plus hyperinsulinism produces a coarse facies, hirsutism, and acanthosis nigricans of the skin. Survival is limited with over 60 percent of patients dying by age two. Preventive management includes evaluation for hypoglycemia, for skeletal anomalies (occipital bony defects, scoliosis, valgus deformities of the lower limbs), and for hepatic cholestasis or fibrosis. The muscle hypoplasia, delayed mental development, and orthopedic anomalies mandate early intervention, physical/occupational therapy, and rehabilitative services (Ozbey et al., 1998). Bilateral ovarian tumors were found in one patient (Brisigotti et al., 1993).

Dubowitz syndrome

Dubowitz syndrome was initially confused with Bloom syndrome until it was recognized as a separate entity in 1971 (Tsukahara & Opitz, 1996). Manifestations of pre- and postnatal growth failure, microcephaly, high-pitched voice, skin changes (eczematous), cancer predilection, and immune deficiency are shared with Bloom syndrome. Children with the Dubowitz syndrome have an unusual facial appearance, mental disability with hyperactivity, and infantile feeding problems with overt or submucous cleft palate in 35 percent (Tsukahara & Opitz, 1996; Winter, 1986). Progressive scoliosis (Soyer & McConnell, 1995) and achalasia (Nowicki & Peterson, 1998) have been reported. Dubowitz syndrome is autosomal recessive.

Preventive management for Dubowitz syndrome should include attention to early feeding, evaluation for hypospadias or cryptorchidism (70 percent of males), audiology and middle ear evaluations, and early childhood intervention to optimize potential in children with dull normal intelligence. Developmental disabilities include delayed speech (60 percent), and hyperactivity (40 percent; Gorlin et al., 1990, pp. 304–6). Neoplasms have included leukemia, lymphoma, and neuroblastoma. Peripheral blood cell counts should be obtained in children with infectious illnesses or fatigue, since aplastic anemias have also been described (Winter, 1986; Tsukahara et al., 1996).

Hallermann–Streiff syndrome

Although Hallermann in 1948 and Streiff in 1950 defined the syndrome as a separate entity, François established the diagnostic criteria of microcephaly, cataracts, microphthalmia, sparse hair, skin atrophy, and proportionate growth failure (Cohen, 1991). Mental disability occurs in about 15 percent, and complications include absent or malformed teeth, ocular anomalies (including cataracts and strabismus), narrow upper airway with respiratory embarrassment or obstructive sleep apnea, severe pulmonary infections, vertebral anomalies with scoliosis, hypoplastic genitalia, and cardiac anomalies (Cohen, 1991; Gorlin et al., 1990, pp. 307–9; Jones, pp. 110–11).

Preventive management for Hallermann–Streiff syndrome should concentrate initially on the upper airway and respiratory system. Altered nasopharyngeal anatomy may mandate early tracheostomy, and Cohen (1991) urged that any child with snoring and daytime somnolence have appropriate sleep studies. Anesthesia may be difficult, so rapid induction is not recommended unless the larynx is first visualized. Otolaryngologists should be available in case emergency tracheostomy is required during surgery, and patients should not be extubated until they are fully awake and functional (Cohen, 1991). Ophthalmology and audiology evaluations at age 8–10 months can probably be justified by the high rate of ocular and respiratory problems, and adolescent management should include inspection for genital hypoplasia and scoliosis. Aggressive investigation of upper respiratory infections is necessary because of the risk of sudden death from pulmonary infections.

Niikawa–Kuroki (Kabuki) syndrome

The Niikawa–Kuroki syndrome was described by two Japanese groups in 1981 (Kuroki et al., 1981; Niikawa et al., 1981). The characteristic was likened to a Kabuki theater mask because of the wide palpebral fissures, eversion of the lower eyelids, prominent ears, and down-turned corners of the mouth. Recognition of the malformation pattern in non-Asian patients prompted numerous reports in the literature (Meinecke & Rodewald, 1989; Schrander-Stumpel et al., 1994), and clinical experience suggests this condition to be more common than is suggested by the ~ 100 cases published to date (Wilson, 1998).

Characteristics of the syndrome in Occidental patients include postnatal growth retardation (80 percent), mental disability (86 percent), neonatal hypotonia (33 percent), seizures (29 percent), microcephaly (36 percent), congenital hip dislocation (21 percent), scoliosis (35 percent), chronic otitis (50 percent), cardiovascular anomaly (26–50 percent), urogenital anomaly (31 percent), and hearing loss (26–50 percent; Schrander-Stumpel et al., 1994; Wilson, 1998). Based on these frequencies of complications, preventive management for Niikawa–Kuroki syndrome should include an early echocardiogram and renal sonogram, evaluation for chronic otitis (including periodic audiology screening), evaluation for skeletal anomalies (including dislocated hip in infancy and scoliosis in adolescence), and early intervention/speech therapy services.

Robinow syndrome

Robinow syndrome involves short stature with an unusual "fetal" face, mesomelic shortening of the limbs, and genital anomalies (Butler & Wadlington, 1987). Affected children have a prominent forehead, wide palpebral fissures, hypertelorism, and micrognathia, which gave rise to the term "fetal face syndrome." Most children have a normal birth weight with mild delay in postnatal growth and adult short stature. Over 80 percent of patients have normal intellect (Butler & Wadlington, 1987; Gorlin et al., 1990, p. 798). Genital anomalies in males (micropenis, cryptorchidism) may be severe enough to present as ambiguous genitalia (Turken et al., 1996), but clinical examination should be sufficient for sex assignment. Other complications include dental (96 percent), vertebral (66 percent), rib (36 percent), renal (29 percent) and cardiac (6 percent) anomalies. One child had growth hormone deficiency (Kawai et al., 1997), and there have been complications with anesthesia (MacDonald & Dearlove, 1995). Preventive management should be directed toward dental care, early intervention in selected patients, and sonographic evaluation of the urinary tract during infancy. Care during anesthesia is warranted. Scoliosis (50 percent) and micropenis (94 percent) warrant evaluation during early puberty and adolescence, with provision for orthopedic or endocrine referral as needed.

Rubinstein–Taybi Syndrome

Rubinstein–Taybi syndrome is a sporadic disorder with an incidence of about 1 in 125,000 live births (Hennekam et al., 1993)). The syndrome is characterized by mental disability, unusual facies with a prominent nose, and broad thumbs and great toes (Gorlin et al., 1990, pp. 309–13). Following the clue of an unusual chromosome rearrangement, Hennekam et al. (1993) described a submicroscopic deletion at chromosome band 16p13.3 in 6 of 24 patients with Rubinstein–Taybi syndrome. Subsequently, a gene encoding a transcriptional regulatory protein was found to be deleted or mutated in Rubinstein–Taybi syndrome (McGaughran et al., 1996). The protein participates in cyclic AMP-regulated gene expression, but its relationship to the growth and developmental problems in Rubinstein–Taybi syndrome is not yet established.

Complications of Rubinstein–Taybi syndrome include a turbulent infantile course with feeding problems, constipation, and poor weight gain in 70–80 percent of patients (Stevens et al., 1990). The syndrome includes predisposition to eye anomalies (strabismus, cataracts, colobomata), upper respiratory infections with chronic otitis, and cardiac anomalies including septal defects, coarctation, and pulmonic stenosis (Stevens & Bhakta, 1995). There may be keloid formation (Hendrix & Greer, 1996), instability of the patellofemoral joints (Mehlman et al., 1998), and delayed recovery from anesthesia (Dunkley & Dearlove, 1996). The average IQ is 51, with seizures and abnormal behaviors being common. Adults may have urinary tract infections, constipation, scarring, and predisposition to tumors of the central nervous system (Miller & Rubinstein, 1995). Preventive management should include an early echocardiogram, frequent vision and hearing screens, surveillance for urinary tract infections, aggressive evaluation of respiratory infections, and neurologic referral for headaches or seizures. Early intervention and supportive services for children with mental disabilities and potential behavior/school problems are indicated.

Russell–Silver syndrome

Russell–Silver syndrome was described initially by Silver in 1953 and Russell in 1954. More than 150 cases of pre- and postnatal growth retardation with head sparing (pseudohydrocephaly), triangular facies, body asymmetry, urogenital anomalies, and precocious puberty or premature estrogenization of the vaginal mucosa have been reported (Patton, 1988; Gorlin et al., 1990, pp. 316–19). The dysmorphologic findings of prominent forehead, triangular face, fifth finger clinodactyly, and cafe-au-lait spots are nonspecific and perhaps best described as a Russell–Silver phenotype rather than a particular syndrome. Mild developmental delay or mental deficiency has been defined in about 35 percent (Patton, 1988; Gorlin et al., 1990, pp. 316–19). There is often catch-up growth later in life, so adult heights may be better than predicted.

Preventive management for Russell–Silver syndrome should include neonatal evaluation for hypoglycemia, partly because these are small-for-gestational-age infants and partly because altered pituitary function has been reported (Cassidy et al., 1986). Motor delay is common because of muscle hypoplasia, so referral for early intervention is beneficial even though the majority have normal cognitive function. Dental care should be emphasized because of teeth crowding (Rubenstein & Vitsky, 1988) and orthopedic evaluation may be required for hemihypertrophy or a higher risk of slipped capital femoral epiphysis (Limbird, 1989). Growth hormone deficiency has been reported in several affected children, and subcutaneous administration of growth hormone increased height and muscle mass (Albanese & Stanhope, 1993; Azcona et al., 1998). Ureteral valves, hydronephrosis, and horseshoe kidney have been described in Russell–Silver syndrome, so clinicians should consider renal sonograms in the neonatal period. Testicular tumors, craniopharyngioma, and Wilms tumor have been reported, and patients with hemihypertrophy should have abdominal ultrasound studies performed every 6–12 months. Close monitoring of puberty and genital development is needed in adolescence, since cryptorchidism and hypospadias are present in over 35 percent of males (Patton, 1988).

Seckel syndrome

Patients with Seckel syndrome have a prominent nose and midface because of microcephaly and micrognathia. The original two patients (Seckel, 1960) probably had different conditions (Gorlin et al., 1990, pp. 313–16), illustrating the heterogeneity of the Seckel phenotype. Children with skeletal dysplasia involving short limbs, short fingers, or axial skeletal anomalies have been categorized as having osteodysplastic primordial dwarfisms; these children have similar pre- and postnatal growth delay, facial anomalies, and mental deficiency to those with Seckel syndrome. Like the Bloom and Dubowitz syndromes, Seckel syndrome has autosomal recessive inheritance. In addition to microcephaly, there may be brain anomalies such as intracranial aneurysms (D'Angelo et al., 1998; Shanske & Marion, 1998). It is also possible that congenital brain lesions producing microcephaly and its resulting facial changes may resemble the Seckel phenotype.

Preventive management should be directed toward early intervention, dental care because of enamel hypoplasia or malocclusion, and evaluation for genital (cryptorchidism, clitoromegaly) and skeletal (congenital hip dislocation) anomalies. About 50 percent of patients will develop craniosynostosis secondary to their microcephaly, and operative correction might be considered in high-functioning children who develop cranial asymmetry.

Noonan syndrome

Terminology

Noonan syndrome was described by Jacqueline Noonan, a pediatric cardiologist (Noonan & Ehmke, 1963). The short stature, hypertelorism, anteverted ear lobes due to fetal cystic hygroma, webbed neck, cubitus valgus, characteristic pectus, and hypogonadism prompted use of the term "male Turner syndrome" because of resemblance to women with a 45,X karyotype. Both sexes are affected in Noonan syndrome and the karyotype is normal. Noonan clinical features may occur together with neurofibromatosis in Watson syndrome (Carey, 1998), together with myopathy and malignant hyperthermia in King syndrome, and together with ichthyosis in cardiofaciocutaneous syndrome (Gorlin et al., 1990, p. 804). The implied genetic heterogeneity may be emphasized by using the term "Noonan phenotype."

Historical diagnosis and management

The disorder has been recognized since 1883, and more than 300 cases have been reported. Allanson (1989) illustrated the changing facial appearance of Noonan syndrome patients over time, providing a challenge for early diagnosis.

Incidence, etiology, and differential diagnosis

Noonan syndrome is quite common, having an incidence of 1 in 1000–2500 (Allanson, 1987). The etiology is unknown, although pathogenesis includes an abnormality of fetal lymphatic circulation that produces a cystic hygroma reminiscent of Turner syndrome. The fetal hygroma may cause the postnatal webbed neck, anteverted ear lobes, and chest deformities (Fig. 10.1, color plate). Direct transmission from parent to child has been observed in 30 percent of the septal defect, atrial septal defect, pulmonic stenosisautosomal dominant inheritance. Genetic linkage studies have been successful in some families and have highlighted one locus on the long arm of chromosome 12.

Differential diagnosis includes the syndromes mentioned above which have Noonan syndrome features plus other findings like café-au-lait spots, myopathy, or ichthyosis. Some cases of Watson syndrome (Noonan–neurofibromatosis features) have alterations of the neurofibromatosis type 1 gene on chromosome 17 (Tassabehji et al., 1993). The Aarskog syndrome (with short stature and hypertelorism), Costello syndrome with mucosal papillomas (see above), the Williams syndrome (with short stature and coarse facies), and the LEOPARD syndrome (with Lentigines, Echocardiographic findings, Pulmonic stenosis, Retarded growth and Deafness) may cause confusion. Females with Noonan syndrome may be misdiagnosed as having Turner syndrome until the different heart lesion and the karyotype are appreciated.

Diagnostic evaluation and medical counseling

Although it is expected to be normal, a karyotype should be performed in all but the most typical cases of Noonan syndrome. The heterogeneous Noonan phenotype can be mimicked by several chromosomal disorders including Turner syndrome. A normal life span with frequently normal intelligence warrants optimistic medical counseling for the parents of a child with Noonan syndrome. An echocardiogram is needed in early infancy to evaluate the degree of pulmonary valve dysplasia and cardiomyopathy in the 67–87.5 percent of patients with congenital heart anomalies (Noonan checklist, part 1). The degree of pulmonary valve dysplasia has significant impact on prognosis, since dilation of severely dysplastic valves is difficult (Burch et al., 1993). Although the cardiomyopathy of Noonan syndrome is not associated with sudden death (Burch et al., 1993), it can be lethal.

Family and psychosocial counseling

A thorough history and partial physical examination should be conducted on parents of children with Noonan syndrome to rule out the possibility of parental transmission (Mendez & Opitz, 1985). Sharland et al. (1993), in a study of 117 families containing 144 individuals with Noonan syndrome, concluded that a parent with typical Noonan features has a 50 percent risk of transmitting the disorder and a 14 percent risk of having a child expressing the full syndrome. If either parent has a few features of the syndrome but is atypical, then a 5 percent recurrence risk of a second child with the full features of Noonan syndrome can be given (Sharland et al., 1993). The data of Allanson (1989) would suggest that childhood photographs of the parents would be helpful in deciding if they had features of Noonan syndrome. Family studies have demonstrated that maternal transmission is 2–3 fold more common than paternal transmission, probably reflecting the hypogonadism and decreased fertility of males with Noonan syndrome.

Parent representatives are useful in supporting families, both in affirming the significant potential of children with Noonan syndrome and in helping with advocacy for early intervention and school placement. Parent support groups are listed on the Noonan checklist, part 1

Natural history and complications

The major complications of Noonan syndrome involve the heart, eyes, ears, teeth, trunk, coagulation system, and musculoskeletal system, as listed on part 1 of the checklist. Problems with feeding can be severe, with 24 percent of patients requiring tube feedings. Although some patients experience motor and speech delays, the outlook for overall intelligence and learning is excellent, with 80–90 percent having normal intelligence and only 11 percent requiring special education. Ocular problems such as ptosis, strabismus, and amblyopia (Lee et al., 1992), together with chronic otitis media or anomalies of the ear ossicles (Qiu et al., 1998), may produce vision and hearing impairment. Dental malocclusion is common and cherubism (cystic enlargement of the jaws) is occasionally seen in Noonan syndrome (Levine et al., 1991). Study of 11 affected males showed that 3 had delayed puberty with delay of sexual function (Elsawi et al., 1994). The men had normal fertility unless

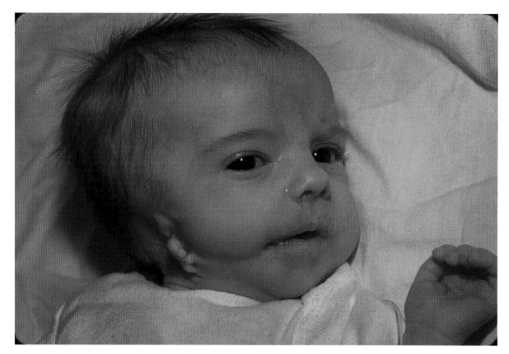

Fig. 1.3   A 3-month-old male with hemifacial microsomia illustrating an anomalous ear, small jaw, and lateral cleft on the right.

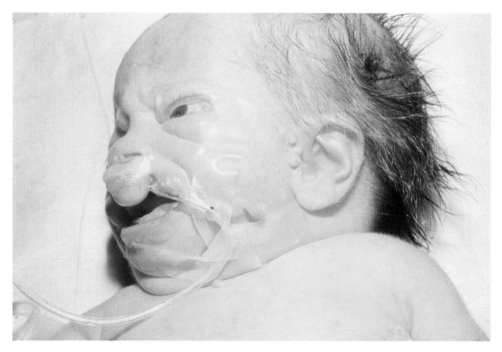

Fig. 1.4   A 2-month-old female with Goldenhar syndrome illustrating cleft lip and palate, anomalous ear, preauricular skin tags, facial skin tags, small jaw, and a coloboma (cleft) of the upper eye lid. Note the more extensive malformations seen in syndromes, in contrast to the patient in Fig. 1.3 with hemifacial microsomia.

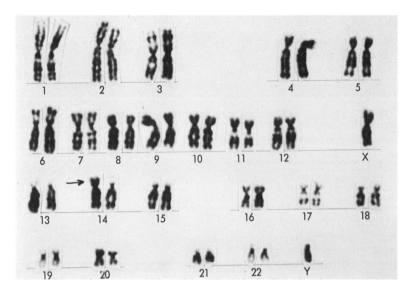

Fig. 1.5   A standard karyotype illustrating extra material on chromosome 14 (arrow) that is derived from chromosome 21. The patient has a 14/21 translocation that yields three doses of chromosome 21 and produces the phenotype of Down syndrome.

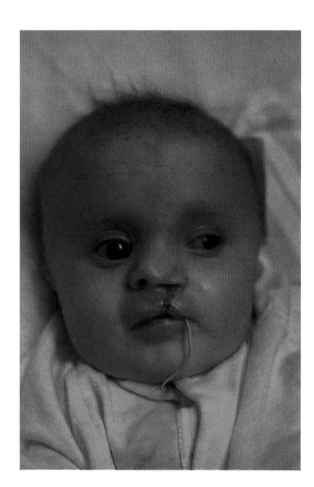

Fig. 5.1   A 9-month-old male with CHARGE association illustrating cleft lip and palate, coloboma and deviation of the eye.

Fig. 6.1   A 2.5-year-old female with fetal
            alcohol syndrome illustrating a flat
            philtrum and thin upper lip.

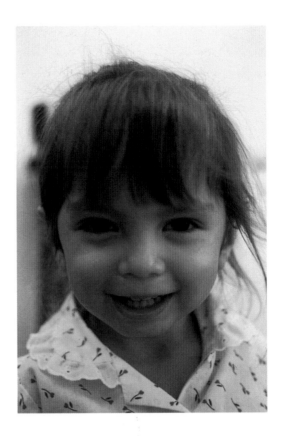

Fig. 7.1   A 2-year-old female with trisomy
            13 illustrating small eyes,
            prominent nose, umbilical hernia,
            and unusually long survival.

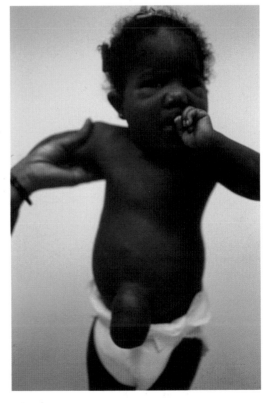

Fig. 7.2   An infant female with trisomy 18
            illustrating the typical clenched fists,
            club feet, prominent heels, and
            convex plantar surfaces (rocker-
            bottom feet).

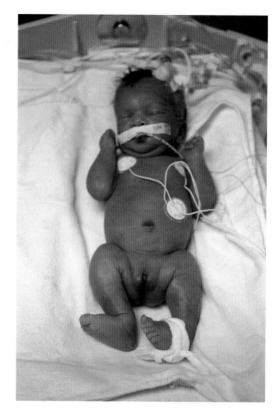

Fig. 7.3   A 6-month-old male with Down
            syndrome illustrating the facial gestalt
            with upslanting palpebral fissures.

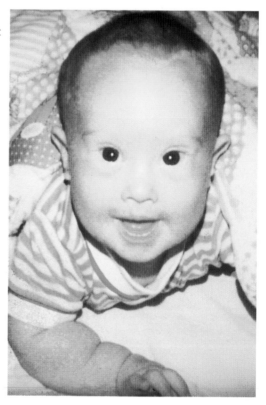

Fig. 8.1   A 4-month-old female with
            Turner syndrome illustrating
            unusual ears, hypoplastic nipples,
            and a broad-appearing chest.

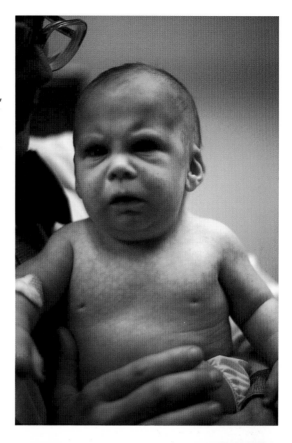

Fig. 8.2   A 6-year-old male with fragile X
            syndrome illustrating the subtle
            facial gestalt with prominent ears
            and jaw.

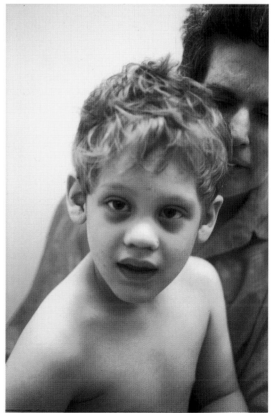

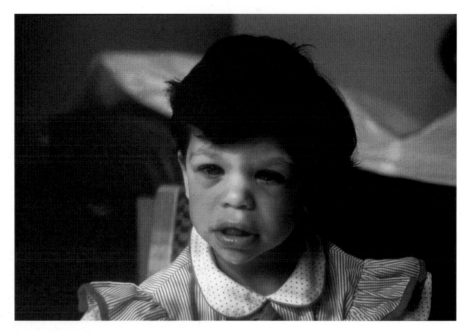

Fig. 9.1   A 3-year-old female with Williams syndrome illustrating the facial gestalt with increased subcutaneous tissue and prominent lips.

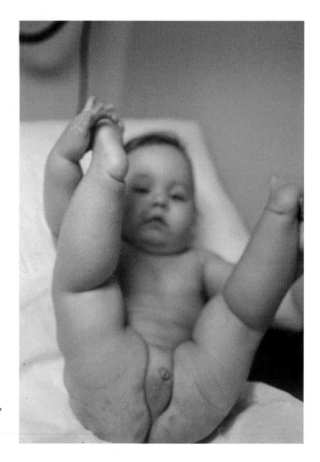

Fig. 9.2   A 9-month-old male with Prader–Willi syndrome illustrating almond-shaped palpebral fissures, down-turned corners of the mouth, mild obesity, and hypogonadism.

Fig. 10.1   A newborn male with Noonan syndrome illustrating a broad nasal root, bilateral ptosis, down-slanting palpebral fissures, and mild pectus excavatum.

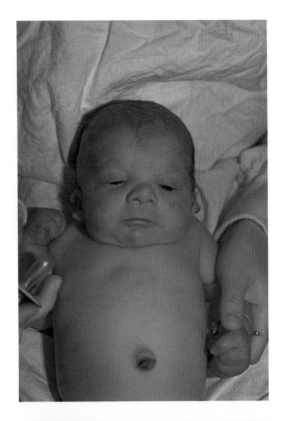

Fig. 11.1   A 2-year-old male with achondroplasia illustrating frontal bossing, shallow nasal bridge, and proximal (rhizomelic shortening) of the limbs.

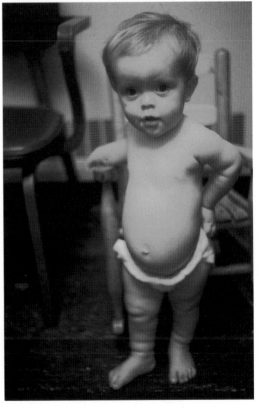

Fig. 12.1   A 10-month-old male with Beckwith–Wiedemann syndrome illustrating a large tongue, protuberant abdomen with large organs, and umbilical hernia.

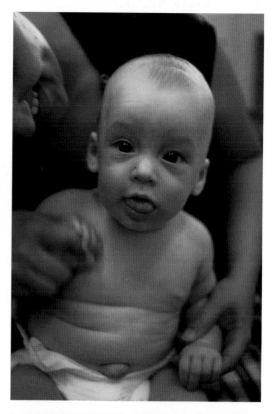

Fig. 14.1   A newborn male with Apert syndrome illustrating a high forehead (acrocephaly) and shallow midface with ocular proptosis due to bilateral coronal synostosis.

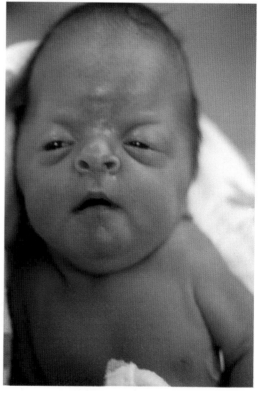

All clinical photographs are published with parental permission.

there was uncorrected bilateral cryptorchidism, in which case they had azoospermia (Elsawi et al., 1994).

The cardiac anomalies in Noonan syndrome often involve the pulmonary valve, as opposed to aortic defects in the Turner or Williams syndromes. Pulmonary hypertension can occur (Tinker et al., 1989), emphasizing the importance of early cardiac assessment. A bleeding diathesis is present in as many as 56 percent of patients, and this has been attributed to partial factor XI deficiency (de Haan et al., 1988; Witt et al., 1988). Lymphedema may occur (Witt et al., 1987), and one case of spontaneous chylothorax was treated with prednisone (Goens et al., 1992). Autoimmune thryoiditis is common, and there is early hepatosplenomegaly of unknown cause. If these abnormalities reflect a generalized immune dysfunction, then neoplastic defenses seem normal except for rare patients with acute lymphoblastic leukemia (Piombo et al., 1993) or neurogenic tumors (Cotton & Williams, 1995; checklist, part 1). In a series of 44 patients having abdominal ultrasounds (George et al., 1993), 11 percent had renal anomalies and 53 percent had splenomegaly, but there were no tumors.

Neurologic complications have been reported in single patients with Noonan syndrome, including moya moya disease (Ganesan & Kirkham, 1997), cerebral infarction (Robertson et al., 1997), and progressive hydrocephalus (Fryns, 1997). These may be related to the bleeding diathesis, and complications have been reported after surgeries (Yellon, 1997).

Noonan syndrome preventive medical checklist

Preventive care for patients with Noonan syndrome should begin with an echocardiogram to define the cardiac anatomy, and evaluation of feeding to promote growth during infancy (checklist, parts 2–4). Chronic otitis, hearing, and visual problems are frequent, so referrals to audiology, ophthalmology, and possibly otolaryngology are recommended. Despite the normal intellectual outlook for many children, early intervention with occupational, physical, and speech therapy is recommended because of frequent motor and language delays. Monitoring of thyroid function is recommended because of autoimmune thyroiditis, and occasional children require cervical spine films if they have unusually short or immobile necks. A creatine phosphokinase (CPK) level as a screen for the possibility of malignant hyperthermia, and a bleeding time are recommended before surgery.

Later childhood and adolescent care should be concerned with optimizing school placement and performance; screening for thyroid, vision, or hearing problems; and close monitoring of nutrition and dentistry. Males need evaluations for cryptorchidism, micropenis, and pubertal development to optimize the chances for later fertility. For this reason and for concerns about stature, referral to endocrinology should be considered at age 6–8 years. One patient had deficient synthesis of growth hormone (Tanaka et al., 1992), and others have shown a good response to growth hormone therapy (Romano et al., 1996).

Brachmann–de Lange syndrome

Terminology

Brachmann–de Lange syndrome combines the name of Cornelia de Lange, an academic pediatrician who described the syndrome in 1933, and W. Brachmann, a young physician-in-training who had reported a case in 1916 (Opitz, 1985). Although Cornelia de Lange named the condition "Typus degenerativus Amstelodamensis," the term "Cornelia de Lange syndrome" or "Brachmann-de Lange syndrome" is now preferred.

Historical diagnosis and management

Awareness of Brachmann–de Lange syndrome was renewed by the report of 6 cases (Ptacek et al., 1963). Severe feeding problems and a propensity for infection undoubtedly led to significant mortality in earlier times.

Incidence, etiology, and differential diagnosis

Most authors feel that the incidence of Brachmann–de Lange syndrome is under-estimated because of early mortality and the occurrence of mildly affected individuals (Opitz, 1985; Opitz, 1994). Estimates of birth incidence range from 1 in 10,000 to 1 in 50,000 (Gorlin et al., 1990, pp. 300–3). Although the majority of cases are sporadic, four cases of monozygotic twins and several families with vertical transmission favor autosomal dominant inheritance with a high frequency of new mutations (Kousseff et al., 1994; Opitz, 1994). Although a majority of cases have a normal karyotype, rare aberrations have highlighted two candidate regions for the hypothesized mutant gene. Rearrangements involving the distal long arm of chromosome 3 produce a phenotype that is similar to the Brachmann–de Lange syndrome. Other patients have had rearrangement of chromosome 9 or deficiency of a chromosome 9-encoded protein – the pregnancy-associated plasma protein A (Opitz, 1994). The linkage of the milder, vertically transmitted form of Brachmann–de Lange syndrome to the chromosome 3q region adds support for a causative locus at 3q (Rizzu et al., 1995).

The differential diagnosis of Brachmann–de Lange syndrome includes the fetal alcohol, duplication 3q, and ring 9 syndromes (Opitz, 1994; Gorlin et al., 1990, pp. 300–3). Growth retardation, problems with feeding, and facial characteristics such as synophrys (fusion of the eyebrows), eye anomalies, thin upper lip, and a long philtrum are seen in the fetal alcohol, dup(3q), and Brachmann–de Lange syndromes. Until a specific laboratory marker becomes available, the diagnosis of

Brachmann-de Lange syndrome is clinical, based on the distinctive facial appearance and pattern of anomalies (de Lange checklist, part 1).

Diagnostic evaluation and medical counseling

The facial appearance is usually sufficient for a diagnosis of Brachmann–de Lange syndrome (Allanson et al., 1997). Tracheomegaly visualized by radiography may be a diagnostic sign (Grunebaum et al., 1996). Chromosomal disorders should be excluded in atypical cases, and a thorough gestational history to exclude alcohol exposure is important. Evaluation of feeding and gastrointestinal function is important in early infancy, since 77 percent of children have problems (de Lange checklist, part 1). In the presence of significant gastroesophageal reflux or vomiting, particularly when accompanied by respiratory distress, chest x-ray and imaging of the gastrointestinal tract should be performed to rule out pyloric stenosis, intestinal malrotation, or diaphragmatic hernia. Congenital heart disease should also be considered, since it occurs in 13–29 percent of patients (checklist, part 1). Cleft lip and palate may also complicate early management. Medical counseling should be concerned with growth, feeding, cardiac, and gastrointestinal problems, with planning for medical and financial services appropriate for children with significant developmental disability.

Family and psychosocial counseling

Until an etiology for Brachmann-de Lange syndrome is defined, an empiric recurrence risk of 2–5 percent can be cited (Gorlin et al., 1990, pp. 300–3). There seems to be a mild form that is autosomal dominant with a 50 percent recurrence risk (Kozma, 1996). The low pregnancy-associated plasma protein A found in a few Brachmann–de Lange pregnancies offers promise as a prenatal diagnostic marker, but no method of prenatal diagnosis is available until this marker is validated (Opitz, 1994). Parents will need supportive counseling regarding the risks of mental disability and growth failure, although recent developmental assessment is more positive than that reported previously (Kline et al., 1993b). Parent support groups are listed on the de Lange checklist, part 1.

Natural history and complications

Problems with feeding, growth, speech, and mental development dominate the natural history of patients with Brachmann–de Lange syndrome (checklist, part 1). During a survey of 310 patients (Jackson et al., 1993), 14 (4.5 percent) of the children died. Causes of death included apnea, aspiration, cardiac anomalies (Mehta & Ambalavanan, 1997), intracranial bleeding with a risk for brain anomalies (Hayashi et al., 1996), and postoperative events (Tsusaki & Mayhew, 1998). The intracranial bleeding occurred in a child with thrombocytopenia, a rare complication of

Brachmann–de Lange syndrome. There is little information on adolescents or adults, but reports document a milder form of Brachmann–de Lange syndrome with reasonable self-help and communication skills (Jackson et al., 1993). Eight individuals have been reported with normal intelligence (IQ > 70; Saal et al., 1993). Nevertheless, most individuals with the syndrome require supervisory care throughout life.

Jackson et al. (1993) reported that the most under-appreciated complication of Brachmann–de Lange syndrome is poor feeding during infancy, often because of gastro-esophageal reflux. Cleft or high-arched palate and narrow external auditory canals place children with Brachmann–de Lange syndrome at greater risk of chronic otitis; conductive and/or sensorineural hearing loss is common (Sataloff et al., 1990). Ophthalmologic problems include high myopia, nystagmus, and ptosis that may cause chin lifting to achieve vision (Levin et al., 1990). Communication may be impaired by visual or hearing problems, and only 4 percent of children had low-normal to normal speech by age 4 (Goodban, 1993). Limb anomalies include small hands and feet, proximally placed thumbs, fifth finger clinodactyly, syndactyly of toes 2/3, and, in about 20 percent, oligodactyly or phocomelia. Flexion contractures of the elbow are common and the acetabular angle is low with coxa valga (Gorlin et al., 1990, pp. 300–3). Internal anomalies of the heart, urinary tract and gastrointestinal tract are common, and genital anomalies include hypospadias, cryptorchidism, bicornuate uterus, and narrow ovaries (checklist, part 1). A higher risk for malignancies may be present (DuVall & Walden, 1996) as with many other malformation syndromes.

Brachmann–de Lange syndrome preventive medical checklist

Opitz (1994) has articulated the need to use the diagnosis of Brachmann–de Lange syndrome as an aid to management rather than as a negative label that precludes services. Attention to feeding and screening for cardiac and urinary tract anomalies are important for infants with Brachmann–de Lange syndrome (checklist, parts 2–4). The high frequency of gastroesophageal reflux, and the known deaths from apnea or aspiration (Jackson et al., 1993), mandate observation and counseling regarding early feeding so appropriate medical or surgical treatment is provided. High risks of chronic otitis and hearing loss require careful monitoring of hearing, as emphasized by Sataloff et al. (1990), so patients develop sufficient communication skills to enable placement of the child in a group home rather than a custodial care facility. Other preventive measures in early childhood include urinalysis to rule out urinary tract infection, dental care for the detection and correction of tooth anomalies, and physical/occupational therapy to minimize the effects of contractures and hip malpositioning. In the older child (checklist, parts 3–4), school performance requires evaluation because of the risks of behavioral (57 percent) or cognitive (75–100 percent) dysfunction. Monitoring of puberty is particularly important in males, in whom hypogonadism may cause ostracism, and depilatory treatments may be useful for hypertrichosis. Growth hormone deficiency has been reported, and very short individuals should have endocrine evaluation with consideration of growth hormone therapy. Schwartz et al. (1990) reported decreased renal concentrating ability, growth hormone deficiency, and variable dysfunction of the hypothalamic-pituitary axis as a cause of genital anomalies in Brachmann–de Lange syndrome. They recommended against growth hormone therapy unless there is significant hypoglycemia. Acute monocytic leukemia and Wilms tumor have been reported in single patients, but it is not clear whether these malignancies were coincidental or part of the syndrome. The older individual with Brachmann–de Lange syndrome should certainly have regular hearing and vision assessments, since myopia and hearing loss are common.

Preventive Management of Noonan syndrome

Clinical diagnosis: Pattern of manifestations including short stature, ptosis, anteverted ear lobes, connective tissue changes (pectus, hernias, joint laxity), cardiac anomalies (pulmonic stenosis, septal defects), hypogonadism, learning differences. Some similarity to Turner syndrome.

Incidence: 1 in 1000–2500 affecting both males and females.

Laboratory diagnosis: None.

Genetics: Autosomal dominant inheritance in some families, conferring an overall 15% recurrence risk for affected individuals to have a fully affected child. If either parent has minor manifestations of the syndrome, a 5 percent recurrence for a fully affected child can be given.

Key management issues: Monitoring for early feeding, growth, vision, hearing, dental cardiac, coagulation, and orthopedic problems. Cognitive disability is usually mild but requires early intervention and school planning.

Growth Charts: Witt et al. (1986).

Parent groups: (TNSSG) Noonan Syndrome Support Group, P. O. Box 145, Upperco MD, 21155, (888) 686-2224, wandar@bellatlantic.net, http://www.noonansyndrome.org

Basis for management recommendations: Derived from the complications below as documented by Allanson (1987), Sharland et al. (1992).

Summary of clinical concerns

General	Learning	Cognitive disability (11–20%) – median IQ 102 (range 64–127), verbal IQ discrepancy (15%), learning differences, **speech problems** (20%)
	Growth	**Failure to thrive** (50%), **short stature** (50%)
	Tumors	**Nevi**, café-au-lait spots (25%), pheochromocytoma, ganglioneuroma
Facial	Eye	**Ptosis** (42%), **strabismus** (63%), **amblyopia** (31%)
	Ear	Posteriorly rotated ears, anteverted lobules, otitis media
	Mouth	**Feeding problems** (76%), **dental anomalies** (35%)
Surface	Neck/trunk	**Webbing of neck** (23–90%), **pectus** (70–95%)
	Epidermal	**Decreased hair growth**, curly or sparse hair
Skeletal	Axial	Cervical spine fusion (2%), **vertebral anomalies** (25%), scoliosis (13%)
	Limbs	**Cubitus valgus** (50%), **increased joint laxity** (50%), club feet (12%)
Internal	Digestive	**Dysphagia** (24%), **hepatosplenomegaly** (26%)
	Pulmonary	Pulmonary lymphangiectasia
	Circulatory	**Cardiac anomalies** (60–80% – pulmonary valve stenosis, atrial septal defect, ventricular septal defect, mitral valve prolapse), **cardiomyopathy** (20%), **lymphatic anomalies** (20%)
	Endocrine	**Antithyroid antibodies** (30%), hypo- or hyperthyroidism
	RES	**Abnormal bleeding** (20–56%), severe hemorrhage (3%), metrorrhagia
	Excretory	Renal anomalies (11%)
	Genital	**Cryptorchidism** (60–77%)
Neural	CNS	Seizures (9%)
	Motor	**Delayed motor skills** (26%)
	Sensory	**Abnormal vision** (55%), **mild hearing loss** (12–40%)
	Muscular	Ill-defined myopathy, malignant hyperthermia

RES, reticuloendothelial system; **bold**: frequency > 20%

Key references

Allanson, J.E. (1987). *Journal of Medical Genetics* 24:9–13.
Sharland, M. et al. (1992). *Archives of Disease in Childhood* 67:178–83.
Witt, D. R., Keena, B. A., Hall, J. G. & Allanson, J. E . (1986). *Clinical Genetics* 30:150–3

Noonan syndrome

Preventive medical checklist (0–1yr)

Patient **Birth Date** / / **Number**

Pediatric	Screen		Evaluate		Refer/Counsel	
Neonatal / / *Newborn screen* ❑ *HB* ❑	ABR	❑	Feeding	❑	Genetic evaluation Developmental pediatrics Genetic counseling	❑ ❑ ❑
1 month / /	Echocardiogram	❑	Feeding	❑	Family support[4] Cardiology	❑ ❑
2 months / / *HB[1]* ❑ *Hib* ❑ *DTaP, IPV* ❑ *RV* ❑	Growth Hearing, vision[2]	❑ ❑	Feeding Otitis	❑ ❑	Early intervention[5] Developmental pediatrics[3] Genetic counseling	❑ ❑ ❑
4 months / / *HB[1]* ❑ *Hib* ❑ *DTaP/IPV* ❑ *RV* ❑	Growth Hearing, vision[2]	❑ ❑	Feeding Otitis	❑ ❑	Early intervention[5] Genetics ENT[3]	❑ ❑ ❑
6 months / / *Hib* ❑ *IPV[1]* ❑ *DTaP* ❑ *RV* ❑	Growth Hearing, vision[2]	❑ ❑	Feeding Otitis Strabismus	❑ ❑ ❑	Family support[4]	❑
9 months / / *IPV[1]* ❑	Audiology Bleeding time CPK[3]	❑ ❑ ❑	Feeding Otitis Strabismus	❑ ❑ ❑	Ophthalmology	❑
1 year / / *HB* ❑ *Hib[1]* ❑ *IPV[1]* ❑ *MMR[1]* ❑ *Var[1]* ❑	Growth Hearing, vision[2] T4, TSH	❑ ❑ ❑	Feeding Otitis Strabismus Neck motion	❑ ❑ ❑ ❑	Family support[4] Early intervention[5] Developmental pediatrics[3] Genetics	❑ ❑ ❑ ❑

Clinical concerns for Noonan syndrome, ages 0–1 year

Feeding problems	Autoimmune thyroiditis	Developmental disability
Eye anomalies (strabismus)	Abnormal bleeding	Learning differences
Chronic otitis	Cardiac anomalies	Poor verbal performance
Mild hearing loss	Cervical spine anomalies	Vertebral/sternal anomalies

Guidelines for the neonatal period should be undertaken *at whatever age* the diagnosis is made; DTaP, acellular DTP; IPV, inactivated poliovirus (oral polio also used); RV, rotavirus; MMR, measles–mumps–rubella; Var, varicella; [1]alternative timing; [2]by practitioner; [3]as dictated by clinical findings – ENT for children with chronic otitis or sleep apnea, CPK prior to surgery; [4]parent group, family/sib, financial, and behavioral issues as discussed in the preface; [5]including developmental monitoring and motor/speech therapy.

Noonan syndrome

Preventive medical checklist (15m–6yrs)

Patient   **Birth Date**   /   /   **Number**

Pediatric	Screen		Evaluate		Refer/Counsel	
15 months / / Hib[1] ☐ MMR[1] ☐ DTaP, IPV[1] ☐ Varicella[1] ☐					Family support[4] Early intervention[5]	☐ ☐
18 months / / DTaP, IPV[1] ☐ Varicella[1] ☐ Influenza[3] ☐	Growth	☐	Otitis Neck motion	☐ ☐		
2 years / / Influenza[3] ☐ Pneumovax[3] ☐ Dentist ☐	Audiology T4, TSH	☐ ☐	Feeding Neck motion	☐ ☐	Family support[4] Developmental pediatrics[3] Genetics ENT[3] Ophthalmology	☐ ☐ ☐ ☐ ☐
3 years / / Influenza[3] ☐ Pneumovax[3] ☐ Dentist ☐	Audiology T4, TSH C-spine x-rays[3] Bleeding time CPK[3]	☐ ☐ ☐ ☐ ☐	Feeding Neck motion	☐ ☐	Family support[4] Preschool transition[5] Genetics	☐ ☐ ☐
4 years / / Influenza[3] ☐ Pneumovax[3] ☐ Dentist ☐	Growth Hearing, vision[2] T4, TSH	☐ ☐ ☐	Nutrition	☐	Family support[4] Preschool program[5] Developmental pediatrics[3] Genetics Ophthalmology[3]	☐ ☐ ☐ ☐ ☐
5 years / / DTaP, IPV[1] ☐ MMR[1] ☐	Audiology Bleeding time CPK[3]	☐ ☐ ☐	Heart Nutrition	☐ ☐	School transition[5] Cardiology[3]	☐ ☐
6 years / / DTaP, IPV[1] ☐ MMR[1] ☐ Dentist ☐	Growth Hearing, vision[3] T4, TSH	☐ ☐ ☐	Nutrition School progress	☐ ☐	Family support[5] Developmental pediatrics[3] Genetics Ophthalmology ENT[3]	☐ ☐ ☐ ☐ ☐

Clinical concerns for Noonan syndrome, ages 1–6 years

Feeding problems	Autoimmune thyroiditis	Developmental disability
Eye anomalies (strabismus)	Abnormal bleeding	Learning differences
Chronic otitis	Cardiac anomalies	Poor verbal performance
Mild hearing loss	Cervical spine anomalies	Vertebral/sternal anomalies

Guidelines for prior ages should be undertaken *at the time of diagnosis*; DTaP, acellular DTP; IPV, inactivated poliovirus (oral polio also used); MMR, measles–mumps–rubella; [1]alternative timing; [2]by practitioner; [3]as dictated by clinical findings – ENT for children with chronic otitis or sleep apnea, CPK prior to surgery, endocrinology for those with severe short stature; [4]parent group, family/sib, financial, and behavioral issues as discussed in the preface; [5]including developmental monitoring and motor/speech therapy.

Noonan syndrome

Preventive medical checklist (6+ yrs)

Patient   **Birth Date** / /   **Number**

Pediatric	Screen	Evaluate	Refer/Counsel
8 years / / *Dentist* ❑	Growth ❑ Hearing, vision[2] ❑ T4, TSH ❑	Nutrition ❑	School options ❑ Developmental pediatrics[3] ❑ Genetics ❑ Endocrinology[3] ❑
10 years / /	Hearing, vision[2] ❑ T4, TSH ❑	Nutrition ❑ Phallus size ❑ School progress ❑	Genetics ❑ Ophthalmology ❑ ENT[3] ❑
12 years / / *Td[1], MMR, Var* ❑ *CBC* ❑ *Dentist* ❑ *Scoliosis* ❑ *Cholesterol* ❑	Hearing, vision[2] ❑ T4, TSH ❑ Bleeding time ❑ CPK[3] ❑	Nutrition ❑ Puberty ❑ Heart ❑ Phallus size ❑	Family support[4] ❑ School options ❑ Developmental pediatrics[3] ❑ Genetics ❑ Cardiology[3] ❑
14 years / / *CBC* ❑ *Dentist* ❑ *Cholesterol* ❑ *Breast CA* ❑ *Testicular CA* ❑	Hearing, vision[2] ❑ T4, TSH ❑	School progress ❑ Nutrition ❑ Puberty ❑ Phallus size ❑	
16 years / / *Td[1]* ❑ *CBC* ❑ *Cholesterol* ❑ *Sexual[5]* ❑ *Dentist* ❑	Hearing, vision[2] ❑ T4, TSH ❑	Nutrition ❑ Puberty ❑	Vocational planning ❑ Developmental pediatrics[3] ❑ Genetics ❑
18 years / / *CBC* ❑ *Sexual[5]* ❑ *Cholesterol* ❑ *Scoliosis* ❑	Hearing, vision[2] ❑ T4, TSH ❑	School progress ❑	Vocational planning ❑
20 years[6] / / *CBC* ❑ *Sexual[5]* ❑ *Cholesterol* ❑ *Dentist* ❑	Bleeding time ❑ CPK[3] ❑	Work, residence ❑	Family support[4] ❑ Cardiology[3] ❑

Clinical concerns for Noonan syndrome, ages 6+ years

Vision problems	Cardiac anomalies	Learning differences
Mild hearing loss	Abnormal bleeding	Vertebral/sternal anomalies
Dental malocclusion	Cryptorchidism, micropenis	Joint laxity
Autoimmune thyroiditis	Lymphatic abnormalities	Malignant hyperthermia

Guidelines for prior ages should be undertaken *at the time of diagnosis*; Td, tetanus/diphtheria; MMR, measles–mumps–rubella; Var, varicella; [1]alternative timing; [2]by practitioner; [3]as dictated by clinical findings – ENT for children with chronic otitis or sleep apnea, CPK prior to surgery, endocrinology for those with severe short stature; [4]parent group, family/sib, financial, and behavioral issues as discussed in the preface; [5]birth control, STD screening if sexually active; [6]repeat every decade.

Preventive Management of Brachmann–De Lange syndrome

Clinical diagnosis: Pattern of manifestations including a characteristic facial appearance with joined eyebrows (synophrys), down-turned corners of the mouth; small hands and feet with potentially missing digits; internal anomalies of the heart, gastrointestinal and urinary systems, growth failure and moderate/severe developmental disability.

Incidence: 1 in 10,000 to 50,000 live births.

Laboratory diagnosis: None.

Genetics: Sporadic disorder of unknown etiology; minimal recurrence risk.

Key management issues: Monitoring for early feeding problems and gastroesophageal reflux, screening for cardiac and urinary tract anomalies, monitoring of hearing and vision, dental care, physical/occupational therapy to minimize the effects of contractures and hip malpositioning, depilatory treatments for hypertrichosis, early intervention and speech therapy.

Growth Charts: Kline et al. (1993).

Parent groups: Cornelia de Lange Syndrome Foundation, 302 W. Main St. #100, Avon CT, 06001-3681, cdisintl@iconn.net, http://www.cdisoutreach.org.

Basis for management recommendations: Derived from the complications below as documented by Jackson et al. (1993), Kousseff et al. (1994), Opitz (1994).

Summary of clinical concerns

General	Learning	**Cognitive disability** (87% with IQ < 60), **learning differences** (100%), **speech delay** (75–100%)
	Behavior	Behavior problems (excessive screaming, stereotypic movements, tantrums, biting) dietary behavior problems[1]
	Growth	**Low birth weight** (72%), failure to thrive, **short stature** (86–96%), poor feeding (lack of interest in food, regurgitation, projectile vomiting)
	Tumors	Acute monocytic leukemia Wilms tumor
Facial	Eye	**Eye anomalies** – 57% (myopia, 60%, ptosis, 45%, nystagmus, 37%)
	Ear	**Narrow ear canals** (30%), **chronic otitis** (60%)
	Nose	Choanal atresia
	Mouth	Cleft lip/palate (13–21%), **high palate** (59–86%), **anomalous teeth** (86%)
Surface	Neck/trunk	**Nuchal webbing** (11–33%), **low hairline** (92%)
	Epidermal	**Hypertrichosis** (78–97%)
Skeletal	Cranial	**Microbrachycephaly** (50–98%)
	Limbs	**Limb anomalies** (56–99% – proximal thumbs 80%, reduction defects 20–27%, syndactyly of toes 2–3 86%), limb deficiencies, **contractures** (32–84%)
Internal	Digestive	**Gastroesophageal reflux** (27%), **gastrointestinal anomalies** (49–71% – pyloric stenosis, malrotation, diaphragmatic hernia)
	Pulmonary	**Respiratory infections** (25%)
	Circulatory	**Cardiac anomalies** (13–29% – ventricular septal defect, atrial septal defect, pulmonic stenosis)
	Endocrine	Growth hormone deficiency
	RES	Thrombocytopenia
	Excretory	Ureteral reflux (12%), urinary tract infections
	Genital	Hypospadias (11–33%), **cryptorchidism** (73%)
Neural	CNS	Seizures (14–20%)
	Sensory	Chronic otitis, **hearing loss** (20–27%), **vision deficits**

RES, reticuloendothelial system; **bold:** frequency > 20%

Key references

Jackson, L. G. et al. (1993). *American Journal of Medical Genetics* 47:940–6.

Goodban, M.T. (1993). *American Journal of Medical Genetics* 47:1059–63.

Kline, A.D., M. Barr & L.G. Jackson. (1993). *American Journal of Medical Genetics* 47:1042–9.

Kousseff, B. G. et al. (1994). *Archives of Pediatrics and Adolescent Medicine* 148:749–55.

Opitz, J.M. (1994). *Archives of Pediatrics and Adolescent Medicine* 148:1206–7.

Brachmann–De Lange syndrome

Preventive medical checklist (0–1yr)

Patient Birth Date / / **Number**

Pediatric	Screen	Evaluate	Refer/Counsel
Neonatal / / *Newborn screen* ❑ *HB* ❑	ABR ❑ Renal sonogram ❑	Feeding, reflux ❑ Eye anomaly ❑ Palate ❑ Genitalia ❑	Genetic evaluation ❑ Feeding specialist ❑
1 month / /	Echocardiogram ❑	Feeding, reflux ❑ Glaucoma ❑ Otitis ❑ Contractures ❑	Family support[4] ❑ Feeding specialist ❑ Cardiology ❑ Ophthalmology[3] ❑
2 months / / *HB[1]* ❑ *Hib* ❑ *DTaP, IPV* ❑ *RV* ❑	Growth ❑ Hearing, vision[2] ❑	Feeding, reflux ❑ Otitis ❑ Contractures ❑	Early intervention[5] ❑ Developmental pediatrics ❑ Genetic counseling ❑ Gastroenterology[3] ❑
4 months / / *HB[1]* ❑ *Hib* ❑ *DTaP/IPV* ❑ *RV* ❑	Growth ❑ Hearing, vision[2] ❑	Feeding, reflux ❑ Otitis ❑ Contractures ❑	Early intervention[5] ❑ Genetics ❑
6 months / / *Hib* ❑ *IPV[1]* ❑ *DTaP* ❑ *RV* ❑	Growth ❑ Hearing, vision[2] ❑	Glaucoma ❑ Feeding, reflux ❑ Otitis ❑ Contractures ❑	Family support[4] ❑ Feeding specialist[3] ❑
9 months / / *IPV[1]* ❑	Audiology ❑	Feeding, reflux ❑ Otitis ❑	Ophthalmology[3] ❑ ENT[3] ❑
1 year / / *HB* ❑ *Hib[1]* ❑ *IPV[1]* ❑ *MMR[1]* ❑ *Var[1]* ❑	Growth ❑ Hearing, vision[2] ❑ Urinalysis, BP ❑	Nutrition ❑ Feeding, reflux ❑ Otitis ❑	Family support[4] ❑ Early intervention[5] ❑ Developmental pediatrics ❑ Genetics ❑ Dietician[3] ❑

Clinical concerns for Brachmann–De Lange syndrome, ages 0–1 year

Feeding problems, reflux	Cardiac anomalies	Developmental disability
Eye anomalies	GI tract anomalies	Speech delay
Cleft or high palate	Limb anomalies	Behavioral problems
Otitis media, hearing loss	Urinary tract anomalies	Microcephaly
Dental anomalies	Genital anomalies	Irritability, seizures

Guidelines for the neonatal period should be undertaken *at whatever age* the diagnosis is made; DTaP, acellular DTP; IPV, inactivated poliovirus (oral polio also used); RV, rotavirus; MMR, measles–mumps–rubella; Var, varicella; [1]alternative timing; [2]by practitioner; [3]as dictated by clinical findings; [4]parent group, family/sib, financial, and behavioral issues as discussed in the preface; [5]including developmental monitoring and motor/speech therapy.

Brachmann–De Lange syndrome

Preventive medical checklist (15m–6yrs)

Patient		Birth Date / /	Number

Pediatric	Screen	Evaluate	Refer/Counsel
15 months / / Hib[1] ❏ MMR[1] ❏ DTaP, IPV[1] ❏ Varicella[1] ❏			Family support[4] ❏ Early intervention[5] ❏
18 months / / DTaP, IPV[1] ❏ Varicella[1] ❏ Influenza[3] ❏	Growth ❏ Hearing, vision[2] ❏	Feeding ❏	Feeding specialist[3] ❏
2 years / / Influenza[3] ❏ Pneumovax[3] ❏ Dentist ❏	Growth ❏ Hearing, vision[2] ❏ Audiology ❏ Urinalysis, BP ❏	Feeding ❏ Otitis ❏ Contractures ❏	Family support[4] ❏ Developmental pediatrics ❏ Genetics ❏ ENT[3] ❏ Ophthalmology[3] ❏
3 years / / Influenza[3] ❏ Pneumovax[3] ❏ Dentist ❏	Growth ❏ Hearing, vision[2] ❏ Audiology ❏ Urinalysis, BP ❏	Feeding ❏ Otitis ❏ Contractures ❏ Nutrition ❏	Preschool transition[5] ❏ Family support[4] ❏ Dietician[3] ❏
4 years / / Influenza[3] ❏ Pneumovax[3] ❏ Dentist ❏	Growth ❏ Hearing, vision[2] ❏	Nutrition ❏ Behavior ❏	Family support[4] ❏ Preschool program[5] ❏ Developmental pediatrics ❏ Genetics ❏ Ophthalmology[3] ❏
5 years / / DTaP, IPV[1] ❏ MMR[1] ❏	Hearing, vision[2] ❏ Audiology ❏ Urinalysis, BP ❏	Nutrition ❏ Behavior ❏ Glaucoma ❏	School transition[5] ❏
6 years / / DTaP, IPV[1] ❏ MMR[1] ❏ Dentist ❏	Growth ❏ Hearing, vision[2] ❏	School progress ❏ Nutrition ❏ Behavior ❏	Family support[4] ❏ Developmental pediatrics ❏ Genetics ❏ Ophthalmology[3] ❏ ENT[3] ❏ Endocrinology[3] ❏

Clinical concerns for Brachmann–De Lange syndrome, ages 1–6 years

Feeding problems, reflux	Cardiac anomalies	Developmental disability
Eye anomalies	GI tract anomalies	Speech delay
Cleft or high palate	Limb anomalies	Behavioral problems
Otitis media, hearing loss	Urinary tract anomalies	Microcephaly
Dental anomalies	Genital anomalies	Irritability, seizures

Guidelines for prior ages should be undertaken *at the time of diagnosis*; DTaP, acellular DTP; IPV, inactivated poliovirus (oral polio also used); MMR, measles–mumps–rubella; [1]alternative timing; [2]by practitioner; [3]as dictated by clinical findings; [4]parent group, family/sib, financial, and behavioral issues as discussed in the preface; [5]including developmental monitoring and motor/speech therapy.

Brachmann–De Lange syndrome

Preventive medical checklist (6+ yrs)

Patient   **Birth Date** / /   **Number**

Pediatric	Screen	Evaluate		Refer/Counsel	
8 years / / *Dentist* ❏	Urinalysis, BP ❏	Nutrition	❏	School options Developmental pediatrics Genetics	❏ ❏ ❏
10 years / /	Hearing, vision[2] ❏	School progress Nutrition Phallus size	❏ ❏ ❏	Ophthalmology[3] ENT[3]	❏ ❏
12 years / / *Td[1], MMR, Var* ❏ *CBC* ❏ *Dentist* ❏ *Scoliosis* ❏ *Cholesterol* ❏	Urinalysis, BP ❏	Nutrition Puberty Phallus size Behavior	❏ ❏ ❏ ❏	Family support[4] School options Developmental pediatrics Genetics	❏ ❏ ❏ ❏
14 years / / *CBC* ❏ *Dentist* ❏ *Cholesterol* ❏ *Breast CA* ❏ *Testicular CA* ❏	Hearing, vision[2] ❏	School progress Nutrition Puberty Behavior	❏ ❏ ❏ ❏		
16 years / / *Td[1]* ❏ *CBC* ❏ *Cholesterol* ❏ *Sexual[5]* ❏ *Dentist* ❏	Hearing, vision[2] ❏ Urinalysis, BP ❏	School progress Nutrition Behavior	❏ ❏ ❏	Vocational planning	❏
18 years / / *CBC* ❏ *Sexual[5]* ❏ *Cholesterol* ❏ *Scoliosis* ❏	Hearing, vision[2] ❏	Nutrition Behavior	❏ ❏	Vocational planning Developmental pediatrics Genetics	❏ ❏ ❏
20 years[6] / / *CBC* ❏ *Sexual[5]* ❏ *Cholesterol* ❏ *Dentist* ❏	Hearing, vision[2] ❏ Urinalysis, BP ❏	Nutrition Behavior Work, residence	❏ ❏ ❏	Family support[4]	❏

Clinical concerns for Brachmann–De Lange syndrome, ages 6+ years

Failure to thrive	Dental anomalies	Cognitive disability
Recurrent infections	Hypertrichosis	Behavioral problems
Otitis media, hearing loss	Genital anomalies	

Guidelines for prior ages should be undertaken *at the time of diagnosis*; Td, tetanus/diphtheria; MMR, measles–mumps–rubella; Var, varicella; [1]alternative timing; [2]by practitioner; [3]as dictated by clinical findings; [4]parent group, family/sib, financial, and behavioral issues as discussed in the preface; [5]birth control, STD screening if sexually active; [6]repeat every decade.

11

Syndromes with disproportionate growth failure (dwarfism)

Skeletal dysplasias are distinguished by disproportionate short stature and bony anomalies with more than 100 disorders now recognized. The combined prevalence of skeletal dysplasias is 2–4 per 10,000 births (Orioli et al., 1986). Skeletal radiography is the cardinal diagnostic study, allowing the recognition of skeletal dysplasia and classification according to affected skeletal regions and accessory anomalies. Several of the more common or prototypic skeletal dysplasias are listed in Table 11.1. Pediatricians may be involved with perinatal management of dwarfism recognized by prenatal ultrasound studies, with management of neonatal lethal dysplasias where death occurs from thoracic dysplasia and asphyxia, or with long-term preventive management of children and adults with dwarfism.

Many skeletal dysplasias are compatible with a normal life span, but have complications affecting the membranous and cartilaginous bony skeletons, brain, spinal cord, eyes, teeth, heart, and bone marrow (Apajasalo et al., 1998). As a rule, affected children have a head that is large in proportion to the body with platybasia or other cranial deformities; these impose risks for hydrocephalus, foramen magnum/atlanto-axial abnormalities, and spinal cord injury. Bony foramina or inner ear ossicles may be affected, producing hearing and vision problems. Frequent fractures and/or limb deformities often require orthopedic monitoring, and many skeletal disorders are generalized connective tissue diseases with lax joints, easy bruising, bluish sclerae, or mitral valve prolapse. Some skeletal disorders with exuberant or ectopic bone formation will produce bone marrow failure with bleeding or infection. Those with significant short stature require special appliances to aid ambulation, driving, and daily living.

Less common skeletal dysplasias

The early diagnosis and preventive management of skeletal dysplasias can vastly improve the length and quality of life for affected children. Prevention for disorders that are representative of skeletal dysplasia categories will be discussed briefly (Table 11.1), followed by detailed discussion of achondroplasia and osteogenesis imperfecta.

Table 11.1 Skeletal dysplasias and dystrophies

Syndrome	Incidence	Frequent abnormalities (in addition to dwarfism)
Lethal dwarfisms		
Thanatophoric dwarfism	1 in 25,000 live births	Short limbs, small thorax, craniosynostosis, cleft palate
Short rib-polydactyly syndromes	∼ 50 cases	Short limbs, small thorax, polydactyly, genital a.
Chondrodysplasias		
Achondroplasia	1 in 25,000 live births	Short limbs, frontal bossing, spinal compression, hypotonia
Cleidocranial dysplasia	∼ 700 cases	Macrocephaly, large fontanelle, absent clavicles, dental a.
Diastrophic dysplasia	∼ 130 cases	Short limbs, heart a., progressive scoliosis, dislocated hip, cervical spinal cord compression, heart a., speech problems
Spondyloepiphyseal dysplasia	1 in 100,000 live births	Myopia, vitreoretinal degeneration, scoliosis, odontoid hypoplasia
Chondrodysplasias with unusual features		
Cartilage-hair hypoplasia	∼ 100 cases	Short limbs, immune deficiency, Hodgkin's disease, lymphomas
Ellis van Crevald syndrome	∼ 250 cases	Short limbs, cardiac a., small nails, genitourinary a.
Chondrodysplasia punctata	∼ 200 cases	Short limbs, cataracts, ichthyosis, ocular a., cardiac a.,
Recognized metabolic alterations		
Osteogenesis imperfectas	1 in 20,000	Multiple fractures, blue sclerae, hearing loss, bowed limbs
Pseudohypoparathyroidism	∼ 200 cases	Short digits, hypocalcemia, bowed limbs, hypothyroidism
Hypophosphatasia	1 in 100,000	Craniosynostosis, seizures, eye a., dental a., orthopedic a.
Other skeletal disorders		
Osteopetrosis	∼ 600 cases	Pancytopenia, blindness, deafness, fractures, renal disease (rare)
Fibrodysplasia ossificans progressiva	∼ 550 cases	Exogenous bone deposition, hearing loss, respiratory failure

Notes:
a., anomalies.

Lethal neonatal dwarfism

Preventive management is less relevant to patients with lethal forms of dwarfism except in the sense of early diagnosis to guide parental expectation and counseling. More than 20 types of lethal dwarfism are known, with neonatal photographs and radiographs being crucial for specific diagnosis and accurate genetic counseling. Thanatophoric (death-bringing) dwarfism is the most common example, with an incidence of about 1 in 25,000. Affected infants have the appearance of severely affected achondroplasts, with frontal bossing, shallow nasal bridge, and short extremities. Most cases have been sporadic, and the disorder is allelic with achondroplasia in that both involve mutations within the fibroblast growth factor receptor-3 gene (Tavormina et al., 1995). Skeletal survey is important, since certain autosomal recessive disorders (e.g., dwarfism with a snail-like pelvis – Schneckenbecken dysplasia) may produce a similar phenotype. Rare patients survive beyond 1 year of age, and will need monitoring for craniosynostosis, cleft palate, and congenital heart disease.

Another group of neonatal-lethal skeletal dysplasias are the short rib-polydactyly syndromes of Saldino–Noonan, Naumoff, and Majewski (Gorlin et al., 1990, pp. 218–20; Jones, 1997, pp. 336–7). Although distinguished by radiographic features and accessory anomalies, all three syndromes exhibit autosomal recessive inheritance, short ribs with thoracic dysplasia, and neonatal death. Cleft lip/palate, cardiac anomalies, pre- or postaxial polydactyly, gastrointestinal anomalies, renal anomalies, and ambiguous or hypoplastic genitalia may occur in one or more of these syndromes, and polyhydramnios or fetal hydrops may occur. In these and other complex skeletal disorders, the role of primary care is to ensure that adequate imaging studies and subspecialty consultation are obtained so that precise diagnosis and counseling are possible.

Cartilage-hair hypoplasia

Individuals with cartilage-hair hypoplasia may have a normal facial appearance with sparse hair and short, bowed limbs (Makitie et al., 1995). The disorder is an example of the T-cell and B-cell immunologic deficiencies that may be associated with short-limb dwarfism. Susceptibility to varicella and other viral illnesses has been attributed to diminished response to phytohemagglutinin in vitro and delayed allograft rejection in vivo. Preventive management includes the avoidance of live vaccines (e.g., polio except for Salk vaccine) and prophylaxis, where indicated, for chronic infections. There is an increased risk for cancer, with 6% of patients having Hodgkin disease, lymphoma, or leukemia (Gorlin et al., 1990, pp. 186–8; Jones, 1997, pp. 384–5).

Chondrodysplasia punctata

Patients with radiographic stippling (chondrodysplasia punctata) were first described by Conradi in 1914 and Hünermann in 1931 (Spranger et al. (1971).

Chondrodysplasia punctata describes focal or punctate calcifications of infantile cartilage that occur primarily but not exclusively in the epiphyses. The epiphyses do not exhibit clinical abnormalities but appear stippled on x-ray, as if someone dabbed at them with a white paintbrush. As a clinical sign, chondrodysplasia punctata occurs in many disorders including Zellweger syndrome, Smith–Lemli–Opitz syndrome, trisomy 18, fetal warfarin syndrome, or even hypothyroidism. As a disease entity, chondrodysplasia punctata refers to at least four genetically distinct skeletal dysplasias (Wilson et al., 1988).

Autosomal recessive chondrodysplasia punctata is the most severe, with short limbs, microcephaly, unusual facies (frontal bossing, shallow nasal bridge), bilateral cataracts (80 percent), ichthyosis or alopecia (27 percent), and contractures (48 percent). This disorder is caused by altered biogenesis of peroxisomes (see Chapter 19). Autosomal dominant chondrodysplasia punctata is milder, with normal limb lengths, mental development, and survival. X-linked dominant chondrodysplasia punctata exhibits unilateral scoliosis (100 percent), joint contractures (46 percent), cataracts (46 percent), and stippling of epiphyses. Ichthyosis or erythroderma (95 percent) may occur in patches and whorls as predicted by random inactivation of normal/abnormal X chromosome alleles (Happle, 1979). X-linked recessive chondrodysplasia punctata denotes a small group of male patients who have visible X chromosome deletions. These males have symmetric short stature with typical facial changes (shallow nasal bridge, short nose) and hypoplastic distal phalanges (Curry et al., 1984). The disorder results from the deletion of an arylsulfatase gene, and it has been demonstrated that warfarin is an inhibitor of this gene (Franco et al., 1995).

Once nonspecific stippling has been excluded, the diagnosis of the autosomal recessive or X-linked dominant forms of chondrodysplasia punctata is made by the demonstration of plasmalogen or peroxisomal enzyme deficiency. The X-linked recessive form can be recognized by chromosomal or molecular analysis, but the autosomal dominant form remains a clinical diagnosis. Preventive management should include ophthalmologic and orthopedic follow-up, with recognition that the autosomal recessive form often involves chronic pulmonary infections that are lethal in early childhood.

Cleidocranial dysplasia

Cleidocranial dysplasia is an autosomal dominant disorder with short stature and skeletal and oral anomalies. More than 700 cases have been described, including one by Meckel in 1760 and a potentially affected Neanderthal skeleton (Gorlin et al., 1990, pp. 249–53). Patients have a large anterior fontanelle and relative macrocephaly in the neonatal period, when a skeletal radiographic survey can be obtained for diagnosis (Jones, 1997, pp. 408–9). Wormian bones of the skull, absent clavicles, decreased ossification of the pubis, spina bifida occulta, and cone-shaped epiphyses of the distal phalanges comprise a distinctive radiographic pattern (Gorlin et al., 1990, pp. 249–53). The inheritance is autosomal dominant, and the causative gene has been isolated for one form of this heterogeneous condition – it encodes an osteoblast-specific transcription factor (Lee et al., 1997).

Complications of cleidocranial dysplasia include conductive hearing loss, high palate, dental anomalies such as supernumerary teeth or lack of tooth eruption, syringomyelia (Vari et al., 1996), and increased motion of the upper limbs due to the absent clavicles. Care should be taken not to extract baby or supernumerary teeth until permanent teeth can be demonstrated. Preventive management should include early audiologic testing, regular dental care, and orthopedic referral as required for skeletal abnormalities. Interestingly, the patients and their parents are often unaware of the absent clavicles, despite anomalies of the sternocleidomastoid, trapezius, and pectoralis major muscles.

Diastrophic dwarfism

Diastrophic dwarfism was described in 1960 and consists of short limb dwarfism with cleft palate and skeletal deformities. A "hitchhiker thumb" and a cystic malformation of the outer ear, together with progressive scoliosis, club feet, and mesomelic (middle limb segment) dwarfism comprise a diagnostic pattern. Diastrophic dwarfism is representative of a family of disorders, all involving mutations in a sulfate transporter protein that brings sulfate into osteoid cells. The rare, lethal dwarfisms atelosteogenesis type II and achondrogenesis type 1B also involve mutations in the sulfate transporter, which is expressed in many tissues but seems most critical for cartilage development (Horton, 1996).

Complications of diastrophic dysplasia in addition to the aforementioned skeletal deformities include infantile respiratory distress because of micrognathia and tracheomalacia, progressive cervical kyphosis with compression of the cervical spinal cord, congenital heart disease, and dislocation or subluxation of the hips (Gorlin et al., 1990, pp. 193–6; Jones, 1997, pp. 376–7). Preventive management should include careful assessment of the airway in neonates, with interventions ranging from prone positioning to tracheostomy. A hoarse cry is predictive of laryngeal hypoplasia and early respiratory problems, which may be lethal for 25 percent of patients (Gorlin et al., 1990, pp. 193–6). An initial skeletal radiographic survey can evaluate both cardiac status and bony deformities, with careful evaluation for congenital dislocation of the hip. Narrow auditory canals and platybasia may cause frequent otitis media, so audiologic screening together with physical and occupational therapy are important. Regular orthopedic visits are needed for the treatment of scoliosis and possible compression of the cervical cord. Patients with cleft palate may require speech therapy because of problems with articulation, but intelligence is normal. The growth of patients with diastrophic dysplasia has been plotted by Makitie & Kaitila (1997).

Ellis–van Crevald syndrome

The most common form of dwarfism among the Amish, Ellis–van Crevald syndrome is an autosomal recessive disorder that occurs in other populations as well. It is recognized by its unusual pattern of short limbs, polydactyly, club feet, natal teeth, ectodermal dysplasia with hypoplastic nails, congenital heart disease, and genitourinary anomalies. Preventive management should include early echo- and electrocardiogram, recognizing that 50–60 percent will have cardiac anomalies and that there is a significant incidence of sudden cardiac arrest (Gorlin et al., 1990, pp. 201–4; pp. 374–5). Evaluation of the eyes for cataracts and dental care is important, since many patients have missing or supernumerary teeth. Periodic urinalyses and evaluation of the genitalia are important because of genitourinary anomalies such as cryptorchidism, hypospadias, and hydronephrosis.

Fibrodysplasia ossificans progressiva (FOP)

Most cases of FOP are sporadic, but a few instances of familial transmission have suggested autosomal dominant inheritance. Congenital malformations include the absence of digits and thumb anomalies, short femora, and small cervical vertebrae. Most of the complications result from ectopic bone formation, including restriction of limb and pectoral girdle motion, chest wall fixation with respiratory failure, traumatic fractures, spinal deformity, and conductive or sensorineural hearing loss (Einhorn & Kaplan, 1994; Shah et al., 1994). Mental deficiency occurs but is unusual. Preventive management should concentrate on the evaluation of auditory and respiratory function, with early intervention and inclusive school programs for those with mental disability.

Hypophosphatasia

Decreased activity of alkaline phosphatase produces an autosomal recessive disorder with a phenotype similar to that of vitamin D-deficient rickets. Numerous mutations have been defined in the gene for tissue-nonspecific alkaline phosphatase (Henthorn & Whyte, 1992). The severity is variable, with infantile, childhood, and adulthood forms. Prenatal polyhydramnios and neonatal craniotabes, large fontanelle, short limbs, hypercalcemia, hypotonia, and thoracic dysplasia typifies the severe infantile form, and survival is limited to a few days. Moderately affected infants present as failure to thrive with irritability, vomiting, polyuria, and constipation that may reflect hypercalcemia. The radiographic changes of rickets may not be recognized until age 2 or 3, although the diagnosis can be made based on a low serum alkaline phosphatase level and increased urinary phosphoethanolamine.

The adult form may exhibit only osteomalacia and episodes of bone pain; pseudo-fracture of the femur with loss of mobility is a frequent adult presentation. Preventive management (Watanabe et al., 1993) will include surveillance for feeding problems, growth delay, cranial anomalies (craniosynostosis, seizures), ocular anomalies (keratopathy, conjunctival calcification), dental anomalies (premature tooth loss, periodontal disease), decreased renal function (nephrocalcinosis), and bony deformities (genu valgum, osteoporosis). There is no specific therapy, but remissions may occur in later childhood accompanied by increases in alkaline phosphatase activity.

Osteopetrosis

Osteopetrosis includes mild and severe forms with autosomal recessive or autosomal dominant inheritance (Carolino et al., 1998). More than 400 cases of the severe, recessive Albers–Schonberg disease have been reported, many dying in infancy or early childhood. Increased bone deposition encroaches on bone marrow and osteal foramina to produce pancytopenia, hepatosplenomegaly, blindness, deafness, and cranial nerve paralysis. Monitoring of vision, hearing, peripheral blood counts, and dental care is important for preventive management. Bone marrow transplant has been helpful in several patients (Gerritsen et al., 1994), but calcium diuresis has not been useful (van Lie Peters et al., 1993). One form of autosomal recessive osteopetrosis involves a mutation in the gene for carbonic anhydrase (Hu et al., 1994). Affected patients have renal tubular acidosis and dull mentality in addition to features of Albers–Schonberg syndrome.

Autosomal dominant osteopetrosis is more benign, and does not manifest until early childhood. Complications include fractures after minor trauma, conductive hearing loss, ablation of the sinuses, and frequent osteomyelitis of the mandible (necessitating thorough oral examinations at each pediatric visit together with regular dental care). Elevation of acid phosphatase may be a helpful diagnostic screen, and preventive management should focus on audiology and orthopedic assessment.

Pseudohypoparathyroidism (Albright hereditary osteodystrophy)

Described by Albright and colleagues in 1942, pseudohypoparathyroidism presents with radiographic, renal, and serum calcium changes suggestive of hypoparathyroidism, but involves normal levels of parathormone (Gorlin et al., 1990, pp. 139–43; Jones, 1997, pp. 444–5). The disorder exhibits marked variability, exemplified by patients with normal calcium levels who were once distinguished by the term "pseudo-pseudo-hypoparathyroidism." Inheritance is usually autosomal dominant, with predominance of affected females, but autosomal recessive forms have been described. A small deletion in the chromosome 2q37 region has been found in some patients (Phelan et al., 1995), and mutations in the Gs alpha gene have been characterized (Wilson et al., 1994) in some but not all (Shapira et al., 1996). Phenotypic variation according to parental origin of the mutation is implied, and genomic imprinting may account for the striking clinical variability of the disorder (Wilson et al., 1994).

Complications include short stature (60 percent), mental disability (70 percent of hypocalcemic patients, 30 percent of normocalcemic patients), ocular cataracts, enamel hypoplasia of the teeth, short digits with bowing of the long bones, osteopenia with bone cysts, hypothyroidism, and ectopic calcification in the basal ganglia and choroid plexus. Less common complications include anosmia (because Gs proteins are involved in olfactory signal transduction), hearing loss (Garty et al., 1994), growth hormone deficiency (Manfredi et al., 1993), and spinal stenosis (Okada et al., 1994).

The diagnosis of pseudohypoparathyroidism is based on compatible clinical manifestations plus the laboratory findings of hypocalcemia, hyperphosphatemia, and increased levels of parathormone. Preventive management should include the treatment of hypocalcemia to avoid seizures or ectopic calcification, periodic ophthalmologic and audiologic evaluations to rule out cataracts and hearing loss, monitoring of growth and thyroid hormone levels, periodic skeletal examination to recognize early bowing or limb deformities, and monitoring of gait and urinary function to exclude spinal stenosis. Patients should also have early intervention and speech/physical therapy/occupational therapy to maximize developmental potential, regular dental care, and nutritional counseling to prevent obesity.

Spondyloepiphyseal dysplasia congenita (SED)

Spranger and Wiedemann first described spondyloepiphyseal dysplasia congenita (SED) in 1966 (Gorlin et al., 1990, pp. 221–3; Jones, 1997, pp. 358–9). The incidence of SED is about 1 in 100,000 births, and it exhibits autosomal dominant inheritance. SED, Strudwick spondylometaphyseal dysplasia, and lethal hypochondrogenesis comprise a family of chondrodysplasias with flattened vertebrae and mutations in the type II collagen gene (Spranger et al., 1994).

Short stature is severe in SED, with other complications including kyphoscoliosis, myopia, vitreoretinal degeneration, and hypoplasia of the odontoid bone with potential atlantoaxial instability. Cleft or high palate is also common, and some patients develop coxa vara and hip degeneration as adults. The skeletal changes of SED may be seen in congenital hypothyroidism or Down syndrome (Eberle, 1993; Ioan et al., 1993), and one patient with SED presented with nephrotic syndrome (Bogdanovic et al., 1994). The heterogeneity of SED emphasizes the need for early genetic referral for proper diagnosis and counseling. Preventive management should include early and regular ocular and orthopedic consultation, with monitoring for retinal detachment, cervical spine compression, or atlanto-axial instability. Evaluation of the cervical spine and extreme caution are indicated for patients undergoing anesthesia (Redl, 1998). Thyroid functional screening should be performed in early childhood to rule out hypothyroidism.

Achondroplasia

Terminology

"Achondroplasia," coined by Parrot in 1878, is a well-established but incorrect term, since cartilage is not completely lacking in the disorder (Gorlin et al., 1990, pp. 171–5). Hypochondroplasia, like achondroplasia, results from mutations in the gene for the fibroblast growth factor-3 receptor (Bellus et al., 1995). Patients with hypochondroplasia have a relatively normal face and milder skeletal changes than patients with achondroplasia.

Incidence, etiology, and differential diagnosis

The incidence of achondroplasia is between 1 in 16,000 and 1 in 25,000 births, while that for hypochondroplasia is about 10-fold less. Both disorders result from mutations in different portions of the fibroblast growth factor-3 receptor gene. Thanatophoric dysplasia, a lethal form of dwarfism discussed above, comprises the fourth member of this allelic group (homozygous achondroplasia is also distinctive). Differential diagnosis involves the separation of achondroplasia from other forms of short-limbed dwarfism. Patients with achondroplasia have rhizomelic (proximal) limb shortening, prominent forehead with shallow nasal bridge, and characteristic splayed or "trident" fingers. Skeletal radiographs will demonstrate characteristic changes in the lumbar vertebrae and pelvis (e.g., unusual iliac wings). Thanatophoric dysplasia can be distinguished at birth by its more severe facial changes, limb shortening, and thoracic narrowing which results in death.

Diagnostic evaluation and medical counseling

The diagnosis of achondroplasia is made by clinical examination (Fig. 11.1, color plate) and skeletal radiographic survey. DNA analysis could be pursued in uncertain cases, but this is not usually required. Inheritance of achondroplasia, hypochondroplasia, and thanatophoric dysplasia is autosomal dominant, with homozygous achondroplasia representing one of the autosomal dominant conditions where a double dose of the abnormal allele causes a more severe phenotype. About 75 percent of achondroplastic patients represent new mutations, explaining why the majority of patients have a normal family history. The chief concerns to be mentioned during medical counseling are the average adult height of 110–45 centimeters and the risks for early hydrocephalus or spinal cord compression. For achondroplasia and particularly hypochondroplasia, medical counseling can be optimistic in view of the normal intelligence, normal lifespan, and remarkable physical adaptation exhibited by these individuals. Individuals with hypochondroplasia do have a 10 percent incidence of cognitive disability.

Family and psychosocial counseling

The majority of patients with achondroplasia will be born to normal parents, provoking a crisis similar to that surrounding the birth of a child with Down syndrome. Genetic referral is essential for evaluation and counseling. As with other situations involving a newborn with congenital anomalies, timely and unrushed explanation of the diagnostic approach is important, followed by supportive counseling once the diagnosis seems probable. For normal parents, the recurrence risk will be negligible but not zero due to the possibility of germinal mosaicism (Reiser et al., 1984). Couples with achondroplasia have a 50 percent risk of having a child with achondroplasia, a 25 percent risk of having a child with lethal homozygous achondroplasia, and a 25 percent risk of having a normal or "average-sized" child. The diagnosis of achondroplasia is increasingly made by fetal ultrasound, allowing earlier preparation and counseling of the parents.

Positive literature on achondroplasia and other dwarfing conditions is available from the Little People of America (see the achondroplasia checklist, part 1). Discussion with other average-sized parents can be invaluable in fostering acceptance of the child with dwarfism. Some parents will need time before confronting the reality forced by support groups, but the exposure to medical or psychosocial resources and the positive images promoted for their child warrant continued encouragement to realize the advantages offered by Little People of America (achondroplasia checklist, part 1). Most regions of the United States and Canada have local chapters.

Natural history and complications

Although intellectual potential is normal, complications of the central nervous system are of foremost concern for infants with achondroplasia. The large head, platybasia, and small foramen magnum cause these children to be at risk for compression of the brain stem and upper spinal cord (Ryken & Menezes, 1994; Pauli et al., 1995; Tasker et al., 1998). The cervicomedullary compression may present as recurrent apnea, central sleep apnea, unusually severe hypotonia and developmental delay, or sudden death (Pauli et al., 1984; Waters et al., 1993). This compression may also be associated with hydrocephalus, causing increased intracranial venous pressure from presumed constriction of jugular venous return (checklist, part 1).

The lower spinal canal is also narrow, producing cord and nerve root compression from vertebral bone spurs, disc prolapse, or deformed vertebral bodies later in life. The interpedicular distances narrow as one progresses to the lower spine, causing kyphosis (20 percent) and/or scoliosis (7 percent). Limbs may become bowed due to ligamentous laxity, resulting in genua vara (15 percent) or varus foot deformity. Of 100 achondroplastic patients over age 18, 75–97 percent had a history of ear infections and 11–72 percent had significant hearing loss (Glass et al., 1981; Shohat et al., 1993). Studies of younger patients showed frequencies of conductive hearing loss as great as 50 percent, with mixed or sensorineural hearing loss being less common (Gorlin et al., 1990, pp. 171–5).

Other complications of achondroplasia include restrictive lung disease with risks for hypoxia or infection, and mild glucose intolerance (Jones, 1997, pp. 346–7). Females have an increased incidence of uterine fibroids with menorrhagia, and their narrow pelvis requires delivery by Cesarean section under general anesthesia (Allanson & Hall, 1986). Little has been written about the psychiatric burdens of dwarfism, but anecdotal evidence of depression in these individuals warrants attention to their affect and mood during medical assessments.

In hypochondroplasia, short stature and macrocephaly are less pronounced than in achondroplasia, and there is developmental disability in 10 percent. Limb bowing and lumbar lordosis also occur, but rarely require treatment. Chronic otitis or hearing loss has not been documented, but Cesarean section may be required for the delivery of pregnant females. Thus, by virtue of early lethality or benign natural history, few preventive measures can be employed for the other allelic disorders of the fibroblast growth factor-3 receptor.

Achondroplasia preventive medical checklist

Preventive management is critical during infancy to prevent major disability or death, which can result from cervicomedullary spinal compression (checklist, parts 2–4). Clinicians should follow head circumference and motor development, using charts specific for achondroplasia to account for the macrocephaly and motor delay seen in these children (Horton et al., 1978). Parents should be warned about the possibility of spontaneous or sleep-related apnea, and monitors provided when appropriate. If there is apnea or disproportionate variation in head circumference or growth, then structural and functional evaluations of the foramen magnum region are indicated. Skull tomograms or CT scans to evaluate foramen magnum diameter can be compared with age-specific standards (Committee on Genetics, 1995a). Sleep studies to evaluate respiratory abnormalities from medullary compression should be performed. Somatic evoked potentials, which measure the time required for back-and-forth impulse transmission through the foramen magnum, may also be helpful in demonstrating functional spinal cord compression. Those children with demonstrated abnormalities should be followed with an apnea monitor and considered for surgery to enlarge the foramen magnum. There is currently some controversy about the timing and utility of surgical intervention (Pauli et al., 1995a). The medical advisory board for Little People of America can be helpful in these decisions, and are available for consultation at national conventions.

Another early concern is to begin preventive management for the skeletal system so that later bony deformities, arthritis, and lower spinal cord compressions can be minimized. Because of their disproportionate macrocephaly and joint laxity, children with achondroplasia need additional support during infancy. The head should be supported during handling and devices that artificially prop the infant or give poor support should be avoided. Such devices include umbrella strollers, baby walkers, and certain types of infant swings. Normal infant activity will not cause damage and should not be restricted. The degree of kyphosis and other joint deformities should be monitored during childhood, and aggressive dietary management should be initiated to avoid obesity that predisposes to nerve root compression and degenerative arthritis. A frequency of ear infections and hearing loss that is comparable to that of Down syndrome suggests the same monitoring of auditory function should apply – yearly audiology until the child is 3–4 years old. Newer therapies for dwarfism include growth hormone supplementation and surgical leg-lengthening procedures. Both are expensive, and the latter includes risks of infection or bony deformity (Ganel & Horoszowsky, 1996). There is evidence of response to growth hormone supplementation (Yamate et al., 1993; Gross, 1996; Shohat et al., 1996).

Osteogenesis imperfecta

Terminology

Sillence et al. (1979) delineated four major types of osteogenesis imperfecta, and more than a dozen additional syndromes include bone fragility as a component feature (Gorlin et al., 1990, pp. 156–66; Jones, 1997, pp. 486–7). Most common is type I osteogenesis imperfecta with short stature, fractures, blue sclerae, and normal life span. Perinatal lethal osteogenesis imperfecta is designated as type II, with types III (prominent limb bowing) and IV (normal sclerae) being intermediate in severity.

Incidence, etiology, and differential diagnosis

The estimated prevalence of the major types of osteogenesis imperfecta is about 1 in 20,000 individuals (Gorlin et al., 1990, pp. 156–66). Types I, III and IV were long known to exhibit autosomal dominant inheritance, while type II was considered autosomal recessive. Now it is realized that all major types of osteogenesis imperfecta involve mutations in the genes for type I collagen, with type II osteogenesis imperfecta caused by new mutations in critical regions of the collagen molecule.

Occasional type II families in which normal parents have several affected children are thought to represent germinal mosaicism. Differential diagnosis includes numerous syndromes with osteogenesis imperfecta plus unusual features like craniosynostosis (Cole–Carpenter syndrome), microcephaly (Buyse–Bull syndrome), or Marfanoid habitus (Miegel syndrome). These disorders are discussed by Gorlin et al. (1990, pp. 156–66).

Diagnostic evaluation and medical counseling

The presence of osteopenia, fractures, blue sclerae, and hearing loss is strongly suggestive of osteogenesis imperfecta, particularly when there is a family history. Skeletal radiographs are often diagnostic, but biochemical and molecular analysis of type I collagen provide the most definitive diagnosis when an abnormality can be detected. Although DNA testing can be performed from blood samples, the variety of mutations in the osteogenesis imperfectas is too great to allow comprehensive screening. A better algorithm for testing is to analyze type I collagen synthesis from cultured fibroblasts in the hope of finding deficient or altered $\alpha 1$ or $\alpha 2$ chains. If an abnormality of type I collagen biosynthesis is detected, then mutational screening of appropriate $\alpha 1$ or $\alpha 2$ procollagen gene regions can proceed based on the clinical and biochemical phenotype (Prockop & Kivirikko, 1995).

Since mutations in either procollagen gene have been detected in all four types of osteogenesis imperfecta and in two types of Ehlers–Danlos syndrome, clinical correlation is still required for diagnosis and prognosis. Type II osteogenesis imperfecta often produces thickened limb bones that can be recognized by skeletal radiography; early recognition is important because of very short, deformed limbs, and the limited life span and developmental potential. Survival of patients with type II osteogenesis imperfecta is often determined by the severity of rib fractures and deformities as related to respiratory sufficiency. The poor outlook for these children is magnified by the recent demonstration of impaired nerve cell migration in the brain due to prenatal vascular changes (Verkh et al., 1995). Children with type III osteogenesis imperfecta also exhibit increased mortality. Milder disease in children typical of types I or IV osteogenesis imperfecta warrants optimistic medical counseling, particularly since the frequency of fractures decreases after puberty.

Family and psychosocial counseling

Normal parents of children with type II osteogenesis imperfecta have a surprisingly high recurrence risk of 6% based on the incidence of germinal mosaicism. Parents of children with other types of osteogenesis imperfecta should be evaluated carefully, since affected individuals may not exhibit fractures or blue sclerae. Skeletal radiographs may be warranted to separate affected parents with a 50 percent recurrence risk from unaffected parents with a negligible recurrence risk. Genetic referral and counseling is essential for these families.

Cole (1993) emphasized the psychosocial effects of osteogenesis imperfecta that result from the stigmatization of individuals as different from their peers. The altered lifestyle enforced by brittle bones will depend on the severity of disease and the number of affected family members, and strategies are available to aid families adjust to their social and work environment (Cole, 1993). Parent group organizations (checklist, part 1) are very helpful in providing information on psychosocial adjustment and diagnostic testing.

Natural history and complications

The complications of osteogenesis imperfecta vary greatly by type (checklist, part 1). Patients with type II disease are often recognized prenatally, and exhibit extremely short stature with multiple prenatal fractures. Their sclerae will be dark gray or blue, and the skeletal and central nervous system complications are extremely severe. Patients with other types of osteogenesis imperfecta may be difficult to recognize in the neonatal period. Many present in early childhood for evaluation of short stature or recurrent fractures.

The usual phenotype in osteogenesis imperfecta consists of short stature with relative macrocephaly, small nose and chin with blue sclerae and abnormal teeth, joint laxity with dislocations, limb bowing, or kyphoscoliosis, hearing loss that increases with age, and easy bruisability. Less common complications include basilar impression with brain stem damage (Sawin & Menezes, 1997), communicating hydrocephalus with basilar impression of the skull, seizures, aortic root dilatation or mitral valve prolapse (Wong et al., 1995), abdominal pain with constipation from acetabular protrusion (Lee et al., 1995), and renal calculi. Rarely, patients may have complications typical of weakened connective tissue such as retinal detachment (Madigan et al., 1994) or aortic or cerebral aneurysm (Moriyama et al., 1995; Wong et al., 1995; Narvaez et al., 1996).

Osteogenesis imperfecta preventive medical checklist

Preventive management for the osteogenesis imperfectas will primarily focus on the skeletal, nervous, and vascular systems (checklist, parts 2–4). A complete skeletal radiologic survey should be performed as soon as the diagnosis is suspected, both for diagnosis and to evaluate bony deformities that may require treatment. Key issues in early management include appropriate developmental support in children with propensity to fractures, avoidance of immunization sites in fracture-prone areas, and close monitoring with dentistry for signs of excessive tooth wear or misalignment because of fragile teeth (dentinogenesis imperfecta).

Binder et al. (1993) described the value of comprehensive rehabilitation of children with osteogenesis imperfecta, emphasizing gain of head and trunk control using physical supports such as internal and external bracing. Even children with severe osteogenesis imperfecta, limited by joint contractures, impaired balance, and low endurance, showed continued improvement after 10 years of physical rehabilitation. Referrals to orthopedic and physical medicine should accompany regular pediatric evaluation of skeletal growth and alignment, and early intervention is important for reasons of physical and occupational therapy.

Charnas & Marini (1993) emphasized the potential complications of communicating hydrocephalus, basilar skull invagination (Sawin & Menezes, 1997), skull fracture, spinal cord compression, and seizures in osteogenesis imperfecta, and suggested that neurologic evaluation be performed in all patients with severe disease. Neurologic assessment should be part of the regular pediatric examination as indicated on the checklist (parts 2–4), with periodic neurology referrals for patients with severe disease. Symptoms of basilar invagination included headache (76 percent), lower cranial nerve dysfunction (68 percent), hyperreflexia (56 percent), quadriparesis (48 percent), ataxia (32 percent), nystagmus (28 percent), and scoliosis (20 percent; Sawin & Menezes, 1997). Basilar invagination was a significant cause of death for patients with more severe forms of osteogenesis imperfecta, along with restrictive lung disease and congestive heart failure secondary to severe kyphoscoliosis (McAllion & Paterson, 1996; Paterson et al., 1996).

Short stature is the rule for osteogenesis imperfecta, and Marini et al. (1993) demonstrated a blunted response to growth hormone provocation tests in 18 of 28 children with osteogenesis imperfecta. They also demonstrated increased growth velocity in several children after the administration of growth hormone therapy, so endocrinology referral should be considered in children with severe short stature. Early and regular assessment of hearing and vision is also recommended because of sensorineural hearing loss, retinal detachment, and myopia that is frequent in osteogenesis imperfecta. Although congenital heart disease is not common, later aortic dilatation and mitral valve prolapse warrant careful cardiac examination during pediatric follow-up and formal cardiac assessment in adolescence or early adulthood (checklist, part 4).

Newer therapies for the severe osteoporosis that accompanies osteogenesis imperfecta include intravenous pamidronate and biphosphonates (Bembi et al., 1997; Brumsen et al., 1997; Marini & Gerber, 1997; Shaw, 1997). Therapy may be associated with hypercalcemia (Williams et al., 1997).

Preventive Management of Achondroplasia

Clinical diagnosis: Pattern of skeletal changes including short stature with disproportionately short limbs, prominent forehead, shallow nasal bridge, lordotic posture, broad hands and feet.
Incidence: 1 in 16,000–25,000 live births.
Laboratory diagnosis: DNA analysis to demonstrate characteristic mutations in the fibroblast growth factor-3 receptor.
Genetics: Autosomal dominant inheritance predicting a 50% recurrence risk for affected individuals; achondroplast couples also have a 25% risk for severely affected homozygotes.
Key management issues: Monitor head circumference, muscle tone, and development to recognize cervicomedullary spinal compression; consider foramen magnum measurement by CT scan; dietary counsel and weight control to minimize later bony deformities, arthritis, and lower spinal cord compression; prevention of chronic otitis and hearing loss; alertness for depression.
Growth charts: Horton et al. (1978), Committee on Genetics (1995).
Parent groups: Little People of America, P.O. Box 745, Lubbock TX, 79408, (888) 572-2001, http://www.lpaonline.org; Restricted Growth Association, P.O. Box 8, Countesthorpe, Leicestershire, LE8 5ZS UK, 44 1(16) 247-8913.
Basis for management recommendations: Consensus guidelines from the Committee on Genetics (1995) and the complications below as documented by Pauli et al. (1995), Ryken & Menezes (1994).

Summary of clinical concerns

General	Life cycle	Sudden infant death (5%)
	Behavior	Risk for depression in older individuals
	Growth	**Short stature** (males average 130 cm, females average 123 cm)
Facial	Face	Frontal bossing, shallow nasal bridge
	Ear	**Otitis media** (75–97%)
Surface	Neck/trunk	Neck injuries, cervical cord compression
Skeletal	Cranial	Macrocephaly, platybasia, narrow foramen magnum
	Axial	Spinal stenosis, **kyphosis** (20%), scoliosis (7%)
	Limbs	Rhizomelic shortening, genu vara (15%), **joint laxity**, **arthritis**, joint injuries
Internal	Pulmonary	Restrictive disease ($< 3\%$), apnea
	Endocrine	Mild glucose intolerance
	Genital	**Narrow pelvis**, uterine fibroids, metrorrhagia
Neural	CNS	Altered CSF circulation, hydrocephalus, cervical cord compression, sleep apnea
	Sensory	Chronic otitis, Hearing loss (11–72%)

RES, reticuloendothelial system, GI, gastrointestinal system; **bold: frequency > 20%**

Key references

Committee on Genetics, (1995). *Pediatrics* 95:443–51.
Horton, W. A. et al. (1978). *Journal of Pediatrics* 93:435–8.
Pauli, R. M. et al. (1995). *American Journal of Human Genetics* 56:732–44.
Ryken, T.C. & Menezes, A. H. (1994). *Journal of Neurosurgery* 81:43–8.

Achondroplasia

Preventive medical checklist (0–1yr)

Patient		Birth Date / /	Number	

Pediatric	Screen		Evaluate		Refer/Counsel	
Neonatal / / *Newborn screen* ☐ *HB* ☐	Skeletal x-rays ☐ Head sonogram ☐		Skeleton ☐		Genetic evaluation ☐	
1 month / /	Growth ☐ Head size ☐		Skeleton ☐ Muscle tone ☐ Otitis ☐		Family support[4] ☐	
2 months / / *HB[1]* ☐ *Hib* ☐ *DTaP, IPV* ☐ *RV* ☐	Growth ☐ Head size ☐ Hearing, vision[2] ☐		Skeleton ☐ Muscle tone ☐		Early intervention[5] ☐ Genetic counseling ☐ Careful anesthesia ☐	
4 months / / *HB[1]* ☐ *Hib* ☐ *DTaP/IPV* ☐ *RV* ☐	Growth ☐ Head size ☐ Hearing, vision[2] ☐		Skeleton ☐ Muscle tone ☐ Otitis ☐		Early intervention[5] ☐	
6 months / / *Hib* ☐ *IPV[1]* ☐ *DTaP* ☐ *RV* ☐	Growth ☐ Head size ☐ Hearing, vision[2] ☐ Head MRI[3] ☐		Skeleton ☐ Muscle tone ☐ Sleep apnea ☐		Family support[4] ☐ Neurosurgery[3] ☐	
9 months / / *IPV[1]* ☐	Audiology ☐		Otitis ☐		Careful anesthesia ☐	
1 year / / *HB* ☐ *Hib[1]* ☐ *IPV[1]* ☐ *MMR[1]* ☐ *Var[1]* ☐	Growth ☐ Head size ☐ Hearing, vision[2] ☐ Head, spine MRI[3] ☐		Skeleton ☐ Muscle tone ☐ Sleep apnea ☐ Otitis ☐		Family support[4] ☐ Early intervention[5] ☐ Genetics ☐ Orthopedics ☐ Neurology, ENT[3] ☐	

Clinical concerns for Achondroplasia, ages 0–1 year

Macrocephaly	Dental anomalies	Developmental delay
Chronic otitis	Apnea, sudden death	Hydrocephalus
Hearing loss	Kyphosis	Stenosis of foramen magnum
Short stature		Hypotonia, joint laxity

Guidelines for the neonatal period should be undertaken *at whatever age* the diagnosis is made; DTaP, acellular DTP; IPV, inactivated poliovirus (oral polio also used); RV, rotavirus; MMR, measles–mumps–rubella; Var, varicella; [1]alternative timing; [2]by practitioner; [3]as dictated by clinical findings – head and/or foramen magnum MRI for extreme hypotonia, focal signs, excessive head growth, sleep problems; [4]parent group, family/sib, financial, and behavioral issues as discussed in the preface; [5]including developmental monitoring and motor/speech therapy.

Achondroplasia

Preventive medical checklist (15m–6yrs)

Patient   **Birth Date**   /   /   **Number**

Pediatric	Screen		Evaluate		Refer/Counsel	
15 months / / Hib[1] ☐ MMR[1] ☐ DTaP, IPV[1] ☐ Varicella[1] ☐	Hearing[2]	☐			Family support[4] Early intervention[5]	☐ ☐
18 months / / DTaP, IPV[1] ☐ Varicella[1] ☐ Influenza[3] ☐	Hearing[2]	☐	Skeleton Muscle tone Sleep apnea	☐ ☐ ☐		
2 years / / Influenza[3] ☐ Pneumovax[3] ☐ Dentist ☐	Hearing[2]	☐	Skeleton, hips Muscle tone Sleep apnea	☐ ☐ ☐	Genetics Home adaptation[3]	☐ ☐
3 years / / Influenza[3] ☐ Pneumovax[3] ☐ Dentist ☐	Hearing[2] Growth Head size Audiology	☐ ☐ ☐ ☐	Skeleton, hips Muscle tone Sleep apnea	☐ ☐ ☐	Family support[4] Orthopedics Neurology[3] ENT[3]	☐ ☐ ☐ ☐
4 years / / Influenza[3] ☐ Pneumovax[3] ☐ Dentist ☐	Hearing[2] Growth Head size	☐ ☐ ☐	Skeleton, hips Gait, bowing Neuro exam	☐ ☐ ☐	Family support[4] Genetics Orthopedics[3] Physical medicine[3] Neurology[3]	☐ ☐ ☐ ☐ ☐
5 years / / DTaP, IPV[1] ☐ MMR[1] ☐	Hearing[2] Audiology	☐ ☐	Skeleton, spine Gait, bowing Neuro exam	☐ ☐ ☐	Orthopedics[3] Physical medicine[3] Dietician[3]	☐ ☐ ☐
6 years / / DTaP, IPV[1] ☐ MMR[1] ☐ Dentist ☐	Growth Head size Hearing, vision[2]	☐ ☐ ☐	Skeleton, spine Gait, bowing Neuro exam	☐ ☐ ☐	Family support[5] Orthopedics Neurology[3] Endocrinology[3]	☐ ☐ ☐ ☐

Clinical concerns for Achondroplasia, ages 1–6 years

Macrocephaly	Dental anomalies	Developmental delay
Chronic otitis, hearing loss	Kyphosis	Hydrocephalus
Short stature	Hypotonia, joint laxity	Stenosis of foramen magnum

Guidelines for prior ages should be undertaken *at the time of diagnosis*; DTaP, acellular DTP; IPV, inactivated poliovirus (oral polio also used); MMR, measles–mumps–rubella; [1]alternative timing; [2]by practitioner; [3]as dictated by clinical findings – head and/or foramen magnum MRI for extreme hypotonia, focal signs, excessive head growth, sleep problems; endocrinology for those with severe short stature; adaptation of toilets, etc., for size; [4]parent group, family/sib, financial, and behavioral issues as discussed in the preface; [5]including developmental monitoring and motor/speech therapy.

Achondroplasia

Preventive medical checklist (6+ yrs)

Patient		Birth Date / /		Number	

Pediatric	Screen	Evaluate		Refer/Counsel	
8 years / / *Dentist* ❑		Skeleton Neurology exam	❑ ❑	Genetics Careful anesthesia Diet, exercise Endocrinology[3]	❑ ❑ ❑ ❑
10 years / /	Growth ❑ Head size ❑ Hearing, vision[2] ❑	Skeleton Obesity	❑ ❑	Orthopedics[3] Neurology[3] Dietician[3]	❑ ❑ ❑
12 years / / *Td[1], MMR, Var* ❑ *CBC* ❑ *Dentist* ❑ *Scoliosis* ❑ *Cholesterol* ❑		Skeleton Puberty Neurology exam	❑ ❑ ❑	Family support[4] Diet, exercise Genetics	❑ ❑ ❑
14 years / / *CBC* ❑ *Dentist* ❑ *Cholesterol* ❑ *Breast CA* ❑ *Testicular CA* ❑	Growth ❑ Head size ❑	Skeleton Puberty Menstruation	❑ ❑ ❑	Orthopedics[3] Neurology[3] Nutrition[3]	❑ ❑ ❑
16 years / / *Td[1]* ❑ *CBC* ❑ *Cholesterol* ❑ *Sexual[5]* ❑ *Dentist* ❑	Hearing, vision[2] ❑	Skeleton Puberty Neurology exam	❑ ❑ ❑	Genetics Diet, exercise	❑ ❑
18 years / / *CBC* ❑ *Sexual[5]* ❑ *Cholesterol* ❑ *Scoliosis* ❑	Growth ❑ Head size ❑			Reproductive counsel[3]	❑
20 years[6] / / *CBC* ❑ *Sexual[5]* ❑ *Cholesterol* ❑ *Dentist* ❑	Hearing, vision[2] ❑	Scoliosis Spinal nerves Arthritis Menstruation	❑ ❑ ❑ ❑	Family support[4] Orthopedics[3] Neurology[3] Diet, exercise Dietician[3]	❑ ❑ ❑ ❑ ❑

Clinical concerns for Achondroplasia, ages 6+ years

Obesity	Spinal nerve compression	Uterine fibroids
Hearing loss	Lower cord compression	Menorrhagia
Dental crowding	Scoliosis	Arthritis

Guidelines for prior ages should be undertaken *at the time of diagnosis*; Td, tetanus/diphtheria; MMR, measles–mumps–rubella; Var, varicella; [1]alternative timing; [2]by practitioner; [3]as dictated by clinical findings – endocrinology for those with severe short stature, reproductive issues include necessity of cesarean section for affected women; [4]parent group, family/sib, financial, and behavioral issues as discussed in the preface; [5]birth control, STD screening if sexually active; [6]repeat every decade.

Preventive Management of Osteogenesis Imperfecta

Clinical diagnosis: Four major phenotypes including type I osteogenesis imperfecta with short stature, fractures, deafness, and blue sclerae; type II with severe dwarfism, thick bones, deformed craniofacies, small chest and infantile death; type III with prominent limb bowing; and type IV with normal sclerae, fractures, and mild limb bowing.

Incidence: 1 in 20,000 live births.

Laboratory diagnosis: Cell culture demonstrating deficiency of type I collagen synthesis, DNA diagnosis defining characteristic mutations in type I collagen (all 4 clinical types).

Genetics: Autosomal dominant inheritance with a 50% risk for transmitting the disease. Significant frequencies of germline mosaicism yield a 5–6% risk recurrence risk for normal parents.

Key management issues: Monitoring of skeletal growth and contour with initial skeletal radiologic survey; hearing assessments; avoidance of immunization sites near fractures; dental evaluations for signs of excessive tooth wear or misalignment; comprehensive rehabilitation with physical supports such as internal and external bracing; early intervention is important for reasons of physical and occupational therapy.

Growth charts: None.

Parent groups: Osteogenesis Imperfecta Foundation, 804 W. Diamond Ave. Suite 210, Gaithersburg MD, 20878, (800) 981-2663, bonelink@aol.com; Canadian Osteogenesis Imperfecta Society, 128 Thornhill Crescent, Chatham ON, Canada, N7L 4M3, (519) 436-0025, mkearney@kent.net; National Osteoporosis Society, P. O. Box 10, Radstock, Bath BA3 3YB UK, (01761) 471771.

Basis for management recommendations: Derived from the complications listed below as documented by Binder et al. (1993), Charnas & Marini (1993), Sillence et al. (1979).

Summary of clinical concerns

General	Life cycle	Infant mortality (90% by 1 month in type II)
	Growth	**Short stature**
	Tumors	Osteosarcoma
Facial	Eye	Blue sclerae, embryotoxon, retinal detachment
	Mouth	**Dental anomalies** (tooth discoloration, opalescent teeth (type IV), shortened dental roots, mandibular bone cysts)
Surface	Neck/trunk	
	Epidermal	**Easy bruisability** (75%)
Skeletal	Cranial	Macrocephaly, Wormian bones, platybasia
	Axial	**Kyphosis, scoliosis** (20%)
	Limbs	**Multiple fractures**, short limbs (type II), limb bowing (type III), joint laxity, joint dislocations
Internal	Digestive	Abdominal pain, constipation
	Pulmonary	Restricted lung volume from rib fractures (type II)
	Circulatory	Aortic root dilatation (12%), mitral valve prolapse (9%)
	Excretory	Renal calculi
Neural	CNS	**Basilar impression** (25%), hydrocephaly, cerebral aneurysm, spinal cord compression, seizures
	Sensory	**Sensorineural hearing loss** (50%)

RES, reticuloendothelial system, GI, gastrointestinal system; **bold:** frequency > 20%

Key references

Binder, H. et al. (1993). *American Journal of Medical Genetics* 45:265–9.
Charnas, L. R. & Marini, J. C. (1993). *Neurology* 43:2603–8.
Prockop, D. J. & Kivirikko, K. I. (1995). *Annual Review of Biochemistry* 64:403–34.
Sillence, D. O., Senn, A. & Danks, D. M. (1979). *Journal of Medical Genetics* 16:101–16

Osteogenesis Imperfecta

Preventive medical checklist (0–1yr)

Patient   **Birth Date**   /   /   **Number**

Pediatric	Screen		Evaluate		Refer/Counsel	
Neonatal / / *Newborn screen* ❑ *HB* ❑	Skeletal x-rays Head size	❑ ❑	Skeleton Fractures	❑ ❑	Genetic evaluation Orthopedic evaluation Physical medicine[3]	❑ ❑ ❑
1 month / /			Skeleton Fractures Heart	❑ ❑ ❑	Family support[4] Cardiology[3] Physical medicine[3]	❑ ❑ ❑
2 months / / *HB[1]* ❑ *Hib* ❑ *DTaP, IPV* ❑ *RV* ❑	Growth Head size Hearing, vision[2]	❑ ❑ ❑	Skeleton Fractures	❑ ❑	Early intervention[5] Genetic counseling Careful anesthesia	❑ ❑ ❑
4 months / / *HB[1]* ❑ *Hib* ❑ *DTaP/IPV* ❑ *RV* ❑	Growth Head size Hearing, vision[2]	❑ ❑ ❑	Skeleton Fractures	❑ ❑	Physical medicine[3] Early intervention[5]	❑ ❑
6 months / / *Hib* ❑ *IPV[1]* ❑ *DTaP* ❑ *RV* ❑	Growth Head size Hearing, vision[2]	❑ ❑ ❑	Skeleton Fractures	❑ ❑	Family support[4] Orthopedic evaluation Physical medicine[3] Neurology[3]	❑ ❑ ❑ ❑
9 months / / *IPV[1]* ❑	Audiology	❑			Ophthalmology[3]	❑
1 year / / *HB* ❑ *Hib[1]* ❑ *IPV[1]* ❑ *MMR[1]* ❑ *Var[1]* ❑	Growth Head size Hearing, vision[3]	❑ ❑ ❑	Skeleton Fractures, heart Neuro exam	❑ ❑ ❑	Family support[4] Early intervention[5] Genetics Orthopedics[3] Physical medicine[3]	❑ ❑ ❑ ❑ ❑

Clinical concerns for Osteogenesis Imperfecta, ages 0–1 year

Fractures	Atlantoaxial instability	Joint laxity
Eye anomalies (retina)	Cardiac anomalies	Limb bowing
Hearing loss	Dental anomalies	Orthopedic problems

Guidelines for the neonatal period should be undertaken *at whatever age* the diagnosis is made; DTaP, acellular DTP; IPV, inactivated poliovirus (oral polio also used); RV, rotavirus; MMR, measles–mumps–rubella; Var, varicella; [1]alternative timing; [2]by practitioner; [3]as dictated by clinical findings; [4]parent group, family/sib, financial, and behavioral issues as discussed in the preface; [5]including developmental monitoring and motor/speech therapy.

Osteogenesis Imperfecta

Preventive medical checklist (15m–6yrs)

Patient **Birth Date** / / **Number**

Pediatric	Screen		Evaluate		Refer/Counsel	
15 months / / *Hib*[1] ☐ *MMR*[1] ☐ *DTaP, IPV*[1] ☐ *Varicella*[1] ☐					Family support[4] Early intervention[5]	☐ ☐
18 months / / *DTaP, IPV*[1] ☐ *Varicella*[1] ☐ *Influenza*[3] ☐					Careful anesthesia	☐
2 years / / *Influenza*[3] ☐ *Pneumovax*[3] ☐ *Dentist* ☐	Growth Head size Hearing, vision[2] Audiology	☐ ☐ ☐ ☐	Skeleton Fractures AAI Neuro exam	☐ ☐ ☐ ☐	Family support[4] Genetics Orthopedics[3] Physical medicine[3]	☐ ☐ ☐ ☐
3 years / / *Influenza*[3] ☐ *Pneumovax*[3] ☐ *Dentist* ☐	Growth Head size Audiology C-spine x-rays	☐ ☐ ☐ ☐	Skeleton Fractures AAI Heart Neuro exam	☐ ☐ ☐ ☐ ☐	Family support[4] Preschool transition[5] Orthopedics[3] Physical medicine[3]	☐ ☐ ☐ ☐
4 years / / *Influenza*[3] ☐ *Pneumovax*[3] ☐ *Dentist* ☐	Growth	☐	Skeleton Fractures AAI Gait, bowing Neuro exam	☐ ☐ ☐ ☐ ☐	Family support[4] Preschool program[3,5] Orthopedics[3] Physical medicine[3] Careful anesthesia	☐ ☐ ☐ ☐ ☐
5 years / / *DTaP, IPV*[1] ☐ *MMR*[1] ☐	Audiology	☐	Skeleton Fractures	☐ ☐	School transition[3,5] Orthopedics[3] Physical medicine[3]	☐ ☐ ☐
6 years / / *DTaP, IPV*[1] ☐ *MMR*[1] ☐ *Dentist* ☐	Growth Hearing, vision[3]	☐ ☐	Skeleton Fractures Gait, bowing Neuro exam	☐ ☐ ☐ ☐	Family support[4] Genetics Orthopedics[3] Ophthalmology[3]	☐ ☐ ☐ ☐

Clinical concerns for Osteogenesis Imperfecta, ages 1–6 years

Fractures	Atlantoaxial instability	Joint laxity
Eye anomalies (retina)	Cardiac anomalies	Limb bowing
Hearing loss	Dental anomalies	Orthopedic problems

Guidelines for prior ages should be undertaken *at the time of diagnosis*; DTaP, acellular DTP; IPV, inactivated poliovirus (oral polio also used); MMR, measles–mumps–rubella; C-spine, cervical spine; AAI, atlantoaxial instability; [1]alternative timing; [2]by practitioner; [3]as dictated by clinical findings; [4]parent group, family/sib, financial, and behavioral issues as discussed in the preface; [5]including developmental monitoring and motor/speech therapy.

Osteogenesis Imperfecta

Preventive medical checklist (6+ yrs)

Patient   **Birth Date** / /   **Number**

Pediatric	Screen	Evaluate	Refer/Counsel	
8 years / / *Dentist* ❑			Genetics Orthopedics[3] Physical medicine[3]	❑ ❑ ❑
10 years / /	Growth ❑ Hearing, vision[2] ❑	Skeleton ❑ Fractures ❑ Neurology exam ❑	Ophthalmology[3] Careful anesthesia	❑ ❑
12 years / / *Td[1], MMR, Var* ❑ *CBC* ❑ *Dentist* ❑ *Scoliosis* ❑ *Cholesterol* ❑	C-spine x-rays[3] ❑	Skeleton ❑ Fractures ❑ AAI ❑ Gait, bowing ❑ Neurology exam ❑	Family support[4] Orthopedics[3] Physical medicine[3] Genetics	❑ ❑ ❑ ❑
14 years / / *CBC* ❑ *Dentist* ❑ *Cholesterol* ❑ *Breast CA* ❑ *Testicular CA* ❑	Growth ❑ Echocardiogram[3] ❑	Skeleton ❑ Fractures ❑ Heart ❑ Neurology exam ❑	Cardiology[3]	❑
16 years / / *Td[1]* ❑ *CBC* ❑ *Cholesterol* ❑ *Sexual[5]* ❑ *Dentist* ❑	Hearing, vision[2] ❑	Skeleton ❑ Fractures ❑ Neurology exam ❑	Genetics Orthopedics[3] Physical medicine[3]	❑ ❑ ❑
18 years / / *CBC* ❑ *Sexual[5]* ❑ *Cholesterol* ❑ *Scoliosis* ❑		Skeleton ❑ Fractures ❑ AAI ❑ Gait, bowing ❑ Neuro exam ❑		
20 years[6] / / *CBC* ❑ *Sexual[5]* ❑ *Cholesterol* ❑ *Dentist* ❑	Hearing, vision[2] ❑	Skeleton ❑ Fractures ❑ Heart ❑ Neuro exam ❑	Family support[4] Orthopedics[3] Physical medicine[3]	❑ ❑ ❑

Clinical concerns for Osteogenesis Imperfecta, ages 6+ years

Eye anomalies (retina)	Aortic dilatation	Fractures
Hearing loss	Mitral valve prolapse	Atlantoaxial instability
Short stature	Joint laxity	Arthritis

Guidelines for prior ages should be undertaken *at the time of diagnosis*; Td, tetanus/diphtheria; MMR, measles–mumps–rubella; Var, varicella; C-spine, cervical spine; AAI, atlantoaxial instability; [1]alternative timing; [2]by practitioner; [3]as dictated by clinical findings; [4]parent group, family/sib, financial, and behavioral issues as discussed in the preface; [5]birth control, STD screening if sexually active; [6]repeat every decade.

12

Overgrowth syndromes

Syndromes with increased growth are listed in Table 12.1. Several, including Beckwith–Wiedemann syndrome, exhibit increased fetal growth with a high birth weight. Others, like cerebral gigantism or Sotos syndrome, are more remarkable for accelerated postnatal growth. Often there is neuropathology manifested by macrocephaly, dilated ventricles, structural brain anomalies, or early hypotonia. Predisposition to neoplasia accompanies many overgrowth disorders, exemplified by the occurrence of Wilms tumor in Beckwith–Wiedemann, Sotos, and hemihyperplasia syndromes. Accelerated skeletal maturation during childhood is also common, suggesting that growth factors acting early in life provide a common pathogenetic mechanism.

Overgrowth is also found in certain chromosomal disorders (e.g., fragile X syndrome), metabolic disorders (e.g., pseudohypoparathyroidism and the mucopolysaccharidoses), or hamartosis syndromes that also have predisposition to cancer (e.g., neurofibromatosis type 1). These disorders are discussed in other chapters. Obesity may also be considered a form of overgrowth, and increased caloric intake may produce increased statural growth and skeletal maturation during childhood. The growth acceleration induced by hyperphagia is usually transient, however, as exemplified by the short adult stature in Prader–Willi syndrome. Here syndromes with sustained growth acceleration due to unknown etiologies are discussed, including detailed consideration of Beckwith–Wiedemann syndrome.

Less common growth disorders

Börjeson–Forssman–Lehmann syndrome

Börjeson–Forssman–Lehmann syndrome is an X-linked recessive disorder that involves facial, skeletal, and genital anomalies in addition to mental disability. Overgrowth in this condition consists mainly of obesity, since 80 percent of patients eventually display short stature (Gorlin et al., 1990, pp. 351–2; Jones et al, 1997, pp. 584–5). Skeletal anomalies include thickened calvaria, narrow spinal canal, epiphyseal dysplasia, and short distal phalanges. Neurologic problems

Table 12.1 Overgrowth syndromes

Syndrome	Inheritance	Incidence	Frequent abnormalities in addition to overgrowth
Hemihyperplasia	Sporadic	>200 cases	Asymmetry, neoplasms
Beckwith–Wiedemann	AD[a]	1 in 17,000 live births	Cerebral, facial, cardiac, visceromegaly, GI, skeletal, endocrine, urinary tract, genital
Perlman		~30 cases	Visceromegaly, renal hamartomas, nephroblastomatosis, Wilms tumor
Sotos	Sporadic	>200 cases	Macrocephaly, hypotonia, accelerated osseous maturation
Weaver	AD	~20 cases	Macrocephaly, characteristic facies, accelerated osseous maturation developmental disability, joint contractures, hernias
Marshall–Smith	Sporadic	~20 cases	Macrocephaly, hypotonia, accelerated osseous maturation, failure to thrive, early death
Simpson–Golabi–Behmel	XLR	~30 cases	Macrocephaly, polydactyly, vertebral anomalies, cardiac conduction defects, genitourinary anomalies, early death
Cohen	AR	~80 cases	Microcephaly, hypotonia, obesity, ocular anomalies, tall stature, genital anomalies, happy affect
Börjeson–Forssman–Lehmann	XLR	~20 cases	Macrocephaly, hypotonia, obesity, hypogonadism

Notes:

[a] With variable penetrance and genomic imprinting; AD, autosomal dominant; AR, autosomal recessive; XLR, X-linked recessive; GI, gastrointestinal.

include microencephaly, hypotonia, seizures (50 percent), and, in the eye, nystagmus and ptosis. Certain of the genital anomalies (small penis, atrophic testes) may reflect pituitary dysfunction, with later alterations in puberty (delay, immaturity, gynecomastia). Female heterozygotes may have mild mental disability and ovarian failure. Preventive management should include early intervention, nutritional counseling to minimize obesity, regular ophthalmologic evaluations, and monitoring of puberty with possible referral to endocrinology.

Cohen syndrome

Cohen syndrome is an autosomal recessive disorder that includes hypotonia, obesity, facial anomalies, chorioretinal dystrophy, and skeletal anomalies (Cohen et al., 1973; Gunay-Aygun et al., 1997). The facial appearance includes down-slanting palpebral fissures, prominent incisors, open mouth, and a short philtrum. Because patients with hypotonia often keep their mouths open, this non-specific characteristic has undoubtedly led to many reported cases that do not actually have the syndrome (Gorlin et al., 1990, pp. 349–50). Complications include overgrowth (20 percent) or short stature (68 percent), hypotonia (92 percent), microcephaly (50–60 percent), mental disability (IQ 30–80), seizures (6 percent), cardiac defects (10 percent), chorioretinopathy with altered electroretinograms, delayed puberty (80 percent), cryptorchidism (31 percent), and hyperextensible joints with narrow hands and fingers (Gorlin et al., 1990, pp. 349–50). Several observers have described a happy, pleasant affect. North et al. (1995a) reported identical twin females with Cohen syndrome who manifested macrocephaly and tall stature early in life with subsequent precocious puberty.

Preventive management for Cohen syndrome should include early intervention for hypotonia and mental disability, baseline ophthalmologic evaluation, nutritional counseling for the prevention of obesity, and adolescent monitoring for delayed/precocious puberty or scoliosis because of joint laxity. Schlictemeier et al. (1994) reported a patient with cerebral thrombosis and a coagulation disorder involving protein S and C deficiencies who had several features of Cohen syndrome.

Hemihyperplasia

Gorlin et al. (1990, pp. 323–9) stressed the use of hemihyperplasia rather than hemihypertrophy because the disorder may be limited to a single tissue (i.e., bone) rather than involving overgrowth of multiple tissues. The hallmark of hemihyperplasia is asymmetry of the face or limbs (Cohen, 1995). Most patients exhibit asymmetry at birth, but discrepancies in limb lengths may not be noticed until later childhood or during puberty. A large number of tissues and regions may be abnormal in association with hemihyperplasia, even though many patients have isolated asymmetry. Abnormalities of the skin (nevi, hemangiomas, ichthyosis), eye (strabismus), mouth (enlarged teeth or tongue), heart (congenital defects), limbs (macrodactyly, polydactyly, club foot, hip dysplasia), viscera (hepatic cysts, polycystic kidneys), genitalia (hypospadias, cryptorchidism), and the central nervous system (macrocephaly, mental deficiency, seizures) may be seen (Gorlin et al., 1990, pp. 323–9). Of particular importance are neoplasms such as Wilms tumor, adrenocortical carcinoma, hepatoblastoma, and neuroblastoma, which occur in 3.8 percent of patients with hemihyperplasia (Hoyme et al., 1987).

Preventive management should include periodic measurement of limb girths and lengths, early intervention, and ophthalmologic referral. The predisposition to tumors warrants surveillance similar to that recommended for Beckwith–Wiedemann syndrome: abdominal ultrasound as soon as the diagnosis is established and followed at 3–6 month intervals until skeletal growth has ceased. Additional preventive measures should include orthopedic monitoring for scoliosis or disturbances in gait, cardiac evaluation with specialty referral if a murmur is detected, and regular dental care.

Marshall–Smith syndrome

This rare syndrome consists of accelerated skeletal maturation with facial and skeletal changes (Gorlin et al., 1990, pp. 340–2; Jones, 1997, pp. 252–3). The clinical course is severe, with hypotonia, failure to thrive, and death before age 3 years in most cases. Facial anomalies include prominent forehead, shallow orbits, large-appearing eyes with blue sclerae and macrocorneae, prominent eyebrows, high-arched palate, unusual ears, and micrognathia. Some patients have a small nose with choanal atresia, and there may be stridor because of a small larynx or laryngomalacia. The extremities and fingers appear long, and patients have unusual posturing with extension of the neck and scoliosis. Occasional anomalies include cardiac defects (patent ductus arteriosus, atrial septal defect), umbilical hernia or omphalocele, and pachygyria of the brain. One patient had an inflammatory rectal polyp that presented with hematochezia (Washington et al., 1993). Preventive management should focus on early intervention for motor and speech delay, hearing and audiology testing, cardiac evaluation with echocardiographic studies if surgery is required, and a baseline head MRI scan to define brain anomalies. Long-term survivors with Marshall–Smith syndrome have been reported (Sperli et al., 1993).

Perlman syndrome

Perlman et al. (1973) reported the combination of fetal gigantism, renal hamartomas, nephroblastosis, and Wilms tumor. Grundy et al. (1992) and Fahmy et al., (1998) emphasized the differences between Perlman and Beckwith–Wiedemann syndromes that mainly concern the abdominal wall and urogenital systems. Gorlin et al. (1990, p. 327) view Perlman syndrome as part of the spectrum of Beckwith–Wiedemann syndrome, and a similar strategy for preventive management is appropriate (see below).

Simpson–Golabi–Behmel syndrome

This X-linked recessive overgrowth disorder was first reported by Simpson and colleagues in 1973 and further delineated by Opitz, Golabi, Rosen, and Behmel (Gorlin et al., 1990, pp. 343–5; Jones, 1997, pp. 168–9). Affected children have high birth weights with subsequent overgrowth and mild mental deficiency. The neonatal course is turbulent, with an infant mortality rate of 50 percent due to cardiac defects, cor pulmonale, respiratory infections, or severe hypoglycemia. Other complications include colobomata, strabismus, cleft palate, macroglossia, cardiac structural or conduction defects, vertebral anomalies with scoliosis, pectus excavatum, inguinal or umbilical hernias, cystic kidneys, urinary tract anomalies, cryptorchidism, and intestinal malrotation (Gorlin et al., 1990, pp. 343–5). Diaphragmatic hernias have also been reported (Chen et al., 1993).

Preventive management for Simpson–Golabi–Behmel syndrome should include neonatal assessment of blood glucose, cardiopulmonary, and urinary tract status. Because of the high rate of infant mortality, baseline electrocardiogram, echocardiogram, skeletal radiologic survey, and abdominal ultrasound can be justified. For patients with a short, broad neck or with torticollis, cervical spine films should be repeated during early childhood. Ophthalmologic evaluation should be performed in the first year, and periodic urinalysis obtained because of possible urinary tract anomalies. Adolescents should be monitored for scoliosis and other skeletal deformities.

After genetic mapping localized the gene for Simpson–Golabi–Behmel syndrome to the Xq26 region, Pilia et al. (1996) characterized deletions in a glypican 3 gene using DNA from two patients with X-autosome translocations. As deduced from DNA sequencing and RNA studies, the glypican 3 gene encodes an extracellular proteoglycan that is expressed in embryonic mesoderm. Alterations in glypican 3 may cause accelerated growth because it forms a complex with insulin-like growth factor-2 (Pilia et al., 1996).

Weaver syndrome

Weaver syndrome is a very rare condition with overgrowth, accelerated skeletal maturation, and distinctive facies (Weaver et al., 1974). The syndrome has been described in siblings, but this may represent germline mosaicism since some cases exhibit autosomal dominant inheritance (Fryer et al., 1997). Typical craniofacial changes include macrocephaly, flattened occiput, hypertelorism, small palpebral fissures, bulbous nasal tip, and abnormal ears. Complications include brain anomalies (cysts of the septum pellucidum, dilated ventricles), delayed motor development, difficulty in swallowing and feeding, skeletal anomalies such as club foot or flat feet, and inguinal or umbilical hernia. An increased risk for neoplasms has not been documented. Preventive management should include early intervention, evaluation of feeding, evaluation for limb deformities, and monitoring of nutrition since some patients exhibit a voracious appetite.

Beckwith–Wiedemann syndrome

Terminology

Beckwith in 1963 and Wiedemann in 1964 reported several patients with macroglossia, omphalocele, and visceromegaly that comprise Beckwith–Wiedemann syndrome (Fig. 12.1, color plate; Gorlin et al., 1990, pp. 323–9; Jones, 1997, pp. 164–5).

Incidence, etiology, and differential diagnosis

The incidence of Beckwith–Wiedemann syndrome is about 1 in 15,000 births (Weng et al., 1995). The disorder is usually sporadic, but occasional familial transmission is now explained by autosomal dominant inheritance subject to incomplete penetrance and genomic imprinting. Rare cases of Beckwith–Wiedemann syndrome resulted from a duplication of the chromosome 11p15 region, while others involved a deletion of this same region. It was soon demonstrated that the duplications always involved the paternally inherited chromosome 11, while deletions involved the maternally inherited chromosome (Weng et al., 1995; Weksberg & Squire, 1996). The implied alteration of parental imprinting has been confirmed by showing that the insulin-like growth factor-2 gene within the chromosome 11p15 region is expressed aberrantly in patients with Beckwith–Wiedemann syndrome (Ohlsson et al., 1993). The number of genes involved and the pathogenesis by which altered gene expression produces the syndrome remain to be defined.

Differential diagnosis includes other disorders with high birth weight, particularly diabetic embryopathy. The latter condition may also produce neonatal polycythemia, hypoglycemia, and hypocalcemia; it should be excluded by maternal history or evaluation. Children with mucopolysaccharidosis often have visceromegaly, increased early growth, and large tongues, but only the most severe forms would present neonatally. Skeletal survey and urine mucopolysaccharide/oligosaccharide screens should differentiate these disorders from Beckwith–Wiedemann syndrome. Infantile hypothyroidism can present with umbilical hernia and macroglossia. Wilms tumor with renal and genital abnormalities (Drash syndrome) can be discriminated by the presence of mutations in the WT-1 Wilms tumor gene.

Diagnostic evaluation and medical counseling

Monitoring of blood glucose should be performed in the infantile period, and a high-resolution karyotype is worthwhile to detect the minority of Beckwith–Wiedemann children with overt chromosomal anomalies. DNA testing is becoming increasingly useful to detect uniparental inheritance of one or more genes at band 11p15, but is still in the experimental stage (Weksberg & Squire, 1996). Uniparental inheritance of the 11p15 region from the father has been demonstrated in 20 percent of sporadic cases (Henry et al., 1993). The constellation of macrosomia, glabellar hemangioma, ear pits, and abdominal wall anomaly allows a definitive clinical diagnosis in most cases.

Family and psychosocial counseling

Except for those with unrecognized hypoglycemia or respiratory insufficiency due to macroglossia, the excellent prognosis for infants with Beckwith–Wiedemann syndrome warrants optimistic medical counseling. Because of the complex inheritance, a careful family history complete with parental birth weights and neonatal histories is important. Adults have few manifestations of the syndrome, so childhood histories and photographs are useful to exclude the diagnosis. For sporadic cases with normal parents, a 5 percent recurrence risk is appropriate, based on the possibility of imprinting/transmission effects (Elliott et al., 1994). There is little information on reproduction of affected individuals, but women with the syndrome have a higher risk for transmission than men (Elliott et al., 1994).

Parental support is most crucial during the neonatal and infantile periods, when the children may undergo operations or evaluation for respiratory insufficiency (Menard et al., 1995). Parent support groups are available (Beckwith–Wiedemann checklist, part 1).

Natural history and complications

The complications of Beckwith–Wiedemann syndrome (checklist, part 1) derive from anomalies in the orofacial, cardiac, abdominal, gastrointestinal, endocrine, and skeletal regions or systems. Affected pregnancies may be accompanied by proteinuric hypertension, preterm labor, or polyhydramnios, and there have been molar changes in placentas (McCowan & Becroft, 1994). The birth weight is usually high, followed by increased postnatal growth in 33–88 percent of patients and hemihyperplasia in 24–33 percent.

The facial appearance is distinctive with a glabellar hemangioma, malar flattening, and a large tongue. Omphalocele and intestinal stenoses or atresias are the most dramatic neonatal anomaly; one infant had meconium ileus scrotal rupture caused by omphalocele and jejunal atresia (Salle et al., 1992). Macroglossia is a frequent and severe neonatal problem that may cause respiratory obstruction, hypoxemia, apnea, feeding problems, and speech difficulties. Neonatal hypoglycemia relates to pancreatic islet cell hyperplasia, and there is a general visceromegaly, including nephromegaly. Cardiac anomalies have included septal defects, aortic coarctation and pulmonic stenosis, and generalized cardiomegaly (Gorlin et al., 1990, pp. 323–9). Less frequent complications include seizures, hydrocephalus, umbilical and inguinal hernias, cleft palate, polydactyly, and urinary tract anomalies. Of most concern for preventive management are the risks of abdominal tumors (DeBaun & Tucker, 1998) and of hypoxemia or apnea from tongue obstruction. Children with nephromegaly may have higher risks for tumors (DeBaun et al., 1998).

Once neonatal metabolic and morphologic abnormalities have been treated, the outlook for growth and development in the Beckwith–Wiedemann syndrome is excellent. Six of 74 patients in one series died during infancy; all were premature infants (Elliott et al., 1994). Most patients have normal intelligence, but 12 percent have mild mental deficiency with or without microcephaly. Rarely, hypothyroidism may occur with low levels of thyroxine-binding globulin (Leung, 1985).

Beckwith–Wiedemann syndrome preventive medical checklist

In the newborn period, abdominal and renal ultrasounds should be obtained to assess bowel atresias or stenoses, cystic kidneys, and ureteral obstruction that occasionally presents as the "prune belly" anomaly. Weng et al. (1995) recommended a baseline abdominal CT scan followed by abdominal ultrasound studies every 3 months up until age 7, then every 6 months until skeletal growth is complete (checklist, parts 2–4). Serum alpha-fetoprotein (AFP) measurements have been elevated in the presence of tumors or hypothyroidism, and yearly measurements are recommended (Weng et al., 1995). Abdominal palpation is also important, and some advocate training parents to perform this evaluation. Urinalysis may reveal tumor cells, and is indicated for surveillance of nephroblastoma (Wilms tumor) as well as for monitoring of infections in patients with urinary tract anomalies. Vaughan et al. (1995) reported the favorable outcomes of 13 children with abdominal tumors including Wilms tumor, hepatoblastoma, bladder rhabdomyosarcoma, and adrenocortical tumor. The disease-free survival rate of 100 percent after 9 years (average age at diagnosis was 3.5 years) underlines the recommendations for ultrasound screening of the liver, urinary tract, and adrenal glands every 3–6 months (checklist, parts 2–4 – Vaughan et al., 1995; DeBaun et al., 1998).

Although the macroglossia of Beckwith-Wiedemann syndrome often resolves without visible sequellae in the adult, Menard et al. (1995) reported that early, partial glossectomy in a series of 11 patients lessened the degree of anterior open bite and mandibular prognathism. Respiratory obstruction and hypoxemia from macroglossia can be significant, so referral to a multidisciplinary craniofacial surgery team should be considered. Rimell et al. (1995) reported that only 2 of their 13 patients required infantile tracheostomy because of macroglossia, while 7 of 13 required tonsillectomy and adenoidectomy for relief of upper airway obstruction during childhood. They recommended that anterior tongue reduction be considered for dental malocclusion, articulation errors, and cosmetic purposes, with tonsillectomy and adenoidectomy being indicated for later obstructive symptoms (Rimell et al., 1995).

The expected normal intelligence diminishes the need for special school and financial planning by families affected with the Beckwith–Wiedemann syndrome, but early intervention is still useful to monitor growth, development, hearing, and speech problems. Occasional children will have feeding difficulties, developmental delay (especially speech problems), and failure to thrive because of macroglossia, while others will have borderline mental disability. Most children will probably be discharged from early intervention services after demonstrating normal physical and intellectual development.

Sotos syndrome

Terminology

Sotos syndrome, also known as cerebral gigantism, was originally described in five children with overgrowth, macrocephaly acromegaloid features with advanced bone age, hypotonia, and a distinctive facial appearance in early childhood (Sotos et al., 1964; Allanson & Cole, 1996).

Incidence, etiology, and differential diagnosis

The incidence of Sotos syndrome is unknown, but the > 200 reported cases (Cole & Hughes, 1990) suggest a prevalence of at least 1 in 20–30,000 individuals. Only about half of the cases reviewed by four clinical geneticists (Cole & Hughes, 1994) proved to have the disorder, and there is no objective laboratory test to confirm the diagnosis. No consistent chromosomal changes have been described in conjunction with Sotos syndrome, and the advanced paternal age (Cole & Hughes, 1994) together with sporadic occurrence suggests the possibility of a *de novo* genetic mutation. Since abnormalities of pubertal development (see below) together with cognitive disability reduces reproductive fitness, a small number of offspring are available to examine the possibility of genetic transmission from affected individuals.

Other overgrowth syndromes such as Weaver syndrome may be confused with Sotos syndrome, as may familial macrocephaly (Cole & Hughes, 1994). Any condition with early growth acceleration may prompt consideration of the disorder, but the striking neonatal hypotonia and characteristic facial appearance should exclude other possibilities in the differential.

Diagnostic evaluation and medical counseling

The diagnosis of Sotos syndrome is clinical through noting the pattern of neonatal hypotonia; the distinctive facial appearance with dolichocephaly, prominent forehead, oval-shaped face, down-slanting palpebral fissures, and hypertelorism (Allanson & Cole, 1996); the large hands and feet; the pre- and postnatal growth acceleration. A karyotype may be considered in patients with cognitive disability as overgrowth can be seen in certain chromosomal disorders. Hand radiographs to verify an accelerated bone age offers an additional diagnostic criterion. Medical counseling can be optimistic since most children do better than their early hypotonia and motor delay might predict. The cognitive potential may also be underestimated because the over-sized child appears so much older than their actual age.

Family and psychosocial counseling

Most cases are sporadic, and the few literature reports of autosomal dominant or autosomal recessive inheritance were not thought convincing by Cole & Hughes

(1994). The elevated paternal age would be consistent with a new autosomal dominant mutation, and it will be interesting to monitor offspring of the affected patients that have been registered for study (Cole & Hughes, 1994). The recurrence risk is extremely low for parents whose child has verified Sotos syndrome, and no sibships suggestive of germline mosacism have been documented.

Natural history and complications

Despite their increased size at birth, the incidence of forceps (7.5 percent) or Cesarean section (7.5 percent) deliveries does not seem increased in children with Sotos syndrome despite their large head size (Cole & Hughes, 1990). Obstetric complications are therefore unlikely causes of the neonatal hypotonia with subsequent motor, speech, and cognitive delays. Birth length is more increased than weight, and over 50 percent have a large head circumference at birth. The head circumference quickly joins the height and weight in being over the 97th centile in most children, although adult height is channeled back towards the mean in females because of early puberty.

Medical complications include early feeding problems due to hypotonia with 40 percent requiring tube feedings (Cole & Hughes, 1994). Problems relating to the early hypotonia may include strabismus, chronic otitis, constipation, clumsiness (with an increased frequency of fractures), and orthopedic problems such as flat feet or scoliosis. Eye anomalies (cataracts, strabismus, nystagmus, myopia); congenital heart defects (patent ductus arteriosus, septal defects); urological anomalies; and malignancies (neuroblastoma, hepatocellular carcinoma, non-Hodgkins lymphoma, leukemia and osteochondroma) also occur at increased frequency (Gorlin et al., 1990, pp. 332–6; Nance et al., 1990; Hersh et al., 1992; Cole & Hughes, 1994; Maino et al., 1994; Hammadeh et al., 1995; Koenekoop et al., 1995; Corsello et al., 1996). Posterior spinal fusion was successful in one case of scoliosis (Suresh, 1991). Neurologic findings include paradoxically brisk deep tendon reflexes and brain anomalies including dilated cerebral ventricles (without functional hydrocephalus), anomalies of the corpus callosum, and periventricular leukomalacia (Schaefer et al., 1997). The range of developmental quotients in 41 children was 40 to 129, with a mean of 78 (Cole & Hughes, 1994). No specific language deficits have been defined, but a range of behavioral problems has been reported by teachers and parents including tantrums, withdrawal, sleep difficulties, and hyperactivity (38 percent – Rutter & Cole, 1991; Finegan et al., 1994). Behavioral problems may not exceed those of comparably delayed and over-sized children (Finegan et al., 1994).

Sotos syndrome preventive medical checklist

Recommendations for preventive management include attention to feeding and stooling problems in the first year; ophthalmologic, urologic, and cardiac assessment during early infancy; early intervention with physical, speech, and occupational therapy; monitoring of growth, hearing, and skeletal development in early childhood through adolescence; and school planning with anticipation of potential behavioral problems (due to inappropriate expectations or actual hyperactivity). The low frequency and different types of tumors do not lend themselves to the regimen of abdominal ultrasounds followed for Beckwith–Wiedemann syndrome, but physicians and parents should be alert for symptoms.

Preventive Management of Beckwith–Wiedemann syndrome

Clinical diagnosis: Pattern of manifestations including large birth weight, facial hemangiomas, ear creases, macroglossia, omphalocele, and visceromegaly; later overgrowth with predisposition to abdominal tumors and hemihypertrophy.

Laboratory diagnosis: Neonatal hypoglycemia is frequent, with some cases due to uniparental inheritance or chromosomal rearrangement in the 11p15 region.

Genetics: Multifactorial disorder with minimal recurrence risk; genetic factors indicated by occasional concordant twins.

Key management issues: Neonatal monitoring of blood glucose, serial abdominal/renal ultrasounds and serum alpha-fetoprotein measurements to screen for urinary tract anomalies and tumors, routine abdominal palpation and urinalysis to screen for tumors and urinary infections, monitoring for respiratory obstruction with aggressive treatment of hypoxemia (partial glossectomy, tonsillectomy, adenoidectomy, tracheotomy), early intervention to monitor growth, development, hearing, and speech problems.

Growth charts: None.

Parent groups: Beckwith–Wiedemann Support Group, 3206 Braeburn Circle, Ann Arbor, MI 48108, (800) 837-2976, A800BWSN@aol.com.

Basis for management recommendations: Complications listed below as documented by Elliot et al. (1994), Weng et al. (1995). The timing of abdominal ultrasound examinations is particularly controversial, with recommendations ranging from annually to every three months.

Summary of clinical concerns

General	Learning	Cognitive disability (4–12%)
	Growth	**Large birth weight** (39–77%), **macrosomia** (33–88%), **hemihyperplasia** (24–33%)
	Tumors	Abdominal (4–7.5% – Wilms tumor, hepatoblastoma, adrenocortical carcinoma)
Facial	Face	Maxillary hypoplasia, flat nasal bridge
	Ear	Ear pits, creases (66–76%), chronic otitis
	Mouth	Oromotor dysfunction, macroglossia (82–100%), cleft palate (2.5%)
Surface	Neck/trunk	Diastasis recti (33%)
	Epidermal	Nevus flammeus (63%)
Skeletal	Limbs	Advanced bone age, polydactyly (4%), hemihyperplasia
Internal	Digestive	**Visceromegaly** (57%), **omphalocele** (34–76%), imperforate anus, malrotation (5%), **umbilical hernia** (24–49%)
	Pulmonary	Hypoventilation, hypoxia
	Circulatory	Cardiac defects (6.5–18% – atrial septal defect, ventricular septal defect, patent ductus arteriosus, hypoplastic left heart, tetralogy of Fallot)
	Endocrine	**Hypoglycemia** (30–63%), pancreatic islet hyperplasia, hypocalcemia (4.6%)
	RES	Polycythemia (20%)
	Excretory	**Renal anomalies** (59–100%), **nephromegaly** (45%), renal diverticula, hydronephrosis (7%), obstructive uropathy, urinary tract infections
	Genital	Hypospadias, cryptorchidism, bicornuate uterus
Neural	CNS	Seizures, hydrocephalus
	Motor	Occasional motor delays
	Sensory	Conductive hearing loss

RES, reticuloendothelial system; **bold: frequency > 20%**

Key references

Elliott, M. R. et al. (1994). *Clinical Genetics* 46:168–74.
Menard, R.M., Delaire, J. & Schendel, S. A. (1995). *Plastic & Reconstructive Surgery* 96:27–33.
Weng, E.Y., Mortier, G. R. & Graham, J. M., Jr. (1995). *Clinical Pediatrics* 34:317–26.

Beckwith–Wiedemann syndrome

Preventive medical checklist (0–1yr)

Patient   **Birth Date**   /   /   **Number**

Pediatric	Screen	Evaluate	Refer/Counsel
Neonatal / / *Newborn screen* ❑ *HB* ❑	Renal sonogram ❑ Abdominal sono ❑ Glucose, calcium ❑ Karyotype ❑	Macroglossia ❑ Airway ❑ Feeding, apnea ❑	Genetic evaluation ❑ ENT[3] ❑ Oral surgery[3] ❑
1 month / /	Growth ❑ Serum glucose ❑ Abdominal sono ❑	Airway, heart ❑ Feeding, apnea ❑ Abdominal exam ❑	Family support[4] ❑ Cardiology[3] ❑
2 months / / *HB[1]* ❑ *Hib* ❑ *DTaP, IPV* ❑ *RV* ❑	Hearing, vision[3] ❑ Glucose, Ca ❑ Serum AFP ❑	Airway, heart ❑ Feeding, apnea ❑ Abdominal exam ❑	Early intervention[3,5] ❑ Genetic counseling ❑
4 months / / *HB[1]* ❑ *Hib* ❑ *DTaP/IPV* ❑ *RV* ❑	Hearing, vision[2] ❑ Glucose, Ca ❑ Abdominal sono ❑	Airway, heart ❑ Feeding, apnea ❑ Abdominal exam ❑	Early intervention[3,5] ❑ Genetics ❑ ENT[4] ❑ Oral surgery[4] ❑
6 months / / *Hib* ❑ *IPV[1]* ❑ *DTaP* ❑ *RV* ❑	Growth ❑ Hearing, vision[2] ❑ Serum AFP ❑ Abdominal sono ❑	Airway ❑ Feeding, apnea ❑ Abdominal exam ❑	Family support[4] ❑
9 months / / *IPV[1]* ❑	Abdominal sono ❑	Airway ❑ Feeding, apnea ❑ Abdominal exam ❑	ENT[3] ❑ Oral surgery[3] ❑
1 year / / *HB* ❑ *Hib[1]* ❑ *IPV[1]* ❑ *MMR[1]* ❑ *Var[1]* ❑	Growth ❑ Hearing, vision[3] ❑ Serum AFP, T4 ❑ Abdominal sono ❑	Airway ❑ Feeding, apnea ❑ Abdominal exam ❑	Family support[4] ❑ Early intervention[3,5] ❑ Genetics ❑

Clinical concerns for Beckwith–Wiedemann syndrome, ages 0–1 year

Hydrocephalus	Cardiac anomalies	Hypoglycemia, hypocalcemia
Macroglossia, macrosomia	Urogenital anomalies	Polycythemia
Omphalocele, umbilical hernia	Hemihyperplasia	Feeding problems
	Wilms tumor	Airway obstruction, apnea

Guidelines for the neonatal period should be undertaken *at whatever age* the diagnosis is made; DTaP, acellular DTP; IPV, inactivated poliovirus (oral polio also used); RV, rotavirus; MMR, measles–mumps–rubella; Var, varicella; [1]alternative timing; [2]by practitioner; [3]as dictated by clinical findings – abdominal sonogram every 3 months until age 7, then every 6 months until completion of skeletal growth, ENT and oral surgery for children with macroglossia, airway obstruction; [4]parent group, family/sib, financial, and behavioral issues as discussed in the preface; [5]including developmental monitoring and motor/speech therapy.

Beckwith–Wiedemann syndrome

Preventive medical checklist (15m–6yrs)

Patient **Birth Date** / / **Number**

Pediatric	Screen	Evaluate		Refer/Counsel	
15 months / / *Hib[1]* ☐ *MMR[1]* ☐ *DTaP, IPV[1]* ☐ *Varicella[1]* ☐	Abdominal sono ☐	Airway Feeding, apnea Abdominal exam	☐ ☐ ☐	Family support[4] Early intervention[5]	☐ ☐
18 months / / *DTaP, IPV[1]* ☐ *Varicella[1]* ☐ *Influenza[3]* ☐	Serum AFP ☐ Abdominal sono ☐	Airway Feeding, apnea Abdominal exam	☐ ☐ ☐		
2 years / / *Influenza[3]* ☐ *Pneumovax[3]* ☐ *Dentist* ☐	Audiology ☐ Serum AFP, T4 ☐ Abdominal sono ☐	Feeding, apnea Abdominal exam Limb lengths	☐ ☐ ☐	Family support[4] Genetics ENT[5] Oral surgery[5]	☐ ☐ ☐ ☐
3 years / / *Influenza[3]* ☐ *Pneumovax[3]* ☐ *Dentist* ☐	Growth ☐ Audiology ☐ Serum AFP, T4 ☐ Abdominal sono ☐	Feeding, apnea Abdominal exam Limb lengths	☐ ☐ ☐	Family support[5] Preschool transition	☐ ☐
4 years / / *Influenza[3]* ☐ *Pneumovax[3]* ☐ *Dentist* ☐	Hearing, vision[2] ☐ Serum AFP, T4 ☐ Abdominal sono ☐ Urinalysis, BP ☐	Abdominal exam Limb lengths	☐ ☐	Family support[5] Preschool program[3,5] Developmental pediatrics[3] Genetics ENT, oral surgery[3]	☐ ☐ ☐ ☐ ☐
5 years / / *DTaP, IPV[1]* ☐ *MMR[1]* ☐	Hearing, vision[2] ☐ Serum AFP, T4 ☐ Abdominal sono ☐ Urinalysis, BP ☐	Abdominal exam Limb lengths	☐ ☐	School transition	☐
6 years / / *DTaP, IPV[1]* ☐ *MMR[1]* ☐ *Dentist* ☐	Growth ☐ Hearing, vision[2] ☐ Serum AFP, T4 ☐ Abdominal sono ☐ Urinalysis, BP ☐	School progress Abdominal exam Limb lengths Scoliosis	☐ ☐ ☐ ☐	Family support[4] Developmental pediatrics[3] Genetics ENT[3] Oral surgery[3]	☐ ☐ ☐ ☐ ☐

Clinical concerns for Beckwith–Wiedemann syndrome, ages 1–6 years

Hydrocephalus Macroglossia, macrosomia Omphalocele, umbilical hernia	Cardiac anomalies Urogenital anomalies Hemihyperplasia Wilms tumor	Hypoglycemia, hypocalcemia Polycythemia Feeding problems Airway obstruction, apnea

Guidelines for prior ages should be undertaken *at the time of diagnosis*; DTaP, acellular DTP; IPV, inactivated poliovirus (oral polio also used); MMR, measles–mumps–rubella; [1]alternative timing; [2]by practitioner; [3]as dictated by clinical findings – abdominal sonogram every 3 months until age 7, then every 6 months until completion of skeletal growth, ENT and oral surgery for children with macroglossia, airway obstruction; [4]parent group, family/sib, financial, and behavioral issues as discussed in the preface; [5]including developmental monitoring and motor/speech therapy.

Beckwith–Wiedemann syndrome

Preventive medical checklist (6+ yrs)

Patient   **Birth Date** / /   **Number**

Pediatric	Screen	Evaluate	Refer/Counsel
8 years / / _Dentist_ ❏	Serum AFP ❏ Abdominal sono ❏ Urinalysis, BP ❏	Abdominal exam ❏ Limb lengths ❏	School options ❏ Developmental pediatrics[3] ❏ Genetics ❏
10 years / /	Growth ❏ Serum AFP ❏ Abdominal sono ❏ Urinalysis, BP ❏	School progress ❏ Abdominal exam ❏ Limb lengths ❏ Scoliosis ❏	ENT[3] ❏ Oral surgery[3] ❏
12 years / / _Td[1], MMR, Var_ ❏ _CBC_ ❏ _Dentist_ ❏ _Scoliosis_ ❏ _Cholesterol_ ❏	Serum AFP ❏ Abdominal sono ❏ Urinalysis, BP ❏	Abdominal exam ❏ Limb lengths ❏	Family support[4] ❏ School options ❏
14 years / / _CBC_ ❏ _Dentist_ ❏ _Cholesterol_ ❏ _Breast CA_ ❏ _Testicular CA_ ❏	Urinalysis, BP ❏	School progress ❏ Abdominal exam ❏ Limb lengths ❏ Scoliosis ❏	
16 years / / _Td[1]_ ❏ _CBC_ ❏ _Cholesterol_ ❏ _Sexual[5]_ ❏ _Dentist_ ❏	Urinalysis, BP ❏	Abdominal exam ❏ Limb lengths ❏ Scoliosis ❏	Vocational planning[3] ❏
18 years / / _CBC_ ❏ _Sexual[5]_ ❏ _Cholesterol_ ❏ _Scoliosis_ ❏	Urinalysis, BP ❏	School progress ❏ Abdominal exam ❏ Limb lengths ❏	Vocational planning[3] ❏
20 years[6] / / _CBC_ ❏ _Sexual[5]_ ❏ _Cholesterol_ ❏ _Dentist_ ❏	Urinalysis, BP ❏	Abdominal exam ❏ Limb lengths ❏ Scoliosis ❏ Work, residence[3] ❏	Family support[4] ❏

Clinical concerns for Beckwith–Wiedemann syndrome, ages 6+ years

Conductive hearing loss   Urinary tract anomalies   Learning differences
Abdominal tumors   Cryptorchidism   Hemihyperplasia, scoliosis
Malocclusion, overbite   Sleep apnea, cor pulmonale

Guidelines for prior ages should be undertaken *at the time of diagnosis*; Td, tetanus/diphtheria; MMR, measles–mumps–rubella; Var, varicella; [1]alternative timing; [2]by practitioner; [3]as dictated by clinical findings – abdominal sonogram every 3 months until age 7, then every 6 months until completion of skeletal growth, ENT and oral surgery for children with macroglossia, airway obstruction; [4]parent group, family/sib, financial, and behavioral issues as discussed in the preface; [5]birth control, STD screening if sexually active; [6]repeat every decade.

Preventive Management of Sotos syndrome

Clinical diagnosis: Pattern of manifestations including neonatal hypotonia, pre- and postnatal overgrowth, macrocephaly, characteristic facial appearance (frontal bossing, sparse frontal hair, down-slanting palpebral fissures, prominent jaw), accelerated bone age, and cognitive disability.

Incidence: Unknown but a prevalence of 1 in 20–30,000 can be estimated based on over 200 reported cases.

Laboratory diagnosis: None.

Genetics: Sporadic occurrence with minimal recurrence risk for parents of affected children; risks for affected individuals to transmit the syndrome are presumed low but not defined.

Key management issues: Monitoring of feeding and stooling during the first year; ophthalmologic, urologic, and cardiac assessment during early infancy; early intervention, monitoring of growth, hearing, and skeletal development; and school planning with anticipation of potential behavioral problems.

Growth Charts: Growth profiles are presented by Cole and Hughes (1994).

Parent groups: Sotos Syndrome USA Support Association, Three Danada Sq. E. #235, Wheaton IL, 60187, (888) 246-SSSA, sssa@well.com, http://www.well.com/user/sssa/

Basis for management recommendations: Derived from the complications below as documented by Cole and Hughes (1990; 1994).

Summary of clinical concerns

General	Learning	**Cognitive disability** (IQ range 40–129, mean 78), learning differences
	Behavior	**Hyperactivity** (38%), tantrums, withdrawal
	Growth	**Accelerated growth** with macrocephaly and macrosomia
	Tumors	Neuroblastoma, hepatocellular carcinoma, lymphomas
Facial	Face	Frontal bossing, high hairline, down-slanting palpebral fissures
	Eye	Strabismus, cataracts, nystagmus
	Ear	**Chronic otitis** (72%)
	Mouth	High palate, early tooth eruption, **worn and discolored teeth** (75%)
Surface	Neck/trunk	**Sparse frontal hair** (98%), thin or brittle nails (58%)
Skeletal	Cranial	**Macrocephaly** (50% at birth, virtually 100% later), dolichocephaly
	Axial	Kyphoscoliosis (8%)
	Limbs	**Flat feet** (46%), **accelerated bone age** (84%), **large hands and feet** (80%), hip dislocation
Internal	Digestive	**Poor feeding** (40% tube feeding as neonates), constipation
	Circulatory	Cardiac anomalies (15% – patent ductus arteriosus, atrial septal defect)
	Excretory	Ureteral reflux, urinary tract infections
Neural	CNS	**Seizures** (50%, often with fevers), **brain anomalies** (ventricular dilation, 63%, anomalies of the corpus callosum, generous extracerebral fluid spaces, periventricular leukomalacia)
	Motor	**Neonatal hypotonia** (88%) **brisk reflexes** (78%), **poor coordination** (100%)
	Sensory	Hearing and vision deficits

Bold: frequency > 20%

Key references

Cole, T. R. & Hughes, H. E. (1990). *Journal of Medical Genetics* 27:571–6.

Cole, T. R. & Hughes, H. E. (1994). *Journal of Medical Genetics* 31:20–32.

Finegan, J. K. et al. (1994). *Journal of the American Academy of Child & Adolescent Psychiatry* 33:1307–15.

Hersh, J. H. et al. (1992). *Journal of Pediatrics* 120:572–4.

Rutter, S. C. & Cole, T. R. (1991). *Developmental Medicine & Child Neurology* 33:898–902.

Schaefer, G. B. et al. (1997). *American Journal of Medical Genetics* 68:462–5.

Sotos syndrome

Preventive medical checklist (0–1yr)

Patient		Birth Date / /		Number

Pediatric	Screen	Evaluate		Refer/Counsel	
Neonatal / / Newborn screen ❏ HB ❏		Feeding Hip dislocation Head size Heart	❏ ❏ ❏ ❏	Feeding specialist[3] Genetic evaluation	❏ ❏
1 month / /		Feeding Constipation Head size Heart	❏ ❏ ❏ ❏	Family support[4] Feeding specialist[3] Cardiology[3]	❏ ❏ ❏
2 months / / HB[1] ❏ Hib ❏ DTaP, IPV ❏ RV ❏	Growth ❏ Hearing, vision[2] ❏	Feeding Constipation Head size	❏ ❏ ❏	Early intervention[5] Feeding specialist[3] Developmental 　pediatrician Genetic counseling	❏ ❏ ❏ ❏
4 months / / HB[1] ❏ Hib ❏ DTaP/IPV ❏ RV ❏	Growth ❏ Hearing, vision[2] ❏	Feeding Constipation Head size	❏ ❏ ❏	Early intervention[5]	❏
6 months / / Hib ❏ IPV[1] ❏ DTaP ❏ RV ❏	Growth ❏ Hearing, vision[2] ❏	Feeding Constipation Head size Strabismus	❏ ❏ ❏ ❏	Family support[4]	❏
9 months / / IPV[1] ❏	Audiology ❏ Urinalysis ❏	Otitis Constipation Strabismus	❏ ❏ ❏	Ophthalmology	❏
1 year / / HB ❏ Hib[1] ❏ IPV[1] ❏ MMR[1] ❏ Var[1] ❏	Growth ❏ Hearing, vision[2] ❏ Bone age ❏	Otitis Head size Strabismus Heart	❏ ❏ ❏ ❏	Family support[4] Early intervention[5] Developmental 　pediatrics Genetics	❏ ❏ ❏ ❏

Clinical concerns for Sotos syndrome, ages 0–1 year

Poor feeding (infancy)	Cardiac anomalies	Developmental delays
Eye anomalies (strabismus)	Hip dislocation	Hypotonia
Chronic otitis	Urinary tract anomalies	Macrocephaly
High palate		Overgrowth

Guidelines for the neonatal period should be undertaken *at whatever age* the diagnosis is made; DTaP, acellular DTP; IPV, inactivated poliovirus (oral polio also used); RV, rotavirus; MMR, measles–mumps–rubella; Var, varicella; [1]alternative timing; [2]by practitioner; [3]as dictated by clinical findings; [4]parent group, family/sib, financial, and behavioral issues as discussed in the preface; [5]including developmental monitoring and motor/speech therapy.

Sotos syndrome

Preventive medical checklist (15m–6yrs)

Patient		Birth Date / /	Number

Pediatric	Screen	Evaluate	Refer/Counsel
15 months / / Hib[1] ☐ MMR[1] ☐ DTaP, IPV[1] ☐ Varicella[1] ☐	Growth ☐ Hearing, vision[2] ☐	Head size ☐ Otitis ☐ Strabismus ☐	Family support[4] ☐ Early intervention[5] ☐
18 months / / DTaP, IPV[1] ☐ Varicella[1] ☐ Influenza[3] ☐	Growth ☐ Hearing, vision[2] ☐	Head size ☐ Strabismus ☐	Ophthalmology ☐
2 years / / Influenza[3] ☐ Pneumovax[3] ☐ Dentist ☐	Growth ☐ Audiology ☐ Urinalysis ☐	Otitis ☐ Strabismus ☐ Scoliosis ☐	Family support[4] ☐ Dentistry ☐ Genetics ☐ ENT[3] ☐
3 years / / Influenza[3] ☐ Pneumovax[3] ☐ Dentist ☐	Growth ☐ Hearing, vision[2] ☐	Otitis ☐ Strabismus ☐	Family support[4] ☐ Preschool transition[5] ☐ Ophthalmology[3] ☐
4 years / / Influenza[3] ☐ Pneumovax[3] ☐ Dentist ☐	Growth ☐ Hearing, vision[2] ☐	Scoliosis ☐ Flat feet ☐	Family support[4] ☐ Preschool program[5] ☐ Dietician ☐ Developmental pediatrics ☐ Genetics ☐
5 years / / DTaP, IPV[1] ☐ MMR[1] ☐	Growth ☐	Salivation ☐ Feeding ☐ Obesity ☐	School transition[5] ☐ Ophthalmology[3] ☐
6 years / / DTaP, IPV[1] ☐ MMR[1] ☐ Dentist ☐	Growth ☐ Hearing, vision[2] ☐	School progress ☐ Behavior ☐	Family support[4] ☐ Developmental pediatrics ☐ Genetics ☐

Clinical concerns for Sotos syndrome, ages 1–6 years

Eye anomalies (strabismus)	Cardiac anomalies	Cognitive disability
Chronic otitis	Flat feet	Behavior problems
High palate	Scoliosis	Macrocephaly, seizures
Dental problems	Urinary tract anomalies	Overgrowth

Guidelines for prior ages should be undertaken *at the time of diagnosis*; DTaP, acellular DTP; IPV, inactivated poliovirus (oral polio also used); MMR, measles–mumps–rubella; [1]alternative timing; [2]by practitioner; [3]as dictated by clinical findings; [4]parent group, family/sib, financial, and behavioral issues as discussed in the preface; [5]including developmental monitoring and motor/speech therapy.

Sotos syndrome

Preventive medical checklist (6+ yrs)

Patient		Birth Date / /	Number	

Pediatric	Screen		Evaluate		Refer/Counsel	
8 years / / *Dentist* ❑	Growth Hearing, vision[2]	❑ ❑	Puberty Scoliosis, flat feet Heart	❑ ❑ ❑	School options Developmental pediatrics Genetics	❑ ❑ ❑
10 years / /	Growth Hearing, vision[2]	❑ ❑	School progress Puberty	❑ ❑	Ophthalmology[3]	❑
12 years / / *Td[1], MMR, Var* ❑ *CBC* ❑ *Dentist* ❑ *Scoliosis* ❑ *Cholesterol* ❑	Growth Urinalysts	❑ ❑	Puberty Scoliosis, flat feet Behavior	❑ ❑ ❑	Family support[4] School options Developmental pediatrics Genetics	❑ ❑ ❑ ❑
14 years / / *CBC* ❑ *Dentist* ❑ *Cholesterol* ❑ *Breast CA* ❑ *Testicular CA* ❑	Growth Hearing, vision[2]	❑ ❑	School progress Behavior	❑ ❑	Dietician Endocrinology[6]	❑ ❑
16 years / / *Td[1]* ❑ *CBC* ❑ *Cholesterol* ❑ *Sexual[5]* ❑ *Dentist* ❑	Growth Hearing, vision[2] Urinalysis	❑ ❑ ❑	Scoliosis, flat feet Behavior Heart	❑ ❑ ❑	Vocational planning Developmental pediatrics Genetics Ophthalmology[3]	❑ ❑ ❑ ❑
18 years / / *CBC* ❑ *Sexual[5]* ❑ *Cholesterol* ❑ *Scoliosis* ❑	Growth Hearing, vision[2]	❑ ❑	Behavior	❑	Vocational planning	❑
20 years[6] / / *CBC* ❑ *Sexual[5]* ❑ *Cholesterol* ❑ *Dentist* ❑	Growth Hearing, vision[2] Urinalysis	❑ ❑ ❑	Scoliosis, flat feet Behavior Work, residence	❑ ❑ ❑	Family support[4] Ophthalmology[3]	❑ ❑

Clinical concerns for Sotos syndrome, ages 6+ years

Eye anomalies (strabismus)	Cardiac anomalies	Cognitive disability
Chronic otitis	Flat feet	Behavior problems
High palate	Scoliosis	Macrocephaly, seizures
Dental problems	Urinary tract anomalies	Overgrowth

Guidelines for prior ages should be undertaken *at the time of diagnosis*; Td, tetanus/diphtheria; MMR, measles–mumps–rubella; Var, varicella; [1]alternative timing; [2]by practitioner; [3]as dictated by clinical findings; [4]parent group, family/sib, financial, and behavioral issues as discussed in the preface; [5]birth control, STD screening if sexually active; [6]repeat every decade.

13

Hamartosis syndromes

Hamartomas are overgrowths of normal tissue. They are similar to tumors in their potential for continuous growth and in their lack of normal tissue organization (dysplasia). Hamartomas are different from choristomas, which are composed of tissue that is alien to its body region, and from teratomas, which are true neoplasms arising from embryonic cells. Hamartosis syndromes, epitomized by neuro-fibromatosis, are characterized by hamartomas, dysharmonic growth, and neoplastic potential (Table 13.1).

In general, hamartosis syndromes affect the central nervous system (seizures, brain tumors, neurosensory abnormalities), oral cavity (tumors, nevi), heart (tumors), skeleton (limb length discrepancies, scoliosis, bony deformities), and epidermis (nevi, café-au-lait spots, surface tumors). Hamartosis syndromes are often associated with high risk of cancer, and produce physical deformities that require supportive counseling and family support. The more common syndromes – Gardner syndrome, neurofibromatosis-1, and tuberous sclerosis – exhibit autosomal dominant inheritance that is compatible with the causative gene being a tumor suppressor. The cloning and characterization of the responsible gene has provided strong support for this hypothesis in all three syndromes. Since several of the genetic hamartomatous syndromes have high rates of new mutation, it is reasonable to expect that apparently sporadic disorders such as the Klippel–Trenaunay–Weber or Proteus syndromes (Table 13.1) will prove to be single-gene mutations as well. Hall (1988) suggested that the latter conditions may represent somatic mutations, accounting for the variable distributions of lesions and the lack of familial transmission.

Less common syndromes

Bannayan–Riley–Ruvalcaba Syndrome

The combination of macrocephaly with hemangiomas, lipomas, and pigmented macules was reported by Riley & Smith (1960), Ruvalcaba et al. (1980), Bannayan (1971), Stephan et al. (1975), and Zonana et al. (1976). Gorlin et al. (1992) followed the suggestion of Saul & Stevenson (1986) that these autosomal dominant disorders

Table 13.1 Hamartosis syndromes

Syndrome	Incidence	Inheritance	Complications
Basal cell carcinoma (Gorlin)	~500 cases	AD	Nevoid basal cell carcinomas, eye anomalies, jaw cysts, skeletal changes (scoliosis), other cancers
Bannayan–Riley–Ruvalcaba	AD	~100 cases	Macrocephaly, lipomas, hemangiomas, intestinal polyps, joint laxity, penile spots
Epidermal nevus	~100 cases	AD	Epidermal nevi, hemangiomas, café-au-lait spots, colobomata, nystagmus, hemihyperplasia, limb deformities, cognitive disability, seizures
Gardner (familial polyposis of the colon)	1 in 12,000 live births	AD	Skin cysts, bony osteomas, colonic polyps, colon cancer, retinal changes, adrenal, hepatic and thyroid cancers
Klippel–Trenauney–Weber Sturge–Weber angiomatosis	~1000 cases	Sporadic	Hemangiomas, skeletal asymmetry, eye anomalies, limb anomalies; seizures, cerebrovascular anomalies, and cognitive disability with Sturge–Weber angiomatosis.
Mafucci	~150 cases	Sporadic	Hemangiomas, enchondromas, skeletal deformities, other cancers
Neurofibromatosis-1	1 in 2500 live births	AD	Café-au-lait spots, neurofibromas, skeletal anomalies, seizures, cognitive disability
Neurofibromatosis-2	1 in 100,000 live births	AD	Hearing loss due to acoustic neuromas
Peutz–Jeghers	~300 cases	AD	Skin and mouth pigmentation, intestinal polyposis, cancer
Tuberous sclerosis	1 in 10,000	AD	Hypomelanotic nodules, facial angiofibromas, intracranial ependymomas and astrocytomas, cardiac rhabdomyomas, renal angiomyolipomas, seizures, cognitive disability

Note:
AD, autosomal dominant.

represent variable manifestations of the same genetic disease. The term "Bannayan–Riley–Ruvalcaba syndrome" reflects the contributions of these separate descriptions (Gorlin et al., 1990, p. 336). Complications in addition to the macrocephaly and overgrowth include hypotonia, mental disability, seizures (25 percent), intestinal polyps (45 percent), joint laxity, scoliosis, and enlarged testes (Gorlin et al., 1990, pp. 336–7). Although most of the tumors are benign lipomas, hemangiomas, or lymphangiomas, they may grow aggressively and erode normal tissues. Malignant tumors (thyroid or breast cancers) have also been noted, and the Bannayan–Riley–Ruvalcaba syndrome could be viewed as a hamartosis syndrome.

Pigmented macules on the penis may provide a subtle aid to diagnosis in affected males. Many patients have had abnormal muscle biopsy with fat accumulation in type I fibers. Fryburg et al. (1994) reported a patient with long-chain-3-hydroxycoenzyme-A-dehydrogenase and Bannayan–Riley–Ruvalcaba syndrome. Ophthalmologic examination may be helpful diagnostically, showing visible corneal nerves and prominent Schwalbe lines. Preventive measures should include early intervention with physical and occupational therapy for hypotonia and developmental delay, examination for mass lesions, and monitoring of the hematocrit to rule out anemia. Malignant transformation of intestinal polyps has not been reported, but they may be associated with anemia and melena or protein-losing enteropathy (Gorlin et al., 1990, pp. 336–8). Thyroid functions should be monitored periodically, since Gorlin et al. (1992) reported autoimmune thyroiditis in 7 of 12 patients from one family.

Epidermal nevus syndrome

Anomalies of the central nervous system, eye, skin, and skeletal system are found in the epidermal nevus syndrome. Multiple linear nevi are the most characteristic finding, as recognized by the term "linear sebaceous nevus syndrome." This term is inaccurate because sebaceous elements are usually not present in the nevi (Gorlin et al., 1990, pp. 362–6). Most cases have been sporadic, but rare instances of vertical transmission suggest the possibility of autosomal dominant inheritance with a high rate of new mutations. Happle (1995) emphasized that the entity called "epidermal nevus syndrome" is heterogeneous. Epidermal nevi have been associated with various anomalies including lipoepidermoid cysts of the eye, ipsilateral hypoplasia of the breast, or limb defects, and it is not clear which of these combinations falls within the pioneering description of Solomon & Esterly (1975).

Frequent complications of the epidermal nevus syndrome include cognitive disability, seizures, facial asymmetry, ocular anomalies, oral lesions, and skeletal anomalies (Grebe et al., 1993; Dodge & Dobyns, 1995). Review of 74 cases established a correlation between epidermal nevi on the head and complications of the central nervous system (Grebe et al., 1993). Preventive management should focus on early intervention and supportive counseling appropriate for a disorder with a 50 percent risk for significant mental disability. Periodic vision screening and ophthalmology visits are needed to detect the 33 percent of patients that have ocular anomalies (Gorlin et al., 1990, pp. 362–6). Regular monitoring of growth and skeletal development should be conducted, since congenital anomalies of the vertebrae and limbs occur, along with hemihyperplasia and scoliosis secondary to asymmetry. Oral inspection and dental care should include surveillance for clefts or hypoplastic teeth. Neoplasms occur with increased frequency, including Wilms tumor, gastric carcinoma, breast cancer, and astrocytoma.

Gardner syndrome

Pediatric health care providers will definitely encounter children with Gardner syndrome, based on its prevalence of 1 in 1400 to 1 in 12,000 individuals (Gorlin et al., 1990, pp. 366–71). Although the disorder is relatively common, its usual presentation after puberty limits the utility of a specific pediatric checklist. Major features of Gardner syndrome include cystic tumors in bone (osteomas), skin (epidermoid cysts), and the colon (familial adenomatous polyposis). Patients with isolated familial adenomatous polyposis coli (APC) were originally thought to have a different disorder. However, the presence of subtle jaw lesions in most patients with APC suggests that it forms a spectrum with Gardner syndrome. This hypothesis was confirmed when the causative FAP gene was characterized at chromosome band 5q21 (Kinzler & Vogelstein, 1992). Davies et al. (1995) performed DNA analysis on 84 individuals from 36 families with Gardner syndrome, and found a correlation between associated anomalies (congenital hypertrophy of the retinal epithelium, orofacial osteomas) and the position of the mutation within the FAP gene. Patients with mutations 5′ to exon 9 had virtually no retinal changes, while those with mutations 3′ to exon 9 had a higher frequency of orofacial osteomas. Thus, the nature of the FAP gene mutation determines whether one has polyposis only or polyposis plus associated features.

Overall, the frequencies of osteomas and skin cysts in FAP are each about 50 percent, and that of congenital hypertrophy of the retinal pigment epithelium is 85 percent (Gorlin et al., 1990, pp. 366–71). Either lesion may precede the appearance of intestinal polyps. Only 5 percent of patients experience malignant degeneration of intestinal polyps before puberty, with a mean age for diagnosis of colon cancer of 37 years. The risk of colon cancer eventually reaches 100 percent, and the chief preventive management concern is early diagnosis so that surgical options can be considered. Some patients opt for a total colectomy, while others are willing to undergo regular colonoscopy with excision of polyps. Regular dental care is needed because supernumerary teeth and multiple osteomas of the jaws may occur. There is increased risk of other neoplasms, including adrenal, hepatic, skin, and, in females, thyroid cancers.

Nevoid basal cell carcinoma (Gorlin) syndrome

Over 500 cases of Gorlin syndrome have been described, and it accounts for 1 in 200 patients who develop basal cell carcinomas of the skin. The disorder exhibits autosomal dominant inheritance and has been mapped to chromosome region 9q23–q31 (Chevenix-Trench et al., 1993). The rate of new mutations among 64 families was high (14–81 percent), and there was some evidence for worsening of symptoms with each generation (anticipation – Shanley et al., 1994). Facial, ocular, oral, and skeletal changes predominate in the nevoid basal cell carcinoma syndrome, but the manifestations are protean and can affect most organ systems. Nevoid basal cell carcinomas are the distinguishing feature of the condition, appearing sometimes at birth but usually between puberty and 35 years of age (Gorlin, 1987). There is a distinctive facies in 70 percent of patients, caused by prominence of the forehead and supra-orbital ridges with hypertelorism. Eye anomalies include cataracts, glaucoma, and colobomata with occasional retinitis pigmentosa and detachment. Oral changes include cysts in the jaws (keratocysts), which often develop in the first decade of life. Central nervous system changes such as hydrocephalus or agenesis of the corpus callosum are rare, and there is a 3 percent incidence of mental deficiency (Gorlin, 1987).

Gorlin syndrome has few manifestations in childhood, although central nervous system anomalies causing hydrocephalus have been reported (Snider, 1994). Nevoid basal cell carcinomas may be present before puberty, but they rarely cause problems. It is after adolescence that regular dermatologic evaluations are needed to identify the surprisingly few tumors that become invasive. Although the nevoid tumors occur in areas unexposed to the sun, full protection from sunlight and from other sources of radiation is an obvious recommendation for affected children. Damage from sunlight may be evident in an Australian study, which showed earlier onset and greater multiplicity of the tumors than in patients in England (Shanley et al., 1994). Topical treatment of the lesions with isotretinoin and 5-fluorouracil shows promise for long-term suppression of the basal cell carcinomas (Strange & Lang, 1992). Other preventive measures include regular ophthalmology and dentistry examinations, evaluation of skeletal growth with referral to orthopedics if scoliosis or bony deformities occur, and referral for early intervention/rehabilitative services for the unusual patient with mental disability. As is common in hamartomatous syndromes, other neoplasms besides basal cell carcinomas can occur. Medulloblastomas in early childhood, ovarian or cardiac fibromas, fibrosarcomas after radiation therapy, and a variety of visceral cancers have been reported (Gorlin et al., 1990, pp. 372–80).

Klippel–Trenaunay–Weber and Sturge–Weber syndromes

Multiple hemangiomas with skeletal asymmetry are characteristic of Klippel–Trenaunay–Weber syndrome (Jones, 1997, pp. 512–13). Over 1000 cases have been described, but an incidence figure has not been determined. Major complications include limb or digital enlargement with edema (84 percent), varicose veins (36 percent), and malformations of deep veins such as the popliteal (51 percent), femoral (16 percent), iliac (3 percent) and inferior vena cava (1 percent). Lymphatic abnormalities with edema and digital anomalies suggestive of embryonic circulatory defects (syndactyly, polydactyly) are also seen. Mental development is usually normal unless the craniofacies is involved, when the disorder blends with Sturge–Weber syndrome. Cranial findings in patients with Klippel–Trenaunay–Weber syndrome are quite similar to those of Sturge–Weber angiomatosis when they occur, suggesting that these are different manifestations of the same disorder (Gorlin et al., 1990, p. 408; Williams & Elster, 1992). Both are sporadic with virtually no familial cases described. As mentioned above, Hall (1988) speculated that they are lethal, autosomal dominant disorders that arise in liveborn individuals as somatic mutations.

Preventive management for Klippel–Trenaunay–Weber syndrome consists mainly of physical examination, being alert for complications due to abnormal venous or lymphatic drainage. Limb hypertrophy may lead to scoliosis, so orthopedic referral is useful when skeletal asymmetry is noted. No increased risk of neoplasia has been described, perhaps because limb hypertrophy rather than hemihyperplasia is involved. Patients with severe vascular distortions are at risk for bleeding from platelet trapping (Kasabach–Merritt syndrome) or cellulitis. Visceral hemangiomatosis can affect the lungs, gastrointestinal tract, and urinary tract, but imaging studies are not indicated unless symptoms occur. Protein-losing enteropathy due to intestinal lesions has occurred (Gorlin et al., 1990, pp. 380–3). In general, patients with Klippel–Trenaunay–Weber syndrome should have routine medical care in addition to regular physical examinations and reassurance concerning a normal prognosis for adult size and function.

When a nevus flammeus is found over the trigeminal nerve distribution, with or without hemangiomas elsewhere in the body, the Sturge–Weber pattern of angiomatosis should be suspected. Angiomas of the leptomeninges usually occur on the ipsilateral side, and concurrent cerebrovascular anomalies (46 percent) and/or intracranial calcifications (57 percent) may be present (Gorlin et al., 1990, pp. 408–9; Sujansky & Conradi, 1995). Oakes (1992) followed 30 patients with radiographic evidence of cortical calcification; 87 percent had seizures, 97 percent a port-wine nevus, and 14 percent died from their disease over a follow-up period of at least 10 years. Eye anomalies (glaucoma with buphthalmos, choroidal angioma) and oral anomalies (gingival angiomas, abnormal tooth eruption, macrodontia) are also common, and 30 percent have mental disability. Those with seizures have a higher risk of developmental delay (43 percent versus 0 percent in those without seizures), special education requirements (71 percent versus 0 percent), and emotional or behavioral problems (85 versus 58 percent; Sujansky & Conradi, 1995). Employability was also decreased in those with seizures (46 percent versus 78 percent), but the overall frequency of self-sufficiency (39 percent) and marriage (55 percent) provides an optimistic outlook for patients with Sturge–Weber syndrome. Preventive management for patients with Klippel–Trenaunay–Weber or Sturge-Weber syndrome who have cerebral involvement should include early head MRI scan, ophthalmology, neurology, and early intervention services. The number and severity of neurologic abnormalities will then determine the requirements for subsequent medical, rehabilitative, and scholastic evaluations. Fortunately, there is no increased risk of malignancy in Klippel–Trenaunay–Weber or Sturge–Weber syndrome.

Mafucci syndrome

Mafucci syndrome, like Klippel–Trenaunay–Weber syndrome, involves multiple hemangiomas with risk of skeletal deformities. In addition, there are multiple enchondromas of bone and associated other neoplasms. The enchondromas appear between ages 1 and 5 years, producing greater deformity than is seen in the Klippel–Trenaunay–Weber syndrome, including risk of limb fractures. Beyond surveillance for bleeding or platelet depletion, there is little preventive management for Mafucci syndrome other than surgical referral to manage the cosmetic, vascular, and skeletal complications. Malignant neoplasms have included angiosarcoma, fibrosarcoma, pancreatic and hepatic carcinomas, and brain tumors (Gorlin et al., 1990, pp. 383–5; Jones, 1997, p. 518).

Peutz–Jeghers syndrome

The combination of melanotic nodules on the lips and intestinal polyposis characterizes Peutz–Jeghers syndrome. It is an autosomal dominant disorder with an increased risk of cancer (Gorlin et al., 1990, pp. 399–403; Rebsdorf Pederson, 1994; Evans, 1995; Spigelman et al., 1995). The oral pigmentation most frequently involves the lips (98 percent), but also is seen on the buccal mucosa (88 percent), palate (less common), or tongue (rare). Pigment also appears on the skin, varying from a few macules to large pigmented areas. The polyps are benign hamartomas that occur in the jejunum (65 percent), ileum (55 percent), large intestine (36 percent), stomach (23 percent), or duodenum (15 percent – Gorlin et al., 1990, p. 399). More than 70 percent of patients experience some type of symptom (pain, melena) from the polyps, with an age of onset between a few weeks and 82 years (mean age, 29 years). The skin and oral pigmentation is usually present during infancy, but may appear as late as the eighth decade (Gorlin et al., 1990, p. 399; Spigelman et al., 1995; Jones, 1997, pp. 520–1).

Preventive management of Peutz–Jeghers syndrome should include a thorough evaluation of the gastrointestinal tract once the diagnosis is made. The intestinal polyps are hamartomas rather than cancers, but malignant transformation has been clearly documented (Evans, 1995; Spigelman et al., 1995). While earlier authors recommended removal of polyps only if they were responsible for intussusception, current policy is to surgically excise them when feasible (Spigelman et al., 1995). Endoscopic techniques have greatly lessened the need for repeated abdominal surgery, and most recommend "top and tail" endoscopy to be performed every two years, with removal of polyps greater than 0.5 cm in size (Spigelman et al., 1995). Unfortunately, there is also increased risk of neoplasm at other sites, including ovarian, breast, testicular or pancreatic cancers. Since these tumors occur at high frequency (10–14 percent risk of ovarian tumors in females), abdominal ultrasound screening every 3–6 months should be considered in these patients. In the Danish Polyposis Register (Rebsdorf Pederson et al., 1994), pelvic examination, cervical smear, and breast and testicular examinations are carried out annually after age 30 years.

Proteus syndrome

Cohen & Hayden (1979) first recognized Proteus syndrome as a separate disorder. As the name implies, the patients may suffer considerable distortions in appearance due to localized overgrowth and hamartomas. Hemangiomas, lipomas, and lymphangiomas may occur, and fibrous growths on the foot may form the characteristic "moccasin" lesion that is preserved in the skeleton of Joseph Merrick, the "Elephant Man" (Cohen, 1987). Other complications include increased growth, strabismus, skeletal abnormalities such as scoliosis, kyphosis, dislocated hips, and striking overgrowth of digits or toes. Mental deficiency (55 percent) and seizures (13 percent) also occur (Gorlin et al., 1990, pp. 403–6; Jones, 1997, pp. 514–15). Preventive management should consist of early intervention and developmental assessment, ophthalmology referral during the first year, evaluation of skeletal growth for orthopedic problems, and periodic examinations to detect early cancers. Neoplasms of the parotid gland, testis, and breast have been reported, and more evidence of carcinogenesis can be anticipated in this unusual hamartosis syndrome (Gorlin et al., 1990, pp. 403–6).

Neurofibromatosis-2

As discussed in Gorlin et al. (1990, pp. 392–3), several types of neurofibromatosis can be distinguished according to the type and distribution of hamartomatous lesions. Neurofibromatosis-1 is a common and well-known disorder (see below), while neurofibromatosis-2 is rare (incidence 1 in 40 to 100,000 births) and notable for the presence of vestibular schwannomas along the 8th cranial nerve (NIH Consensus Development Conference, 1991; MacCollin et al., 1993). The term "acoustic neuroma" has been discarded because the tumors derive from Schwann cells and are distributed along the vestibular branch of the eighth nerve. Additional complications include cataracts at a young age and other types of brain tumors, including meningiomas and gliomas. Like neurofibromatosis-1, neurofibromatosis-2 is an autosomal dominant disorder with associated neurofibromas and plexiform neurofibromas; axillary freckling and café-au-lait spots rarely occur.

Lisch nodules of the irides are also unusual in neurofibromatosis-2, but epiretinal membranes are a unique ophthalmologic finding (Kaye et al., 1992). The gene responsible for neurofibromatosis-2 has been cloned and is a tumor suppressor that interacts with the cytoskeleton (MacCollin et al., 1993).

Preventive management for neurofibromatosis-2 should focus on the detection of vestibular schwannomas, since these tumors cause the most severe problems in the disorder. The usual presentation is hearing loss noted in late adolescence or early adulthood. However, a study of 204 patients with vestibular schwannomas showed a broader range of symptoms: unilateral hearing loss in 93 percent, tinnitus in 61 percent, imbalance in 36 percent, aural fullness in 24 percent, and headache in 5 percent (Leonetti, 1995). In that study, 20 percent of patients were completely deaf at the time of diagnosis (Leonetti, 1995). Variability in the time of presentation mandates early and frequent auditory evoked response and audiology screening once the diagnosis of neurofibromatosis-2 is made, along with annual MRI scan of the brain to measure the tumor size. Since affected individuals may have few cutaneous lesions, children of a parent with neurofibromatosis-2 (i.e., those at 50 percent risk) may deserve a baseline head MRI scan and annual hearing assessments until their genetic status is defined. Unless there are hearing deficits, it is best to wait until age 10 for the head MRI so that anesthesia can be avoided. Conversely, parents of affected individuals should also be warned about the symptoms, even though there is a substantial new mutation rate of 50 percent. DNA diagnosis will be helpful in determining the appropriate management of asymptomatic individuals once it is widely available.

When a vestibular schwannoma is documented, surgery is usually indicated except in debilitated patients. Of 40 older patients with vestibular schwannomas, about 10 percent showed sufficient tumor progression to require limited surgery to debulk the lesions (Leonetti, 1995). The preservation of hearing after surgery correlates with the size of the schwannoma(s), emphasizing the importance of early detection (Leonetti, 1995). Follow-up is critical, with brain imaging and hearing tests as frequent as every 3 months, depending on the patient's age and the rate of tumor progression (NIH Consensus Development Conference, 1991). Support groups may help patients deal with the prospects and complications (facial nerve palsies, distortions in appearance) of frequent surgery. They may be located through Exceptional Parent magazine or the Alliance of Genetic Support Groups, and include: Acoustic Neuroma Association, P.O. Box 12402, Atlanta, GA 30355, (404) 237–8023, anausa@aol.com, http://www.anausa.org; Acoustic Neuroma Association of Canada, P.O. Box 369, Edmonton AB, Canada, T5J 2J6, (800) 561–2622, anac@compusmart.ab.ca; The British Acoustic Neuroma Association, Oak House, Ransom Wood Business Park, Southwell Road West, Mansfield, Nottinghamshire NG21 0HJ (01623) 632–143 http://www.ukan.co.uk/bana/info.htm.

Neurofibromatosis-1

Terminology

Although the disorder was first described in 1849, von Recklinghausen's identification of neural elements in neurofibromatosis gained him credit for recognizing the disease in 1882 (Gorlin et al., 1990, pp. 392–9). The classical description was of type 1 neurofibromatosis with multiple café-au-lait spots and neurofibromas, which accounts for 90 percent of all cases (Riccardi, 1981). Neurofibromatosis-2 with acoustic neuromas, discussed above, is the other recognized form of neurofibromatosis. Other forms of neurofibromatosis have been proposed but are not well delineated (Riccardi, 1981). Isolation of the genes responsible for type 1 (neurofibromin gene on chromosome 17) and type 2 (merlin tumor suppressor on chromosome 22) has established these disorders as separate entities (Xu et al., 1990; MacCollin et al., 1993). Proof that other neurofibromatosis types are not simply due to variable expressivity of type 1 awaits further molecular studies.

Incidence, etiology, and differential diagnosis

The prevalence of neurofibromatosis-1 is between 1 in 2500 and 1 in 3000 births, with about 50 percent representing new mutations. The disorder exhibits autosomal dominant inheritance with virtually 100 percent penetrance if findings such as café-au-lait spots are scored. The responsible gene has been cloned and encodes a protein called neurofibromin; neurofibromin is homologous to components of the G protein signal transduction pathway and seems to function as a tumor suppressor. The neurofibromin gene is located on chromosome 17. Large deletions of the gene are common, as detected by fluorescent in situ hybridization (FISH), and these patients often have additional dysmorphology and more café-au-lait spots than others with neurofibromatosis-1 (Leppig et al., 1996). The germ-line mutation of one neurofibromin allele (one hit) may cause a proliferation of skin (café-au-lait spots) or Schwann cells (neurofibromas), since the second normal neurofibromin allele is retained in neurofibromas (Stark et al., 1995). Loss of heterozygosity (second hit) may occur in the malignant tumors associated with neurofibromatosis-1 (Wilms tumor, neuroblastoma, leukemia, adrenal carcinomas), but that remains to be demonstrated.

The differential diagnosis is between other hamartoses such as Bannayan–Riley–Ruvalcaba syndrome (macrocephaly, lipomas, pigmented lesions), LEOPARD syndrome with multiple lentigines, or Proteus syndrome with lipomas, epidermal nevi, and asymmetric gigantism of the limbs or face. Cohen (1987) presented compelling evidence that Joseph Merrick, the "Elephant Man," had Proteus syndrome rather than neurofibromatosis-1 (see above). This distinction is reassuring to patients with a common disease (neurofibromatosis-1), although the severe deformities of Joseph Merrick remain a worrisome symbol for patients with the extremely rare Proteus syndrome. Among the other forms of neurofibromatosis, neurofibromatosis-2 is important to differentiate because of its different preventive management oriented toward vestibular schwannomas (see above). There is also an autosomal dominant disorder that involves multiple café-au-lait spots without other findings of neurofibromatosis-1; genetic linkage studies using DNA probes surrounding the neurofibromin gene demonstrated that the phenotype of multiple café-au-lait spots is caused by mutation at a different locus (Charrow et al., 1993).

Diagnostic evaluation and medical counseling

Crowe et al. (1956) developed a criterion of six café-au-lait spots larger than 1.5 cm when selecting patients for their classic study of neurofibromatosis-1. This criterion is widely accepted for a diagnosis of the disease, although six spots more than 0.5 cm diameter before puberty is accepted. A National Institutes of Health Consensus Development Conference (1988) established a broader criterion, wherein the requisite number of café-au-lait spots was one of seven findings, any two of which would confirm the clinical diagnosis of neurofibromatosis-1. The other findings included: (1) two neurofibroma or one plexiform neuroma, (2) axillary or inguinal freckling, (3) optic glioma, (4) two or more Lisch nodules, (5) a distinctive osseous lesion (e.g., pseudoarthrosis), and (6) a first-degree relative with neurofibromatosis. Molecular confirmation of the diagnosis is technologically feasible but not commercially available because of the large neurofibromin gene and the variety of mutations (Xu et al., 1990).

In asymptomatic patients, optimistic medical counseling is warranted based on the 40 percent of patients with neurofibromatosis-1 who never have complications. However, Riccardi (1981) emphasized that a milder disease course involving pigmented lesions can quickly change to one with incapacitating neurologic deficits from encroaching tumors. It is thus important to inform patients about the risks of learning disabilities, of neurologic deficits or asymmetries secondary to tumor growth, and of vascular lesions with hypertension. Realistic mention of complications should aid in accomplishing the regular physical examinations that are the crux of preventive management of neurofibromatosis-1.

Family and psychosocial counseling

A common scenario for this autosomal dominant disease with a 50% new mutation rate is for normal couples to have a child affected with neurofibromatosis-1. If one parent has macrocephaly or other findings suggestive of neurofibromatosis, then examination for café-au-lait spots, head MRI scan, and ophthalmology slit-lamp examination for Lisch spots may detect the diagnosis. Individuals with the disease have a 50 percent risk to transmit the disorder with each pregnancy, and variable expressivity dictates that mildly affected parents may have severely affected offspring and vice versa. Most states have active neurofibromatosis organizations that can be helpful for family counseling and support, particularly in relieving the specter of deformity that may dominate lay images of the disease. Parent support groups are listed on the neurofibromatosis checklist, part 1.

Natural history and complications

As mentioned above, 40 percent of patients avoid complications beyond café-au-lait spots. The diagnosis may be difficult to recognize in the neonatal period, and most individuals with neurofibromatosis-1 avoid early complications. Macrocephaly is relatively common (30 percent), and seizures or hydrocephalus may occur. The asymmetry and disfigurement of plexiform neuromas that occur in about 30 percent of children may cause difficult management problems when the tumors cannot be surgically dissected free of nerve roots.

Optic gliomas are common in neurofibromatosis-1, and are often multifocal. Fortunately, the tumors are less invasive of the optic nerves than optic gliomas in patients without neurofibromatosis-1. Equally troubling are spinal neurofibromas that may recur in patients with neurofibromatosis-1. Seppala et al. (1995) described 22 patients with spinal neurofibromas that occurred mainly in the cervical region. These tumors were associated with a significant decrease in life span for the affected patients with neurofibromatosis-1.

Neurofibromatosis-1 commonly affects the skeleton, with dislocations, pseudo-arthroses, scoliosis, and underdevelopment of the maxilla and mandible being common (Neurofibromatosis checklist, part 1). The long bones may contain cyst-like lesions that are useful for diagnosis but seem not to cause pain or fractures. Schotland et al. (1992) reported a family with neurofibromatosis-1 in whom the multiple bone fibromas raised the question of coincidental fibrous dysplasia. Vascular lesions such as renal artery stenosis and congenital cardiac lesions do occur, and hypertension may be a problem during adulthood. Some patients develop arteriovenous fistulae of the spinal column, adding another reason for vigilance concerning neck or back pain and altered gait (Cluzel et al., 1994). Akbarnia et al. (1992) found that 23 of 220 patients with neurofibromatosis-1 had scoliosis, the majority because of dystrophic vertebrae.

About 40 percent of neurofibromatosis-1 patients have cognitive disability, with speech delay and selective learning differences. The children may also have neurosensory deficits from optic glioma (4 percent) or aural neurofibromas. Neurofibromas of the external ear canal and pinna were found in 28 of 434 patients with neurofibromatosis-1, but only two of these patients had tumors in the middle ear

(Smullen et al., 1994). These findings contrasted with the invasive vestibular schwannomas and hearing loss experienced by 6 patients with neurofibromatosis-2 in the same study (Smullen et al., 1994). However, neurofibromatosis-1 patients are at risk for neoplasms in most body regions, with examples of benign (neurofibromas), malignant by position (plexiform neurofibromas), or true malignant tumors (neurofibrosarcomas, Wilms tumor, leukemias, pancreatic or adrenal carcinomas).

Neurofibromatosis-1 preventive medical checklist

Parts 2–4 of the checklist incorporate health care recommendations for neurofibromatosis endorsed by the Committee on Genetics, American Academy of Pediatrics (1995). Although some authors have recommended brain imaging studies as soon as the diagnosis of neurofibromatosis-1 is made (Riccardi, 1981), the general consensus is to await such symptoms as seizures, increased head circumference, or precocious puberty before obtaining a head MRI scan. Since there is increased risk for optic gliomas and other intracranial tumors, and since benign or malignant tumors can arise in many other body locations, aggressive radiologic evaluations should be pursued when changes are revealed by periodic history review and physical examination. Once tumors such as optic gliomas or acoustic neuromas are discovered, their management will depend on their rate of growth and the disability inflicted on the patient. Since these tumors are usually multifocal, surgical intervention should be saved for symptoms of severe neurosensory dysfunction or of increased intracranial pressure. Leonetti (1995) discusses the advantages of medical management or of limited debulking operations in acoustic neuroma, and conservative approaches aimed at preserving nerve function are particularly important for children.

Regular physical examinations noting the distribution of café-au-lait spots and neurofibromas are useful, including drawings or photographs of lesions. Because neurosensory or skeletal alterations may be harbingers of tumor growth, regular hearing/vision assessment by the physician with annual ophthalmology and audiology screening is recommended through adulthood. Note on part 4 of the checklist that annual rather than biennial examinations are recommended for the patient with neurofibromatosis-1 after age 6. Puberty is particularly important to monitor, since precocious puberty and accelerated tumor growth during puberty are established phenomena. Lesions may also grow during pregnancy.

Early intervention, speech evaluation, and preschool evaluation of cognitive performance are important because of the frequent occurrence of learning disabilities in neurofibromatosis-1 (Hofman et al., 1994). Skeletal asymmetry and scoliosis may compromise motor function, and job training is important in patients with cognitive disabilities. Hypertension may occur through a narrowing of the renal artery or pheochromocytomas, so annual monitoring of blood pressure is also recommended. A neurofibromatosis clinic in reasonable proximity is an excellent resource for the coordinated subspecialty management that neurofibromatosis-1 patients may require.

Tuberous sclerosis

Terminology

The term "tuberous sclerosis" was coined in 1880 by Bourneville (Gorlin et al., 1990, pp. 410–15). The fibrotic tumors in brain ("tubers") cause seizures and mental retardation that, together with "adenoma sebaceum," comprise the classic diagnostic recognized by Vogt in 1908 (Hunt, 1993). In fact, the term "adenoma sebaceum" is incorrect, because the facial lesions are actually angiofibromas. "Epiloa" is also an outdated term derived from Greek roots meaning epilepsy and mindlessness (Hunt, 1993). Clinical findings in tuberous sclerosis include reddish-yellow plaques on the forehead ("forehead plaque"), leathery plaques in the lumbosacral area ("shagreen patches"), and diffuse regions of skin hyper/hypopigmentation ("confetti skin lesions"). The variability of clinical findings and evidence of genetic heterogeneity in tuberous sclerosis have led to the term "tuberous sclerosis complex" (Roach et al., 1992, 1998).

Incidence, etiology, and differential diagnosis

Although incidence figures as low as 1 per 100,000 have been cited for tuberous sclerosis, improvements in clinical detection suggest the true incidence is 1 per 8,000–23,000 births (Gorlin et al., 1990, pp. 410–15; Hunt, 1993; Jones, 1997, pp. 506–7). Tuberous sclerosis is an autosomal dominant disorder, and genetic linkage studies identified two genes in chromosome regions 9q34 and 16p13.3. The TSC1 gene on chromosome 9 acts as a growth suppressor analogous to neurofibromin (Green et al., 1994), and the TSC2 gene on chromosome 16, like that for neurofibromin, appears to function in a G-protein mediated signal transduction pathway (Anonymous, 1993). Interestingly, contiguous gene deletions affecting the TSC2 tuberous sclerosis and nearby polycystic kidney disease gene on chromosome 16 have occurred in patients with both diseases (Brook-Carter et al., 1994); the subset of tuberous sclerosis patients with early and severe renal cystic disease may arise from such deletions.

The major clinical findings of seizures, facial angiofibromas, ungual fibromas, hypopigmented macules, cardiac or renal tumors, and neural (brain, retina) hamartomas comprise a distinctive clinical picture for tuberous sclerosis. Differential diagnosis would include other disorders with brain and skin lesions, such as Sturge–Weber angiomatosis or neurofibromatosis, congenital infection with toxoplasma or cytomegalovirus, and facial xanthomas or milia.

Table 13.2 Diagnostic criteria for tuberous sclerosis

Major features
Facial angiofibromas or forehead plaque
Nontraumatic ungual or periungual fibroma
Hypomelanotic macules
Shagreen patch (connective tissue nevus)
Multiple retinal nodular hamartomas
Cortical tuber
Subependymal nodule or giant cell astrocytoma[a]
Cardiac rhabdomyoma, single or multiple
Lymphangiomyomatosis
Renal angiomyolipoma

Secondary features
Multiple, randomly distributed pits in the dental enamel
Hamartomatous rectal polyps
Bone cysts
Cerebral white matter radial migration lines
Gingival fibromas
Nonrenal hamartoma
Retinal achromatic patch
"Confetti" skin lesions
Multiple renal cysts

Source: Roach et al. (1998).

Diagnostic evaluation and medical counseling

Diagnostic criteria for tuberous sclerosis have been formulated by a subcommittee of the National Tuberous Sclerosis Association and a recent consensus conference (Roach et al., 1992, 1998). A major problem with the diagnosis in childhood is that features such as facial angiofibromas, ungual fibromas, renal angiomyolipomas, and even calcified subependymal nodules may not be present during infancy. Periodic diagnostic assessment is thus required for individuals at risk. With this caveat in mind, major diagnostic criteria for tuberous sclerosis are listed in Table 13.2. Some findings require histologic and/or radiographic confirmation before qualifying as criteria, while others (facial angiofibromas, ungual fibromas, retinal astrocytomas, shagreen patches, or hypomelanotic nodules) can be diagnosed only by physical examination. For a definite diagnosis, two major features or one major feature plus two minor features are required (Roach et al., 1998). Patients with fewer features can be considered as probable or suspect for tuberous sclerosis, with the implication that younger patients need careful follow-up. Examination with ultraviolet light A (Wood's lamp) is much more sensitive in detecting the white macules in light-skinned people (Janniger & Schwartz, 1993).

Medical counseling must take into account the 60–80 percent of patients that have mental or learning disabilities, but many affected individuals are asymptomatic. Brain involvement with tumors, heterotopias, seizures, and developmental disability often accompanies the presentation in early childhood, and these patients will require the full spectrum of psychosocial and medical counseling appropriate for children with severe handicaps. Behavioral abnormalities such as childhood autism or later schizophrenia are frequent, and changes in behavior should be mentioned as a mandate for brain imaging.

Family and psychosocial counseling

Affected individuals will have a 50 percent risk of transmitting tuberous sclerosis with each pregnancy. The difficulty in genetic counseling is to distinguish whether parents of an obviously affected child are themselves affected. Cassidy et al. (1983) demonstrated that full investigation of at-risk family members is required for accurate counseling. For asymptomatic but affected individuals, skin examination (96 percent positive), cranial CT scan (67 percent), skull radiographs (46 percent), hand/foot radiographs (39 percent), fundoscopic examination (33 percent), and renal ultrasound study (30 percent) were most useful in making the diagnosis (Cassidy et al., 1983; Gorlin et al., 1990, pp. 410–15). Thorough ascertainment of family members has revised prior estimates of the new mutation rate from 70 percent to less than 50 percent (Gorlin et al., 1990, pp. 410–15). Parents who have no signs of tuberous sclerosis after complete evaluation can be assigned a low recurrence risk, but the difficulty of ruling out the diagnosis should be discussed.

Considerable psychosocial support is needed for families with severely affected infants, since these children will have extensive mental and physical disabilities. Patients with facial lesions (facial angiofibromas, forehead plaques) may require cosmetic surgery, dermatologic treatment, and psychiatric support because of their altered appearance. Parent groups are listed on the tuberous sclerosis checklist, part 1.

Natural history and complications

Complications of tuberous sclerosis affect the nervous system most severely with seizures in 88–93 percent, mental deficiency in 60–80 percent, and intracranial calcifications in 56 percent (Gorlin et al., 1990, pp. 410–15; Hunt, 1993). Tonic-clonic (41 percent) and infantile spasms (30 percent) are the most common types of seizures, but myoclonic, absence, and akinetic seizures also occur. Seizures have an early onset, with 20 percent starting before age 3 months, 46 percent starting before age 3–7 months, and only 4 percent occurring after age 5 years in a survey of 300 affected families (Hunt, 1993). Cranial calcification of subependymal hamartomas is progressive, with 15 percent of patients by age 1 year, 35 percent by age 5 years, and 50–60 percent by age 14 years exhibiting this finding (Gorlin et al., 1990, pp. 410–15). Behavioral changes are common, including hyperactivity (28 percent), impaired social interaction (43 percent), repetitive behaviors (25 percent), and aggressive behaviors with attacks on other people (28 percent) or self-injury (29 percent – Hunt, 1993).

Other symptomatic findings include intracranial hypertension from cranial giant cell astrocytomas that occur in 6–14 percent of patients (Roach & Delgado, 1995). Cardiac rhabdomyomas occur in 30–67 percent of patients, and sympto-matic infants have significant mortality (Gorlin et al., 1990, pp. 410–15). These cardiac tumors may also resolve over time. Endocrine abnormalities rarely occur, but can include acromegaly or precocious puberty. Cystic disease of the lung (hon-eycomb lung) occurs predominantly in females, causing symptoms after the third decade with a five-year mortality rate of 67 percent.

Lesions of tuberous sclerosis that are generally asymptomatic include the hypo-melanotic macules, facial angiofibromas, and ungual fibromas of the skin; renal angiomyolipomas or cysts; and miscellaneous hamartomas in organs such as pan-creas, liver, and testes. Retinal hamartomas are of two types, presenting as gray-yellow semitranslucent lesions (55 percent) or opaque, nodular lesions (45 percent). Some patients have both types, but few have visual problems (Gorlin et al., 1990, pp. 410–15). The phalanges and, less frequently, the long bones may exhibit asymptomatic cysts or periosteal new bone formation on radiographs. Some patients have overgrowth of one digit, and one presented with an acromegaly (Gorlin et al., 1990, pp. 410–15).

Tuberous sclerosis preventive medical checklist

Preventive management of tuberous sclerosis will be directed toward early evalua-tion of neurologic, ophthalmologic, cardiac, dermatologic, and developmental problems (checklist, parts 2–4). If the disease is recognized at birth, head ultra-sound or MRI studies can be justified to determine the presence and size of epen-dymomas or giant cell astrocytomas. Changes in behavior, alterations in head circumference, and symptoms of intracranial hypertension warrant additional head MRI studies, and contrast may be helpful in recognizing the more trouble-some giant-cell astrocytomas (Roach & Delgado, 1995). The latter tumors should be removed when accessible, particularly if they are expanding or symptomatic (Roach & Delgado, 1995). Epilepsy begins early and takes many forms, so pediat-ric neurology referral is important for diagnosis and treatment. Anticonvulsant therapy tends to be complex, and surgical treatment has a role in severe cases (Bebin et al., 1993). Sleep disturbances appear frequent in patients with epilepsy, so sleep studies may be considered (Bruni et al., 1995). The high risk of mental disability justifies early intervention with regular speech, occupational and physical therapy assessments. Financial, psychosocial, and genetic counseling should be facilitated and re-emphasized in subsequent visits; thorough educational evaluations and job training are also essential.

Preventive management for problems outside the nervous system should include a cardiac evaluation with ultrasound as soon as the diagnosis is made. Renal ultrasound to detect angiomyolipomas or cysts can also be justified at the time of diagnosis, and should be repeated to monitor tumors and cysts or after episodes of hematuria. Referral to urology is useful for enlarging cysts or other renal symptoms, since decompression of the cysts has been associated with reversal of hypertension and renal failure (Wood et al., 1992). Moulis et al. (1992) reported a patient with tuberous sclerosis and colon carcinoma, commenting on the high frequency of intestinal polyps in those patients who have been investigated. It is therefore wise to alert adult patients to report hematochezia and recognize that oral, gastric, and intestinal hamartomas occur in these patients (Moulis et al., 1992). Zimmer-Galler & Robertson (1995) provide evidence that retinal hamartomas can manifest in previously normal regions and progress. Regular evaluation of the heart, limbs, skin, and oral cavity is indicated, along with periodic referrals to neurology, ophthalmology, and dentistry. These same management strategies should extend through adolescence, with vigilance for precocious puberty. The occurrence of cystic lung disease in adulthood warrants periodic chest radiographs and auscultation after age 20. Anticipation of airway lesions or seizures is important during anesthesia for patients with tuberous sclerosis (Lee et al., 1994).

Preventive Management of Neurofibromatosis-1

Clinical diagnosis: Criteria include 6 spots café-au-lait more than 0.5 cm diameter before puberty, two neurofibroma or one plexiform neuroma, axillary or inguinal freckling, optic glioma, two or more Lisch nodules, or osseous lesions such as pseudoarthroses (NIH Consensus Development Conference, 1988).

Incidence: 1 in 2500–3000 live births.

Laboratory diagnosis: Mutations in the neurofibromin gene on chromosome 17 are the gold standard for diagnosis, but routine DNA testing is not available.

Genetics: Autosomal dominant inheritance with 50% of patients representing new mutations. Affected individuals have a 50% risk for transmission to offspring.

Key management issues: Regular physical examinations documenting the location and size of café-au-lait spots and neurofibromas; brain scanning for findings such as seizures, increasing head circumference, or precocious puberty; aggressive radiologic evaluations when changes are noted in other body regions; monitoring of puberty, skeletal growth, and blood pressure; early intervention, speech evaluation, and preschool evaluation of cognitive performance.

Growth charts: None available.

Parent groups: National Neurofibromatosis Foundation, 95 Pine St., 16th Floor, New York NY, 10005, (800) 323-7988, nnff@aol.com; http://www.nf.org; Neurofibromatosis Society of Ontario, 923 Annes Street Whitby ON, Canada L1N5K7, (905)430-6141;The Neurofibromatosis Association, 82 London Road, Kingston-upon-Thames, Surrey KT2 6PX, (0181) 547-1636 http://www/cressida.demon.co.uk/neuro/

Basis for management recommendations: Guidelines endorsed by the Committee on Genetics, American Academy of Pediatrics (1995).

Summary of clinical concerns

General	Learning	**Cognitive disability** (40% – 8–9% with IQ < 70), **learning differences** (25%), **speech problems** (30–40%)
	Growth	Short stature
	Tumors	Neurofibromas (15%), **skin angiomas** (53%), malignancy of various types (6%), neurofibrosarcomas (3–12%)
Facial	Eye	Eye anomalies (congenital glaucoma, corneal opacity, retinal detachment, optic atrophy, ptosis), **Lisch nodules** (28%), strabismus, proptosis
	Mouth	**Oral changes** (66% – oral neurofibromas, macroglossia, large lingual papillae, malpositioned teeth)
Surface	Epidermal	**Café-au-lait spots** (99%), **axillary freckling** (81%), pruritis
Skeletal	Cranial	Macrocephaly (30%) Craniofacial deformities
	Axial	Scoliosis (5%)
	Limbs	Pseudoarthrosis (3%), hemihyperplasia, dislocations (hip, radius, ulna)
Internal	Digestive	Constipation (10%)
	Circulatory	Pulmonary stenosis
		Aortic stenosis, renal artery stenosis (2%)
	Endocrine	Precocious puberty
Neural	CNS	Hydrocephalus (1%), seizures (5%)
	Motor	Plexiform neuromas (30%)
	Sensory	Optic glioma (4%), visual deficits

Bold: frequency > 20%

Key references

Cohen, M. M., Jr. (1987). *Proceedings of the Greenwood Genetics Center* 6:187–92.

Committee on Genetics, American Academy of Pediatrics (1995) *Pediatrics* 96:368–71.

Hofman, K. J. et al. (1994). *Journal of Pediatrics* 124:A1–S8.

National Institute of Health (NIH) Consensus Development Conference Statement: neurofibromatosis (1988) *Neurofibromatosis* 1:172–8.

Obringer, A. C. et al. (1989). *American Journal of Diseases of Children* 143:717–19.

Neurofibromatosis-1

Preventive medical checklist (0–1yr)

Patient		Birth Date / /		Number	
Pediatric	**Screen**	**Evaluate**		**Refer/Counsel**	
Neonatal / / *Newborn screen* ❑ HB ❑	Head sonogram ❑	Proptosis ❑ Skin ❑ Skeleton[3] ❑		Neurofibromatosis-1 clinic ❑ Genetic evaluation ❑	
1 month / /	Head size ❑ Hearing, vision[2] ❑ Head MRI[3] ❑	Skin ❑		Family support[4] ❑	
2 months / / HB[1] ❑ Hib ❑ DTaP, IPV ❑ RV ❑	Head size, BP ❑ Hearing, vision[2] ❑	Skin ❑		Early intervention[5] ❑ Developmental pediatrics ❑ Genetic counseling ❑ Neurofibromatosis-1 clinic ❑	
4 months / / HB[1] ❑ Hib ❑ DTaP/IPV ❑ RV ❑	Head size, BP ❑ Hearing, vision[2] ❑	Skin ❑		Early intervention[5] ❑	
6 months / / Hib ❑ OPV[1] ❑ DTaP ❑ RV ❑	Head size, BP ❑ Hearing, vision[2] ❑ Skeletal x-rays[3] ❑	Proptosis ❑ Skin ❑ Skeleton[3] ❑		Family support[4] ❑	
9 months / / IPV[1] ❑	Head size, BP ❑ Hearing, vision[2] ❑				
1 year / / HB ❑ Hib[1] ❑ IPV[1] ❑ MMR[1] ❑ Var[1] ❑	Head size, BP ❑ Hearing, vision[2] ❑ Audiology ❑	Proptosis ❑ Skin ❑ Skeleton[3] ❑		Family support[4] ❑ Early intervention[5] ❑ Neurofibromatosis-1 clinic ❑ Ophthalmology[3] ❑	

Clinical concerns for Neurofibromatosis-1, ages 0–1 year

Facial asymmetry	Renal artery stenosis	Developmental disability
Sensorineural hearing loss	Hypertension	Learning differences
Vision deficits (optic glioma)	Skeletal dislocations	Short stature
Cataracts, strabismus	Benign tumors	Constipation, hydrocephalus

Guidelines for the neonatal period should be undertaken *at whatever age* the diagnosis is made; DTaP, acellular DTP; IPV, inactivated poliovirus (oral polio also used); RV, rotavirus; MMR, measles–mumps–rubella; Var, varicella; BP, blood pressure, [1]alternative timing; [2]by practitioner; [3]as dictated by clinical findings – head MRI for seizures, visual problems, orthopedics evaluation for asymmetry, pseudoarthroses, dislocations; [4]parent group, family/sib, financial, and behavioral issues as discussed in the preface; [5]including developmental monitoring and motor/speech therapy.

Neurofibromatosis-1

Preventive medical checklist (15m–6yrs)

Patient   **Birth Date**   /   /   **Number**

Pediatric	Screen	Evaluate	Refer/Counsel
15 months / / Hib[1] ☐ MMR[1] ☐ DTaP, IPV[1] ☐ Varicella[1] ☐	Head size, BP ☐ Hearing, vision[2] ☐		Family support[3] ☐ Early intervention[4] ☐
18 months / / DTaP, IPV[1] ☐ Varicella[1] ☐ Influenza[3] ☐	Head size, BP ☐ Hearing, vision[2] ☐	Skin ☐	
2 years / / Influenza[3] ☐ Pneumovax[3] ☐ Dentist ☐	Head size, BP ☐ Hearing, vision[2] ☐ Audiology ☐	Proptosis ☐ Skin ☐ Skeleton[3] ☐	Family support[4] ☐ Neurofibromatosis-1 clinic ☐ Ophthalmology ☐ Sunscreen ☐
3 years / / Influenza[3] ☐ Pneumovax[3] ☐ Dentist ☐	Head size, BP ☐ Hearing, vision[2] ☐ Audiology ☐	Proptosis ☐ Skin ☐ Skeleton[3] ☐	Family support[4] ☐ Preschool transition[5] ☐ Neurofibromatosis-1 clinic ☐ Ophthalmology[3] ☐ Sunscreen ☐
4 years / / Influenza[3] ☐ Pneumovax[3] ☐ Dentist ☐	Growth ☐ Head size ☐ Hearing, vision[2] ☐ BP ☐	Proptosis ☐ Skin ☐ Skeleton[3] ☐	Family support[4] ☐ Preschool program[5] ☐ Neurofibromatosis-1 clinic ☐ Ophthalmology[3] ☐ Orthopedics[3] ☐
5 years / / DTaP, IPV[1] ☐ MMR[1] ☐	Hearing, vision[2] ☐ Audiology ☐ Head MRI[3] ☐ BP ☐	Proptosis ☐ Skin ☐ Skeleton[3] ☐	School transition[5] ☐ Ophthalmology ☐ Sunscreen ☐
6 years / / DTaP, IPV[1] ☐ MMR[1] ☐ Dentist ☐	Growth ☐ Hearing, vision[2] ☐ BP ☐	School progress ☐ Puberty ☐ Skin ☐ Skeleton[3] ☐	Family support[4] ☐ Neurofibromatosis-1 clinic ☐ Ophthalmology[3] ☐ Orthopedics[3] ☐

Clinical concerns for Neurofibromatosis-1, ages 1–6 years

Facial asymmetry	Renal artery stenosis	Developmental disability
Sensorineural hearing loss	Hypertension	Learning differences
Vision deficits (optic glioma)	Skeletal dislocations	Short stature
Cataracts, strabismus	Benign tumors	Constipation, hydrocephalus

Guidelines for prior ages should be undertaken *at the time of diagnosis*; DTaP, acellular DTP; IPV, inactivated poliovirus (oral polio also used); MMR, measles–mumps–rubella; BP, blood pressure; [1]alternative timing; [2]by practitioner; [3]as dictated by clinical findings – head MRI for seizures, visual problems, precocious puberty, orthopedics evaluation for asymmetry, pseudoarthroses, scoliosis, dislocations; [4]parent group, family/sib, financial, and behavioral issues as discussed in the preface; [5]including developmental monitoring and motor/speech therapy.

Neurofibromatosis-1

Preventive medical checklist (6+ yrs)

Patient   **Birth Date** / /   **Number**

Pediatric	Screen		Evaluate		Refer/Counsel	
8 years / / *Dentist* ❑	Hearing, vision[2] BP	❑ ❑	Puberty Skin Skeleton[3]	❑ ❑ ❑	School options Neurofibromatosis-1 clinic Ophthalmology[3]	❑ ❑ ❑
10 years / /	Growth Hearing, vision[2] BP	❑ ❑ ❑	School progress Puberty Skin Skeleton[3]	❑ ❑ ❑ ❑	Ophthalmology Orthopedics[3] Sunscreen	❑ ❑ ❑
12 years / / *Td[1], MMR, Var* ❑ *CBC* ❑ *Dentist* ❑ *Scoliosis* ❑ *Cholesterol* ❑	Hearing, vision[2] Head MRI[3] BP	❑ ❑ ❑	Puberty Skin Skeleton[4]	❑ ❑ ❑	Family support[4] School options Ophthalmology[3] Neurofibromatosis-1 clinic	❑ ❑ ❑ ❑
14 years / / *CBC* ❑ *Dentist* ❑ *Cholesterol* ❑ *Breast CA* ❑ *Testicular CA* ❑	Growth Hearing, vision[2] BP	❑ ❑ ❑	School progress Skin Skeleton[3]	❑ ❑ ❑	Ophthalmology[3] Orthopedics[3]	❑ ❑
16 years / / *Td[1]* ❑ *CBC* ❑ *Cholesterol* ❑ *Sexual[5]* ❑ *Dentist* ❑	Hearing, vision[2] BP	❑ ❑	Skin Skeleton[3]	❑ ❑	Vocational planning Ophthalmology[4] Neurofibromatosis-1 clinic Sunscreen	❑ ❑ ❑ ❑
18 years / / *CBC* ❑ *Sexual[5]* ❑ *Cholesterol* ❑ *Scoliosis* ❑	Hearing, vision[2] BP	❑ ❑	School progress Skin Skeleton[3]	❑ ❑ ❑	Vocational planning Ophthalmology[3]	❑ ❑
20 years[6] / / *CBC* ❑ *Sexual[5]* ❑ *Cholesterol* ❑ *Dentist* ❑	Hearing, vision[2] Head MRI[3] BP	❑ ❑ ❑	Skin Skeleton[3] Work, residence	❑ ❑ ❑	Family support[4] Neurofibromatosis-1 clinic Ophthalmology[3] Orthopedics[3]	❑ ❑ ❑ ❑

Clinical concerns for Neurofibromatosis-1, ages 6+ years

Facial asymmetry	Hypertension	Cognitive disability
Sensorineural hearing loss	Skeletal dislocations	Learning differences
Vision deficits (optic glioma)	Benign tumors	Short stature
Malposition, macroglossia	Malignant tumors	Seizures

Guidelines for prior ages should be undertaken *at the time of diagnosis*; Td, tetanus/diphtheria; MMR, measles–mumps–rubella; Var, varicella; BP blood pressure; [1]alternative timing; [2]by practitioner; [3]as dictated by clinical findings – head MRI for seizures, visual problems, precocious puberty, orthopedics evaluation for asymmetry, pseudoarthroses, scoliosis, dislocations; [4]parent group, family/sib, financial, and behavioral issues as discussed in the preface; [5]birth control, STD screening if sexually active; [6]repeat every decade.

Preventive Management of Tuberous Sclerosis

Clinical diagnosis: Manifestations include fibrotic tumors in brain ("tubers") that cause seizures and mental disability, adenoma sebaceum on the face, hypopigmented ("ash leaf") spots best seen with a Woods lamp, reddish-yellow plaques on the forehead ("forehead plaque"), leathery plaques in the lumbosacral area ("shagreen patches"), and diffuse regions of skin hyper/hypopigmentation ("confetti skin lesions" – Roach et al., 1992; 1998).

Incidence: 1 in 8,000–23,000 live births.

Laboratory diagnosis: Mutations in the tuberin gene can be identified in some patients.

Genetics: Affected individuals will have a 50 percent risk of transmitting tuberous sclerosis with each pregnancy; parents may require renal and cardiac ultrasound studies to discern if they are subclinically affected.

Key management issues: Monitoring for neurologic, ophthalmologic, cardiac, dermatologic, and developmental problems, head MRI studies for changes in behavior, alterations in head circumference, or symptoms of intracranial hypertension, echocardiographic and renal ultrasound studies to detect angiomyolipomas or cysts, referral to urology for new or persisting renal symptoms, early intervention with school planning.

Parent groups: National Tuberous Sclerosis Foundation 8181 Professional Pl. Suite 120, Landover, MD 20785-2226, (800) 225-6872, ntsa@ntsa.org, http://www.ntsa.org; Tuberous Sclerosis Canada (Sclérose Tubéreuse), 2443 New Wood Dr., Oakville ON, Canada L6H 5Y3, (800) 347-0252, jillian.dasilva@ablelink.org, http://www.skynet/~adamse/

Basis for management recommendations: Derived from the complications below as documented by Hunt (1993), Roach & Delgado (1995).

Summary of clinical concerns

General	Learning	**Cognitive disability** (60–80%), **learning differences, speech problems** (69%)
	Behavior	Autism, schizophrenia
	Tumors	Multiple hamartomas, **angiofibromas** (70%), astrocytomas (6–14%), colon carcinoma
Facial	Eye	**Retinal hamartomas** (50–87%)
	Mouth	Enamel pits (70–90%), fibromas of mucosa (11%)
Surface	Epidermal	**Poliosis** (white hair – 20%), **depigmented nodules** (90%), **shagreen patches** (36%)
Skeletal	Cranial	Thickened calvarium, frontal bone exostoses
	Limbs	**Phalangeal cysts** (60%), periosteal new bone formation, **periungual fibromas** (15–20%)
Internal	Digestive	Angiomas of liver and spleen, colonic polyps
	Pulmonary	Pulmonary, lymphangio-myomatosis (1%)
	Circulatory	**Cardiac rhabdomyomas** (30–67%)
	Endocrine	Precocious puberty, hamartomas of the thyroid, pancreas
	Excretory	**Renal tumors** (60–67%), renal cysts
Neural	CNS	**Ventricular dilatation** (50%), **brain calcifications** (35%), **seizures** (88–93%)

Bold: frequency > 20%

Key references

Hunt, A. (1993). *Journal of Intellectual Disability Research* 37:41–51.
Janniger, C.K. & Schwartz, R. A. (1993). *Cutis* 51:167–74.
Roach, E. S.& Delgado, M. R. (1995). *Dermatologic Clinics* 13:151–61.
Roach, E. S. et al. (1992). *Journal of Child Neurology* 7:221–4.
Roach, E. S. et al. (1998). *Journal of Child Neurology* 13:624–8.

Tuberous Sclerosis

Preventive medical checklist (0–1yr)

Patient **Birth Date** / / **Number**

Pediatric	Screen	Evaluate		Refer/Counsel	
Neonatal / / *Newborn screen* ❏ *HB* ❏	Echocardiogram ❏ Renal sonogram ❏ Head sonogram ❏	Heart Skin Seizures	❏ ❏ ❏	Genetic evaluation Neurology	❏ ❏
1 month / /		Heart Skin Seizures	❏ ❏ ❏	Family support[4]	❏
2 months / / *HB[1]* ❏ *Hib* ❏ *DTaP, IPV* ❏ *RV* ❏		Heart Skin Seizures	❏ ❏ ❏	Early intervention[5] Developmental pediatrics Genetic counseling	❏ ❏ ❏
4 months / / *HB[1]* ❏ *Hib* ❏ *DTaP/IPV* ❏ *RV* ❏		Heart Skin Seizures	❏ ❏ ❏	Early intervention[5] Neurology	❏ ❏
6 months / / *Hib* ❏ *IPV[1]* ❏ *DTaP* ❏ *RV* ❏	Hearing, vision[2] ❏	Heart Skin Seizures	❏ ❏ ❏	Family support[4] Neurology	❏ ❏
9 months / / *IPV[1]* ❏				Ophthalmology	❏
1 year / / *HB* ❏ *Hib[1]* ❏ *IPV[1]* ❏ *MMR[1]* ❏ *Var[1]* ❏	Hearing, vision[2] ❏	Heart Skin, limbs Seizures	❏ ❏ ❏	Family support[4] Early intervention[3] Developmental pediatrics Neurology	❏ ❏ ❏ ❏

Clinical concerns for Tuberous Sclerosis, ages 0–1 year

Retinal hamartomas	Cardiac rhabdomyomas	Developmental disability
Facial angiofibromas	Renal angiomyolipomas	Learning differences
Dental enamel pits	Renal cysts	Intracranial calcifications
Ungual fibromas	Limb overgrowth	Seizures

Guidelines for the neonatal period should be undertaken *at whatever age* the diagnosis is made; DTaP, acellular DTP; IPV, inactivated poliovirus (oral polio also used); RV, rotavirus; MMR, measles–mumps–rubella; Var, varicella; [1]alternative timing; [2]by practitioner; [3]as dictated by clinical findings; [4]parent group, family/sib, financial, and behavioral issues as discussed in the preface; [5]including developmental monitoring and motor/speech therapy.

Tuberous Sclerosis

Preventive medical checklist (15m–6yrs)

Patient   **Birth Date** / /   **Number**

Pediatric	Screen	Evaluate		Refer/Counsel	
15 months / / *Hib[1]* ☐ *MMR[1]* ☐ *DTaP, IPV[1]* ☐ *Varicella[1]* ☐	Head MRI[3] ☐			Family support[4] Early intervention[5]	☐ ☐
18 months / / *DTaP, IPV[1]* ☐ *Varicella[1]* ☐ *Influenza[3]* ☐	Hearing, vision[2] ☐	Heart Skin, limbs Seizures	☐ ☐ ☐		
2 years / / *Influenza[3]* ☐ *Pneumovax[3]* ☐ *Dentist* ☐	Hearing, vision[2] ☐	Heart Skin, limbs Seizures	☐ ☐ ☐	Family support[4] Developmental pediatrics Genetics Neurology[3] Ophthalmology[3]	☐ ☐ ☐ ☐ ☐
3 years / / *Influenza[3]* ☐ *Pneumovax[3]* ☐ *Dentist* ☐	Hearing, vision[2] ☐	Heart Skin, limbs Seizures	☐ ☐ ☐	Family support[4] Preschool program[5] Neurology[3] Ophthalmology[3]	☐ ☐ ☐ ☐
4 years / / *Influenza[3]* ☐ *Pneumovax[3]* ☐ *Dentist* ☐	Hearing, vision[2] ☐ Urinalysis, BP ☐	Heart Skin, limbs Seizures	☐ ☐ ☐	Family support[4] Preschool program[5] Developmental pediatrics Genetics Neurology[3] Ophthalmology[3]	☐ ☐ ☐ ☐ ☐ ☐
5 years / / *DTaP, IPV[1]* ☐ *MMR[1]* ☐		Heart Skin, limbs Seizure	☐ ☐ ☐	School transition Neurology Ophthalmology	☐ ☐ ☐
6 years / / *DTaP, IPV[1]* ☐ *MMR[1]* ☐ *Dentist* ☐	Hearing, vision[2] ☐ Renal sonogram[3] ☐	School progress Puberty Heart Skin, limbs	☐ ☐ ☐ ☐	Family support[5] Developmental pediatrics Genetics Neurology[3] Ophthalmology[3]	☐ ☐ ☐ ☐ ☐

Clinical concerns for Tuberous Sclerosis, ages 1–6 years

Retinal hamartomas	Cardiac rhabdomyomas	Developmental disability
Facial angiofibromas	Renal angiomyolipomas	Learning differences
Dental enamel pits	Renal cysts	Intracranial calcifications
Ungual fibromas	Limb overgrowth	Seizures

Guidelines for prior ages should be undertaken *at the time of diagnosis*; DTaP, acellular DTP; IPV, inactivated poliovirus (oral polio also used); MMR, measles–mumps–rubella; BP, blood pressure; [1]alternative timing; [2]by practitioner; [3]as dictated by clinical findings; [4]parent group, family/sib, financial, and behavioral issues as discussed in the preface; [5]including developmental monitoring and motor/speech therapy.

Tuberous Sclerosis

Preventive medical checklist (6+ yrs)

Patient		Birth Date / /		Number	

Pediatric	Screen	Evaluate		Refer/Counsel	
8 years / / *Dentist* ❑		Puberty Heart Skin, limbs	❑ ❑ ❑	School options Developmental pediatrics Genetics	❑ ❑ ❑
10 years / /	Hearing, vision[2] ❑ Urinalysis, BP ❑	School progress Puberty Heart Skin, limbs	❑ ❑ ❑ ❑	Neurology[3] Ophthalmology[3]	❑ ❑
12 years / / *Td[1], MMR, Var* ❑ *CBC* ❑ *Dentist* ❑ *Scoliosis* ❑ *Cholesterol* ❑		Puberty Heart Skin, limbs	❑ ❑ ❑	Family support[4] Developmental pediatrics Genetics	❑ ❑ ❑
14 years / / *CBC* ❑ *Dentist* ❑ *Cholesterol* ❑ *Breast CA* ❑ *Testicular CA* ❑	Hearing, vision[2] ❑	School progress Puberty Heart Skin, limbs	❑ ❑ ❑	Neurology[3] Ophthalmology[3]	❑ ❑
16 years / / *Td[1]* ❑ *CBC* ❑ *Cholesterol* ❑ *Sexual[5]* ❑ *Dentist* ❑	Renal sonogram[3] ❑	Puberty Heart Skin, limbs	❑ ❑ ❑	Vocational planning Developmental pediatrics Genetics	❑ ❑ ❑
18 years / / *CBC* ❑ *Sexual[5]* ❑ *Cholesterol* ❑ *Scoliosis* ❑	Hearing, vision[2] ❑ Urinalysis, BP ❑	School progress Heart Skin, limbs	❑ ❑ ❑	Vocational planning Neurology[3] Ophthalmology[3]	❑ ❑ ❑
20 years[6] / / *CBC* ❑ *Sexual[5]* ❑ *Cholesterol* ❑ *Dentist* ❑	Chest x-ray ❑ (females) Urinalysis, BP ❑ Renal sonogram[3] ❑	Heart Lung Skin, limbs Work, residence	❑ ❑ ❑ ❑	Family support[4] Neurology[3] Ophthalmology[3]	❑ ❑ ❑

Clinical concerns for Tuberous Sclerosis, ages 6+ years

Retinal hamartomas	Cardiac rhabdomyomas	Cognitive disability
Facial angiofibromas	Renal hamartomas, cysts	Seizures
Dental enamel pits	Cystic lung disease	Intracranial calcifications
Ungual fibromas	Limb overgrowth	Precocious puberty

Guidelines for prior ages should be undertaken *at the time of diagnosis*; Td, tetanus/diphtheria; MMR, measles–mumps–rubella; Var, varicella; BP blood pressure; [1]alternative timing; [2]by practitioner; [3]as dictated by clinical findings; [4]parent group, family/sib, financial, and behavioral issues as discussed in the preface; [5]birth control, STD screening if sexually active; [6]repeat every decade.

Part V

Management of craniofacial syndromes

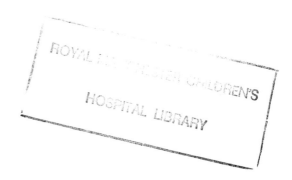

14

Craniosynostosis syndromes

Premature fusion of the cranial sutures occurs as a primary event in more than 70 craniosynostosis syndromes (Gorlin et al., 1990, p. 520; Wilkie & Wall, 1996; Jones, 1997, pp. 412–430). Craniosynostosis also occurs as a secondary or occasional event in conditions such as rickets or thalassemia, resulting in an aggregate frequency of 0.4–0.6 per 1000 births (Gorlin et al., p. 520). Preventive care is particularly important in the craniosynostosis syndromes, since altered cranial growth can have a severe impact on cognitive, visual, and auditory functions. Patients with fused cranial sutures share many problems with impact on surgical and preventive management regardless of their specific syndrome diagnosis. For this reason, a common craniosynostosis checklist is provided in this chapter that can be used for the Saethre–Chotzen, Apert, Crouzon, Pfeiffer, and Carpenter syndromes. The craniosynostosis checklist can also be used for less common disorders if their unique features are added to the complications table (part 1) and checklist pages (parts 2–4).

Patients with significant cranial asymmetry (plagiocephaly) and suspected synostosis should be promptly referred to a craniofacial surgery team, since early treatment may avoid the need for surgery or avoid severe complications. Standards for the evaluation and treatment of craniofacial malformations have been developed by the American Cleft Palate–Craniofacial Association (1993).

Cohen (1975, 1979, 1995) emphasized the fundamental principle that it is the pattern of accessory malformations, *not* the affected sutures, that allows differentiation among the craniosynostosis syndromes (Table 14.1). For example, patients with the Apert, Pfeiffer, or Crouzon syndrome may have premature synostosis of the coronal sutures, but the digital syndactyly (Apert), broad thumbs (Pfeiffer), or normal hand findings (Crouzon) guide the diagnosis (Table 14.1). Families with craniosynostosis syndromes often exhibit variable expressivity with one or multiple sutures affected (Cohen, 1975, 1979, 1995). When several sutures are fused, patients present with the severe Kleeblattschädel or clover-leaf skull anomaly.

Despite their clinical delineation as discrete syndromes, molecular analysis

Table 14.1 Craniosynostosis syndromes

Syndrome	Incidence	Inheritance	Accessory findings
Antley–Bixler	10–20 cases	AR	Midface hypoplasia, radiohumeral synostosis, heart a., genital a.
Apert	1 in 100,000 live births	AD	Midface hypoplasia, syndactyly
Baller–Gerold	10–20 cases	AR	Radial ray a., imperforate anus
Carpenter	~50 cases	AR	Preaxial polydactyly, obesity, short stature, mental deficiency
Crouzon	1 in 25,000 live births	AD	Ocular proptosis, shallow orbits
Jackson–Weiss	~100 cases	AD	Short first metatarsal bones
Pfeiffer	~100 cases	AD	Broad thumbs and toes, syndactyly
Saethre–Chotzen	>1 in 25,000 live births	AD	Facial asymmetry, ptosis, brachydactyly, syndactyly

Note:
AD, autosomal dominant; AR, autosomal recessive; a., anomalies.

indicates that seemingly different craniosynostosis phenotypes may be caused by mutations in the same gene. Mutations in the fibroblast growth factor receptor 2 (FGFR2) gene have been described in Apert, Crouzon, Jackson–Weiss, and Pfeiffer syndromes (Gorry et al., 1995; Wilkie & Wall, 1996; De Moerlooze & Dickson, 1997). In some instances, identical FGFR2 mutations are found in phenotypically different syndromes (Park et al., 1995). Variable expressivity or second-site mutations are postulated to explain why the same FGFR2 gene mutation produces limb anomalies in one patient but not in another (Gorry et al., 1995; Park et al., 1995).

Less common syndromes

Antley–Bixler syndrome

Antley–Bixler syndrome is a multiple-system disorder involving craniosynostosis, limb anomalies, urogenital anomalies, and congenital cardiac defects (Antley & Bixler, 1975). Craniofacial anomalies are often quite severe due to synostosis of the coronal and lambdoidal sutures (Gorlin et al., 1990, pp. 533–4; Poddevin et al., 1995; Jones, 1997, pp. 428–9), with a large anterior fontanelle, frontal bossing, midface hypoplasia, choanal atresia, and shallow nasal bridge produce a distinctive facies with a high incidence of respiratory obstruction. The skeleton is abnormal, with thin, gracile bones, frequent fractures, bowing of the limbs, deformed chest cage, narrow pelvis, vertebral anomalies, and congenital hip dislocations.

Urogenital anomalies may include renal aplasia/duplication, ureteral obstruction, vaginal atresia, and fused labia minor. Other anomalies include radiohumeral synostosis, imperforate anus, cardiac defects, and lumbar meningomyelocele (Gorlin et al., 1990, p. 534). LeHeup et al. (1995) reported two patients with severe renal and anal anomalies. Respiratory obstruction often leads to death during infancy.

Preventive management will include multidisciplinary craniofacial assessment with definition of airway function. Otolaryngology, maxillofacial surgery, plastic surgery, and neurosurgery evaluations are important for the treatment of possible craniosynostosis, choanal atresia, and airway compromise. Assessment of thoracic morphology may be useful in aiding respiratory function. Screening for congenital dislocation of the hips, skeletal radiographic survey, and orthopedic evaluation should also be considered during infancy. Additional neonatal evaluations should include echocardiography, renal ultrasound, and examination of the genital and perineal areas for anomalies. Apnea is the usual cause of death, so tracheostomy and apnea monitoring may be needed if home care can be achieved. The long-term prognosis is not established, but the many complications warrant early intervention and nutrition services.

Apert syndrome

Apert syndrome consists of craniosynostosis and syndactyly of the hands and feet (Table 14.1). It is an autosomal dominant disorder produced by mutations in the fibroblast growth factor receptor 2 gene. Premature fusion of the coronal sutures and the absence of true sagittal suture formation cause a deformed cranium with mid-face hypoplasia. Upward growth of the cranium produces a "tower skull" (acrocephaly), and there is midface hypoplasia due to malformation of the sphenoid bones and the cranial base (Fig. 14.1, color plate). Infants have a huge fontanelle, extending from the lower forehead to the occiput. The nasal bridge is depressed and the nasal septum may be deviated. Stenosis or atresia of the posterior choanae may occur and produce respiratory distress or cor pulmonale in the young child. Palatal anomalies (cleft soft palate, highly arched palate) together with maxillary retrusion and prognathism cause dental misalignment (Gorlin et al., 1990, pp. 520–4; Jones, 1997, pp. 418–19). Dental eruption may also be delayed.

Patients with Apert syndrome are at risk of upper and lower airway obstruction (Cohen & Kreiborg, 1992). Upper airway compromise is caused by reduced oro- and nasopharyngeal dimensions, causing symptoms of obstructive sleep apnea and cor pulmonale. Moore (1993) reported that upper airway obstruction is more common in Crouzon and Pfeiffer syndromes than in Apert syndrome; surgical treatment including uvulopalatopharyngoplasty, palatal splits, or adenotonsillectomy may be considered for symptomatic patients. Lower airway obstruction can result from tracheal stenosis and lack of tracheal distensibility, causing difficulty in clearing secretions and possible damage from tracheal suctioning (Cohen & Kreiborg, 1992). Cervical spine fusions occur in 68 percent of patients with Apert syndrome, involving the lower spine (C5–C6) rather than the upper cervical spine fusions as seen in Crouzon syndrome (Kreiborg et al., 1992). Because cervical vertebral fusions may further compromise the upper airway, cervical spine films are recommended before attempting intubation for general anesthesia (Kreiborg et al., 1992).

Preventive management of Apert syndrome should focus on early risks for respiratory obstruction and cervical injury because of craniocervical malformations (craniosynostosis checklist, parts 2–4). Management is ideally coordinated with a multidisciplinary craniofacial surgery team if it is available; plastic surgery, otolaryngology, maxillofacial surgery, and neurosurgery should evaluate craniofacial morphology and airway function. Patients with excessively noisy breathing in association with poor weight gain deserve urgent evaluation. Radiography of the cervical spine should be part of the initial evaluation, and surveillance for hydrocephalus and signs of increased intracranial pressure is important pre- and postoperatively (Murovic et al., 1993; Gosain et al., 1996b). Impaired absorption of cerebrospinal fluid was postulated to explain the 23 percent of patients who experienced hydrocephalus after operation, and this complication was associated with intellectual deficit (average IQ 72.5; Murovic et al., 1993).

Management during and after craniofacial surgery should include the coordination of brain imaging and neurosensory studies with careful observation of feeding and growth. Cohen & Kreiborg (1993) reported a unique growth pattern for patients with Apert syndrome, consisting of increased size of all parameters at birth, deceleration of linear growth during childhood, and deceleration of the head circumference from above the 50th centile at birth to within or at −2 standard deviations in young adulthood. Otitis media and congenital fixation of the stapedial foot plate are common causes of hearing loss, so auditory evoked response and audiology monitoring are required. Regular eye examinations are needed for the detection of optic atrophy or strabismus, and early intervention is important in view of the risks of neurosensory and cognitive problems. In addition to congenital cervical spine fusion described above, there is progressive calcification and fusion of the cervical spine and limb bones in Apert syndrome (Gorlin et al., 1990, pp. 520–4). Periodic evaluation for symptoms of cervical spine compression (neck pain, torticollis, altered gait or urination) is also recommended. The crowded teeth produced by maxillary hypoplasia require early and regular dental care.

Baller–Gerold syndrome

Baller–Gerold syndrome is an autosomal recessive condition with variable craniosynostosis, growth deficiency, malformed ears, cleft or highly arched palate, radial ray reduction defects, cardiac anomalies, renal anomalies, and imperforate anus (Gorlin et al., 1990, pp. 535–6; Jones, 1997; pp. 430–1). Craniosynostosis often involves a single suture and is usually milder than encountered in Apert or Crouzon syndrome. Brain anomalies such as microgyria have occurred, and mental deficiency is described in the majority of cases. Appropriate preventive management requires an extensive diagnostic evaluation including radiographic survey of the cranium and appendicular skeleton, echocardiography and renal sonography for the evaluation of internal anomalies, and examination of the limbs and perineal area to rule out radial and anal anomalies. Sudden infant death has been described, so evaluation of the upper airway and respiratory function is important in the neonatal and infantile periods (Gorlin et al., 1990, pp. 535–6).

Carpenter syndrome

Although first described in 1903 by Carpenter, Temtamy (1966) presented a comprehensive review that delineated the Carpenter syndrome. The chief findings are craniosynostosis, preaxial polydactyly of the feet, short stature, obesity, and mental deficiency (Robinson et al., 1985; Gorlin et al., 1990, pp. 531–3). Optic anomalies (microcornea, corneal opacity, optic atropy) and cardiac anomalies (septal defects, tetralogy of Fallot, transposition of the great arteries) are common. Occasional patients have had urinary tract (hydronephrosis, hydroureter) or genital anomalies (cryptorchidism), and inguinal hernias have occurred. Mental deficiency and brain anomalies are frequent, but some patients have had normal intelligence (Frias et al., 1978). External ear anomalies may be associated with conductive hearing loss (Hall et al., 1995).

Preventive management of Carpenter syndrome should begin with multidisciplinary evaluation for craniofacial surgery, including imaging studies of the brain, heart, and renal system. Initial and periodic neurosensory assessments should be conducted, along with early intervention services and psychosocial counseling appropriate for children with disabilities. Periodic urinalyses should be performed because of the increased risk of urinary tract anomalies.

Crouzon syndrome

A syndrome of craniosynostosis, maxillary hypoplasia, and shallow orbits with proptosis was described by Crouzon in 1912 (Gorlin et al., 1990, pp. 524–6). Cohen estimated an incidence of 1 per 25,000 births for Crouzon syndrome (Cohen & Kreiborg, 1992). The disorder exhibits autosomal dominant inheritance, with 44–67 percent of cases representing new mutations (Gorlin et al.,1990, pp. 524–6). Mutations have been defined in the fibroblast growth factor receptor 2 gene, but identical mutations may cause a phenotype of Crouzon syndrome in one patient and Pfeiffer syndrome in another (Gorry et al., 1995). Preference for cysteine substitutions in a particular fibroblast growth factor receptor 2 gene region has been defined (Steinberger et al., 1995). The mechanisms by which altered fibroblast growth factor receptors produce variable patterns of craniosynostosis remain to be defined.

Coronal, sagittal, and lambdoidal synostoses are most common, occurring in 75 percent of cases (Gorlin et al., 1990, pp. 524–6). Many patients will experience airway obstruction during infancy, and may require tracheostomy (Sirotnak et al., 1995). The midface hypoplasia produces shallow orbits with a risk of exposure keratitis to the protruding eyes. Midface hypoplasia contributes to the development of highly arched or cleft palate (3 percent of patients), and probably explains the frequency of conductive hearing deficit (55 percent), mouth breathing (32 percent), and tooth crowding. Deviation of the nasal septum is found in 33 percent of patients (Gorlin et al., 1990, pp. 524–6). There may be jugular foramina synostosis (Martinez-Perez et al., 1996). Cervical vertebral fusions account for 83 percent of cervical spine anomalies, with fusion of the C2–C3 vertebrae occurring in about 20 percent of patients (Anderson et al., 1997). The limbs are usually not affected, but radioulnar synostosis has been described.

Preventive management is outlined on the craniosynostosis checklist, parts 2–4, with attention to proptosis and airway obstruction that may result from midface hypoplasia. Early assessment of craniosynostosis, ear, and eye abnormalities should be coordinated through a craniofacial surgical team, and all families should have genetic evaluation and counseling. Surveillance for airway obstruction, sleep apnea, cervical spine anomalies (particularly before anesthesia), exposure keratitis due to proptosis, and neurosensory deficits is particularly important. Although many patients have normal cognitive outcomes, evaluation of developmental progress should be performed during early pediatric visits and appropriate early intervention services provided for those patients with delay.

Jackson–Weiss syndrome

Jackson–Weiss syndrome can be described as the facies of Crouzon syndrome with foot anomalies (Jackson et al., 1976). There is phenotypic overlap with Pfeiffer and Saethre–Chotzen syndromes, and all three autosomal dominant syndromes have been attributed to mutations in the fibroblast growth factor receptor 2 gene (Gorry et al., 1995). The foot abnormalities include broad great toes, syndactyly of toes 2 and 3, and fusions of the metatarsal bones (Gorlin et al., 1990, pp. 529–30). The midface hypoplasia causes proptosis, and there may be hypertelorism.

Preventive management of patients with Jackson–Weiss syndrome will be similar to that of patients with Crouzon syndrome described below, with screening for ophthalmologic or auditory problems and craniofacial evaluation for reconstructive and dental problems. Most reported families exhibit normal intelligence with variable expression of the limb anomalies (e.g., Stankovic et al., 1994). Precautions concerning airway management and postoperative hydrocephalus will be similar to those for Apert and Crouzon syndromes, but early intervention services will usually not be needed.

Pfeiffer syndrome

The Pfeiffer syndrome of craniosynostosis with broad thumbs and broad great toes was described in 1964 (Pfeiffer, 1969). It is an autosomal dominant condition, with major findings including maxillary hypoplasia, mandibular prognathism, ocular proptosis, short fingers and toes, fused cervical and lumbar vertebrae, and occasional mental deficiency (Cohen, 1993; Moore et al., 1995a). Cervical spine fusion was common and complex in one series of patients with Pfeiffer syndrome (Moore et al., 1995b), and sacrococcygeal anomalies also occurred. Less common complications include optic nerve hypoplasia, hearing deficits, supernumerary teeth, and other skeletal anomalies (club feet, radioulnar or radiohumeral synostosis, short humeri). Jones et al. (1993) reported an atypical coloboma in a patient with Pfeiffer syndrome. Bilateral coronal synostosis with tower skull is most common, but unilateral synostosis with cranial asymmetry can occur. Multiple sutural fusion producing the clover leaf skull anomaly has also been described. Some patients with Pfeiffer syndrome have severe ocular proptosis, and these patients often have an early death (Cohen, 1993).

Preventive management should begin in the neonatal period with thorough craniofacial and skeletal evaluations. Brain MRI scanning and skeletal radiographic survey should be considered based on physical findings. Ophthalmologic referral and auditory evoked response studies will be needed during infancy to rule out optic atrophy, strabismus, and hearing loss. If motor milestones are delayed, referral for early intervention should be considered. As with other craniosynostosis syndromes, regular dental care is needed for the evaluation of tooth crowding and supernumerary teeth. Evaluation of neck mobility and cervical spine fusion should be performed before surgery, and the potential for lumbar vertebral fusion warrants surveillance for back pain or gait disturbances that might indicate cord compression (Saldino et al., 1972).

Saethre–Chotzen syndrome

Recognized by Saethre in 1931 and Chotzen in 1932, Saethre–Chotzen syndrome has a very broad pattern of malformations affecting the craniofacies and skeleton (Gorlin et al., 1990, pp. 527–8; Reardon & Winter, 1994). Facial asymmetry with unilateral ptosis and partial cutaneous syndactyly are common features of the syndrome.

Saethre–Chotzen syndrome is thought to be more common than Crouzon syndrome, which has an estimated incidence of 1 in 25,000 births (Jones, 1997, pp. 412–13). The disorder exhibits autosomal dominant inheritance and has been mapped to a locus at chromosome band 7p21.2 (Rose et al., 1994). The differential diagnosis of craniosynostosis syndromes is summarized in Table 14.1. Craniofacial findings such as asymmetry and low hairline, and skeletal anomalies such as syndactyly, brachydactyly, and clinodactyly of the fifth fingers are distinguishing features of Saethre–Chotzen syndrome.

The diagnosis of Saethre–Chotzen syndrome is based on clinical examination and radiographic findings. Cranial radiographs and imaging studies will determine the extent and distribution of craniosynostosis, and reveal unusual complications such as hydrocephalus. Examination of the extremities will discover brachydactyly or partial syndactyly that distinguish the disorder from Apert, Crouzon, or Pfeiffer syndrome (Table 14.1).

Because of the multiple craniofacial problems in patients with Saethre–Chotzen syndrome, multidisciplinary evaluation by a craniofacial surgery team is optimal for medical management and counseling. The low risk for mental deficiency warrants optimistic counseling, and a good cosmetic outcome can be anticipated with modern surgery. Pediatric involvement is important to ensure the monitoring of hearing and vision (see below).

Normal parents of children with Saethre–Chotzen syndrome will have a minimal recurrence risk, although germinal mosaicism has been described (Gorlin et al., 1990, pp. 524–6). Affected patients will have a 50 percent recurrence risk, and gene testing is not yet routinely available for prenatal diagnosis. All families should be referred for genetic counseling, which will attend to possible guilt on the part of parents who transmit their disease. Ideally, genetic and psychosocial counseling will be included in the services of a multidisciplinary craniofacial surgery team. An optimistic outlook is usually warranted, since enormous improvements in craniofacial surgery have produced dramatic cosmetic benefits for most patients. Families will require support and counseling appropriate for major surgery and hospitalization.

Major complications of Saethre–Chotzen syndrome

Craniosynostosis is more variable in Saethre–Chotzen syndrome, and its onset may be delayed until later life. Asymmetric involvement is common, and fusion of the metopic suture may produce trigonocephaly (Cohen, 1975). Other anomalies include a low frontal hairline, ptosis or strabismus of the eyes, blepharophimosis, low-set ears with hearing deficit, highly arched or cleft palate, and dental anomalies including tooth crowding, enamel hypoplasia, or malocclusion. Mental deficiency and epilepsy have been reported, but mental development is usually normal.

Skeletal abnormalities may include syndactyly, asymmetry of the fingers, broad great toes and thumbs, and defects of the cervical or lumbar spine. Anomalies of other systems include short stature, cardiac defects, congenital adrenal hyperplasia, renal anomalies, and cryptorchidism. The degree and extent of sutural fusion will determine whether the orbits, optic nerves, conjunctiva, or auditory nerves are compressed, with risk of vision and hearing loss (Ensink et al., 1996).

As with other craniosynostosis syndromes, the first step in preventive care for Saethre–Chotzen syndrome is to define the nature and extent of craniofacial anomalies (craniosynostosis checklist, parts 2–4). Brain imaging and skull radiographs are recommended for all patients for whom craniosynostosis is suspected. Significant anomalies mandate the coordinated involvement of neurosurgery, plastic surgery, and otolaryngology specialists immediately after the craniosynostosis is documented. Many children may benefit from helmets to correct cranial asymmetry if management is initiated during infancy. Regular evaluation of hearing and vision, with early audiology and ophthalmology assessments, is required. Inspection of the eyes for irritation due to protrusion and exposure may prevent damaging keratitis. Protective drops and irrigation may be required. If cervical spine anomalies are detected, then lateral radiographs for atlanto-axial instability should be obtained in the 3–5-year-old age range.

Preventive management consists of multidisciplinary craniofacial and skeletal evaluation in the newborn period, with consideration of brain MRI scan and skeletal radiographic survey. Early and periodic audiology screening is worthwhile, and ophthalmology referral will be needed during infancy to rule out strabismus. Evaluation of the cervical spine before anesthesia and regular dental care are also recommended. Later preventive management should include the monitoring of hearing and vision, evaluation for symptoms of cervical spine compression or instability, and regular dental and ophthalmology evaluations. Many patients have had progressive joint fusions and restrictions, so range-of-motion evaluation should be part of regular examinations.

Preventive Management of Craniosynostosis syndromes

Clinical diagnosis: Craniosynostosis alone (Crouzon syndrome) or with syndactyly (Apert syndrome), broad thumbs (Pfeiffer syndrome), digital anomalies (Saethre–Chotzen syndrome), or polydactyly (Carpenter syndrome); many patients have a shallow midface with ocular proptosis. The sutural involvement is not specific for a particular syndrome.

Laboratory diagnosis: Several craniosynostosis syndromes have been associated with mutations in the fibroblast growth factor-2 gene, but DNA diagnosis is not routinely available.

Genetics: Apert, Crouzon, Saethre-Chotzen, and Pfeiffer syndrome are autosomal dominant, while Carpenter syndrome is autosomal recessive.

Key management issues: Multidisciplinary management by a craniofacial surgery team; monitoring for hydrocephalus, airway obstruction, sleep apnea, and growth failure; screening of hearing, vision, and dental status; protection from exposure keratitis in protruding eyes; screening for cervical spine fusion/instability; range-of-motion evaluations for joint fusions and restrictions; orthopedic, cardiac, and urogenital assessment in some patients, early intervention for potential neurosensory and cognitive problems.

Growth Charts: None available – growth may be impacted by airway obstruction.

Parent groups: Apert Support and Informaton network, P. O. Box 1184, Fair Oaks CA, 95628, (650) 961-1092, apertnet@ix.netcom.com; Let's Face It, P.O. Box 29972, Bellingham WA, 98228-1972, (360) 676-7325, letsfaceit@faceit.org, http://www.faceit.org/~faceit/

Basis for management recommendations: Derived from the complications below as documented by Reardon & Winter (1994).

Summary of clinical concerns

General	Learning	Cognitive disability, particularly in those with hydrocephalus
	Behavior	Psychosis (rare)
	Growth	Short stature
Facial	Face	Midface hypoplasia, flat forehead, beaked nose
	Eye	Proptosis with corneal injury, strabismus, lacrimal duct anomalies, ptosis, blepharophimosis, optic atrophy
	Ear	Otitis media, congenital fixation of the stapedial foot plate (Apert syndrome)
	Nose	Upper respiratory obstruction (deviation of nasal septum, shallow nasal bridge, stenosis or atresia of the posterior choanae)
	Mouth	Mouth breathing, high or cleft palate, dental anomalies (malocclusion, crowded teeth, supernumerary teeth, enamel hypoplasia)
Surface	Epidermal	Acne vulgaris in Apert, acanthosis nigricans in Crouzon
Skeletal	Cranial	Craniosynostosis of coronal, metopic, lamdoidal sutures, huge fontanelle acrocephaly, brachycephaly
	Axial	Cervical vertebral fusion, instability. Cervical spine fusions occur in 68% of patients with Apert syndrome
	Limbs	Syndactyly of digits 2–5 (Apert), syndactyly fingers 2 and 3 with broad thumbs (Saethre-Chotzen), broad thumbs (Pfeiffer), polydactyly (Carpenter), limited joint movement due to synostosis
Internal	Pulmonary	Respiratory obstruction, hypoxemia
	Circulatory	Cardiac anomalies (septal defects, tetralogy of Fallot, transposition of the great arteries)
	Excretory	Renal anomalies (hydronephrosis, hydroureter)
	Genital	Cryptorchidism
Neural	CNS	Hydrocephalus, seizures, sleep apnea
	Sensory	Conductive hearing loss, visual deficits

Bold: frequency > 20%

Key references

Cohen, M. M., Jr. (1995). *American Journal of Medical Genetics* 56:334–9.
Reardon, W. & Winter, R. M. (1994). *Journal of Medical Genetics* 31:393–6.

Craniosynostosis syndromes

Preventive medical checklist (0–1yr)

Patient   **Birth Date** / /   **Number**

Pediatric	Screen		Evaluate		Refer/Counsel	
Neonatal / / *Newborn screen* ❏ *HB* ❏	Hearing, vision[2] Skull x-rays Head sonogram	❏ ❏ ❏	Craniosynostosis Airway, apnea Palate Limbs	❏ ❏ ❏ ❏	Genetic evaluation Craniofacial team	❏ ❏
1 month / /	Head size Head MRI[3] Hearing, vision[2]	❏ ❏ ❏	Airway, apnea Head symmetry Eyes	❏ ❏ ❏	Family support[4] Careful anesthesia	❏ ❏
2 months / / *HB[1]* ❏ *Hib* ❏ *DTaP, IPV* ❏ *RV* ❏	Growth Head size Hearing, vision[2]	❏ ❏ ❏	Head symmetry Eyes Limbs	❏ ❏ ❏	Early intervention[3,5] Genetic counseling	❏ ❏
4 months / / *HB[1]* ❏ *Hib* ❏ *DTaP/IPV* ❏ *RV* ❏	Head size Hearing, vision[2]	❏ ❏	Airway, apnea Head symmetry Eyes Limbs	❏ ❏ ❏ ❏	Early intervention[3,5] Genetics	❏ ❏
6 months / / *Hib* ❏ *IPV[1]* ❏ *DTaP* ❏ *RV* ❏	Growth Head size Hearing, vision[2] Cervical spine[3]	❏ ❏ ❏ ❏	Head symmetry Eyes Limbs	❏ ❏ ❏	Family support[4] Craniofacial team	❏ ❏
9 months / / *IPV[1]* ❏	Head size Hearing, vision[2]	❏ ❏	Head symmetry Eyes Limbs	❏ ❏ ❏		
1 year / / *HB* ❏ *Hib[1]* ❏ *IPV[1]* ❏ *MMR[1]* ❏ *Var[1]* ❏	Growth Head size Hearing, vision[2] Audiology Cervical spine[3]	❏ ❏ ❏ ❏ ❏	Head symmetry Eyes Limbs Sleep apnea	❏ ❏ ❏ ❏	Family support[4] Early intervention[3,5] Genetics Craniofacial team Sleep study[3]	❏ ❏ ❏ ❏ ❏

Clinical concerns for Craniosynostosis syndromes, ages 0–1 year

Craniosynostosis	Cervical spine fusion	Learning differences
Hearing, vision loss	Exposure keratitis	Hydrocephalus
Deviated nasal septum	Cardiac anomalies	Headaches, seizures
Proptosis, optic atrophy	Limb, urogenital anomalies	Airway obstruction, sleep apnea

Guidelines for the neonatal period should be undertaken *at whatever age* the diagnosis is made; the craniofacial team should include ophthalmology, ENT, plastic, and neurosurgery; DTaP, acellular DTP; IPV, inactivated poliovirus (oral polio also used); RV, rotavirus; MMR, measles–mumps–rubella; Var, varicella; [1]alternative timing; [2]by practitioner; [3]as dictated by clinical findings; [4]parent group, family/sib, financial, and behavioral issues as discussed in the preface; [5]including developmental monitoring and motor/speech therapy.

Craniosynostosis syndromes

Preventive medical checklist (15m–6yrs)

Patient   **Birth Date** / /   **Number**

Pediatric	Screen		Evaluate		Refer/Counsel	
15 months / / *Hib[1]* ☐ *MMR[1]* ☐ *DTaP, IPV[1]* ☐ *Varicella[1]* ☐	Head size Hearing, vision[2]	☐ ☐	Head symmetry Eyes Limbs	☐ ☐ ☐	Family support[3] Early intervention[4]	☐ ☐
18 months / / *DTaP, IPV[1]* ☐ *Varicella[1]* ☐ *Influenza[3]* ☐	Head size Hearing, vision[2] Cervical spine[3]	☐ ☐ ☐	Head symmetry Eyes Limbs	☐ ☐ ☐	Careful anesthesia	☐
2 years / / *Influenza[3]* ☐ *Pneumovax[3]* ☐ *Dentist* ☐	Head size Hearing, vision[2] Audiology Cervical spine[3]	☐ ☐ ☐ ☐	Head symmetry Eyes Limbs	☐ ☐ ☐	Family support[4] Genetics Craniofacial team	☐ ☐ ☐
3 years / / *Influenza[3]* ☐ *Pneumovax[3]* ☐ *Dentist* ☐	Growth Head size Hearing, vision[2] Audiology	☐ ☐ ☐ ☐	Head symmetry Eyes Limbs Sleep apnea	☐ ☐ ☐ ☐	Family support[4] Preschool transition[5] Craniofacial team Sleep study[3]	☐ ☐ ☐ ☐
4 years / / *Influenza[3]* ☐ *Pneumovax[3]* ☐ *Dentist* ☐	Growth Hearing, vision[2]	☐ ☐	Head symmetry Eyes Limbs	☐ ☐ ☐	Family support[3] Preschool program[3,5] Genetics Craniofacial team	☐ ☐ ☐ ☐
5 years / / *DTaP, IPV[1]* ☐ *MMR[1]* ☐	Hearing, vision[2] Audiology	☐ ☐	Airway Sleep apnea	☐ ☐	School transition[3,5] Craniofacial team Genetics	☐ ☐ ☐
6 years / / *DTaP, IPV[1]* ☐ *MMR[1]* ☐ *Dentist* ☐	Growth Hearing, vision[2] Cervical spine[3]	☐ ☐ ☐	School progress Head symmetry Eyes Limbs	☐ ☐ ☐ ☐	Family support[4] Genetics Craniofacial team Careful anesthesia	☐ ☐ ☐ ☐

Clinical concerns for Craniosynostosis syndromes, ages 1–6 years

Craniosynostosis	Cervical spine fusion	Learning differences
Hearing, vision loss	Exposure keratitis	Hydrocephalus
Deviated nasal septum	Cardiac anomalies	Headaches, seizures
Proptosis, optic atrophy	Limb, urogenital anomalies	

Guidelines for prior ages should be undertaken *at the time of diagnosis*; the craniofacial team should include ophthalmology, ENT, plastic, and neurosurgery; DTaP, acellular DTP; IPV, inactivated poliovirus (oral polio also used); MMR, measles–mumps–rubella; [1]alternative timing; [2]by practitioner; [3]as dictated by clinical findings; [4]parent group, family/sib, financial, and behavioral issues as discussed in the preface; [5]including developmental monitoring and motor/speech therapy.

Craniosynostosis syndromes

Preventive medical checklist (6+ yrs)

Patient   **Birth Date** / /   **Number**

Pediatric	Screen	Evaluate		Refer/Counsel	
8 years / / *Dentist* ❑	Hearing, vision[2] ❑	Airway Sleep apnea	❑ ❑	School options Sleep study[3] Genetics	❑ ❑ ❑
10 years / /	Growth ❑ Hearing, vision[2] ❑	School progress Head symmetry Eyes Limbs	❑ ❑ ❑ ❑	Craniofacial team	❑
12 years / / *Td[1], MMR, Var* ❑ *CBC* ❑ *Dentist* ❑ *Scoliosis* ❑ *Cholesterol* ❑	Hearing, vision[2] ❑	Airway Sleep apnea	❑ ❑	Family support[4] School options Genetics Careful anesthesia	❑ ❑ ❑ ❑
14 years / / *CBC* ❑ *Dentist* ❑ *Cholesterol* ❑ *Breast CA* ❑ *Testicular CA* ❑	Growth ❑ Hearing, vision[2] ❑	School progress Head symmetry Eyes Limbs	❑ ❑ ❑ ❑	Craniofacial team	❑
16 years / / *Td[1]* ❑ *CBC* ❑ *Cholesterol* ❑ *Sexual[5]* ❑ *Dentist* ❑	Hearing, vision[2] ❑	Airway Sleep apnea	❑ ❑	Vocational planning Genetics	❑ ❑
18 years / / *CBC* ❑ *Sexual[5]* ❑ *Cholesterol* ❑ *Scoliosis* ❑	Hearing, vision[2] ❑	School progress Head symmetry Eyes Limbs	❑ ❑ ❑ ❑	Vocational planning Craniofacial team	❑ ❑
20 years[6] / / *CBC* ❑ *Sexual[5]* ❑ *Cholesterol* ❑ *Dentist* ❑	Hearing, vision[2] ❑	Head symmetry Eyes, limbs Sleep apnea	❑ ❑ ❑	Family support[4] Craniofacial team Sleep study[3]	❑ ❑ ❑

Clinical concerns for Craniosynostosis syndromes, ages 6+ years

Craniosynostosis	Airway obstruction	Learning differences
Hearing, vision loss	Sleep apnea	Hydrocephalus
Deviated nasal septum	Exposure keratitis	Headaches
Proptosis, optic atrophy	Limb anomalies	Seizures

Guidelines for prior ages should be undertaken *at the time of diagnosis*; the craniofacial team should include ophthalmology, ENT, plastic, and neurosurgery; Td, tetanus/diphtheria; MMR, measles–mumps–rubella; Var, varicella; [1]alternative timing; [2]by practitioner; [3]as dictated by clinical findings; [4]parent group, family/sib, financial, and behavioral issues as discussed in the preface; [5]birth control, STD screening if sexually active; [6]repeat every decade.

15

Branchial arch and face/limb syndromes

Branchial arch syndromes

Branchial arches are critical for the development of the lower portion of the crani-ofacies, the muscles of the pharynx and jaw, the cardiac conotruncal region, and the salivary, thymus, and parathyroid glands. In addition, branchial arch meso-derm merges with neural crest cells to form an ectomesenchyme that is important for the development of the cranial nerves. The embryonic derivatives of the bran-chial arches explain the anomalies seen in children with branchial arch syndromes: craniofacial anomalies of the mandible, maxilla, palate and ears; palatal, salivary gland, and pharyngeal muscle hypoplasias that cause oromotor dysfunction and feeding difficulties; and cranial nerve, optic, otic, and cardiac anomalies that include neurosensory and cognitive deficits. Preventive management is enor-mously important for children with branchial arch syndromes, since many of their feeding, neurosensory, and learning problems can be anticipated and treated.

Table 15.1 summarizes the clinical manifestations of several branchial arch syn-dromes. The Goldenhar syndrome–hemifacial microsomia spectrum is the most common, and will be discussed in detail after a review of other branchial arch syn-dromes.

Branchio-oculo-facial syndrome

Hall et al. (1983) first described an autosomal dominant syndrome consisting of hemangiomatous branchial clefts, eye anomalies, nasolacrimal duct obstruction, and on occasion limb or renal anomalies. The branchial clefts may appear as cysts, fistulas, hemangiomas, or cutis aplasia in the lateral neck region, and some patients have had upper lip clefts (Gorlin et al., 1990, pp. 728–9; Jones, 1997, pp. 246–7). Eye anomalies may be severe and include microphthalmia, cataracts, strabismus, colo-bomata of the irides or retinae, and eyelid anomalies resulting from nasolacrimal duct obstruction and lacrimal gland infection (dacryocystitis). The external ear anomalies may be associated with conductive hearing loss, a risk that is accentuated

Table 15.1 Branchial arch syndromes

Syndrome	Incidence	Heredity	Complications
Branchio-oculo-facial	∼20 cases	AD	Branchial cysts, eye a. (strabismus, cataracts, colobomata), ear a., cleft lip/palate, renal a.
Branchio-oto-renal (BOR)	1 in 40,000 live births	AD	Ear a., urinary tract a., branchial cysts and fistulas
Goldenhar	1 in 5600	MF	Hemifacial microsomia, cranial asymmetry, eye a. (epibulbar dermoids, lipoepidermoid cysts), micrognathia, cleft lip/palate, cardiac a., limb a., vertebral a., renal a.
Miller	∼20 cases	AD	Malar, mandibular, pharyngeal hypoplasia, eye a., hearing loss, postaxial limb a., cardiac and genital a.
Nager	∼40 cases	AR, AD	Malar, mandibular, pharyngeal hypoplasia, eye a., hearing loss, thumb and radial a., cardiac and renal a.
Townes–Brocks	∼30 cases	AD	External ear a., hearing loss, digital a., imperforate anus
Treacher–Collins	1 in 50,000 live births	AD	Malar, mandibular, pharyngeal hypoplasia, eye a. (colobomata, strabismus, amblyopia), hearing loss, airway obstruction.
Wildervanck	∼100 cases	?AD ?XLR	Klippel–Feil a., abducens palsy with Duane syndrome, hearing loss, facial asymmetry, facial palsy

Note:
MF, multifactorial; AD, autosomal dominant; AR, autosomal recessive; XLR, X-linked recessive inheritance; a., anomaly.

if cleft palate is present. Cystic kidneys and unilateral renal agenesis have been reported, with the broad spectrum of anomalies leading McCool & Weaver (1994) to suggest that branchio-oculo-facial syndrome may derive from a contiguous gene deletion.

Preventive management should include early ophthalmology referral with probing, massage, and/or surgery to ensure patency of the nasolacrimal ducts. Audiology screening later in infancy and monitoring of developmental progress are important because some patients have had mental disability. Although renal anomalies have been rare, initial renal ultrasound, periodic screening by urinalysis, and aggressive evaluation after urinary tract infections seems wise.

Branchio-oto-renal (BOR) syndrome

Melnick et al. (1976) reported a new type of branchial arch syndrome involving anomalies of the external ear including preauricular pits, hearing loss, branchial cysts, and renal anomalies. The condition is autosomal dominant with an estimated incidence of 1 in 40,000 births (Gorlin et al., 1990, pp. 657–9). Kumar et al. (1994) reported linkage to the long arm region of chromosome 8. The branchial cysts or fistulas occur in 60 percent of patients, and may present with draining fluid or infection on the lower cervical region (Chitayat et al., 1992; Chen et al., 1995). Anomalies of the external, middle, and internal ear have been described, with 75 percent of patients having hearing loss, of which 30 percent is conductive, 20 percent sensorineural, and 50 percent mixed (Gorlin et al., 1990, pp. 657–9; Millman et al., 1995). Symptomatic urinary tract anomalies occur in about 10 percent of patients, but some studies revealed 75–100 percent of patients to have structural anomalies and 33 percent to have functional anomalies (Wildervanck, 1962; Rowley, 1969; Leung & Robson, 1992). Renal anomalies may include lethal renal agenesis with Potter sequence and pulmonary hypoplasia (Chitayat et al., 1992).

Preventive management for the condition should include early auditory evoked response assessment of hearing with imaging of the middle and inner ear if sensorineural hearing loss is documented. Although the hearing loss is not progressive in most instances, periodic audiologic assessment is warranted during childhood and adolescence. The urinary tract anatomy should be evaluated by an early renal ultrasound, with periodic urinalyses, blood urea nitrogen, and creatinine studies to assess for infection, proteinuria, and evidence of glomerular lesions. Intravenous pyelogram and voiding cystourethrogram studies should be considered in patients with urinary tract infections, since urinary tract anomalies may be subtle.

Miller syndrome

Patients with Miller syndrome bear facial resemblance to those with Treacher Collins syndrome, but have postaxial limb defects. The face is similar to that in Treacher Collins or Nager syndrome, but ectropion of the lower lids is often more striking. Inheritance is autosomal dominant, and the occurrence of thumb anomalies together with ulnar defects re-emphasizes the question of overlap among Miller, Nager, and Treacher Collins syndromes (Preis et al., 1995; Table 15.1). Preventive management involves multidisciplinary craniofacial assessment, evaluation for airway obstruction, screening for vision or hearing loss, and monitoring of nutrition and growth so that feeding problems can be addressed. Palatal agenesis has been reported as a feature of Nager and Miller syndromes (Jackson et al., 1989). Conical teeth are reported, so dental evaluation is important (Gorlin et al., 1990, pp. 654–5). Less frequent cardiac (patent ductus arteriosus, ventricular septal defect) and genital anomalies (cryptorchidism, micropenis) should also be targeted during physical examination. The postaxial defects tend to be agenesis of a digit, but shortened radius and ulna or radioulnar synostosis have been reported.

Nager syndrome

Nager syndrome consists of abnormal thumbs in addition to mandibulofacial dysostosis reminiscent of that in Treacher Collins syndrome. Nager syndrome exhibits autosomal recessive rather than autosomal dominant inheritance expected for Treacher Collins syndrome. Delineation of the two syndromes is complicated, since vertical transmission of thumb anomalies and typical facial dysostosis is evident in some families (Bonthron et al., 1993). Molecular analysis should soon reveal whether thumb anomalies are an occasional manifestation of Treacher Collins syndrome or whether Nager syndrome exhibits genetic heterogeneity (Anonymous, 1996).

Micrognathia is often more severe in Nager syndrome, requiring multidisciplinary craniofacial management as outlined for Treacher Collins syndrome. Airway obstruction and feeding problems may be more acute than in Treacher Collins syndrome, and some patients have a Robin sequence with cleft palate or velopalatine insufficiency. The palatal anomalies and frequent laryngeal hypoplasia require even greater attention to speech, with the same annual screening for hearing and vision recommended for Treacher Collins syndrome (Meyerson & Nesbit, 1987). Early intervention services should be considered, but intelligence is usually normal. Cardiac and renal anomalies are sufficiently frequent to consider an echocardiogram and renal sonogram as part of the initial diagnostic evaluation. Children with more severe hand defects will need orthopedic and occupational therapy assessments. Radial aplasia, radioulnar synostosis, and limited extension of the elbows may occur (Gorlin et al., 1990, pp. 652–3).

Townes–Brocks syndrome

Townes & Brocks (1972) reported a syndrome consisting of external ear anomalies, limb anomalies, and imperforate anus. Inheritance is autosomal dominant, and two separate patients with coincident inversion and translocation suggest that the gene is located at chromosome band 16q12.1 (Serville et al., 1993). The ear anomalies range from overturned helices ("lop" ear) to microtia with preauricular tags. Sensorineural hearing loss is common (Rossmiller & Pasic, 1994), and the limb anomalies can include triphalangeal or hypoplastic thumbs, abnormal wrist bones, hypoplastic third toes, and cone-shaped epiphyses (Gorlin et al., 1990, pp. 661–2). Imperforate anus or anal stenosis may be present, and cardiac or urogenital anomalies are sometimes found (Kurnit et al., 1978). Preventive management should include early auditory evoked response and later audiologic monitoring, radiographic skeletal survey with particular attention to the preaxial regions of the upper limbs, and consideration of renal sonogram to document the urinary tract anatomy. Evaluation of the genitalia is important, since males have had hypospadias and cryptorchidism.

Treacher Collins syndrome

Treacher Collins syndrome was recognized in the 1800s, but named by the classic description of Treacher Collins (1960). The disorder is also referred to using the eponyms of Franceschetti & Klein (1949) or by the term coined in their article: mandibulofacial dysostosis (Dixon, 1995). It has an incidence of about 1 in 50,000 births, with over 400 cases reported (Jahrsdoerfer & Jacobson, 1995). The most distinctive clinical manifestations are flattened cheeks (malar hypoplasia) and notched eyelids, as indicated by the title of Treacher Collins' article. The frontal, malar, and mandibular bones are underdeveloped, with hypoplasia of the supraorbital ridges, zygomatic process, and mandibular condyles. Malformed external ears, down-slanting palpebral fissures, colobomata (clefts) of the eyelids and pupils, hypoplasia of the alae nasae, and choanal atresia are additional characteristics. Cognitive development is usually normal if hearing loss is anticipated and treated; at least 50 percent of patients have pure conductive hearing loss as a result of external and middle ear anomalies (Pron et al., 1993; Marres et al., 1995). The syndrome exhibits autosomal dominant inheritance, with at least 60 percent representing new mutations; genetic counseling is thus an important aspect of initial management. A gene of unknown function has been identified as the cause of at least one form of Treacher Collins syndrome through analysis of transcribed gene segments in the chromosome region 5q32–33.1 (Anonymous, 1996; Dixon, 1995, 1998).

Preventive care for patients with Treacher Collins syndrome begins with craniofacial and auditory assessment (Posnick, 1997). The occurrence of choanal atresia, palatal clefts, an obtuse cranial base angle, and pharyngeal hypoplasia may make intubation difficult and accounts for instances of neonatal death (Bryden et al., 1995). Mandibular lengthening may lessen upper airway obstruction (Moore et al., 1994). As with other craniofacial syndromes, a craniofacial surgery team is best consulted for the management of the facial anomalies; microsurgical techniques for restoring facial asymmetry may be particularly useful in branchial arch syndromes (Siebert et al., 1996).

Visual abnormalities are also common in Treacher Collins syndrome, with strabismus in 37 percent, amblyopia in 33 percent, refractive errors in 58 percent, and anisometropia in 17 percent (Hertle et al., 1993). Annual referral to ophthalmology and ear-nose-throat/audiology are thus recommended, at least until middle childhood. Hypoplasia of pharyngeal muscles may cause feeding problems requiring referral to nutritional and gastrointestinal specialists. Airway obstruction and sleep apnea may also cause poor feeding and decreased growth. Patients with extensive hospitalizations and surgeries, including those with failure to thrive and developmental delay, will benefit from early intervention referrals and neurosensory/developmental assessments. The normal intellectual potential provides incentive for scrupulous preventive management and an optimistic outlook for parental counseling.

Wildervanck syndrome

The Wildervanck syndrome consists of the Klippel–Feil anomaly, hearing loss, and abducens nerve palsy (Gorlin et al., 1990, pp. 659–61; Jones, 1997, pp. 254–5). The abducens palsy produces a Duane syndrome (inability of eye abduction, retraction of the globe and narrowing of the palpebral fissures during eye adduction). Because the majority of affected individuals are female, autosomal dominant inheritance with sex limitation, X-linked recessive inheritance with male lethality, and multifactorial inheritance mechanisms have been considered (Gorlin et al., 1990, pp. 659–61). Fewer than 100 cases are documented in the literature.

Additional eye anomalies include epibulbar dermoid cysts and lens subluxation, and anomalies may occur in the external, middle, and/or internal ear. The hearing loss may be sensorineural, conductive, or mixed, and stenotic canals have been reported. Cardiac anomalies have been reported (Gupte et al., 1992). Cervical vertebral fusion with restricted neck mobility is common, and other vertebral and rib anomalies may occur. Preventive management should include early auditory evoked response studies, ophthalmology referral, and radiography of the axial skeleton with flexion/extension views of the cervical spine. Inner ear anomalies may be severe, so cochlear imaging should be considered when there is sensorineural hearing loss (Keeney et al., 1992). As with other forms of cervical vertebral fusion, periodic radiographic assessment for atlantoaxial instability, basilar impression, and cervical vertebral arthritis should be performed. Some patients may require assessment by the craniofacial surgery team because of facial asymmetry or paralysis, and others will need early intervention services, since mental disability has been described.

Goldenhar syndrome and related defects

Terminology

Goldenhar (1952) published an influential paper that related eye and ear anomalies to the mandibular hypoplasia that was well known as "hemifacial microsomia." Unilateral hypoplasia of the jaw with external ear anomalies denoted by the latter term was appreciated in the late 1800s. The publication of Goldenhar (1952) initiated a large body of work that delineated a syndrome consisting of craniofacial, ocular, otic, skeletal, cardiac, and renal anomalies (Gorlin et al., 1990, pp. 641–9; Jones, 1997, pp. 642–3). The extreme variability of clinical manifestations has led to several names, including "hemifacial microsomia," "oculoauriculovertebral dysplasia," "facioauriculovertebral spectrum," "first and second branchial arch syndrome," and "Goldenhar complex" (see Figs 1.3 and 1.4, color plates). From a practical standpoint, it is useful to think of Goldenhar syndrome as a variable spectrum of major anomalies similar to those occurring in associations; the pattern of minor anomalies, facial resemblance, and Mendelian or chromosomal inheritance typical of other malformation syndromes is lacking in this disorder.

Incidence, etiology, and differential diagnosis

Estimates of the incidence of Goldenhar syndrome vary between 1 in 3500 and 1 in 26,000 births; Gorlin et al. (1990, p. 641) espoused the figure of 1 in 5600 births derived from the classic study of Grabb (1965). The disorder exhibits multifactorial inheritance, with rare families showing vertical transmission consistent with autosomal dominant inheritance. Environmental influences are represented by the ability to induce hemifacial microsomia in the rat by exposure to teratogens (Poswillo, 1973). Genetic models include the mouse mutant first arch and the mandibulofacial dysostosis produced by transgenic knock-out or overexpression of certain homeotic genes (e.g., Balling et al., 1989). A patient with terminal deletion of chromosome 22 had manifestations of Goldenhar syndrome (Herman et al., 1988). The variable clinical manifestations of Goldenhar syndrome undoubtedly reflect etiologic heterogeneity, ranging from *in utero* vascular accidents to pure Mendelian disorders.

Differential diagnosis of the branchial arch syndromes can be appreciated by perusing Table 15.1. The most important diagnostic consideration is to exclude Mendelian syndromes such as the branchio-oto-renal or Treacher Collins syndrome. Trisomy 18 may present with hemifacial microsomia and epibulbar dermoids, but the pattern of other anomalies should allow discrimination from Goldenhar syndrome. The VATER association of vertebral, anorectal, tracheoesophageal fistula, radial, and renal anomalies has considerable overlap with Goldenhar syndrome, and each disorder is primarily a pattern of major anomalies without a characteristic facies. In most cases, the facial asymmetry and ocular findings of Goldenhar syndrome discriminate it from VATER association. Some patients with Goldenhar syndrome will have the broad nasal region and hypertelorism characteristic of frontonasal dysplasia (Cohen, 1971); this conjunction probably reflects the occurrence of cranial malformations in some patients with Goldenhar syndrome (Wilson, 1983).

Diagnostic evaluation and medical counseling

The diagnosis of Goldenhar syndrome should be considered in the presence of unilateral mandibular hypoplasia and ear anomalies, with or without ocular cysts. The initial diagnostic evaluation for children with Goldenhar syndrome depends on the severity and extent of malformation. For children with hemifacial microsomia (unilateral jaw and ear involvement), minimal diagnostic evaluation is needed beyond contact with craniofacial surgery specialists to determine a schedule for repair. Part of the craniofacial evaluation will be auditory evoked response and imaging studies to determine the extent of middle/inner anomalies and hearing loss. For children with hemifacial microsomia and multiple other anomalies that occur with Goldenhar syndrome, an extensive diagnostic evaluation is required. Skeletal radiologic survey for cranial, vertebral, and limb anomalies; echocardiography to evaluate septal defects, transposition, or tetralogy of Fallot; and renal sonography to evaluate the urinary tract anatomy are important. Children with anophthalmia/microphthalmia, frontonasal dysplasia, or severe cranial asymmetry (plagiocephaly) require cranial imaging studies to evaluate brain structure. Syringomyelia has been reported in one case (Tekkok, 1996). Ophthalmology, otolaryngology, and nutritional evaluations are often needed because of anomalies and/or feeding problems that accompany pharyngeal and salivary gland hypoplasia that is common in Goldenhar syndrome. Airway obstruction may also occur and contribute to poor growth. Chromosomal studies may be considered in patients with severe and extensive anomalies, but a normal result is expected for children with Goldenhar syndrome.

Family and psychosocial counseling

Most families will not have other affected relatives, allowing genetic counseling for a 1–2 percent recurrence risk appropriate for multifactorial inheritance. A family history is important to rule out unusual instances of autosomal dominant inheritance. Although an optimistic prognosis for growth and mental development is appropriate for most children, clinicians must consider early feeding problems and the demands of multiple surgeries in providing support for families. Children with anophthalmia, encephaloceles, or severe cranial asymmetry are at risk for mental disability, so the provision of early intervention services and other supportive counseling is needed for their families. The clinical variability of Goldenhar syndrome mandates care in arranging appropriate family contacts. Parent groups are listed on the Goldenhar syndrome checklist, part 1.

Natural history and complications

Complications of Goldenhar syndrome are listed on the checklist, part 1. As denoted by the alternative name "first and second branchial arch syndrome," the core problems affect the mandibular, maxillary, auditory, and pharyngeal structures. There is facial asymmetry in 20 percent, mainly reflecting unilateral mandibular aplasia. Malformations of the external ear range from a small and simplified pinna to complete absence of the pinna and ear canal. The pinna may be represented by ear tags, and it is common to find extra cartilaginous tags along a line between the ear and the corner of the mouth. Conductive, sensorineural, or mixed hearing loss is present in at least 15 percent of cases due to stenosis of the ear canal, malformations of the ossicles, and basilar skull anomalies.

The eye and central nervous system are commonly affected, with ocular epibulbar dermoids (milky-white masses with defined edges, 50 percent of patients), lipoepidermoid cysts (yellowish, diffuse masses, 25 percent of patients), and anophthalmia/microphthalmia. Ocular motility disorders such as strabismus or Duane syndrome occur in 25 percent of patients. The implication of microphthalmia/anophthalmia for mental disability (Cohen, 1971) fits with an abnormality of neural tissue development in some patients with Goldenhar syndrome: mental retardation (5–15 percent), microcephaly, encephalocele, lissencephaly, holoprosencephaly, and abnormalities of cranial nerves I–VI and XIII–X have been described (Gorlin et al., 1990, pp. 641–9).

Oral complications include macrostomia because of lateral clefts, agenesis of the salivary glands (a prominent skin tag near the tragus is predictive of parotid gland agenesis), hypoplasia of the tongue and pharyngeal muscles, delayed development of teeth, and velopalatine insufficiency. Cleft palate with or without cleft lip may occur, and asynchrony of palatal motion may correlate with facial nerve palsies.

Vertebral anomalies are the best known skeletal complications, but anomalous ribs, thumb and radial ray defects, talipes equinovarus, and skull defects have all been noted (checklist, part 1). Cervical vertebral fusions occur in 20–35 percent of patients, and these may lead to interference with the articulation of the atlas and basilar skull (basilar impression – Gosain et al., 1994). Visceral anomalies include cardiac defects (Morrison et al., 1992), pulmonary hypoplasia, renal anomalies (Rollnick et al., 1987), and gastrointestinal defects including imperforate anus.

Goldenhar syndrome preventive medical checklist

As discussed above, the initial evaluation for patients with severe and extensive anomalies of Goldenhar syndrome should include imaging studies of the brain, heart, urinary tract, and skeleton (checklist, parts 2–4). Careful examination of craniofacial morphology and facial movement is needed, with early referral to craniofacial surgery, otolaryngology, and ophthalmology specialists. Monitoring of head growth (for hydrocephalus, microcephaly), of hearing (conductive or sensorineural deficits), and of vision (strabismus, Duane syndrome) is important during infancy and childhood. If renal sonography demonstrates abnormalities of the urinary tract, then periodic urinalyses are needed. Because cervical vertebral fusions are common, cervical spine films are recommended at age 3–5 years when ossification is complete; those with fusions should be followed for symptoms of atlantoaxial instability (neck pain, altered gait, enuresis) or, in adulthood, for cervical osteoarthritis. Gosain et al. (1994) found that posterior inclination of the odontoid relative to the foramen magnum signaled a higher risk for basilar impression. These patients require periodic neurology referral and consideration of CT or MRI scans of the neck.

Later preventive management of Goldenhar syndrome (checklist, part 4) involves the monitoring of hearing, vision, cervical mobility, urinary function, and dentition. Patients with severe cranial asymmetry or brain anomalies will need developmental assessment and possible early intervention/special and inclusive education services. Nutritional problems will usually resolve after the first year as pharyngeal muscles mature, but some patients will require evaluation by nutrition and gastroenterology specialists. Many patients are at risk of airway obstruction, and appropriate precautions should be taken before anesthesia. The occurrence of palatal dysfunction and dental anomalies often requires speech therapy and regular evaluation by dentistry.

Face/limb syndromes

Table 15.2 lists several syndromes that involve altered development of the craniofacies and limbs. Most are poorly understood, although molecular studies are in progress for many of them (Moore, 1995). All have a fairly low prevalence, and their preventive management will be summarized briefly.

Acrocallosal syndrome

The acrocallosal syndrome consists of pre- or postaxial polydactyly and absence or hypoplasia of the corpus callosum (Schinzel, 1979). It has some similarity to Greig syndrome but is not allelic (Brueton et al., 1992). Consanguinity and occurrence in sibs has suggested autosomal recessive inheritance, but most cases have been isolated (Gorlin et al., 1990, pp. 800–1). All patients have had mental disability, so early intervention and appropriate family counseling are important for management. An early onset of seizures with hypotonia is predictive of a severe neurologic prognosis (Thyen et al., 1992). Cleft lip/palate has been found in 15 percent, mandating evaluation for chronic otitis and audiology screening in these patients. Occasional brain anomalies include cortical atrophy and cystic lesions, with 75 percent of patients having seizures (Gorlin et al., 1990, pp. 800–1).

Coffin–Siris syndrome

Coffin–Siris syndrome is a difficult diagnosis to make because of overlap with conditions such as the fetal hydantoin syndrome. The disorder was described as the combination of coarse facial features, growth failure, and hypoplastic fifth fingers (Coffin & Siris, 1970). Affected sibs are among 30 reported cases, but most instances are isolated (Gorlin et al., 1990, pp. 831–2). Hypoplastic fingernails and

Table 15.2 Craniofacial-limb anomaly syndromes

Syndrome	Incidence	Inheritance	Complications
Acrocallosal	~25 cases	?AR	DD, agenesis of the corpus callosum, polydactyly, cleft palate
Coffin–Lowry	~100 cases	XLR	DD, coarse face, down-slanting palpebral fissures, broad fingers. soft hands
Coffin–Siris	~30 cases	?AR	DD, coarse face, sparse hair, strabismus, cardiac defects, cleft palate, short fingers, absent nails
Cryptophthalmos (Fraser)	~150 cases	AR	DD, eye a. (cryptophthalmos, microphthalmia), ear a., digital syndactyly, urogenital a.
Fryns	~50 cases	AR	Lethal, coarse face, cleft palate, short fingers, absent nails, diaphragmatic hernia, gastrointestinal a., renal a.
Greig	~50 cases	AD	Frontal bossing, hypertelorism, broad thumbs and great toes, polydactyly
Meckel	~200 cases	AR	Lethal, posterior encephalocele, polydactyly, cystic liver and kidneys
Moebius	~200 cases	Sporadic	DD (15 percent), facial nerve palsies, mask-like face, digital defects
Orofacialdigital Type I	~200 cases	XLD	DD (40 percent), lobulated tongue, oral frenula, midline cleft lip, cleft palate, syndactyly, brachydactyly, cystic kidneys, hydrocephalus
Orofacialdigital, Type II	~50 cases	AR	DD, lobulated tongue, midline cleft lip, polydactyly, syndactyly
Orofacialdigital, Type III	~10 cases	AR	DD, lobulated tongue, dental a., postaxial polydactyly, "see-saw winking"
Orofacialdigital, Type IV	~20 cases	AR	DD, cleft lip, dental a., polydactyly, syndactyly, tibial dysplasia
Orofacialdigital, Type V	~20 cases	AR	Median cleft lip, polydactyly
Orofacialdigital, Type VI	~20 cases	AR	DD (severe), cleft lip, ocular a., polydactyly, cardiac a., cerebellar a.
Otopalatodigital	~200 cases	XLR	DD (mild), frontal bossing, down-slanting palpebral fissures, broad thumbs, great toes
Roberts pseudo-thalidomide	~100 cases	AR	DD (severe), cleft lip/palate, cataracts, preaxial limb deficiencies, urogenital a.

Notes:

DD, developmental disability; AD, autosomal dominant; AR, autosomal recessive; XLD, X-linked dominant; XLR, X-linked recessive.

the coarse face explain the resemblance to fetal hydantoin syndrome, and one of us (G.W.) has seen a patient with suggestive features who was subsequently recognized as having fetal alcohol syndrome. A karyotype should be performed to exclude chromosomal disorders. Follow-up will usually be necessary to establish the diagnosis, since growth deficiency, sparse scalp hair, delayed osseous maturation, joint laxity, and hypotonia are virtually constant features (Gorlin et al., 1990, pp. 831–2). Occasional anomalies include cardiac anomalies (30 percent of patients), cleft palate, strabismus, Dandy–Walker malformation of the brain, and agenesis of the corpus callosum. Once the diagnosis is established (usually by exclusion), ophthalmology, cardiology, neurology, and early intervention referrals should be made. The possibility of autosomal recessive inheritance should be mentioned, along with psychosocial counseling and planning appropriate for children with severe disabilities. Patients with cleft palate will need monitoring for chronic otitis and hearing loss.

Cryptophthalmos (Fraser) syndrome

Cryptophthalmos syndrome is probably more common than is reflected by the 100 reported cases, since not all affected children have the characteristic eye findings (Fraser, 1962; Thomas et al., 1986). The diagnosis is easy when the eyes are hidden by overlying skin, although this can occur as an isolated anomaly (Gorlin et al., 1990, pp. 816–18). Cryptophthalmos syndrome exhibits autosomal recessive inheritance, with only 50 percent of patients surviving infancy. Thomas et al. (1986) proposed cryptophthalmos, syndactyly, abnormal genitalia, and an affected sib as major criteria for diagnosis, with nasal, external ear, laryngeal, palatal, umbilical, or renal anomalies as minor criteria. Ocular anomalies include colobomata, epibulbar dermoids, and absent lacrimal or meibomian glands in addition to the cryptophthalmos (Thomas et al., 1986). Nasal hypoplasia with clefts of the alae nasae, pulmonary hypoplasia (Stevens et al., 1994), cleft lip and palate, dental malocclusion, and auricular anomalies are common, with malformed ear ossicles and conductive hearing loss. Genital anomalies (80 percent) and unilateral or bilateral renal agenesis (80 percent) also occur, with 10–15 percent having anomalies of the urinary tract. A broad range of skeletal anomalies includes cranial asymmetry, parietal foramina, and syndactyly of the digits (Thomas et al., 1986; Gorlin et al., 1990, pp. 816–18). Mental deficiency occurs in at least 80 percent of patients, and 20 percent have central nervous system anomalies such as encephalocele or Dandy–Walker cyst.

Preventive management for the cryptophthalmos syndrome should include imaging studies of the cranium and brain during the neonatal period, along with renal sonography and skeletal radiographic survey. Most patients will need ophthalmologic evaluation and plastic surgery, and frequent inspection for conjunctivitis, blepharitis, and keratitis is an important aspect of pediatric care. Auditory evoked response and later audiologic monitoring of hearing is recommended, and the occurrence of laryngeal stenosis may require otolaryngologic evaluation for airway obstruction respiratory problems. Examination of the genitalia may suggest urologic referral, and a gonadoblastoma was documented in one patient (Greenberg et al., 1986). Early intervention services are important, particularly in view of the neurosensory and hearing deficits. Supportive counseling for the parents regarding a potentially lethal and handicapping disorder is often needed in the newborn period, and genetic counseling regarding the 25 percent recurrence risk should be given once the initial shock of diagnosis has subsided.

Fryns syndrome

Fryns syndrome (Fryns, 1979) is an autosomal recessive disorder that consists of facial, limb, ocular, digestive tract, and urogenital anomalies. Most patients have a diaphragmatic eventration or hernia, with coincident gastointestinal anomalies such as omphalocele, intestinal atresias, or imperforate anus. The face is typical with coarse features, malformed ears, micrognathia, macrostomia, and a short neck. Corneal clouding and cleft palate are often present. Renal anomalies include renal agenesis, cystic kidney, hydronephrosis, and ureteral cysts; genital anomalies include bicornuate uterus, cryptorchidism, and saddle scrotum (Gorlin et al., 1990, p. 733). Myoclonic seizures were reported in one patient (Riela et al., 1995).

The clinical course is severe, with 60 percent of affected pregnancies exhibiting polyhydramnios and many cases presenting as stillbirths. Only 14 percent survive the neonatal period, and Van Hove et al. (1995) emphasized the importance of brain imaging studies in assigning a neurologic outcome. Pinar et al. (1994) reported that 72 percent of patients have brain malformations. Recognition of the disorder may avoid unnecessary surgeries and suffering in severely affected patients. Echocardiography and abdominal sonography should be performed in the neonatal period to document anomalies of the heart, diaphragm, and urogenital tracts. Supportive counseling appropriate for infants with a lethal or severe developmental disorder is appropriate, followed by discussion of the 25 percent recurrence risk and the possibility of prenatal diagnosis by ultrasound and measurement of amniotic fluid alpha-fetoprotein levels at 18–20 weeks of pregnancy (Stratton et al., 1993).

Greig syndrome

Greig syndrome involves broad thumbs and first toes, pre- and/or postaxial polydactyly, and an unusual face with frontal bossing, broad forehead, and hypertelorism (Gorlin et al., 1990, pp. 779–80). It is an autosomal dominant disorder, and the occurrence of a balanced translocation in one affected patient allowed characterization of the responsible gene in chromosome region 7p13 (Vortkamp et al., 1991). There are few internal anomalies, so preventive management is directed toward the obvious defects in limb or craniofacial development. Rare patients have had mental disability, and hydrocephalus has been reported (Baraitser et al., 1983).

Meckel syndrome

Meckel syndrome is a lethal, autosomal recessive disorder that has an incidence of between 1 in 3000 and 1 in 50,000 births (Gorlin et al., pp. 724–6). Genetic mapping has assigned a locus for Meckel syndrome within chromosome region 17q21–q24 (Paavola et al., 1995). The presentation is usually striking, with a posterior encephalocele (65–90 percent of patients), postaxial polydactyly (55–75 percent), and a distended abdomen due to large, cystic kidneys (Salonen, 1984). Genital anomalies with micropenis and cryptorchidism, cystic changes in the pancreas and liver, and pulmonary hypoplasia are also frequent. Wright et al. (1994) commented on the clinical variability of Meckel syndrome and the difficulty of deciding on minimal diagnostic criteria. The chief preventive measure is to ensure an accurate diagnosis, so that the parents are aware of their 25 percent recurrence risk.

Moebius syndrome

Moebius syndrome can be separated from a diverse spectrum of face-limb disorders that involve anomalies of the tongue, mouth, facial nerves, and limbs. Gorlin et al. (1990, pp. 666–75) referred to this group as oromandibular-limb hypogenesis syndromes, including the hypoglossia-hypodactylia, Hanhart, Charlie M, and Moebius syndromes. Hall (1971) suggested five categories of oromandibular-limb hypogenesis syndromes, with isolated anomalies such as glossopalatine ankylosis (tongue-tie), Robin sequence, and amniotic band disruptions being included. The practical concern for health care professionals is to recognize that facial palsies and feeding problems may occur in children with oromandibular and limb defects, so that appropriate genetic consultation and neurologic/craniofacial evaluation can be arranged.

More than 200 cases of the Moebius syndrome have been reported, and nearly all, like those of other oromandibular-limb syndromes, were sporadic. Cranial nerve palsies are not confined to the seventh nerve, but also may affect nerves III, V, IX, and XII (Gorlin et al., 1990, pp. 671; Jones, 1997, pp. 230–1). There is micrognathia with a small mouth and hypoplasia of the tongue. Aplasia of the pectoral muscle (Poland sequence), limb anomalies (club foot in 30 percent of patients), and congenital hip dislocation can also occur. Preventive management should focus on oromotor function and dental care, since many patients have failure to thrive because of feeding difficulties. Ophthalmologic referral and monitoring should be conducted during childhood because ptosis, nystagmus, and strabismus may occur. Waterhouse et al. (1993) described a useful surgical technique for strabismus in Moebius syndrome. Mental deficiency occurs in 10–15 percent, and early intervention services should be strongly considered in order to monitor neurosensory, facial nerve, and muscular function. Psychosocial counseling is important for both parents and child, since the mask-like face and inability to smile can cause hardship. Facial function tends to improve with age, and mental deficiency is rarely severe.

Oro-facial-digital syndromes

Like the oromandibular-limb hypogenesis spectrum, the oral-facial-digital syndromes are a heterogeneous group of uncommon disorders that are predominantly sporadic in occurrence. Their distinguishing features are clefts and frenula (bands) affecting the tongue, gums, and palate together with polydactyly and/or syndactyly of the digits. As many as nine oro-facial-digital syndromes have been delineated, of which six are listed in Table 15.2. The chief concern for health care professionals should be appropriate genetic, craniofacial, and dental referral so that a diagnostic and preventive care program can be outlined.

The summary of the oro-facial-digital syndromes in Table 15.2 emphasizes the risk for brain, ocular, oral, lingual, dental, cardiac, renal, and digital anomalies. The initial evaluation should usually include brain imaging, skeletal radiologic survey, and cardiac and/or renal sonography in appropriate patients. Shashi et al. (1995) reported two brothers with absence of the pituitary gland, and Nevin et al. (1994) reported a patient with retinal abnormalities. Most patients will need referral to a craniofacial surgery team, with involvement of dental surgeons and orthodontics for oral care. Those patients with cleft palate will need monitoring for chronic otitis and audiologic screening; clinicians should also consider ophthalmologic referral since nystagmus, strabismus, and alternate winking of the eyes ("see-saw winking") have been described in this syndrome group. If the affected patient is male, then the X-linked dominant type I oro-facial-digital syndrome can be excluded; most families will have a 25 percent recurrence risk befitting autosomal recessive inheritance. Mental disability is often fairly severe, so early intervention and appropriate psychosocial counseling are important. Monitoring of growth with attention to feeding problems is also needed.

Otopalatodigital syndrome

Taybi (1962) first described the otopalatodigital syndrome based on facial changes, short stature, broad thumbs, broad great toes, and irregular digits with broad terminal phalanges. The face is distinctive, with a prominent forehead, down-slanting palpebral fissures, broad nasal root, and down-turned corners of the mouth. The radiographic findings are also quite characteristic, with irregular form and curvature of the fingers and toes, changes in the vertebrae and pelvis, and frontal bossing of the skull (Gorlin et al., 1990, pp. 686–90; Jones, 1997, pp. 270–3). In otopalatodigital syndrome type I, the clinical course is mild and affected males have mild cognitive defects with average IQ in the 75–90 range. A type II otopalatodigital syndrome has been described with more severe skeletal changes and decreased survival; more than 50 percent of affected patients have died before age 6 months. Both syndromes exhibit X-linked recessive inheritance, so molecular analysis will be required to determine if these disorders derive from separate loci, are allelic variations at the same X chromosome locus, or represent variable expressivity of the same genetic mutation. The gene for otopalatodigital syndrome type I has been assigned to chromosome region Xq26–28 (Hoar et al., 1992).

Preventive management of the otopalatodigital syndromes should focus on auditory evoked response and periodic audiology screening for hearing deficits. Preferential speech delays may reflect undetected hearing loss, and early intervention with physical, occupation, and speech therapy is essential for all patients. Cleft palate is a common complication of both otopalatodigital syndromes, providing additional incentive for auditory screening. Apnea secondary to cervical spine anomalies and brain stem compression occurred postoperatively in one patient with otopalatodigital syndrome type II (Clark et al., 1995). Genetic counseling for X-linked recessive inheritance and a 25 percent recurrence risk is indicated, with some female carriers exhibiting facial and digital manifestations of the syndrome.

Roberts pseudothalidomide syndrome

The combination of cleft palate and limb reduction defects recognized by Roberts in 1919 was rediscovered by several different observers (Gorlin et al., 1990, pp. 735–6). Hermann used the term "pseudothalidomide syndrome" to emphasize the limb defects, while Opitz, as was his custom, used the family initials S.C. to denote the condition (Hermann & Opitz, 1977). It is now agreed that pseudothalidomide and SC syndromes share the same spectrum of manifestations with Roberts syndrome. The disorder is autosomal recessive, and chromosome studies often reveal an unusual phenomenon called premature centromere condensation.

Clinical manifestations of Roberts syndrome include microcephaly, cleft lip and palate, cataracts, preaxial digital defects, flexion contractures, and club feet. Allingham-Hawkins & Tomkins (1995) emphasized the heterogeneity of Roberts syndrome, and Van Den Berg & Francke (1993) offered a rating system for severity. Preventive management should include ophthalmologic referral and regular vision screening, craniofacial surgery evaluation for cleft lip and palate, monitoring for chronic otitis and hearing loss, and inspection of the genitalia for cryptorchidism, enlarged penis, or bicornuate uterus. Periodic urinalyses or initial renal sonography should be performed, since horseshoe kidney, polycystic kidneys, and urinary tract anomalies have been reported. Many patients are severely growth retarded and do not survive infancy. Of those who do, 50 percent have mental disability warranting early intervention referral and appropriate school and legal planning. One patient had normal intelligence (Holden et al., 1992). Occasional cardiac anomalies and thrombocytopenia have also been described.

Preventive Management of Goldenhar syndrome

Clinical diagnosis: Pattern of manifestations including mandibular hypoplasia and ear anomalies, often unilateral, with or without ocular cysts. Extreme variability of the craniofacial, ocular, otic, skeletal, cardiac, and renal anomalies led to several names, including "hemifacial microsomia," "oculoauriculovertebral dysplasia," "facioauriculovertebral spectrum," "first and second branchial arch syndrome," and "Goldenhar complex."

Incidence: 1 in 6000 live births.

Laboratory diagnosis: None available although severely affected patients should have karyotypes because the jaw, ear, and ocular anomalies can occur in chromosomal disorders like cri-du-chat.

Genetics: Multifactorial determination with most cases being sporadic; a 2 percent recurrence risk was reported for parents of affected children (Grabb, 1965).

Key management issues: Imaging studies of the brain, heart, urinary tract, and skeleton in extensively affected patients, monitoring of head growth (for hydrocephalus, microcephaly), vision (strabismus, Duane syndrome) hearing (conductive or sensorineural deficits), tooth development, urinary tract (renal anomalies), early intervention particularly for patients with severe cranial asymmetry or microphthalmia, oromotor and speech therapists for problems due to palatal dysfunction and hypoplastic pharyngeal muscles, cautious anesthesia due to risks for cervical spine fusion and airway obstruction.

Growth Charts: No specific charts are available.

Parent groups: Goldenhar Syndrome Research and Information Fund, P. O. Box 61643, St. Petersburg FL, 33714, (813) 522-5772, btorman@pbsnet.com, http://www.GOLDENHAR.com; Ms Nicola Woodgate Goldenhar Syndrome Family Support Group, 9 Hartley Court Gardens, Cranbrook, Kent TN17 3QY UK, http://www.sense.org.uk/sense/ html/dbigolde.htm

Basis for management recommendations:. Derived from the complications below as documented by Rollnick et al. (1987); brain imaging studies should be performed on children with severe plagiocephaly or anophthalmia but are not needed in children with mild manifestations.

Summary of clinical concerns

General	Learning	Cognitive disability (5–15%), learning differences, speech problems
	Growth	Low birth weight, failure to thrive
Facial	Eye	**Strabismus** (25%), **epibulbar dermoids** (50%), **lipoepidermoids** (25%), anophthalmia, microphthalmia
	Ear	**Abnormal pinna** (65%), **preauricular tags** (40%), middle ear anomalies
	Mouth	Dysphagia, decreased salivation, **velopalatal insufficiency** (35%), cleft lip/palate (7–15%), pharyngeal muscle hypoplasia
Surface	Neck/trunk	Skin tags
Skeletal	Cranial	Microcephaly, plagiocephaly, **cranial asymmetry** (20%)
	Axial	**Vertebral anomalies** (30%), **cervical vertebral fusion** (20%), rib anomalies, scoliosis, Klippel–Feil anomaly
	Limbs	Radial anomaly (10%), **club feet** (20%)
Internal	Pulmonary	Pulmonary hypoplasia, abnormal lung lobation, airway obstruction
	Circulatory	**Cardiac anomalies** (5–58% – ventricular septal defects, tetralogy of Fallot, transposition of the great vessels, dextrocardia)
	Excretory	Renal agenesis, hypoplasia, hydronephrosis, double ureter
Neural	CNS	Brain anomalies (encephaloceles, lipomas, teratomas, dermoids, Arnold–Chiari malformation), seizures
	Motor	Cranial nerve anomalies, **facial palsies** (10–20%)
	Sensory	Hearing loss (15%)

Bold: frequency > 20%

Key references

Cohen, M. M., Jr. (1971). *Birth Defects* 7:103–8.
Grabb, W. C. (1965). *Plastic & Reconstructive Surgery* 36:485–508.
Poswillo, D. (1974). *Oral Surgery* 35:302–29.
Rollnick, B. R. et al. (1987). *American Journal of Medical Genetics* 26:361–75.
Wilson, G. N. (1983). *American Journal of Medical Genetics* 14:435–43

Goldenhar syndrome

Preventive medical checklist (0–1yr)

Patient   **Birth Date** / /   **Number**

Pediatric	Screen		Evaluate		Refer/Counsel	
Neonatal / / *Newborn screen* ❑ *HB* ❑	Echocardiogram ❑ Skeletal x-rays ❑ Renal sonogram ❑		Feeding ❑ Airway, apnea ❑ Facial palsies ❑ Ear canals, eyes ❑		Genetic evaluation ❑ Craniofacial team ❑ Cardiology ❑ Feeding specialist ❑	
1 month / /	Growth ❑ Head size ❑ Head MRI[3] ❑		Feeding ❑ Airway, apnea ❑ Facial palsies ❑		Family support[4] ❑ Feeding specialist ❑	
2 months / / *HB[1]* ❑ *Hib* ❑ *DTaP, IPV* ❑ *RV* ❑	Growth ❑ Hearing, vision[2] ❑		Feeding ❑ Airway, apnea ❑		Early intervention[5] ❑ Genetic counseling ❑ Feeding specialist ❑	
4 months / / *HB[1]* ❑ *Hib* ❑ *DTaP/IPV* ❑ *RV* ❑	Growth ❑ Hearing, vision[2] ❑		Feeding ❑ Airway, apnea ❑		Early intervention[5] ❑	
6 months / / *Hib* ❑ *IPV[1]* ❑ *DTaP* ❑ *RV* ❑	Growth ❑ Head size ❑ Hearing, vision[2] ❑		Feeding ❑ Airway, apnea ❑ Facial palsies ❑ Ear canals, eyes ❑		Family support[4] ❑ Craniofacial team ❑ Feeding specialist[3] ❑	
9 months / / *IPV[1]* ❑	Growth ❑ Hearing, vision[2] ❑		Feeding ❑ Airway, apnea ❑			
1 year / / *HB* ❑ *Hib[1]* ❑ *IPV[1]* ❑ *MMR[1]* ❑ *Var[1]* ❑	Growth ❑ Head size ❑ Hearing, vision[2] ❑ Audiology ❑		Feeding ❑ Airway, apnea ❑ Facial palsies ❑ Ear canals, eyes ❑		Family support[4] ❑ Early intervention[5] ❑ Craniofacial team ❑ Feeding specialist[3] ❑	

Clinical concerns for Goldenhar syndrome, ages 0–1 year

Plagiocephaly
Epibulbar dermoids
Anophthalmia
Ear anomalies, hearing loss

Cardiac anomalies
Pulmonary hypoplasia
Renal anomalies
Vertebral anomalies

Developmental disability
Feeding problems
Velopalatal insufficiency
Facial nerve palsies

Guidelines for the neonatal period should be undertaken *at whatever age* the diagnosis is made; the craniofacial team should include ophthalmology, ENT, plastic, and neurosurgery; DTaP, acellular DTP; IPV, inactivated poliovirus (oral polio also used); RV, rotavirus; MMR, measles–mumps–rubella; Var, varicella; BP, blood pressure; C-spine, cervical spine; AAI, atlantoaxial instability; [1]alternative timing; [2]by practitioner; [3]as dictated by clinical findings – head MRI is needed in patients with microphthalmia or plagiocephaly; [4]parent group, family/sib, financial, and behavioral issues as discussed in the preface; [5]including developmental monitoring and motor/speech therapy.

Goldenhar syndrome

Preventive medical checklist (15m–6yrs)

Patient		Birth Date / /		Number	

Pediatric	Screen		Evaluate		Refer/Counsel	
15 months / / *Hib*[1] ❑ *MMR*[1] ❑ *DTaP, IPV*[1] ❑ *Varicella*[1] ❑	Growth Hearing, vision[2]	❑ ❑	Feeding, airway Sleep apnea	❑ ❑	Family support[4] Early intervention[5] Sleep study[3]	❑ ❑ ❑
18 months / / *DTaP, IPV*[1] ❑ *Varicella*[1] ❑ *Influenza*[3] ❑	Hearing, vision[2]	❑	Feeding, airway	❑		
2 years / / *Influenza*[3] ❑ *Pneumovax*[3] ❑ *Dentist* ❑	Growth Hearing, vision[2] Urinalysis, BP	❑ ❑ ❑	Feeding, airway Facial palsies Sleep apnea	❑ ❑ ❑	Family support[4] Genetics Craniofacial team Sleep study[3]	❑ ❑ ❑ ❑
3 years / / *Influenza*[3] ❑ *Pneumovax*[3] ❑ *Dentist* ❑	Hearing, vision[2] Audiology C-spine x-rays[3]	❑ ❑ ❑	Feeding, airway Sleep apnea AAI	❑ ❑	Family support[4] Preschool transition[5] Craniofacial team	❑ ❑ ❑
4 years / / *Influenza*[3] ❑ *Pneumovax*[3] ❑ *Dentist* ❑	Growth Hearing, vision[2] Urinalysis, BP	❑ ❑ ❑	Heart, lungs Scoliosis Sleep apnea	❑ ❑ ❑	Family support[4] Preschool program[5] Genetics Craniofacial team	❑ ❑ ❑ ❑
5 years / / *DTaP, IPV*[1] ❑ *MMR*[1] ❑	Hearing, vision[3] Audiology C-spine x-rays[3]	❑ ❑ ❑	Heart, lungs Scoliosis AAI	❑ ❑ ❑	School transition[5]	❑
6 years / / *DTaP, IPV*[1] ❑ *MMR*[1] ❑ *Dentist* ❑	Growth Hearing, vision[2] Urinalysis, BP	❑ ❑ ❑	School progress Heart, lungs Scoliosis	❑ ❑ ❑	Family support[4] Genetics Craniofacial team	❑ ❑ ❑

Clinical concerns for Goldenhar syndrome, ages 1–6 years

Plagiocephaly
Epibulbar dermoids
Anophthalmia
Ear anomalies, hearing loss

Cardiac anomalies
Pulmonary hypoplasia
Renal anomalies
Vertebral anomalies

Developmental disability
Feeding problems
Velopalatal insufficiency
Facial nerve palsies

Guidelines for the neonatal period should be undertaken *at whatever age* the diagnosis is made; the craniofacial team should include ophthalmology, ENT, plastic, and neurosurgery; DTaP, acellular DTP; IPV, inactivated poliovirus (oral polio also used); MMR, measles–mumps–rubella; Var, varicella; BP, blood pressure; C-spine, cervical spine; AAI, atlantoaxial instability; [1]alternative timing; [2]by practitioner; [3]as dictated by clinical findings – head MRI is needed in patients with microphthalmia or plagiocephaly; [4]parent group, family/sib, financial, and behavioral issues as discussed in the preface; [5]including developmental monitoring and motor/speech therapy.

Goldenhar syndrome

Preventive medical checklist (6+ yrs)

Patient		Birth Date / /		Number	
Pediatric	**Screen**	**Evaluate**		**Refer/Counsel**	
8 years / / *Dentist* ❑	Hearing, vision[2] ❑	Scoliosis ❑ AAI ❑		School options ❑ Genetics ❑	
10 years / /	Growth ❑ Hearing, vision[2] ❑ Urinalysis, BP ❑	School progress ❑ Heart, lungs ❑ Scoliosis ❑		Craniofacial team ❑	
12 years / / *Td[1], MMR, Var* ❑ *CBC* ❑ *Dentist* ❑ *Scoliosis* ❑ *Cholesterol* ❑	Hearing, vision[2] ❑ C-spine x-rays[3] ❑	AAI ❑		Family support[4] ❑ Genetics ❑ School options ❑	
14 years / / *CBC* ❑ *Dentist* ❑ *Cholesterol* ❑ *Breast CA* ❑ *Testicular CA* ❑	Growth ❑ Hearing, vision[2] ❑ Urinalysis, BP ❑	School progress ❑ Heart, lungs ❑ Scoliosis ❑		Craniofacial team ❑	
16 years / / *Td[1]* ❑ *CBC* ❑ *Cholesterol* ❑ *Sexual[5]* ❑ *Dentist* ❑	Hearing, vision[2] ❑	Scoliosis ❑		Genetics ❑	
18 years / / *CBC* ❑ *Sexual[5]* ❑ *Cholesterol* ❑ *Scoliosis* ❑	Hearing, vision[2] ❑ Urinalysis, BP ❑ C-spine x-rays ❑	School progress ❑ AAI ❑		Craniofacial team ❑	
20 years[6] / / *CBC* ❑ *Sexual[5]* ❑ *Cholesterol* ❑ *Dentist* ❑	Hearing, vision[3] ❑ Urinalysis, BP ❑ C-spine x-rays[3] ❑	Heart, lungs ❑ C-spine arthritis ❑ AAI ❑		Family support[4] ❑ Craniofacial team ❑	

Clinical concerns for Goldenhar syndrome, ages 6+ years

Plagiocephaly	Cardiac anomalies	Cognitive disability
Abnormal vision	Renal anomalies	Velopalatal insufficiency
Ear anomalies, hearing loss	Vertebral anomaly, scoliosis	Facial nerve palsies
Absent salivary glands	Cervical spine fusion, AAI	Radial aplasia

Guidelines for the neonatal period should be undertaken *at whatever age* the diagnosis is made; the craniofacial team should include ophthalmology, ENT, plastic, and neurosurgery; Td, tetanus/diphtheria; MMR, measles–mumps–rubella; Var, varicella; BP, blood pressure; C-spine, cervical spine; AAI, atlantoaxial instability; [1]alternative timing; [2]by practitioner; [3]as dictated by clinical findings – head MRI is needed in patients with microphthalmia or plagiocephaly; [4]parent group, family/sib, financial, and behavioral issues as discussed in the preface; [5]including developmental monitoring and motor/speech therapy.

Part VI

Management of connective tissue and integumentary syndromes

16

Connective tissue disorders

Signs and symptoms of connective tissue weakness include joint laxity manifest by increased range of motion and the ability to perform "double-jointed" maneuvers; altered skeletal proportions with elongation of the craniofacies, thorax, and limbs; susceptibility of joints and internal organs to damage during normal function (e.g., joint dislocations, hernias, optic lens dislocations, mitral valve prolapse), and skin fragility manifest by increased bruisability, unusual scarring, and stretch marks. Particular syndrome phenotypes depend on the component of connective tissue that is altered and the spectrum of other developmental abnormalities (Table 16.1). Connective tissue dysplasia is a common feature of many chromosomal, skeletal, and metabolic disorders such as Down syndrome, Williams syndrome, achondroplasia, osteogenesis imperfecta, homocystinuria, and Menkes syndrome. Connective tissue laxity is usually the primary clinical manifestation that draws attention to the patient in the syndromes discussed here, including Marfan and Ehlers–Danlos syndromes, which will be discussed in detail. Syndromes with the opposite finding, tight connective tissue that leads to contractures, will be discussed in Chapter 18.

Inspection of Table 16.1 reveals that connective tissue manifestations in Down syndrome, achondroplasia, or homocystinuria are similar to those of primary connective tissue dysplasias like Marfan or Ehlers–Danlos syndrome. The elongated cranium causes a high palate, resulting in tooth crowding and dental problems. Sparsity of connective tissue in the eyes allows the underlying choroid to show through the sclerae, resulting in a bluish or grayish tinge. Blue sclerae are most typical of the osteogenesis imperfectas, but occur as a general feature in many chromosomal and skeletal diseases. Mitral valve prolapse is a common feature in many normal individuals, but has increased frequency in Down, Williams, or Marfan syndrome. More severe vascular abnormality leads to cystic medial necrosis and aortic regurgitation, as in Marfan syndrome or osteogenesis imperfecta, type I. Some disorders of connective tissue can be understood as defects in particular connective tissue molecules, exemplified by fibrillin defects in Marfan syndrome or type I collagen defects in osteogenesis imperfecta. Respective

Table 16.1 Syndromes with connective tissue abnormality

Syndrome	Incidence	Inheritance	Complications
Syndromes with connective tissue abnormality as a primary manifestation			
Beals	~100 cases	AD	Marfanoid habitus, joint contractures, overturned, "crumpled" ears, ectopia lentis, aortic dilatation, septal defects, scoliosis
Cutis laxa	~100 cases	AR, AD	Lax skin, pulmonary emphysema, bronchiectasis, dilated great arteries, hernias, bladder diverticula, gut diverticula
Ehlers–Danlos, types I–III	1 in 10,000	AD	Joint laxity, elastic skin, "cigarette paper" scars, MVP, scoliosis, hernias, prematurity
Ehlers–Danlos, type IV	1 in 100,000	AD, AR	Thin skin, arterial ruptures and dissections, bowel ruptures, strokes, hemorrhage
Ehlers–Danlos, type V	~20 cases	XLR	Joint laxity, kyphosis, hernia, flat feet
Ehlers–Danlos, type VI	~50 cases	AR	Joint laxity, ocular fragility, elastic skin, scoliosis
Ehlers–Danlos, type VII	~20 cases	AD	Joint laxity, soft skin, hip dislocation
Homocystinuria	1 in 100,000	AR	Restricted joint mobility, ectopia lentis, myopia, retinal detachment, long and thin limbs, pectus, scoliosis, cognitive disability
Larsen	~200 cases	AD, sporadic	Joint laxity, multiple joint dislocations, cleft palate, laryngeal stenosis, cervical vertebral a.
Marfan	1 in 10,000	AD	Joint laxity, tall stature, ectopia lentis, long and thin limbs, aortic dilatation, pectus, scoliosis, hernias, flat feet
Pseudoxanthoma elasticum	1 in 40,000	AD, AR	Joint laxity, skin thickening, myopia, retinal disease, vascular obstruction and hemorrhage
Stickler syndrome	~200 cases	AD	Joint laxity, Marfanoid habitus, myopia, retinal disease, cleft palate, MVP, hearing loss
Syndromes with connective tissue abnormality as a secondary manifestation			
Down	1 in 800	Chromo-somal	Joint laxity, AAI, high palate, MVP, scoliosis, hernias, extra skin folds
Williams	1 in 25,000	Sporadic	Joint laxity, MVP, hernias, scoliosis, bladder diverticuli
Achondroplasia	1 in 16,000	AD	Joint laxity, blue sclerae, scoliosis, prolapsed intervertebral discs
Osteogenesis imperfecta	1 in 20, 000	AD	Joint laxity, blue sclerae, MVP, aortic regurgitation, scoliosis, pectus,
Homocystinuria	1 in 200,000	AR	Tall stature, ectopia lentis, myopia, high palate, arachnodactyly, pectus, flat feet, scoliosis
Menkes			

Note:

AD, autosomal dominant; AR, autosomal recessive, XLR, X-linked recessive.

abnormalities of collagen and elastin are suggested in Down or Williams syndrome, but these complex phenotypes seem to involve more than one connective tissue abnormality, as would be consistent with the duplication/deletion of several genetic loci. Connective tissue abnormality can be viewed as a general feature of altered development, reflecting the large number of interactions between intracellular, adhesion, and extracellular matrix molecules that must occur to construct normal connective tissue. The "pure" connective tissue diseases are thus instructive for preventive health care, since their manifestations are seen in many syndromes and even in normal individuals who wind up on the lax side of the connective tissue spectrum.

Rarer connective tissue disorders

Beals syndrome (congenital contractural arachnodactyly)

Thought to be the disorder originally described by Marfan (Hecht & Beals, 1972), congenital contractural arachnodactyly was described in 1971. It is an autosomal dominant disorder caused by mutations in the fibrillin-2 gene on chromosome 5 (Putnam et al., 1995). Infants may be suspected of having Marfan syndrome, with long and slender limbs (dolichostenomelia), camptodactyly, ulnar deviation of the fingers, and multiple joint contractures (Jones, 1988, pp. 424–5). Rarely, patients may have ectopia lentis and aortic root dilatation (Bawle & Quigg, 1992; Viljoen, 1994). Other findings include micrognathia, congenital heart defects (septal defects), and "crumpled" ears with overturned and irregular helices. Skeletal deformities include kyphoscoliosis and foot deformities.

Preventive management should include cardiologic evaluation and echocardiography when the diagnosis is considered, periodic examination for skeletal deformities, and physical/occupational therapy for joint contractures. Bawle & Quigg (1992) recommended initial and periodic eye and heart examinations as is standard for patients with Marfan syndrome. The joint contractures tend to improve, but the kyphoscoliosis may be progressive (Jones, 1988).

Cutis laxa

The defining manifestation of cutis laxa syndromes is very loose skin that hangs in folds and gives affected patients an aged appearance. Since redundant or loose skin folds are common in disorders such as Down syndrome, one can expect heterogeneity among patients defined by this characteristic.

Although described as a phenotypic finding in the early 1800s, genetic studies allowed delineation of specific cutis laxa syndromes in the latter part of this century (Gorlin et al., 1990, pp. 423–5). The autosomal recessive form is most severe, with growth deficiency and respiratory problems producing childhood morbidity and mortality. The skin appears too large for the body, producing skin folds, narrow palpebral fissures (blepharophimosis), and an aged appearance. Uitto et al. (1993) grouped the cutis laxa syndromes with disorders of premature aging. Abnormal skin fragility or scarring does not occur, but the pulmonary connective tissue seems disproportionately affected with emphysema, pneumonitis, air trapping, respiratory failure, and cor pulmonale. The cardiovascular system is also affected, with tortuous, dilated arteries in the carotid, vertebral, and pulmonary systems. Other complications include diverticulae of the gastrointestinal (pharynx, esophagus, rectum), urinary (bladder), and genital (vagina) tracts. Laxity of the vocal cords may produce a deep voice, and musculoskeletal laxity may produce diaphragmatic, inguinal, or umbilical hernias. One type of recessive cutix laxa is associated with lysyl oxidase deficiency (Khakoo et al., 1997).

Autosomal dominant cutis laxa is much milder, with presentation as skin laxity in middle to later childhood. The chief complications are cosmetic, with exaggerated skin folds, ptosis, accentuation of nasolabial folds, and an aged appearance. Rarely, the same spectrum of serious problems that complicate the autosomal recessive form are seen: hernias, pulmonary stenosis, mitral valve prolapse, bronchiectasis, and tortuosity of the carotid arteries and aorta. Unlike the recessive disorder, where joint laxity seems minimal, patients with autosomal dominant cutis laxa may have joint dislocations and degenerative arthritis.

Preventive management for the cutis laxa syndromes should include surveillance for respiratory problems in the neonatal and infantile periods. Lax pharyngeal tissue poses a risk of obstructive airway disease, and infants may require monitoring for tachypnea as a sign of emphysema or hypoxemia. Imaging studies of the heart and great vessels should be considered in infants with severe cutis laxa, and propensity for pneumonias and bronchiectasis may necessitate therapy to improve pulmonary toilet such as massage or prophylactic antibiotics. The upper airway obstruction, together with hypoxemia, places the affected child at risk of sleep apnea. A history of irregular respirations, stridor, or gasps during sleep plus evidence of growth failure, pectus excavatum, or mouth breathing on examination should prompt sleep studies and referral to otolaryngology. Periodic evaluations for evidence of hernias, bladder or gut diverticulae, and psychosocial needs for cosmetic surgery should be performed.

Homocystinuria

Homocystinuria is one of the metabolic disorders that produces a syndromic appearance. Homocystinuria is a metabolic finding that can arise in conjunction with several enzyme deficiencies; all except those from nutritional deficiency or defective vitamin B_{12} absorption exhibit autosomal recessive inheritance. The most common form of homocystinuria is caused by inherited deficiency of cystathionine-β-synthase. Other causes include alterations in folate and vitamin B_{12} metabolism; these disorders are not associated with a Marfanoid phenotype and connective tissue abnormality.

Tall stature, Marfanoid habitus, ectopia lentis, arachnodactyly, scoliosis, and flat feet are frequent findings in patients with homocystinuria, underlying the importance of plasma amino acid levels when the family history cannot discriminate between autosomal recessive homocystinuria and autosomal dominant Marfan syndrome. Osteoporosis is much more common in homocystinuria, as are thromboembolic events that have made homocystinuria carriers of interest in elucidating risk factors for coronary disease. Other differences from Marfan syndrome include downward rather than upward dislocation of the lens, and neurologic manifestations including mental deficiency (median IQ 64 for those not responding to folic acid supplementation), seizures (21 percent), and psychiatric disorders in up to 50 percent of patients (Gorlin et al., 1990, pp. 132–5).

Preventive management of homocystinuria begins with a diagnostic evaluation that is best coordinated through metabolic disease specialists at an academic center. It is extremely important to evaluate patients with ectopia lentis for homocystinuria, since there is both treatment and presurgical management that may prevent neurologic catastrophes (e.g., Arbour et al., 1988). Once cystathionine-β-synthase deficiency is confirmed as the cause of homocystinuria, the patient can begin a treatment regimen consisting of dietary methionine restriction; pyridoxine, folate, and betaine; and chronic administration of low-dose aspirin or dipyridamol (Skovby, 1993). The reasons for supplementation are that pyridoxine is a co-factor for cystathionine-β-synthase, folate deficiency can interfere with pyridoxine effect, and betaine helps convert homocystine to methionine. The treatment protocol has shown promising results after long-term follow-up (Mudd et al., 1985). Patients who respond to low amounts of pyridoxine are particularly benefited, showing higher mean IQ and fewer thrombotic complications. One patient developed diarrhea and pancreatitis that was responsive to betaine (Ilan et al., 1993). Since dietary methionine levels must be permissive for growth but sufficiently restricted to lower plasma homocystine, regular monitoring through a metabolic disease clinic is recommended. Otherwise, preventive management should include regular ophthalmology, cardiology, and skeletal evaluations as outlined for Marfan syndrome (below). An additional precaution should be anticoagulation, hydration, and oxygenation during surgery so as to lower the risks for thromboembolism (Arbour et al., 1988).

Larsen syndrome

Larsen syndrome consists of increased connective tissue laxity, joint dislocations, club feet, and a flattened face with a shallow nasal bridge (Larsen et al., 1950). The most striking manifestations affect the skeletal system, with dislocation of the radial head (70 percent), dislocation of the tibia onto the femur (80 percent), hip dislocation (80 percent), and club feet (85 percent – Gorlin et al., 1990, pp. 722–3). There may be abnormal segmentation of the carpal and vertebral bones, producing supernumerary bones in the wrist and cervical vertebral anomalies. The latter have been associated with cervical instability and quadriplegia or sudden death. Cardiac anomalies, including septal defects and dilatation of the aorta, have been reported (Kiel et al., 1983). About 15 percent of patients have mental deficiency, and sensorineural or mixed hearing loss does occur (Stanley et al., 1988). Of concern during infancy is laryngotracheomalacia or laryngeal stenosis, which may cause lethal airway obstruction (Crowe et al., 1989).

Preventive management for Larsen syndrome should include careful orthopedic evaluation and skeletal radiographic survey as soon as the diagnosis is suspected. Evaluation of respiratory function including otolaryngologic assessment of the upper airway is critical, particularly before anesthesia and surgery. Evaluation for signs and symptoms of cardiovascular disease should be conducted periodically, and patients should be counseled to avoid high-impact, collision, or highly competitive sports that are apt to cause joint trauma, dislocation, or degeneration. Audiologic screening is worthwhile in early childhood, and development should be monitored, with referral to early intervention if there is delay. For patients with cleft palate, auditory evoked response studies during infancy, followed by examination and audiology screening for chronic otitis, should be performed. If cervical spine fusions are noted on the initial radiographic survey, then screening for atlantoaxial instability before anesthesia or entry into sports programs or school should be considered. The propensity for joint dislocations in the neck and other regions mandates periodic neurologic evaluations for signs of nerve compression; neurologic and orthopedic referral may be needed in some cases.

Pseudoxanthoma elasticum

Pseudoxanthoma elasticum is a disorder of skin, connective tissue, eyes, heart, and blood vessels that usually presents in the second to third decade of life. There are autosomal dominant and autosomal recessive forms of the disease, with an aggregate incidence of about 1 in 40,000 births. A characteristic finding is the "peau d'orange," or orange-peel skin, which represents thickening together with yellow papules. The skin becomes leathery and fragile, sometimes perforating over pressure points. Eye findings include myopia and cataracts, with retinal examination revealing typical "angioid streaks" and later hemorrhage or macular degeneration. Abnormal elastin fibers in the blood vessels lead to calcification, obstruction of vascular flow, and hemorrhage. Clinical manifestations of the vasculopathy include intermittent claudication of the limbs, renovascular hypertension, angina of the coronary or celiac arteries, and hemorrhage into the gut, retina, kidney, uterus, bladder, and central nervous system (Gorlin et al., 1990, pp. 478–82). Intracerebral and subarachnoid hemorrhages may cause neurologic deficits, psychiatric disorders, and seizures during adulthood. Increased joint laxity and vertebral anomalies have been described. Affected children have been recognized (Hacker et al., 1993; Perrot & Mrak, 1993), but usually children are evaluated because a parent or older sib is affected; preventive management should consist of periodic examinations of the eyes, heart, pulses, and skin and testing of the stool for occult blood. Counseling should be given regarding regular medical care as an adult, and the high risks for gastrointestinal hemorrhage during pregnancy (Berde et al., 1983).

Stickler syndrome

Patients with Stickler syndrome may have a Marfanoid habitus (although some have short stature) with vitreoretinal degeneration and detachment, cleft palate, hearing loss, joint laxity, and arthritis (MacDonald et al., 1997). There has been controversy about the delineation of Stickler syndrome, in that Marshall, Wagner, and Weissenbacher–Zweymüller all described similar conditions (Winter et al., 1983). More than 200 patients have been reported, and it is estimated the condition accounts for more than 30 percent of infants with the Robin sequence of micrognathia and cleft soft palate (Gorlin et al., 1990, pp. 288–9). The disorder is autosomal dominant, and mutations in the type II collagen gene have been found in some patients with Stickler syndrome (Brown et al., 1995; MacDonald et al., 1997).

Clinical manifestations of Stickler syndrome are extremely variable (Zlotogora et al., 1992). They can include Robin sequence with risks of respiratory obstruction during early infancy, myopia, chorioretinal degeneration with retinal detachment (70 percent), cataracts, strabismus, flattened midface with cleft palate or velopalatine insufficiency, and multiple skeletal changes. The joint laxity leads to thin, Marfanoid habitus, but at least 25 percent of patients are short rather than tall. The joints may be enlarged and painful, and there may be flattening of the vertebral bodies with hypoplasia of the pelvis. About 10 percent of patients develop scoliosis, and many have joint degeneration in later life. Preventive management should include early assessment of the jaw and palate to diagnose Robin sequence; prone positioning during sleep will allow the jaw to descend and prevent obstructive apnea. Early and aggressive ophthalmology evaluation is needed, with close monitoring by retinal specialists. Patients tend to avoid strenuous activity because of joint pain, but they should be counseled about the possibility of high-impact sports augmenting later joint degeneration. Regular evaluations for alignment of the joints and spine are needed.

Marfan syndrome

Terminology

Several conditions may exhibit the elongated body proportions and tall stature of a Marfanoid habitus, but the presence of these proportions plus ectopia lentis and aortic aneurysm is strongly suggestive of Marfan syndrome. Congenital contractural arachnodactyly (Beals syndrome) and homocystinuria have produced similar phenotypes, and Marfan's original patient is now thought to have been affected with Beals syndrome (Gorlin et al., 1990, pp. 267–73). Affected patients have long, narrow, and hyperextensible fingers ("arachnodactyly") and limbs ("dolichostenomelia"). A degenerative process affecting the aorta and other blood vessels in Marfan syndrome is termed "cystic medial necrosis." Like other findings of the disorder, cystic medial necrosis of the aorta by itself is suggestive but not diagnostic of Marfan syndrome.

Incidence, etiology, and differential diagnosis

The incidence of Marfan syndrome is estimated to be as high as 1 in 10,000 births, and occurs in many ethnic groups. The disorder exhibits autosomal dominant inheritance with 15 percent of patients representing new mutations. Marfan syndrome is caused by mutations at the fibrillin-1 locus on chromosome 15; the large size of the gene and the diverse nature of the mutations has so far not allowed routine DNA diagnostic testing. Isolated ectopia lentis has also been related to a fibrillin-1 mutation (Lonnqvist et al., 1994), and Beals syndrome is caused by mutations in fibrillin-2 on chromosome 5. The differential diagnosis includes other connective tissue dysplasias such as homocystinuria or Beals syndrome; it would have given comfort to Dr. Marfan to realize the many patients reported as having Beals syndrome are thought now to have Marfan syndrome (Pyeritz, 1993). The ear anomalies seen in Beals syndrome and plasma amino acids in patients with no family history should allow differentiation. Interpretation of autopsy or surgical specimens is also difficult, because cystic medial necrosis may occur as an isolated finding or in congenital syphilis. Furthermore, ectopia lentis can occur as an isolated abnormality with autosomal dominant inheritance, and Gorlin et al. (1990, pp. 267–73) tabulated 24 different disorders with mitral valve prolapse. Diagnostic criteria have been published that require at least one major manifestation in patients with an affected first-degree relative and two major manifestations in patients with an unremarkable family history (Pyeritz, 1993; De Paepe et al., 1996). Recently, revised criteria from a Berlin conference required involvement of a third system in addition to major manifestations in two systems before the diagnosis of Marfan syndrome is secure (De Paepe et al., 1996). However, Pyeritz (1993) emphasized the arbitrary and age-sensitive nature of these criteria, asserting that Marfan syndrome is one end of a continuum of connective tissue abnormality that is a challenge for molecular diagnosis and clinical delineation to resolve. Although molecular testing could help delineate this spectrum, it is only available in research laboratories (Burn et al., 1997; Maron et al., 1998).

Diagnostic evaluation and medical counseling

Many patients with Marfan syndrome will not present in the newborn period. Some show signs in later childhood and still others are identified as asymptomatic adults who have an affected relative. Once the diagnosis is suspected, all patients should have an ophthalmologic examination and echocardiography by a cardiologist who is experienced with the condition. The aortic root diameter can be plotted against norms for the patient's age and size, allowing recognition of subclinical dilatation. Optic lens dislocation may not be obvious, and slit lamp exam with a fully dilated pupil may be needed to detect lens hyperkinesia due to laxity of the ciliary ligament (Pyeritz, 1993). Many patients with Marfan syndrome will not have either of these major findings, making decisions about preventive management difficult. If the physician judges the patient is at risk of Marfan syndrome, medical counseling should include prohibition of collision or highly competitive sports, and of isometric exercises that adversely strain cardiac output (Pyeritz, 1993). Emotional stress should also be avoided where possible. Such advice is better accepted after the tragic death of olympic star Flo Hyman, but difficult to enforce in asymptomatic adolescents (Wight & Salem, 1995). Pregnancy is thought to be of higher risk in Marfan syndrome (Elkayam et al., 1995), but Rossiter et al. (1995) reported minimal complications in women whose aortic root was less than 40 mm in width.

Family and psychosocial counseling

Genetic counseling for Marfan syndrome is straightforward numerically but complicated in terms of medical recommendations and patient self-image. All at-risk patients should be referred to a genetic specialist and probably to an experienced cardiologist for detection of subtle manifestations. Affected individuals will have a 50 percent risk of transmitting the condition, and severely affected females should be informed of higher complication rates during pregnancy (Pyeritz, 1981; Rossiter et al., 1995). Fetal diagnosis by ultrasound can sometimes be made in the third trimester of pregnancy, allowing parental adjustment and perinatal planning.

In counseling adults with the Marfan syndrome, clinicians must mention the possibility of aortic aneurysm and sudden death to encourage compliance with preventive measures, but it is also important to emphasize that many patients are asymptomatic throughout life. Silverman et al. (1995) reported marked improvement in the life span of patients with Marfan syndrome; expected survival in 1993 was 72 years, compared to 48 years in 1972. Even severely affected patients requiring aortic surgery could expect a 10-year survival rate of 70 percent. Examination of at-risk adults for suggestive skeletal features is recommended but may elicit disagreements from patients who do not wish to consider the diagnosis. Echocardiography is a useful arbiter, since the results lead directly to a management plan of caution and surveillance (when negative) or of discussion of beta-blocker therapy (when positive). When the diagnostic criteria (De Paepe et al., 1996) are fulfilled, beta-blocker therapy is started even in the absence of aortic dilatation. Parent Support Groups are listed on the Marfan syndrome checklist, part 1.

Natural history and complications

When signs of Marfan syndrome are recognized during infancy or childhood, the outcome is often poor. Graham et al. (1989) reviewed 50 affected infants, of whom 83 percent had serious cardiac abnormalities at birth. Cardiac disease tended to progress in these infants, with 5 of the authors' patients (22 percent) dying in early childhood. Of interest was the presence of congenital hand contractures, many typical skeletal anomalies, and megalocornea in the severely affected infants.

For the more typical patients who present in mid-childhood to adolescence, the spectrum of complications is summarized in the checklist, part 1. Pyeritz & McKusick (1979) provided a classic review of 50 patients with Marfan syndrome. Ocular complications include ectopia lentis (70 percent) and myopia (60 percent); echocardiographic findings (96 percent abnormal) include aortic root enlargement (84 percent) and mitral valve prolapse (58 percent), and skeletal complications include kyphoscoliosis (44 percent), pectus deformity (68 percent), and flat feet (44 percent). Izquierdo et al. (1994) reported a 19 percent incidence of strabismus in Marfan syndrome. On clinical examination, 30 percent had a mid-systolic click typical of mitral valve prolapse, 10 percent had a murmur suggestive of aortic regurgitation, and 6 percent had a murmur suggestive of mitral regurgitation. Most were tall (56 percent greater than 95th centile for age), most had arachnodactyly (88 percent), and some had obvious stretch marks (24 percent). Since these were mostly adults, these frequencies provide a maximal level to expect when examining children and adolescents.

The cardiac symptoms of adolescents and adults with Marfan syndrome include palpitations, dyspnea, and light-headedness associated with mitral valve prolapse (not with arrhythmias), and chest pain related to pneumothorax or aortic dissection (Hirata et al., 1992). Finkbohner et al. (1995) reported recurrences of aortic dissection after surgical repair and emphasized that Marfan syndrome is a disease of the entire aorta. Westaby (1995) reported improvements in surgery for aortic aneurysms using biologic glues and stressed the better outlook for patients afforded by life-long beta-adrenergic blockade. Coselli et al. (1995) stressed the need for life-long follow-up to detect complications after cardiac surgery in Marfan syndrome.

Thoracic surgical management of children may require different approaches (Tsang et al., 1994).

Besides the cardinal ocular, cardiac, and skeletal manifestations, other complications of Marfan syndrome can include a high palate with dental crowding, severe scoliosis with restrictive pulmonary disease and cor pulmonale, unusual lens shape (microspherophlakia) with later predisposition to cataracts, retinal lattice degeneration with rare detachment, increased bruisability but normal healing of skin, and ectasia of the spinal dura with occasional nerve root pain in the neck and pelvic pain due to anterior meningocele (Gorlin et al., 1990, pp. 267–73; Pyeritz, 1993; Schneider et al., 1993). Grahame & Pyeritz (1995) reported locomotor symptoms including spinal pain, arthralgia, ligament injury, and fracture in 96 percent of adults with Marfan syndrome, with no symptoms in children under age 5 years. Women with Marfan syndrome have more severe osteoporosis (Kohlmeier et al., 1993).

Marfan syndrome preventive medical checklist

In neonates with skeletal changes suggestive of Marfan syndrome (elongated limbs and fingers, hand contractures, hernias, pectus), echocardiography and ophthalmologic evaluation should be performed (checklist, parts 2–4; Committee on Genetics, 1996). These same evaluations should be performed on older patients at the time of diagnosis or when affected relatives bring them to attention, providing they have suggestive clinical findings. Regular evaluations of the eyes, heart, and skeletal system then constitute the core of management, including dental and optometric assessments when children are old enough. Because of the risk of scoliosis, adolescents may require evaluation by orthopedics at the time surrounding puberty.

An important and somewhat controversial management strategy is directed toward minimizing the progression of aortic root dilation by treatment with β-adrenergic blocking drugs such as propranolol. Pyeritz (1993) provided a thorough discussion of the difficulties in designing controlled trials testing these drugs, and of the advantages of newer $\beta2$-receptor blocking drugs such as atenolol that have long half-lives and are specific for cardiac tissue. Certain studies have demonstrated slowing of the rate of aortic root dilation by beta-adrenergic blockade (Salim et al., 1994), and many recommend starting beta-blocker therapy once the diagnosis of Marfan syndrome is made. Severely affected children and adults should certainly be considered for atenelol therapy, with monitoring of aortic root size in patients with mild dilation. The varying experience and indications for thoracic surgery in Marfan syndrome (e.g., Hirata et al., 1992; Pyeritz, 1993; Coselli et al., 1995; Finkbohner et al., 1995) emphasize the need for patients to be followed by cardiologists and cardiovascular surgeons who are experienced with the disorder.

Ehlers–Danlos syndrome, types IV, VI, and VII

Ehlers–Danlos syndrome is a heterogeneous group of disorders characterized by remarkable joint laxity, elastic skin, and vascular fragility that may compromise internal organs (Byers, 1994). Steinmann et al. (1993) recounted the prominent place of "elastic men" at fairgrounds. Table 16.1 lists the more common types of Ehlers–Danlos syndrome, indicating that most exhibit autosomal dominant inheritance. Steinmann et al. (1993) questioned whether Ehlers–Danlos syndrome type V is a distinct entity. The former type VIII (with periodontal disease) is now thought to be part of type IV, and the former type IX (occipital horn disease) is classified as a disorder of copper metabolism. Several of the less common types of Ehlers–Danlos syndrome will be discussed before discussing the type I–III group in detail.

Ehlers–Danlos syndrome type IV

The ecchymotic or arterial form of Ehlers–Danlos syndrome (type IV) is the most severe of these disorders. It is an autosomal dominant disorder caused by mutations in type III collagen. Mortality is significant, with 40 percent of affected patients dying before age 40 (Gorlin et al., 1990, pp. 433–5). The skin is not elastic but is thin and translucent with visible venous patterns. There is a subtle facial resemblance among patients, with a thin nose and prominent eyes producing an aged appearance. The weakened vascular tissue is evidenced superficially by varicose veins and internally by aneurysms, dissections, and hemorrhages that may damage a variety of organs. Intestinal ruptures may present as abdominal pain, and bleeding into limbs may produce compartment syndromes. Myocardial infarction may occur in young individuals (Ades et al., 1995), and cerebrovascular hemorrhage and strokes were noted in 19 of 202 (9.4 percent) of individuals with type IV Ehlers–Danlos syndrome (North et al., 1995b).

Preventive management of Ehlers–Danlos syndrome type IV consists of attempts to minimize strain that might provoke bleeding episodes since no curative treatment is available (Steinmann et al., 1993; Nuss & Manco-Johnson, 1995). Strenuous exercise and collision sports should be prohibited, and cough or constipation should be treated with antitussives and laxatives. Anticoagulant therapy and aspirin therapy should be avoided (Steinmann et al., 1993). Appropriate response to bleeding is important, since surgery and angiography have high rates of complications. Vascular fragility can be significant, so medical procedures should avoid intramuscular injections or indwelling catheters. Meldon et al. (1996) reported a case with iliac artery rupture. Because recurrence of colon perforation is so common, colectomy is recommended after the first episode (Steinmann et al., 1993).

Ehlers–Danlos syndrome type VI

Type VI Ehlers–Danlos syndrome is also called the "ocular-scoliotic" type because of ruptured globes, retinal detachment, and severe kyphoscoliosis. It is an autosomal recessive disorder, but the responsible gene has not been characterized. Thoracic cage deformity and hypotonia may cause pulmonary restrictions and episodes of pneumonia during infancy. Early death has been reported. Preventive management consists of frequent musculoskeletal evaluation, regular ophthalmologic referral, and medical counseling to avoid strenuous exercise or collision sports. Infants should be watched for signs of pulmonary compromise or pneumonia, and orthopedic monitoring will often be necessary for progressive scoliosis.

Ehlers–Danlos syndrome type VII

Patients with Ehlers–Danlos syndrome type VII (arthrochalasis multiplex congenita) are most striking for joint hypermobility, multiple subluxations or dislocations, and tearing of ligaments. The disorder is autosomal dominant, and is caused by mutations in type I collagen (different regions of the gene from those causing osteogenesis imperfecta). Infants may have congenital hip dislocation and hypotonia. Motor development is often delayed, and many patients have severe scoliosis. Preventive management consists of avoidance of strenuous activity, with appropriate orthopedic monitoring for dislocations and subluxations.

Ehlers–Danlos syndrome, types I–III

Terminology

Ehlers described patients with lax joints and elastic skin in 1901, while Danlos reported unusual scarring and skin fragility in 1908 (Gorlin et al., 1990, pp. 429–32). Subsequent work has defined many types of Ehlers–Danlos syndrome, as described above and summarized in Table 16.1. Types I–III are very similar, with types II and III essentially being mild forms of type I. Type III has been called the benign, hypermobile form of Ehlers–Danlos syndrome because it lacks skin fragility and "cigarette-paper" scarring (Gorlin et al., 1990, pp. 429–32; Steinmann et al., 1993; Jones, 1997, pp. 482–3).

Incidence, etiology, and differential diagnosis

The overall incidence of Ehlers–Danlos syndromes is estimated to be 1 in 5000 births, with types I and II comprising the majority of cases (Steinmann et al., 1993). Type III is about one-tenth as common as types I and II. All three disorders are autosomal dominant and the causative genes have not been characterized, although there are reports of type V collagen abnormalities in some patients. Based on their overlapping clinical manifestations, it will not be surprising if molecular characterization reveals that types I, II, or III Ehlers–Danlos syndrome can result from mutations in the same gene. Differential diagnosis will include other forms of Ehlers–Danlos syndrome, particularly types IV (with greater risks of hemorrhage and vascular disruption) and VI (with greater risks of globe rupture or retinal detachment – Table 16.1). The normal elasticity of skin in type IV and the lack of typical scarring in types IV and VI should aid in differentiating the disorders. It is important to recognize that a large number of syndromes involve increased laxity of connective tissue (e.g., those in Table 16.1) and that normal families may display increased joint laxity. Clinicians should therefore seek the specific clinical manifestations listed for Ehlers–Danlos syndrome in the checklist, part 1 before labeling a patient with this diagnosis.

Two clinical signs that are helpful in recognizing Ehlers–Danlos syndromes are the Meténier sign (easy eversion of the upper eyelids) and the Gorlin sign (ability to touch the nose with the tongue; Gorlin et al., 1990, pp. 429–31). Signs of joint hypermobility include passive bending of the wrist and thumb to touch the forearm and to wrap one arm behind the back and reach the umbilicus.

Diagnostic evaluation and medical counseling

Most children with types I–III Ehlers–Danlos syndrome present in early childhood because of motor delay from joint laxity and hypotonia. Patients with type I may also present because of increased bruisability, skin fragility, or unusual scarring. There is no specific diagnostic testing for types I–III Ehlers–Danlos syndrome, but skin punch biopsy and fibroblast culture may be considered to rule out types IV (type III collagen defects) or VI. Collagen studies on Ehlers–Danlos syndrome patients are available only through research laboratories. Other evaluations should include ophthalmologic examination as a baseline and to exclude more severe forms of Ehlers–Danlos syndrome. Echocardiography is also warranted after the diagnosis is made so that mitral valve prolapse and congenital heart defects (pulmonic stenosis, septal defects) can be ruled out. The tendencies for bruising and scarring bring some children with Ehlers–Danlos syndrome type I to attention because of suspected child abuse.

Family and psychosocial counseling

Patients with Ehlers–Danlos syndrome types I–III have a 50 percent risk to transmit the condition, and couples should be counseled regarding the risks for prematurity, and bladder or rectal prolapse during pregnancy and delivery (Hordnes, 1994). The normal life span and intelligence in these disorders warrants optimistic counseling with emphasis on periodic evaluation of the eyes and heart. However, Lumley et al. (1994) reported significant psychosocial problems among 41 adults and 7 children with Ehlers–Danlos syndrome. They noted anxiety, depression, anger, sexual difficulties, reproductive concerns, and frustration with the medical care system (Lumley et al., 1994). Psychological intervention was recommended for some families. Parent support groups are listed on the Ehlers–Danlos checklist, part 1.

Natural history and complications

The complications of Ehlers–Danlos syndrome types I–III include prematurity, since the extra-embryonic membranes are fetal in origin and may exhibit fragility. Mothers face an increased risk for postpartum hemorrhage and prolapse of the uterus or bladder (Gorlin et al., 1990, pp. 429–31). Neonates have increased joint mobility but few other complications; infants often come to attention because of developmental delay due to joint laxity and easy bruisability.

As children grow older, their chief complications affect the eyes, heart, skin, and skeleton. The face may be unusual, with occasional blue sclerae and epicanthal folds. Eye anomalies include microcornea, strabismus, angioid streaks, and detachment of the retina. The teeth may have abnormal enamel and dentin formation, with altered tooth morphology. The gums are fragile, and periodontal disease can occur at an early age (Gorlin et al., 1990, pp. 429–31; Pope et al., 1992). Subluxation of the temporomandibular joint may occur. Skin findings include hyperelasticity, gaping wounds from minor trauma, and formation of finely wrinkled, pigmented scars that are likened to cigarette paper. There may be nodules under the skin (pseudotumors), and calcified cysts occur in about 30 percent of patients. Thinning of the skin makes acrocyanosis more prominent in children and varicosities more prominent in adults. Skeletal anomalies include flat feet, genu recurvatum, club feet, and kyphoscoliosis (checklist, part 1). Inguinal or umbilical hernias are more common. Occasional features include reflux nephropathy (Ghosh & O'Bryan, 1995) and peripheral neuropathy (Galan & Kousseff, 1995).

Ehlers–Danlos syndrome types I–III preventive medical checklist

Knowledge of Ehlers–Danlos syndrome types I–III during pregnancy allows planning for the possibility of maternal hemorrhage, bleeding from episiotomy wounds or lacerations, and observation for bladder or rectal prolapse (checklist, parts 2–4). There will be a 50 percent risk of the infant being affected, with a higher risk for prematurity. After birth, the infant should be evaluated for signs of joint laxity and skin elasticity, with ophthalmologic and cardiologic consultation in suspect patients. For children without a family history, ophthalmologic and cardiologic evaluations should be performed once the diagnosis is considered. Fragility of the gums and mild hypotonia may lead to feeding problems, so nutrition and growth, eyes, heart, skin, and joints should be assessed during each pediatric visit. Dental referral should be performed once the child has teeth. Because scoliosis and joint dislocations are common, a baseline orthopedic evaluation may be worthwhile once the child begins walking.

In the adolescent and adult years, surveillance of the eyes, skin, and joints should continue with auscultation for signs of mitral or tricuspid valve prolapse. Patients who have had an earlier echocardiogram to rule out congenital heart lesions can probably be followed symptomatically, but changing auscultatory or clinical signs warrant repeat echocardiography. Counseling to avoid high-impact or collision sports and minimize joint/skin trauma is worthwhile. Bracing and fusions seem to be the most common methods for orthopedic treatment of injured joints (Ainsworth & Aulicino, 1993), including spinal fusions for severe scoliosis (McMaster, 1994).

Preventive Management of Marfan syndrome

Clinical diagnosis: A pattern of manifestations including ectopia lentis and dilatation or aneurysm of the aorta in individuals with tall and thin body build ("Marfanoid habitus"), long, lax fingers ("arachnodactyly"), and limbs ("dolichostenomelia"), other findings of connective tissue weakness such as striae, pectus excavatum, scoliosis, hernias, and flat feet; major manifestations in two organ systems plus minor findings are required for diagnosis (De Paepe et al., 1996).

Incidence: 1 in 10,000 live births.

Laboratory diagnosis: Mutations in the fibrillin gene on chromosome 15 cause Marfan syndrome, but DNA diagnosis is not routinely available.

Genetics: The disorder exhibits autosomal dominant inheritance with 15% of patients representing new mutations. Affected individuals have a 50% risk for transmission to offspring.

Key management issues: Echocardiography and ophthalmologic evaluation at the time of diagnosis; subsequent monitoring of the eyes, heart, and skeletal system, including regular ophthalmology, cardiology, dentistry, dental, and orthopedic evaluations; consideration of β-adrenergic blocking drugs such as propranolol to treat aortic dilation.

Growth Charts: Specific charts available in Pyeritz et al. (1985).

Parent groups: National Marfan Foundation 382 Main Street Port Washington, NY 11050 (516) 883-8712, staff@marfan.ca, http://.marfan.ca; Canadian Marfan Association, Central Plaza PO, 128 Queen St. S., P.O. Box 42257, Mississauga ON, Canada L5M 4Z0, (905)826-3223, marfan@istar.ca; Marfan Association UK, Rochester House, 5 Aldershot Road, Fleet, Hampshire GU13 9NG England, (01252)-810-472, http://www.thenet.co.uk/~marfan/

Basis for management recommendations: Guidelines formulated by the Committee on Genetics, American Academy of Pediatrics (1996).

Summary of clinical concerns

General	Learning	Verbal-performance discrepancy (rare)
	Behavior	Hyperactivity (rare)
	Growth	**Tall stature** (58%), low upper/lower segment ratio (77%), asthenic habitus
Facial	Eye	**Ocular anomalies** (70%) – ectopia lentis (60%), myopia (34%), retinal detachment (6.4%); lens dislocation
	Mouth	**High palate** (40–60%), cleft palate, dental malocclusion, mandibular prognathism, temporomandibular joint disease
Surface	Neck/trunk	**Pectus excavatum** (68%), **inguinal hernia** (22%)
Skeletal	Axial	**Scoliosis** (44%)
	Limbs	**Arachnodactyly** (88%), **flat feet** (44%), joint laxity, recurrent dislocations
Internal	Pulmonary	Reduced vital capacity, pneumothorax (4.4%), emphysema
	Circulatory	**Cardiac dysfunction** (98%), aortic enlargement (84%), mitral valve dysfunction (69%), abnormal echocardiogram (87), mitral prolapse (67–100%), cardiac arrythmias (33%)
Neural	CNS	Sacral meningocele, dural ectasia
	Sensory	Visual deficits (20%)

Bold: frequency > 20%

Key references

Committee on Genetics, American Academy of Pediatrics (1996). *Pediatrics* 98:821–978.
De Paepe, A. et al. (1996). *Proceedings of the Greenwood Genetic Center* 15:127.
Pyeritz, R. E. (1981). *American Journal of Medicine* 71:784–90.
Pyeritz, R. E. et al. (1985).In *Endocrine Genetics and the Genetics of Growth.* New York: Alan R. Liss.
Salim, M. A. et al. (1994). *American Journal of Cardiology* 74:629–33.

Marfan syndrome

Preventive medical checklist (0–1yr)

Patient **Birth Date** / / **Number**

Pediatric	Screen		Evaluate		Refer/Counsel	
Neonatal / / *Newborn screen* ❑ *HB* ❑	Echocardiogram	❑	Palate Eyes Heart, joints	❑ ❑ ❑	Genetic evaluation Cardiology	❑ ❑
1 month / /			Eyes Heart, joints	❑ ❑	Family support[4]	❑
2 months / / *HB[1]* ❑ *Hib* ❑ *DTaP, IPV* ❑ *RV* ❑	Vision[2]	❑	Eyes Heart, joints	❑ ❑	Early intervention[5] Genetic counseling	❑ ❑
4 months / / *HB[1]* ❑ *Hib* ❑ *DTaP/IPV* ❑ *RV* ❑	Vision[2]	❑	Eyes Heart, joints	❑ ❑	Early intervention[4,6]	❑
6 months / / *Hib* ❑ *IPV[1]* ❑ *DTaP* ❑ *RV* ❑	Growth Vision[2]	❑ ❑	Eyes Heart, joints	❑ ❑	Family support[5] Cardiology	❑ ❑
9 months / / *IPV[1]* ❑	Vision[2]	❑	Eyes Heart, joints	❑ ❑		
1 year / / *HB* ❑ *Hib[1]* ❑ *IPV[1]* ❑ *MMR[1]* ❑ *Var[1]* ❑	Growth Vision[2]	❑ ❑	Eyes Heart, joints	❑ ❑	Family support[4] Early intervention[5] Genetics Ophthalmology	❑ ❑ ❑ ❑

Clinical concerns for Marfan syndrome, ages 0–1 year

Myopia, lens dislocation	Mitral valve dysfunction	Sacral meningocele
Retinal detachment	Aortic enlargement	Umbilical, inguinal hernia
Cleft palate	Aortic insufficiency	Joint dislocations
Dental malocclusion	Ventricular arrythmias	Flat feet, pectus

Guidelines for the neonatal period should be undertaken *at whatever age* the diagnosis is made; DTaP, acellular DTP; IPV, inactivated poliovirus (oral polio also used); RV, rotavirus; MMR, measles–mumps–rubella; Var, varicella; [1]alternative timing; [2]by practitioner; [3]as dictated by clinical findings; [4]parent group, family/sib, financial, and behavioral issues as discussed in the preface; [5]including developmental monitoring and motor/speech therapy.

Marfan syndrome

Preventive medical checklist (15m–6yrs)

Patient   **Birth Date**   /   /   **Number**

Pediatric	Screen		Evaluate		Refer/Counsel	
15 months / / *Hib*[1] ❑ *MMR*[1] ❑ *DTaP, IPV*[1] ❑ *Varicella*[1] ❑	Vision[2]	❑	Eyes Heart, joints	❑ ❑	Family support[4] Early intervention[5]	❑ ❑
18 months / / *DTaP, IPV*[1] ❑ *Varicella*[1] ❑ *Influenza*[3] ❑	Vision[2]	❑	Eyes Heart, joints	❑ ❑		
2 years / / *Influenza*[3] ❑ *Pneumovax*[3] ❑ *Dentist* ❑	Growth Vision[2]	❑ ❑	Eyes Heart, joints	❑ ❑	Family support[4] Genetics Cardiology Ophthalmology	❑ ❑ ❑ ❑
3 years / / *Influenza*[3] ❑ *Pneumovax*[3] ❑ *Dentist* ❑	Growth Vision[2]	❑ ❑	Eyes Heart, joints	❑ ❑	Family support[4] Preschool transition[5] Cardiology Ophthalmology Orthopedics	❑ ❑ ❑ ❑ ❑
4 years / / *Influenza*[3] ❑ *Pneumovax*[3] ❑ *Dentist* ❑	Echocardiogram Vision[3]	❑ ❑	Heart, lungs Spine Joints	❑ ❑ ❑	Family support[4] Preschool program[5] Genetics Cardiology	❑ ❑ ❑ ❑
5 years / / *DTaP, IPV*[1] ❑ *MMR*[1] ❑	Growth Echocardiogram Vision[3]	❑ ❑ ❑	Heart, lungs Spine Joints	❑ ❑ ❑	School transition Cardiology Ophthalmology	❑ ❑ ❑
6 years / / *DTaP, IPV*[1] ❑ *MMR*[1] ❑ *Dentist* ❑	Growth Echocardiogram Vision[3]	❑ ❑ ❑	Heart, lungs Spine Joints	❑ ❑ ❑	Family support[4] Genetics Cardiology Ophthalmology Orthopedics[3]	❑ ❑ ❑ ❑ ❑

Clinical concerns for Marfan syndrome, ages 1–6 years

Myopia, lens dislocation	Mitral valve dysfunction	Sacral meningocele
Retinal detachment	Aortic enlargement	Umbilical, inguinal hernia
Cleft palate	Aortic insufficiency	Joint dislocations
Dental malocclusion	Ventricular arrythmias	Flat feet, pectus

Guidelines for prior ages should be undertaken *at the time of diagnosis*; DTaP, acellular DTP; IPV, inactivated poliovirus (oral polio also used); MMR, measles–mumps–rubella; [1]alternative timing; [2]by practitioner; [3]as dictated by clinical findings; [4]parent group, family/sib, financial, and behavioral issues as discussed in the preface; [5]including developmental monitoring and motor/speech therapy.

Marfan syndrome

Preventive medical checklist (6+ yrs)

Patient _____ **Birth Date** / / **Number** _____

Pediatric	Screen		Evaluate		Refer/Counsel	
8 years / / _Dentist_ ❏	Growth Cardiac Echocardiogram Vision[2]	❏ ❏ ❏ ❏	Heart, lungs Spine Joints	❏ ❏ ❏	Avoid collision, high intensity sports Cardiology Ophthalmology Endocrinology[3]	 ❏ ❏ ❏ ❏
10 years / /	Growth Echocardiogram Vision[2]	❏ ❏ ❏	Heart, lungs Spine Joints	❏ ❏ ❏	Genetics Cardiology Ophthalmology Endocrinology[3]	❏ ❏ ❏ ❏
12 years / / _Td[1], MMR, Var_ ❏ _CBC_ ❏ _Dentist_ ❏ _Scoliosis_ ❏ _Cholesterol_ ❏	Echocardiogram Vision[2]	❏ ❏	Heart, lungs Spine Joints	❏ ❏ ❏	Family support[4] Avoid collision, high intensity sports Cardiology Ophthalmology Orthopedics[3]	❏ ❏ ❏ ❏ ❏
14 years / / _CBC_ ❏ _Dentist_ ❏ _Cholesterol_ ❏ _Breast CA_ ❏ _Testicular CA_ ❏	Echocardiogram Vision[2]	❏ ❏	Heart, lungs Spine Joints	❏ ❏ ❏	Cardiology Ophthalmology	❏ ❏
16 years / / _Td[1]_ ❏ _CBC_ ❏ _Cholesterol_ ❏ _Sexual[5]_ ❏ _Dentist_ ❏	Growth Echocardiogram Vision[2]	❏ ❏ ❏	Heart, lungs Spine Joints	❏ ❏ ❏	Avoid collision, high intensity sports Genetics Cardiology Ophthalmology	 ❏ ❏ ❏ ❏
18 years / / _CBC_ ❏ _Sexual[5]_ ❏ _Cholesterol_ ❏ _Scoliosis_ ❏	Echocardiogram Vision[2]	❏ ❏	Heart, lungs Spine Joints	❏ ❏ ❏	Cardiology Ophthalmology	❏ ❏
20 years[6] / / _CBC_ ❏ _Sexual[5]_ ❏ _Cholesterol_ ❏ _Dentist_ ❏	Echocardiogram Vision[2]	❏ ❏	Heart, lungs Spine Joints	❏ ❏ ❏	Family support[4] Avoid collision, high intensity sports Cardiology Ophthalmology Orthopedics[3]	❏ ❏ ❏ ❏ ❏

Clinical concerns for Marfan syndrome, ages 6+ years

Tall stature	Mitral valve dysfunction	Learning differences
Myopia, lens dislocation	Aortic dilation, insufficiency	Inguinal hernia
Retinal detachment	Ventricular arrythmias	Joint dislocations
Dental malocclusion	Spontaneous pneumothorax	Flat feet, pectus, scoliosis

Guidelines for prior ages should be undertaken _at the time of diagnosis_; Td, tetanus/diphtheria; MMR, measles–mumps–rubella; Var, varicella; [1]alternative timing; [2]by practitioner; [3]as dictated by clinical findings; [4]parent group, family/sib, financial, and behavioral issues as discussed in the preface; [5]birth control, STD screening if sexually active; [6]repeat every decade.

Preventive Management of Ehlers–Danlos syndromes

Clinical diagnosis: Pattern of manifestations in types I–III including lax joints, hyperelastic skin, unusual "cigarette paper" scarring, and skin fragility. Examination may elicit Méténier's sign (easy eversion of upper lids) or Gorlin's sign (touching nose with tip of tongue). Types IV and VI are more severe disorders with higher risks for vascular complications and fewer skin findings.

Incidence: 1 in 5,000 live births.

Laboratory diagnosis: Several types of Ehlers–Danlos syndrome have been related to mutations in collagen genes, but DNA diagnosis is not routinely available.

Genetics: Autosomal dominant inheritance with a 50% risk for affected individuals to transmit the disease. Pregnancy risks include premature delivery for affected infants and bladder or rectal prolapse for affected mothers (Hordnes, 1994).

Key management issues: Ophthalmologic and cardiologic evaluation in suspect cases, monitoring of the skin, eyes, teeth, and joints with auscultation for signs of mitral or tricuspid valve prolapse, counseling to avoid high-impact or collision sports, bracing and fusions for injured joints including spinal fusions for severe scoliosis (Ainsworth & Aulicino, 1993), counseling and monitoring for pregnancy risks

Growth Charts: Growth is usually normal, allowing the use of standard growth charts.

Parent groups: Ehlers–Danlos National Foundation, 6399 Wilshire Blvd. #510, Los Angeles CA, 90048, (213) 651-3038, LooseJoint@aol.com, http://www.phoenix.net/~leigh/eds; Ms. Valerie Burrows, Ehlers–Danlos Support Group, 1 Chandler Close, Richmond, North Yorkshire, DL10 5QQ UK, (01748) 823-867, http://www.atv.ndirect.co.uk/ General.htm

Basis for management recommendations: Derived from the complications below as documented by Steinmann et al. (1993) and Gorlin et al. (1990, pp. 429–31).

Summary of clinical concerns

General	Life cycle	Fragile fetal membranes, prematurity
Facial	Face	Broad/shallow nasal bridge, **epicanthal folds** (25%)
	Eye	Ocular anomalies (strabismus, myopia, blue sclerae, retinal detachment)
	Ear	Overturned helices
	Mouth	Dental anomalies, periodontal disease, temporomandibular joint subluxation
Surface	Neck/trunk	**Inguinal hernias** (10–20%), umbilical hernias
	Epidermal	Spheroids (33% – calcified cysts over bony prominences), enhanced scarring, easy bruising
Skeletal	Axial	**Kyphoscoliosis** (15–20%)
	Limbs	Joint laxity, flat feet, **genu recurvatum** (25%), club feet (5%), congenital hip dislocation, joint effusions and dislocations, **osteoarthritis** (20–60%)
Internal	Digestive	Gastrointestinal diverticula, rectal prolapse, constipation
	Circulatory	Cardiac septal defects, bicuspid aortic valve, mitral valve prolapse, tricuspid valve prolapse
	RES	Hematomas, bleeding after surgeries
	Excretory	Bladder prolapse
	Genital	Uterine prolapse
Neural	Motor	Hypotonia, early feeding problems
	Sensory	Vision deficits

RES, reticuloendothelial system; **bold:** frequency > 20%

Key references

Ainsworth, S. R. & Aulicino, P. L. (1993). *Clinical Orthopaedics & Related Research* 286:250–6.

Byers, P. H. (1994). *Journal of Investigative Dermatology* 103 (suppl. 5):47S-52S.

Gorlin, R. J. et al. (1990). *Syndromes of the Head and Neck.* New York: Oxford.

Hordnes, K. (1994). *Acta Obstetricia et Gynecologica Scandinavica* 73:671–3.

Steinmann, B. et al. (1993). In *Connective Tissue and its Heritable Disorders.* New York: Wiley-Liss.

Ehlers–Danlos syndrome, Types I–III

Preventive medical checklist (0–1yr)

Patient		Birth Date / /		Number	
Pediatric	**Screen**	**Evaluate**		**Refer/Counsel**	
Neonatal / / *Newborn screen* ❏ *HB* ❏		Feeding Eyes Hips	❏ ❏ ❏	Genetic evaluation	❏
1 month / /	Vision[2] ❏	Feeding Eyes Hips	❏ ❏ ❏	Family support[4]	❏
2 months / / *HB[1]* ❏ *Hib* ❏ *DTaP, IPV* ❏ *RV* ❏	Vision[2] ❏	Feeding Eyes Hips	❏ ❏ ❏	Early intervention[3,5] Genetic counseling	❏ ❏
4 months / / *HB[1]* ❏ *Hib* ❏ *DTaP/IPV* ❏ *RV* ❏	Vision[2] ❏	Feeding Eyes Joints	❏ ❏ ❏	Early intervention[3,5]	❏
6 months / / *Hib* ❏ *IPV[1]* ❏ *DTaP* ❏ *RV* ❏	Vision[2] ❏	Feeding Eyes Joints	❏ ❏ ❏	Family support[4]	❏
9 months / / *IPV[1]* ❏	Vision[2] ❏	Feeding Eyes Joints	❏ ❏ ❏		
1 year / / *HB* ❏ *Hib[1]* ❏ *IPV[1]* ❏ *MMR[1]* ❏ *Var[1]* ❏	Vision[2] ❏	Heart Feeding Eyes Skin, joints	❏ ❏ ❏ ❏	Family support[5] Early intervention[4,6] Genetics Ophthalmology Cardiology	❏ ❏ ❏ ❏ ❏

Clinical concerns for Ehlers–Danlos syndrome, ages 0–1 year

Hypotonia, motor delays	Cardiac septal defects	Easy bruisability
Feeding problems	Mitral valve prolapse	Bleeding after surgery
Myopia, strabismus	Congenital hip dislocation	Cutaneous fragility
Dental anomalies	Umbilical, inguinal hernia	Enhanced scarring

Guidelines for the neonatal period should be undertaken *at whatever age* the diagnosis is made; DTaP, acellular DTP; IPV, inactivated poliovirus (oral polio also used); RV, rotavirus; MMR, measles–mumps–rubella; Var, varicella; [1]alternative timing; [2]by practitioner; [3]as dictated by clinical findings; [4]parent group, family/sib, financial, and behavioral issues as discussed in the preface; [5]including developmental monitoring and motor/speech therapy.

Ehlers–Danlos syndrome, Types I–III

Preventive medical checklist (15m–6yrs)

Patient		Birth Date / /		Number	
Pediatric	**Screen**	**Evaluate**		**Refer/Counsel**	
15 months / / Hib[1] ❑ MMR[1] ❑ DTaP, IPV[1] ❑ Varicella[1] ❑	Vision[2] ❑	Feeding Eyes Skin, joints	❑ ❑ ❑	Family support[4] Early intervention[5]	❑ ❑
18 months / / DTaP, IPV[1] ❑ Varicella[1] ❑ Influenza[3] ❑	Vision[2] ❑	Feeding Eyes Skin, joints	❑ ❑ ❑		
2 years / / Influenza[3] ❑ Pneumovax[3] ❑ Dentist ❑	Vision[2] ❑	Feeding Eyes Skin, joints	❑ ❑ ❑	Family support[4] Genetics Ophthalmology	❑ ❑ ❑
3 years / / Influenza[3] ❑ Pneumovax[3] ❑ Dentist ❑	Vision[2] ❑	Heart Feeding Eyes Skin, joints	❑ ❑ ❑ ❑	Family support[4] Ophthalmology Orthopedics[3]	❑ ❑ ❑
4 years / / Influenza[3] ❑ Pneumovax[3] ❑ Dentist ❑	Vision[2] ❑	Heart Spine, joints Skin	❑ ❑ ❑	Family support[4] Preschool program[3,5] Genetics Cardiology[4]	❑ ❑ ❑ ❑
5 years / / DTaP, IPV[1] ❑ MMR[1] ❑	Vision[2] ❑	Heart Spine, joints Skin	❑ ❑ ❑		
6 years / / DTaP, IPV[1] ❑ MMR[1] ❑ Dentist ❑	Vision[2] ❑	Heart Spine, joints Skin	❑ ❑ ❑	Family support[5] Ophthalmology[4] Orthopedics[4]	❑ ❑ ❑

Clinical concerns for Ehlers–Danlos syndrome, ages 1–6 years

Hypotonia	Cardiac septal defects	Easy bruisability
Feeding problems	Mitral valve prolapse	Bleeding after surgery
Myopia, strabismus	Congenital hip dislocation	Cutaneous fragility
Dental anomalies	Umbilical, inguinal hernia	Enhanced scarring

Guidelines for prior ages should be undertaken *at the time of diagnosis*; DTaP, acellular DTP; IPV, inactivated poliovirus (oral polio also used); MMR, measles–mumps–rubella; [1]alternative timing; [2]by practitioner; [3]as dictated by clinical findings; [4]parent group, family/sib, financial, and behavioral issues as discussed in the preface; [5]including developmental monitoring and motor/speech therapy.

Ehlers–Danlos syndromes

Preventive medical checklist (6+ yrs)

Patient   **Birth Date**   /   /   **Number**

Pediatric	Screen	Evaluate		Refer/Counsel	
8 years / / *Dentist* ❏	Vision[2] ❏	Heart Spine, joints Skin	❏ ❏ ❏	Avoid collision or high intensity sports[3] Genetics	❏ ❏
10 years / /	Vision[2] ❏	Heart Spine, joints Skin	❏ ❏ ❏		
12 years / / *Td[1], MMR, Var* ❏ *CBC* ❏ *Dentist* ❏ *Scoliosis* ❏ *Cholesterol* ❏	Vision[2] ❏	Heart Spine, joints Skin	❏ ❏ ❏	Family support[4] Genetics Ophthalmology[3] Orthopedics[3]	❏ ❏ ❏ ❏
14 years / / *CBC* ❏ *Dentist* ❏ *Cholesterol* ❏ *Breast CA* ❏ *Testicular CA* ❏	Vision[2] ❏	Heart Spine, joints Skin	❏ ❏ ❏	Avoid collision or high intensity sports[3]	❏
16 years / / *Td[1]* ❏ *CBC* ❏ *Cholesterol* ❏ *Sexual[5]* ❏ *Dentist* ❏	Vision[2] ❏	Heart Spine, joints Skin	❏ ❏ ❏	Genetics	❏
18 years / / *CBC* ❏ *Sexual[5]* ❏ *Cholesterol* ❏ *Scoliosis* ❏	Vision[2] ❏	Heart Spine, joints Skin	❏ ❏ ❏	Avoid collision or high intensity sports[3] Genetics	❏ ❏
20 years[6] / / *CBC* ❏ *Sexual[5]* ❏ *Cholesterol* ❏ *Dentist* ❏	Vision[2] ❏	Heart Spine, joints Skin GI diverticula Arthritis	❏ ❏ ❏ ❏ ❏	Avoid collision or high intensity sports[3] Cardiology[3] Ophthalmology[3] Orthopedics[3]	❏ ❏ ❏ ❏

Clinical concerns for Ehlers–Danlos syndrome, ages 6+ years

Myopia, retinal detachment	Mitral valve prolapse	Easy bruisability
Dental, peridontal disease	Inguinal hernia	Bleeding after surgery
Rectal prolapse	Kyphoscoliosis	Cutaneous fragility
Gastrointestinal diverticula	Genu recurvatum	Enhanced scarring

Guidelines for prior ages should be undertaken *at the time of diagnosis*; Td, tetanus/diphtheria; MMR, measles–mumps–rubella; Var, varicella; GI, gastrointestinal; [1]alternative timing; [2]by practitioner; [3]as dictated by clinical findings; [4]parent group, family/sib, financial, and behavioral issues as discussed in the preface; [5]birth control, STD screening if sexually active; [6]repeat every decade.

17

Integumentary syndromes

Syndromes with primary manifestations affecting the integument comprise a diverse group of relatively rare conditions (Table 17.1). In this chapter, they are categorized as ectodermal dysplasias, albinism, other pigmentary disorders, hemangiomatous disorders, and disorders of radiation sensitivity/accelerated aging. Each disorder will receive a fairly brief description, as only albinism is sufficiently common to be encountered frequently by health professionals.

Ectodermal dysplasias

Hypohidrotic ectodermal dysplasia

Described in the mid-1800s, including mention by Charles Darwin, hypohidrotic ectodermal dysplasia is prototypic of more than 100 disorders that exhibit abnormalities in the hair, teeth, nails, and integumentary glands (Gorlin et al., 1990, pp. 451–4). The incidence is 1 in 100,000 births, with the majority of families exhibiting X-linked recessive inheritance. Genetic mapping studies have defined a locus at the X chromosomal region. Because many disorders have manifestations of ectodermal dysplasia as part of the syndrome spectrum, differential diagnosis is substantial and complex. Referrals to genetics and dermatology specialists are useful for diagnosis and counseling. Decreased numbers of sweat pores can be assessed by a variety of methods, including hypohidrosis by standard sweat testing as performed for diagnosis of cystic fibrosis or by applying starch-iodine mixtures to skin surfaces and noting the distribution and numbers of sweat pores.

Clinical manifestations include a typical face in affected males, with sparse hair, absent or missing eyelashes, frontal bossing with depressed nasal bridge, absence of many permanent teeth, conical maxillary and canine teeth, and protuberant, full lips due to maxillary and dental hypoplasia. The skin is soft and dry, due to the absence of sebaceous glands, and there is scanty body hair. The nails grow slowly and are fragile or spoonshaped. The breasts are hypoplastic, and may be entirely absent in female carriers. Abnormal nasal mucosa and salivary gland function may lead to allergies, sinusitis, and dryness of the mouth. Of most concern in children,

Table 17.1 Integumentary syndromes

Syndrome or disease	Incidence	Inheritance	Complications
Ectodermal dysplasias			
Hypohidrotic ectodermal dysplasia	1 in 100,000	XLR	Sparse hair, dry and hypohidrotic skin, keratitis, sinusitis, absent teeth, conical teeth, high fevers
Ectrodactyly-ectodermal dysplasia-cleft palate (EEC) syndrome	~100 cases	AD	Sparse hair, hypohidrotic skin, photophobia, keratitis, cleft lip/palate, absent teeth, ectrodactyly
Albinism			
Oculocutaneous albinism, type 1	1 in 20,000	AR	Ocular a. (foveal hypoplasia, strabismus, nystagmus), white skin, no tanning
Oculocutaneous albinism, type 2	1 in 20,000	AR	Ocular a. (foveal hypoplasia, strabismus, nystagmus), white skin, no tanning
Ocular albinism	1 in 100,000	XLR, AR	Ocular a. (foveal hypoplasia, strabismus, nystagmus)
Other pigmentary disorders			
Goltz–Gorlin syndrome	~200 cases	XLR	Hyper- or hypopigmented linear streaks on the skin, eye a. (colobomata, strabismus), syndactyly, brachydactyly, urogenital a., cognitive disability
Hypomelanosis of Ito	~50 cases	Chromosomal	Hypopigmented macules and streaks on the skin, microcephaly, seizures, cognitive disability
Incontinentia pigmenti	~200 cases	XLR	Sparse hair, vesicular or pigmented skin, absent teeth, conical teeth, microcephaly, hydrocephalus, seizures, cognitive disability
LEOPARD syndrome	~100 cases	AD	Lentigines, ptosis, hypertelorism, cardiac a., scoliosis, genital a., short stature, cognitive disability
Waardenburg syndrome	~1400 cases	AD	White forelock, dystopia canthorum, heterochromia of the irides, strabismus, sensorineural deafness, Hirschsprung a.
Hemangioma syndromes			
Ataxia-telangiectasia	1 in 100,000	AR	Ataxia, facial and conjunctival telangiectasias, frequent infections, early graying, predisposition to cancer, immune deficiency
Bloom syndrome	~200 cases	AR	Short stature, microcephaly, facial erythema and telangiectasias, hypogonadism, predisposition to cancer, immune deficiency

Table 17.1 (*cont.*)

Syndrome or disease	Incidence	Inheritance	Complications
Osler–Rendu–Weber syndrome	1 in 100,000	AD	Multiple hemorrhagic telangiectasias, pulmonary arteriovenous fistulas, urinary tract bleeding, gastrointestinal bleeding, intracranial bleeding
Rothmund–Thompson syndrome	~150 cases	AR	Short stature, photosensitivity, sparse hair, facial erythema, cataracts, strabismus, dental a., hyper- and hypopigmentation of skin (poikiloderma), hypogonadism, predisposition to sarcomas
Disorders with radiation sensitivity and/or rapid aging			
Cockayne syndrome	~75 cases	AR	Short stature, photosensitivity, sparse hair, retinitis, accelerated aging, early death
Progeria	~75 cases	Sporadic	Short stature, photosensitivity, sparse hair, joint degeneration, atherosclerosis, accelerated aging
Xeroderma pigmentosum	1 in 200,000		Short stature, skin pigmentation, squamous and basal cell carcinomas, early death

Notes:
AR, autosomal recessive; AD, autosomal dominant; XLR, X-linked recessive; a., anomalies.

the hypohidrosis may lead to elevated temperatures during exertion or illness; all families should be counseled about antipyretics and bathing strategies to lower body temperature during these episodes.

Preventive management for hypohidrotic ectodermal dysplasia and related conditions should include early referral to ophthalmology to assess lacrimal gland function and to monitor possible complications such as glaucoma or keratitis. Regular dental evaluation is also important (Boj et al., 1993), and otolaryngologic referral may be needed for the management of atrophic rhinitis, sinusitis, or dysphonia due to atrophy of laryngeal mucosa (Gorlin et al., 1990, pp. 451–4). Cosmetic approaches become important in later childhood and adolescence, with possible need for false teeth or a wig (Boj et al., 1993).

Ectrodactyly-ectodermal dysplasia-clefting (EEC) syndrome

Ectrodactyly, also called "split hand" or "lobster-claw deformity," can occur as an isolated anomaly that exhibits autosomal dominant inheritance. Ectrodactyly, together with ectodermal dysplasia and clefts of the lip and palate, constitutes a rare, autosomal dominant condition with approximately 100 reported cases in the literature (Gorlin et al., 1990, pp. 716–18; Jones, 1997, pp. 294–5). The Hay–Wells syndrome, with ankyloblepharon (adhesions binding together the lateral palpebral fissures), cleft palate and ectodermal dysplasia, is a closely related disorder that also exhibits autosomal dominant inheritance (Jones, 1997, pp. 296–7). The Rapp–Hodgkin syndrome, also autosomal dominant, consists of ectodermal dysplasia, cleft lip/palate, and genital anomalies (Jones, 1997, pp. 543–4). The EEC, Hay–Wells and Rapp–Hodgkin syndromes may well represent variable expressivity of a single autosomal dominant condition; complications and preventive management will be similar for the three conditions.

Complications of the EEC syndrome include sparse hair and eyelashes, eye anomalies (absent lacrimal glands with tearing, photophobia, and keratitis), upper respiratory problems (chronic otitis, conductive hearing loss, abnormal voice to dry vocal cords), oral anomalies (cleft lip/palate, absent or conical teeth), and genitourinary defects (renal duplication, renal aplasia, hydronephrosis, cryptorchidism; Kraemer et al., 1995). In Caucasian patients, the skin and hair are hypopigmented, and there are hypoplastic sebaceous and sweat glands. Preventive management should include ophthalmologic and otolaryngologic referral to ensure monitoring of lacrimal gland and hearing function, dental referral to manage absent or hypoplastic teeth (Tanboga et al., 1992), and a renal sonogram during the initial diagnostic investigation to recognize urinary tract anomalies. Referral to genetics and dermatology for diagnosis and counseling is encouraged, since a variety of syndromes with ectrodactyly and ectodermal dysplasia have been described. As with other forms of ectodermal dysplasia, counseling regarding surveillance for hyperpyrexia in childhood is necessary.

Albinism

Many conditions involve alterations in the production or distribution of melanin, producing light-colored hair, eyes, and/or skin (Sethi et al., 1996; Orlow, 1997; Carden et al., 1998). Tyrosinase deficiency accounts for the classical and most common albinism phenotype, but many other gene products interact to influence melanocyte maturation and distribution (King et al., 1995). Many melanin-regulating genes have been characterized and related to homologous genes in mice skin (King et al., 1995; Sethi et al., 1996; Orlow, 1997; Carden et al., 1998). Albinism is thus a phenotype that has numerous causes ranging from primary albinism associated with severe and diffuse hypopigmentation to associated albinism in syndromes that include localized hypopigmentation as a component feature. Critical to making a diagnosis of albinism is the demonstration of ocular abnormalities such as foveal hypoplasia, strabismus, and nystagmus that reflect a role for melanin in ocular development (King et al., 1995).

Primary albinism can be divided into two categories: oculocutaneous albinism (which affects the hair, skin, and eyes) and ocular albinism (which affects only the eyes). The differences relate to separate derivation of melanocytes in the hair and skin (neural crest origin) and those in the retinal pigmentary epithelium (neurectoderm of the developing optic cup).

Oculocutaneous albinism type 1

Oculocutaneous albinism type 1 includes 4 subtypes with autosomal recessive inheritance. Diagnostic assays are available using the classic hair bulb assay (incubation with tyrosine to produce brown coloration) or molecular analysis that characterizes mutations in the tyrosinase gene (King et al., 1995). Because these assays are not widely used, specific frequencies for the many subtypes of albinism are not known. The general prevalence for albinism ranges from 1 in 10,000 to 1 in 50,000; it is found in all ethnic groups and in all regions of the world.

Heterogeneity of oculocutaneous albinism type 1 includes patients who are tyrosinase-negative and have virtually no pigment throughout their life, patients with residual tyrosinase activity who develop some pigment including distinctive yellow hair, and patients with temperature-sensitive tyrosinase who develop pigment in their distal extremities because these have lower temperature. The latter individuals are analogous to the distal pigment in Siamese cats or Himalayan mice.

Clinical manifestations of oculocutaneous albinism type 1 are generic, albeit milder, for other types of albinism. Melanin within the retinal epithelium and choroid plays an important role in the development of the visual system. As a result, patients with oculocutaneous albinism type 1 have a hypoplastic fovea with reduced visual acuity that cannot be corrected with glasses. There is also misrouting of optic fibers at the chiasm, resulting in alternating strabismus that usually does not develop into amblyopia. Also resulting from the decreased visual acuity and/or developmental abnormalities is nystagmus, which is present from birth in the majority of patients with severe albinism. Absence of melanin pigment in the inner ear also produces changes in the auditory evoked response and enhances patients' susceptibility to noise or drug-induced hearing loss. Occasional patients develop malignant melanoma (Levine et al., 1992).

Tyrosinase-negative oculocutaneous albinism type 1 is distinguished by the absence of pigmentation at birth. Tyrosinase-negative individuals are born with white hair, white skin, and light blue irides that appear pink in certain lights. The hypopigmentation phenotype is constant for all ethnic groups and changes little with age. Exposure to sun usually produces erythema, burning, and little tanning, although patients with residual pigment can tan. As mentioned above, forms of oculocutaneous albinism type 1 that retain partial or temperature-sensitive tyrosinase activity can develop some skin pigment and hair color.

Preventive management of oculocutaneous albinism type 1 includes an early diagnostic evaluation and later protective care. Ocular abnormalities are essential for the diagnosis, and may be documented by visual evoked response testing if foveal hypoplasia and nystagmus are not obvious by clinical inspection. The finding of tyrosinase on hair-bulb assay is helpful for medical counseling in that later acquisition of pigment and less stigmatization can be anticipated. Ophthalmologic examination is essential throughout life, and school arrangements must include provision for large-type texts, appropriate seating, and use of high-contrast visual materials (King et al., 1995; Orlow, 1997). Auditory evoked response studies are not indicated in oculocutaneous albinism unless one of the rare syndromes involving albinism and deafness is suspected. Parents should be counseled about the damaging effects of loud noise, and told to warn health care professionals about the risks of ototoxic antibiotics in their child. The most important protective measures will be to minimize exposure to sun, using sunglasses, long-sleeved clothing, hats, and sunscreens (sun protection factor above 25). Commonsense advice about the occurrence of high-intensity ultraviolet between 10 A.M. and 2 P.M., in certain geographic latitudes, and as reflections from sandy beaches or clouds should be provided.

Oculocutaneous albinism type 2

Formerly distinguished as tyrosinase-positive, "partial," "imperfect," or "incomplete" albinism, oculocutaneous albinism type 2 is caused by a mutation in the P gene, the human homologue of the *pink* gene causing a form of murine albinism (King et al., 1995; Orlow, 1997). This gene is found within the chromosome 15 region that is deleted or abnormally imprinted in the Prader–Willi and Angelman syndromes. Alterations of the P gene explain why some patients with the Prader–Willi and Angelman syndromes have albinoid characteristics such as optic abnormalities, light hair, blue eyes, and pale skin.

Depending on their geographic area, Caucasian individuals with oculocutaneous albinism type 2 vary from minimal (e.g., Scandinavian origin) to moderate (e.g., Mediterranean origin) pigment at birth. The milder patients are hard to distinguish from normal individuals of European descent, who change from blond hair, white skin, and blue eyes as children to darker shades as adults. Most affected individuals of African origin have yellow or yellow-red hair at birth, with blue eyes and white skin (King et al., 1995). In both blacks and whites, affected individuals acquire some pigment with age, including pigmented nevi and freckles with minimal tanning of the skin. Preventive management will be as outlined for oculocutaneous albinism type 1, with ophthalmologic monitoring, provision for visual assistance at school, and protection from sun.

Ocular albinism

Two major types of ocular albinism have been described, and are distinguished by X-linked recessive versus autosomal recessive inheritance. In each disorder, the distinguishing characteristic is hypopigmentation that is limited to the eye. King et al. (1995) emphasized that subclinical cutaneous hypopigmentation is present in individuals with ocular albinism, and that African–American individuals with X-linked ocular albinism may have hypopigmented macules on the skin. The clinical manifestations of ocular albinism are foveal hypoplasia, hypopigmented retina, decreased visual acuity, and nystagmus. The irides are translucent and light blue to brown, with a more normal brown color in African–Americans. Patches of retinal hypopigmentation and iris translucency are found in 80 percent of female carriers of the X-linked form of ocular albinism, but these females rarely have ocular symptoms. Preventive management of individuals with ocular albinism consists of the same ophthalmologic monitoring and school measures mentioned above for oculocutaneous albinism, with alertness for sensorineural deafness, which is occasionally associated (King et al., 1995).

Other pigmentary disorders

Focal dermal hypoplasia (Goltz–Gorlin syndrome)

More than 200 cases of focal dermal hypoplasia have been reported after the initial descriptions of Goltz in 1962 and Gorlin in 1963 (Gorlin et al., 1990, pp. 472–5). Over 90 percent of affected patients are female, raising the possibility of X-linked dominant inheritance with male lethality. Skin findings are distinctive in Goltz–Gorlin syndrome, with linear or reticular hyperpigmented lesions and telangiectases (Pujol et al., 1992; Pereyo et al., 1993). Supernumerary nipples, asymmetry of the breasts, and subcutaneous nodules are also common, and the finger and toenails are often hypoplastic or malformed. Eye anomalies (40 percent of patients) include colobomata of the iris or retina, microphthalmia, strabismus, ectopia lentis, and nystagmus. Mixed hearing loss is fairly common, with cleft palate and hypoplastic, maloccluded teeth being oral manifestations. Only 15 percent have mental disability, which is mild, and brain anomalies including hydrocephalus or Arnold–Chiari malformation have been reported. Skeletal changes include short stature (25 percent), fused or short fingers, absent or extra fingers, scoliosis, congenital hip dislocation, and rib anomalies. Urogenital defects include hydronephrosis, horseshoe kidney, labial hypoplasia, and cryptorchidism. Omphalocele, diaphragmatic hernia, umbilical hernia, and spina bifida are less common anomalies.

Preventive management for Goltz–Gorlin syndrome should include regular ophthalmologic evaluations, early auditory evoked response and audiology assessment, renal sonogram with monitoring for urinary tract infections, regular skeletal examinations screening for congenital dislocated hip and later scoliosis, and regular dental care. Early intervention may be required for developmental delay. Recurrence risks will usually be low, but genetic referral and careful evaluation of parents for minor findings will be needed for precise genetic counseling.

Hypomelanosis of Ito syndrome

Originally recognized by Ito in 1952, the combination of depigmented whorls and macules together with neurologic problems has been called hypomelanosis of Ito syndrome or incontinentia pigmenti achromians (Schwartz et al., 1977). The latter name reflects the idea that the hypomelanosis resembles a negative image of the pigmented lesions in incontinentia pigmenti. Hypomelanosis of Ito is clearly a heterogeneous phenotype with one cause being chromosomal mosaicism (Thomas et al., 1989; Sybert, 1994). In these patients, cell lines of different chromosome constitution are differently pigmented and produce linear markings along body segments (lines of Blaschko). Several different types of chromosomal mosaicism have been documented. Skin biopsy and fibroblast culture may be required to demonstrate the mosaicism, since some patients have normal peripheral blood karyotyping. In other patients with hypomelanosis of Ito syndrome, the presence of macrocephaly and limb asymmetry suggests a hamartosis or overgrowth syndrome analogous to neurofibromatosis. Neurologic problems include micro- or macrocephaly, seizures, and mental disability, which may be more severe than predicted by the degree of mosaicism. Some patients have ocular anomalies (microphthalmia, strabismus, nystagmus, the latter two suggestive of ocular albinism). Preventive management of hypomelanosis of Ito should include regular ophthalmologic assessment, monitoring of growth for asymmetry and of development for learning problems, and skeletal evaluation for limb length discrepancies and scoliosis. The skin lesions may be more apparent by Wood's light examination, and it is important to note that they are not preceded by vesicular or verrucous rashes of the type seen in incontinentia pigmenti.

Incontinentia pigmenti

While vesicular and pigmentary skin lesions are most characteristic of incontinentia pigmenti, more than 50 percent of patients have manifestations outside of the integument (Gorlin et al., 1990, pp. 457–60). The disorder was best defined by the work of Bloch, Sulzberger, and others in the 1920s, and it is sometimes referred to as Bloch–Sulzberger syndrome. Incontinentia pigmenti exhibits X-linked dominant inheritance with high lethality in males that results in over 97 percent of patients being female (Cohen, 1994). Genetic mapping has defined two loci of interest, one at chomosome region Xp11.21 and another near Xq28 (Gorski & Burright, 1993). Some have postulated the existence of an autosomal dominant form of the disorder, or invoked secondary mutations to explain the existence of affected males.

There are three distinctive phases in the clinical course of incontinentia pigmenti (Gorlin et al., 1990, pp. 451–4). The first occurs in infancy, often presenting as an eczematoid rash with eosinophilia that may reach as high as 70–80 percent of the peripheral white blood cell count. The rash is typically vesicular, with clustered or linear lesions that change to papules after the first month of life. Coincident with or shortly after the vesicular phase is the second phase of hyperkeratosis, consisting of warty lesions over the dorsal surfaces of the digits, joints, and limbs. Finally, the third and most characteristic phase appears, with linear or reticular patches of brown/gray pigment. There may be prominent whorls of pigmented and depigmented areas that usually fade in early childhood; remnants of these pigmentary changes can often be found in adults. The pigmentary findings may be confused with the hypomelanosis of Ito spectrum, which includes chromosomal mosaicism as an etiology, or the rare Naegeli syndrome, which exhibits autosomal dominant inheritance. Referral to dermatology and a diagnostic skin biopsy should thus be part of the initial diagnostic evaluation for incontinentia pigmenti.

Other complications are reminiscent of ectodermal dysplasia with sparse hair and conical or absent teeth (Dutheil et al., 1995). The eye anomalies are more severe, with optic atrophy, strabismus, cataract, and retinal detachment. Correlating with optic atrophy are a constellation of central nervous system abnormalities in 35 to 40 percent of patients (Gorlin et al., 1990, pp. 457–60). Mental disability, microcephaly, hydrocephalus, and seizures may occur. Several patients with incontinentia pigmenti have suffered from frequent and unusually severe infections, but no specific defect in immunity has been characterized.

Preventive management for incontinentia pigmenti should include dermatologic and genetic referral during the initial diagnostic evaluation, ophthalmologic referral and monitoring to evaluate strabismus and/or retinal changes, and dental referral to evaluate and treat tooth anomalies. Some children with microcephaly and pigmentary changes will need chromosome studies on peripheral blood and skin fibroblasts to exclude somatic chromosomal mosaicism that is found in hypomelanosis of Ito (see above). Early intervention and psychosocial counseling services should be provided for children with incontinentia pigmenti until mental development is ascertained to be normal. Head circumference should be closely monitored during the first two years of life, since children are at risk for microcephaly or hydrocephalus. CT or MRI scanning of the head should be considered in children with abnormal head circumference or severe developmental delay.

LEOPARD syndrome

"LEOPARD" is an acronym coined by Gorlin et al. (1971) as a mnemonic to describe an autosomal dominant syndrome: Lentigines, Electrocardiographic conduction abnormalities, Ocular hypertelorism, Pulmonary stenosis, Abnormalities of the Genitalia, Retardation of growth, and Deafness. The black-brown macules are usually distributed over the entire body, and may coalesce to form large patches (café-noir spots – Gorlin et al., 1990, pp. 461–2; Jones, 1997, pp. 531–2). Electrocardiographic changes include a superiorly oriented QRS axis with occasional bundle branch or complete heart block. Atrial septal defects in addition to valvular pulmonic stenosis (40 percent of patients) can occur, along with hypertrophic cardiomyopathy. These same cardiac findings occur in Noonan syndrome, as do the facial characteristics (hypertelorism, epicanthal folds, ptosis), short stature, genital anomalies (hypospadias, cryptorchidism), skeletal anomalies (pectus excavatum, cubitus valgus, scoliosis), and mild mental retardation. Since Noonan syndrome can also exhibit autosomal dominant inheritance, it will not be surprising to find that it and LEOPARD syndrome represent different expression of the same genetic disorder. Neither has yet been characterized at the molecular level.

Preventive management for LEOPARD syndrome is identical to that for Noonan syndrome outlined in Chapter 10. In fact, the Noonan syndrome preventive management checklist could be used for children with LEOPARD syndrome. Essentials of prevention include early and regular hearing assessment, echo- and electrocardiography, periodic cardiologic assessment, evaluation of the genitalia and follow-up for micropenis, evaluation for pectus and scoliosis, and referral to early intervention with provision for inclusive education to help children with disabilities. Brain malformations may occur (Agha & Hashimoto, 1995).

Waardenburg syndrome

Waardenburg syndrome is an autosomal dominant disorder that involves hypertelorism, ventromedial hypopigmentation, and sensorineural deafness (Liu et al., 1995; Lee et al., 1996). Two types have been described, the first with dystopia canthorum (lateral displacement of the inner canthi to produce a broad nasal bridge) and the second without. Other pigmentary findings may occur, including heterochromia of the irides (differently colored eyes) and vitiligo. The prevalence has been estimated at 1 in 100,000, but the 1400 case reports cited by Gorlin et al. (1990, pp. 466–9) suggest a higher number. One type of Waardenburg syndrome has been mapped to the 2q35–2q37 chromosome region and shown to involve a mutation of the PAX 3 gene, homologue of the fruit fly *paired* gene that is important in early development (Tassabehji et al., 1995; Read & Newton, 1997; Spritz, 1997).

Clinical manifestations of Waardenburg syndrome include facial changes with poliosis (white forelock), early graying of the hair, dystopia canthorum with increased susceptibility to dacryocystitis, other eye anomalies such as cataracts, strabismus, heterochromia or hypoplasia of the irides, and facial hirsutism with prominent eyebrows (Read & Newton, 1997). Bilateral congenital sensorineural hearing loss is present in 20 percent of type I patients and 50 percent of type II patients, with some patients having malformations of the inner ear. Other abnormalities have included Hirschsprung disease, anal atresia, Sprengel deformity, sacral dimple, spina bifida, and limb defects with elbow and digital contractures. Cleft lip/palate also occurs (Gorlin et al., 1990, pp. 466–9). Homozygous patients with severe manifestations have been reported (Zlotogora et al., 1995).

Preventive management of Waardenburg syndrome should include early hearing assessment with auditory evoked response, then audiology screening, regular ophthalmologic examinations, monitoring of feeding and bowel function to rule out intestinal atresias or Hirschsprung disease, and examination of the skeleton. Patients with thoracic or limb anomalies should have a complete skeletal radiographic survey to identify more subtle defects, and physical therapy may be required to maximize mobility.

Disorders with telangiectasias

Ataxia-telangiectasia

The combination of ataxia with telangiectasias of the ears, conjunctiva, and cheeks is an autosomal recessive disorder with an incidence of about 1 in 100,000 births. The ataxia derives from cerebellar anomalies that include atropy and diminished numbers of Purkinje cells. There are other ocular anomalies such as strabismus, photophobia, and nystagmus, and the face becomes rigid with a staring expression and fixation nystagmus (Gorlin et al., 1990, pp. 469–71). Sinopulmonary infections are recurrent in 75–80 percent of patients, often with decreased amounts of serum immunoglobulin A. Ataxia-telangiectasia could also be categorized as an accelerated aging/neoplasia syndrome, since there is early graying, scleroderma of the skin with poikiloderma (mixed streaks of hypo- and hyperpigmentation), and a predisposition to lymphomas, Hodgkin disease, leukemias, and carcinomas (stomach, skin, liver, ovary, breast; Lynch et al., 1994). Telangiectasias may also affect the oral and nasal mucosa, producing epistaxis.

Preventive management of ataxia-telangiectasia should include regular ophthalmologic examinations, initial neurologic evaluation with consideration of cerebellar imaging, and regular pediatric follow-up with alertness for upper respiratory infections, sinusitis, and lymphoid or solid tumors. Serum immunoglobulin electrophoresis may be useful in deciding whether gamma-globulin therapy may be tried; many patients also have thymic hypoplasia and diminished cellular immunity.

Osler–Rendu–Weber syndrome (hereditary hemorrhagic telangiectasia)

Hereditary hemorrhagic telangiectasia is an autosomal dominant disorder with symptomatology that depends on which organs are afflicted with angiodysplasias. The prevalence of the disorder is about 1 in 100,000 individuals, with accounts of more than 1500 persons in the literature. Infants are rarely affected, and pediatric management will usually concern older children or adolescents. Superficial telangiectasias often occur on the cheeks, ears, and nasal mucosa, with 95 percent of patients experiencing severe epistaxis (Gorlin et al., 1990, pp. 476–8; Jones, 1997, p. 524). The lips, tongue, and gingiva are also frequent sites of telangiectasias, and bleeding from the mouth can be a serious complication. Pulmonary arteriovenous fistulas (15–25 percent of patients), gastrointestinal lesions (20 to 45 percent), urinary tract lesions, and cerebral lesions leading to intracranial hemorrhage and cerebral abscess are other abnormalities that can cause death. As expected for a disorder with multiple telangiectasias, platelet trapping and thrombocytopenia can occur.

Preventive management for Rendu–Weber–Osler syndrome requires careful initial examination for superficial telangiectasias and subsequent monitoring for evidence of internal lesions. Minor traumas such as tooth brushing may elicit superficial bleeding, so counseling regarding gentle grooming techniques and initial management of nose/mouth bleeding with ice and compresses should be provided. Regular urinalysis and stool guaiac screening are useful for the detection of internal bleeding, and regular blood pressure/cardiac assessments should be made for evidence of arteriovenous fistulas. Complaints of chest pain or headache require thorough evaluation to exclude pulmonary or intracranial bleeding.

Rothmund–Thomson syndrome

Rothmund–Thomson syndrome is an autosomal recessive disorder that involves short stature, mixed hyper- and hypopigmentation of the skin (poikiloderma), photosensitivity, eye anomalies, and hypogonadism (Jones, 1997, pp. 148–9). The eye anomalies include cataracts, strabismus, and microcornea. The teeth are also abnormal, with microdontia, supernumerary teeth, and absent teeth (Gorlin et al., 1990, pp. 489–91). Most patients have short stature with thin hair and dysplastic nails. Skeletal anomalies (thumb or radial aplasia), genital anomalies (micropenis in males, scanty menstruation with infertility in females), and predisposition to sarcomas (squamous cell, osteosarcomas) have been described.

Preventive management of Rothmund–Thomson syndrome should include monitoring of growth and genital development, with consideration of endocrinologic evaluation for growth hormone deficiency/supplementation. Dermatologic evaluation of the skin and regular ophthalmologic examinations are important, and cosmetic options may be needed for the sparse hair, eyebrows, and eyelashes.

Cystic lesions and fragility of the bones together with acquired flexion contractures mandate periodic physical therapy and orthopedic evaluation. Patients should avoid exposure to sun and observe the same precautions of long-sleeved clothing and sunscreen recommended for patients with albinism.

Disorders with radiation sensitivity and/or rapid aging

Cockayne syndrome

Cockayne syndrome is a group of disorders that share autosomal recessive inheritance, growth failure, and accelerated aging. Skin fibroblasts from patients with Cockayne syndrome exhibit enhanced death rates when exposed to ultraviolet light. The causative gene for one type of Cockayne syndrome has been identified as a transcription factor that is presumably involved in the regulation of cell growth (Henning et al., 1995). Clinical manifestations include a characteristic face with sunken eyes and a prominent nose, growth delay beginning in the second to third year of life, photosensitivity with erythematous dermatitis appearing on sun-exposed areas, retinitis pigmentosa, and progressive mental disability with microcephaly, ataxia, and demyelination. As the patient reaches mid- to later childhood, the full complement of aging-related disabilities can occur, including diabetes mellitus, hypertension, osteoporosis, and cachexia (Greenhaw et al., 1992). Growth hormone deficiency has been described (Park et al., 1994). Death is inevitable in the severe form, but milder forms have been described.

Preventive management for Cockayne syndrome will include an initial diagnostic evaluation to document retinitis (ophthalmologic evaluation), demyelination (MRI or CT head scan), and skeletal radiographic survey to document thickening of the skull bones, platyspondyly, and osteoporosis. Subsequent management will be chiefly palliative, with maintenance of calories (gastrostomy is often required), avoidance of sunlight, and screening for glycosuria, hypertension, and bony deformities secondary to osteoporosis. Regular ophthalmologic examinations may be helpful in preserving some vision, and early intervention/preschool services provide encouragement and some relief for parents. Fibroblast sensitivity to ultraviolet light can be quantified as an assay for diagnosis and prenatal diagnosis, but these arduous studies can now be replaced by DNA analysis in qualified laboratories.

Xeroderma pigmentosum

Patients with xeroderma pigmentosum also exhibit photosensitivity and damage from sunlight, with progressive freckling and hemangiomatosis. Like Cockayne syndrome, the disorder is autosomal recessive and exhibits a degenerative course with loss of scalp hair, loss of subcutaneous fat, and progressive mental disability.

The most severe problem concerns predisposition to keratosis and skin neoplasms such as basal cell carcinomas, squamous cell carcinomas, and melanomas (Kraemer et al., 1994). Preventive management consists of eye care to minimize photophobia and conjunctivitis, avoidance of sunlight, aggressive diagnosis and treatment of neoplasms, and early intervention/developmental assessments to maximize cognitive function. Variable severity of the disorder reflects the occurrence of numerous complementation groups (i.e., different causative genes), and prenatal diagnosis is available for many families using fibroblast sensitivity to ultraviolet light or DNA analysis.

Progeria (Hutchinson–Gilford syndrome)

Hair loss and accelerated aging are the most dramatic signs of progeria, but growth failure, hearing loss, dental crowding, joint contractures, joint degeneration, and atherosclerotic cardiovascular disease are additional features (Gorlin et al., 1990, pp. 472–5). The face is distinctive with a prominent cranium, absent eyebrows and lashes, small ears, beaked nose, and micrognathia. The head is actually microcephalic, but intelligence is normal. Preventive management of progeria should include early hearing assessment, maintenance of nutrition, regular dental care, and surveillance of joint movement so that contractures and degeneration can be ameliorated with splinting and/or physical therapy (Fernandez-Palazzi et al., 1992). Hearing loss may occur (Hall & Denneny, 1993). Cardiovascular symptoms can appear as early as five years of age, so cholesterol screening and treatment with resins, drugs, or lipophoresis should be carried out from birth. Death usually occurs by age 14 years, but survival to age 45 has been documented (Gorlin et al., 1990, pp. 472–5). Although concordant identical twins and consanguinous parents have been reported, autosomal recessive inheritance is rendered doubtful by the preponderance of sporadic cases. No biochemical assay is available for presymptomatic or prenatal diagnosis.

Part VII

The management of neurologic and neurodegenerative syndromes

Although many malformation syndromes affect the nervous system, some are more distinctive for unusual neurologic or neurodegenerative manifestations. Chapter 18 will discuss syndromes that involve unusual neuromuscular symptoms, such as the arthrogryposes, and Chapter 19 will discuss some chronic metabolic disorders that are associated with neurodegeneration. Selected metabolic disorders with acute presentations are discussed in Chapter 20. The classic reference of Scriver et al. (1995a) provides an encyclopedic and detailed description of inborn errors of metabolism, and this reference should be consulted for detailed therapeutic management.

18

Neurologic syndromes including the arthrogryposes

Abnormalities of development have a disproportionate impact on the more complex body structures, illustrated by the nervous and cardiovascular systems. Most malformation syndromes involve neurologic abnormalities, but this chapter focuses on those notable for pain insensitivity, brain anomalies, or congenital contractures (Table 18.1).

Pain insensitivity syndromes

Familial dysautonomia (Riley–Day syndrome) and the hereditary sensory neuropathies

Riley–Day syndrome has an incidence of 1 in 10–20,000 births in Ashkenazic Jews and is 100-fold more rare in non-Jewish populations (Gorlin et al., 1990, pp. 594–6). It is an autosomal recessive syndrome involving generalized dysfunction of the peripheral nervous system. Many of the clinical manifestations of Riley–Day syndrome overlap with other genetic disorders that are called the hereditary sensory and autonomic neuropathies (HSAN; Thomas, 1992). Four types of HSAN have been delineated (Table 18.1), and other types undoubtedly occur (Axelrod & Pearson, 1984). In contrast to patients with Riley–Day syndrome, those with other types of HSAN may exhibit self-mutilation of the lips and hands (Table 18.1).

The primary genetic lesion is not known for any of these disorders, but several criteria in addition to pain insensitivity allow a probable diagnosis. There is a lack of axon flare after intracutaneous injection of 0.01 ml of 1:10,000 histamine solution, miosis of the pupil after exposure to 0.0625 percent pilocarpine eyedrops, and diminished tear flow (Brunt & McKusick, 1970; Gorlin et al., 1990, pp. 594–6).

Neonatal manifestations of Riley–Day syndrome (Axelrod et al., 1987) include breech presentation (30 percent), premature rupture of membranes (30 percent), and neonatal hypotonia and feeding problems with a poor suck (30–60 percent). In childhood, there is growth delay, diminished deep-tendon reflexes, fixed or frightened facial expression, absent tears, absent tongue papillae, and hypersalivation. There is also indifference to pain but hypersensitivity to touch (dysesthesia),

Table 18.1 Syndromes with brain anomalies and/or arthrogryposis

Syndrome	Incidence	Inheritance	Complications
Syndromes with neuropathy and/or self-mutilation			
Riley-Day	1 in 10,000 live births (J)	AR	Hypotonia, fixed facial expression, keratitis, scoliosis, dysarthric speech, Charcot joints
HSAN I	~50 cases	AD	Sensory neuropathy (feet), foot ulcers, shooting leg pains, deafness, peroneal atrophy
HSAN II	~50 cases	AR	Sensory neuropathy (digits), acro-osteolysis, digital mutilation, hyperhidrosis, Charcot joints
HSAN III Riley–Day	1 in 10,000 live births (J)	AR	Sensorimotor and autonomic neuropathy, hypotonia, fixed facial expression, keratitis, scoliosis, dysarthric speech, Charcot joints
HSAN IV	~25 cases	AR	Sensorimotor/autonomic neuropathy, hyperpyrexia, hypohidrosis, orodigital mutilation
Lesch–Nyhan	~150 cases	XLR	Dystonia, choreoathetosis, hyperuricemia, neurodegeneration, orodigital mutilation
Syndromes with brain anomalies			
Aicardi	~25 cases	XLD	Agenesis of the corpus callosum, lacunar retinal defects, costovertebral a.
FG	~50 cases	XLR	Frontal hair whorl, ptosis, imperforate anus
Walker-Warburg	~50 cases	AR	Lissencephaly, retinal detachment, muscular dystrophy
Syndromes with contractures (arthrogryposis)			
Amyoplasia	1 in 10,000 live births	Sporadic	Limb contractures, micrognathia, muscle atrophy, "policeman's tip" position of hands
Marden–Walker	~50 cases	AR	Limb contractures, immobile facies, blepharophimosis, scoliosis, FTT, DD
Multiple pterygium	~60 cases	AR	Limb and digital contractures, pterygia of neck and limbs, cleft palate, scoliosis, genital a.
Pena–Shokeir I	1 in 10,000 live births	AR	Camptodactyly, club feet, hypertelorism, pulmonary hypoplasia, urogenital a., cardiac a.
Pena–Shokeir II	~25 cases	AR	Hip and knee ankyloses, microcephaly, brain a., cataracts, degenerative course, DD
Popliteal pterygium	~80 cases	AD	Limb and digital contractures, popliteal pterygia, cleft palate, genital a.
Schwartz–Jampel	~50 case	AR	Limb contractures, puckered facies, blepharophimosis, scoliosis, FTT, DD

Table 18.1 (*cont.*)

Syndrome	Incidence	Inheritance	Complications
Whistling face (Freeman–Sheldon)	~65 cases	AD, AR	Distal limb contractures, microstomia and "whistling face," facial immobility, deviated ("windvane") fingers

Notes:

J, Jewish population; AD, autosomal dominant; AR, autosomal recessive; XLR, X-linked recessive; XLD, X-linked dominant; DD, developmental disability; FTT, failure to thrive; a., anomalies.

episodic appearance of erythematous macules over the trunk and limbs, and progressive scoliosis appearing around age 8–9 years (Gorlin et al., 1990, pp. 594–6). Intelligence is normal, but speech is often monotonous or slurred. Other manifestations of neuropathy include sleep apnea (insensitivity to carbon dioxide), Charcot joints (insensitivity to pain), keratitis and corneal ulceration (absent corneal reflex and tears), recurrent aspiration and drooling (diminished gag reflex and dysphagia), and cold hands and feet with poor tolerance of exercise (diminished epinephrine response; Gorlin et al., 1990, pp. 594–6). Intestinal perforation may occur (Applegate & Sargent, 1995). Additional complications of the HSAN group include scarring of the lips and fingers, risks of osteomyelitis and fractures, and severe dental decay with self-extraction of teeth. Preventive management for Riley–Day syndrome and related sensory neuropathies should include early and regular ophthalmologic evaluations to protect against corneal abrasions and vision loss. Feeding and nutrition should be watched closely, with regular chest radiographs to assess chronic aspiration and pneumonia. Sleep studies should be performed in later childhood and adolescence, and regular dental care is needed for malocclusion and crowding in Riley–Day syndrome, or for dental caries in the HSAN group. Anesthesia is accompanied by risks of hypotension and cardiac arrest. Orthopedic referral should be considered in early adolescence because of scoliosis and joint damage from pain insensitivity. Early intervention may be needed because of motor delays, and psychosocial counseling should be facilitated for adolescents because of their somatic and behavioral differences.

Lesch–Nyhan syndrome

Lesch–Nyhan syndrome is an X-linked recessive disorder that causes severe self-mutilation and mental deficiency in affected males (Rossiter & Caskey, 1995). The original description of the disease (Lesch & Nyhan, 1964) was followed shortly by the demonstration of hypoxanthine-guanine phosphoribosyl transferase deficiency as the basic defect (Seegmiller et al., 1967). Molecular analysis is now available, which allows the recognition of female carriers who have a 25 percent risk of having affected sons (Rossiter & Caskey, 1995). More than 150 cases have been reported (Gorlin et al., 1990, pp. 596–8).

Clinical manifestations of Lesch–Nyhan syndrome include a normal neonatal period with onset of hypertonia and motor delay by age 6 months. The neurologic features usually lead to the diagnosis, with opisthotonic posturing, dystonia, and choreoathetosis in most patients. The onset of self-mutilation occurs between ages 4 months and 4 years, involving the lips, fingers, and shoulders. Mental deficiency is often severe, with dysarthric speech and occasional normal intelligence (Gorlin et al., 1990, pp. 596–8). Hyperuricemia can cause orange "sand" or "crystals" in the diaper, with later nephrolithiasis and obstructive uropathy. Subcutaneous or auricular tophi are common, but gouty arthritis is not. Interestingly, patients with partial enzyme deficiencies have hyperuricemia and gouty arthritis without neurologic problems (Rossiter & Caskey, 1995). Other clinical manifestations include propensity for infection, megaloblastic anemia because of folate deficiency, and testicular atrophy (Gorlin et al., 1990, pp. 596–8).

Preventive management for Lesch–Nyhan syndrome consists of pharmacologic therapy for hyperuricemia, hydration to prevent urinary tract stones or damage, and restraints to minimize the injuries from self-mutilation. Early neurologic evaluation and early intervention services are important, although no effective medication for the dystonia or choreoathetosis has been found (Rossiter & Caskey, 1995). Periodic urinalyses, blood urea nitrogen and creatinine, and complete blood counts should be performed to screen for renal or hematologic problems. Hyman (1996) reviewed the behavioral modification, pharmacologic, and physical restraints that have been employed for patients with self-mutilation. Behavior enhancement through positive reinforcement of alternative activities (e.g., crafts rather than hand in mouth), together with elbow restraints that allow freedom of the hands, offer the best options for patients with Lesch–Nyhan syndrome (Rossiter & Caskey, 1995; Hyman, 1996). The anticonvulsants, antidepressants, and neuroleptics that have been tried in other disorders with self-mutilation have not been effective in Lesch–Nyhan syndrome.

Syndromes with brain anomalies

Aicardi syndrome

Aicardi and colleagues characterized a syndrome involving myoclonic epilepsy, brain anomalies including agenesis of the corpus callosum, and chorioretinal defects or "lacunae" in 1969 (Donnenfeld et al., 1989). The disorder affects only females, and is thought to follow X-linked dominant inheritance with male lethality. Several patients have had chromosome anomalies centering on the Xp22.3 region, providing a candidate location for the responsible gene. Other clinical manifestations include persistent hyperplastic primary vitreous (Weissgold et al., 1995), costovertebral defects with absent or malformed ribs, scoliosis, hemivertebrae, and various benign or malignant tumors (Tsao et al., 1993; Trifiletti et al., 1995). Mental disability is usually severe, but survival can be prolonged. Menezes et al. (1994) reported 76 percent survival at age 6 years and 40 percent survival at age 15 years, with 21 percent of the patients being able to walk or crawl and 29 percent having some language ability.

Preventive management of Aicardi syndrome will require an initial evaluation including cranial MRI scan, skeletal radiographic survey, and ophthalmologic examinations. Patients with seizures should have neurologic evaluations, and typical electroencephalographic findings have been reported (Fariello et al., 1977). Anticonvulsant therapy, attention to nutrition with tube feeding or gastrostomy, and early intervention referrals will be needed.

Walker–Warburg syndrome

Walker–Warburg syndrome was delineated using the acronym "HARD E," where the letters stood for Hydrocephalus, Agyria, Retinal Dysplasia, and Encephalocele (Pagon et al., 1978). Walker and Warburg published prior descriptions of affected patients (Dobyns et al., 1989), and Dobyns contributed a classification for related lissencephalies (Dobyns et al., 1985; 1989). Miller–Dieker syndrome and some isolated lissencephalies involve small chromosome 17 deletions (see Chapter 9).

Walker–Warburg patients may have other brain anomalies, including arrhinencephaly, absent corpus callosum, or Dandy–Walker malformation, and the disorder is lethal, with 65 percent dying in the first three months (Gorlin et al., 1990, pp. 592–3). Eye anomalies include microphthalmia, iris hypoplasia, cataracts, retinal hypoplasia with detachment, and optic nerve hypoplasia. Genitourinary anomalies including hydronephrosis and cryptorchidism have also been described. Some patients have a peculiar type of muscular dystrophy which may represent a distinct disorder (Lichtig et al., 1993).

Preventive management consists of an initial evaluation including cranial MRI scan and ophthalmologic examination. Many patients will require neurosurgical intervention (Martinez-Lage et al., 1995). Parents should receive genetic counseling for autosomal recessive inheritance, and prenatal diagnosis has been accomplished by ultrasound. Head growth (with consideration of shunting), nutrition and feeding (with consideration of nasogastric tube or gastrostomy), and urinary tract function should be monitored. Psychosocial counseling and the possibility of hospice care should be provided for families.

Syndromes with congenital contractures (arthrogryposes)

Many different disorders have been grouped under the term "arthrogryposis multiplex congenita." The articles by Hall (1981, 1986, 1997, and in Staheli et al., 1998), who has done fundamental work in delineating the arthrogryposis syndromes, and that by Jones (1997, pp. 688–90) are useful in understanding this complex disease category. An important book is now available that illustrates the value of and methods for multidisciplinary management of arthrogryposis (Staheli et al., 1998).

It should be realized that contractures of the limbs and digits form a spectrum from mildly decreased range of motion, to obvious deformity with webbing across the joint, to severe ankylosis with fixation. The severity of joint limitation and deformity will reflect the degree and duration of fetal immobility, since the rule for fetal limb and lung development is "use it or lose it" (Hall, 1981; 1997). Joint contractures have many genetic and environmental causes, including maternal myasthenia gravis, experimental curare paralysis, agenesis of spinal motor ganglia (e.g., severe Werdnig–Hoffman disease), myopathies presenting in fetal life, and constraint of fetal movement by uterine anomalies or amniotic bands. The webs, joint contractures, muscle atrophy, and pulmonary problems are thus variations on a theme of fetal immotility that occur in several arthrogryposis syndromes (Table 18.1). Several specific conditions will now be discussed, followed by a section on general features of arthrogryposis that outlines preventive management for these various disorders.

Amyoplasia

Children with amyoplasia have decreased muscle mass with specific changes in limb positioning (Hall, 1981). The cause of the disorder is unknown and it is a sporadic condition with a good prognosis (Sells et al., 1996; Niki et al., 1997). The face may be round, with glabellar hemangiomas and micrognathia. The hands are held in the typical "policeman's tip" configuration with the shoulders internally rotated, the wrists flexed, and the palms extended backward. The knees may be flexed or extended and the hips are flexed. Club feet, scoliosis, dimpling over the affected joints, and atrophic muscles are characteristic. Amyoplasia occurs more commonly in twins, where it is usually discordant. The diagnostic evaluation is clinical; muscle biopsies are nonspecific with decreased numbers of muscle fibers (Hall, 1981, 1983; Hall et al., 1983).

Preventive management of amyoplasia should follow the guidelines in the arthrogryposis checklist, parts 2–4. Hall (1981) placed particular emphasis on physical therapy to preserve what little muscle is present. However, it is important for an experienced therapist to be involved, since fractures can occur (Simonian & Staheli, 1995; Staheli et al., 1998). The normal intelligence and frequent improvement in patients with amyoplasia warrant optimistic medical counseling, since 85 percent of patients are ambulatory and achieve independent function (Sells et al., 1996).

Marden–Walker and Schwartz–Jampel syndromes

Marden–Walker and Schwartz–Jampel syndromes exhibit similar manifestations of joint contractures, feeding problems, failure to thrive, abnormalities of the facial muscles, and eye anomalies (Gorlin et al., 1990, pp. 631–4). Schwartz–Jampel syndrome (also known as chondrodystrophic myotonia) involves increased tone of the facial muscles, with a characteristic puckering of the lips and grimace that is present in the neonatal period (Gellis & Feingold, 1973; Kirschner & Pachman, 1976). Marden–Walker syndrome involves decreased tone of the facial muscles, with decreased mobility of the mouth and sagging cheeks (Schrander-Stumpel et al., 1993; Williams et al., 1993; Marden & Walker, 1966). Marden–Walker syndrome also involves earlier onset of contractures and more severe developmental delay than does Schwartz-Jampel syndrome, and the latter condition involves a chondrodysplasia with bowed long bones, acetabular dysplasia, and metaphyseal widening (Gorlin et al., 1990, pp. 631–34). Both conditions exhibit autosomal recessive inheritance. and prenatal diagnosis may be approached through ultrasonography.

Preventive management of Schwartz–Jampel and Marden–Walker syndromes can follow the arthrogryposis checklist, parts 2–4 with attention to certain special concerns. Both conditions will require attention to feeding and nutrition, and specialists in oromotor function may be helpful (Staheli et al., 1998). Anesthesia must be performed by experienced personnel (Ray & Rubin, 1994). Ophthalmologic assessment and follow-up is important because of ptosis, blepharospasm, and/or myopia in Schwarz–Jampel syndrome and ptosis, blepharophimosis, and/or strabismus in Marden–Walker syndrome (Gorlin et al., 1990, pp. 631–4). Renal anomalies may occur (Ben-Neriah et al., 1995). Orthopedic and physical therapy evaluations are emphasized because both syndromes have multiple skeletal changes in addition to joint contractures, including pectus and scoliosis. Mental deficiency occurs in 25 percent of patients with Schwartz–Jampel syndrome and nearly all cases of Marden–Walker syndrome, indicating the importance of early intervention services and developmental assessments. Alertness for aspiration and pneumonias should be maintained, with immunoglobulin A deficiency being reported in Schwartz–Jampel syndrome (Kirschner & Pachman, 1976). Carbamezapine has been beneficial in treating the myotonia of Schwartz–Jampel syndrome (Topaloglu et al., 1993). Marden–Walker syndrome was reported as a connective tissue dysplasia (Marden & Walker, 1966), so periodic evaluation for hernias, easy bruising, stretch marks, and mitral valve prolapse should be performed as with the disorders discussed in Chapter 16.

Multiple and popliteal pterygium syndromes

The multiple pterygium syndrome (Escobar et al., 1978) has been confused with disorders involving a webbed neck (Noonan syndrome, Turner syndrome) and with other forms of arthrogryposis (Gorlin et al., 1990, pp. 626–9). It is distinguished from popliteal pterygium syndrome (Gorlin et al., 1968) by having pterygia (webs) of the neck *and* popliteal region, and by autosomal recessive rather than autosomal dominant inheritance (Table 18.1). Congenital contractures with club feet and scoliosis can occur in either syndrome, as can cleft palate, hearing loss, and webs in the genital region that produce cryptorchidism and scrotal abnormalities (Koch et al., 1992). Cervical vertebral fusion or absent patella may occur in multiple pterygium syndrome, and both syndromes can produce camptodactyly and syndactyly of the digits (Gorlin et al., 1968; Escobar et al., 1978; McCall & Budden, 1992). The popliteal pterygium syndrome has a characteristic finding where a triangle of skin extends over the dorsum of the great toenail (Gorlin et al., 1990, p. 630).

Preventive management of the multiple and popliteal pterygium syndromes can follow the recommendations in the arthrogryposis checklist, parts 2–4, but more aggressive orthopedic and plastic surgical management may be required to mobilize joints and remove webs (Staheli et al., 1998). Urologic evaluation of the genital anomalies may also be needed. Recurrent pneumonias due to severe kyphoscoliosis may lead to early death in multiple pterygium syndrome, but the normal intelligence in patients with these conditions supports an optimistic and aggressive medical outlook (Soekarman et al., 1995).

Pena–Shokeir syndrome types I and II

Pena & Shokeir (1974, 1976) wrote a pivotal description of children with congenital contractures that gave rise to two different eponymic syndromes with autosomal recessive inheritance. Pena–Shokeir type I syndrome involves limb contractures, an unusual facies (hypertelorism, high nasal bridge, malformed ears, micrognathia), and pulmonary hypoplasia; Pena–Shokeir type II syndrome involves limb contractures, microcephaly, unusual facies (enophthalmos, microphthalmia), and brain anomalies (agenesis of the corpus callosum, cerebellar hypoplasia). The type II disorder has also been called cerebro-oculo-facial syndrome (COFS), and has a degenerative course resembling Cockayne syndrome (see Chapter 17).

Pena–Shokeir type I syndrome has an estimated incidence of 1 in 10,000 births, while the type II syndrome is quite rare (Table 18.1). The higher frequency of type I patients is in part due to phenotypic heterogeneity, since a variety of neurologic or muscular injuries that render the fetus immobile can cause the Pena–Shokeir type I phenotype (Hall, 1986; Lidang Jensen et al., 1995). Some prefer the term "fetal akinesia sequence" to indicate that immobility of the fetal limbs results in contractures (arthrogryposis, ankylosis) and that decreased fetal respiratory excursions result in pulmonary hypoplasia (Gorlin et al., 1990, pp. 621–4). In support of this view is the similar phenotype obtained when rodent fetuses are paralyzed in utero (Moessinger, 1983).

Additional manifestations of Pena–Shokeir type I syndrome include webbing of the neck, small chest, and contractures that can involve any of the limb joints or digits (Gorlin et al., 1990, pp. 621–4). Cardiac anomalies (25 percent), urinary tract anomalies (30 percent), and genital anomalies (cryptorchidism in virtually 100 percent, hypospadias in 20 percent, labial hypoplasia in 15 percent) (Hall, 1986; Gorlin et al., 1990, pp. 621–4). Pena–Shokeir type II patients can have cataracts, dislocation or contracture of limb joints, scoliosis, and a degenerative course with wasting of subcutaneous tissue.

Preventive management of the Pena–Shokeir syndrome type I can utilize the arthrogryposis checklist, but type II is a very different disorder that requires mainly palliative management. Genetic counseling regarding the possibility of a 25 percent recurrence risk for normal parents with affected children should be mentioned. For severe cases, fetal ultrasonography can be used for prenatal diagnosis by detecting fetal hydrops or other anomalies.

Whistling face (Freeman–Sheldon) syndrome

The puckered lips and immobile face of the Freeman–Sheldon syndrome are so distinctive that the "whistling face" description should be retained. Not surprisingly, the syndrome was recognized some time ago and has been separated from other forms of "distal" arthrogryposis (Hall et al., 1982a). Most families show vertical transmission consistent with autosomal dominant inheritance, but some pedigrees involve consanguinity typical of autosomal recessive inheritance (Gorlin et al., 1990, pp. 634–6).

Complications of whistling face syndrome include enopthalmos, hypertelorism or strabismus, microstomia with an "H"-like cleft on the chin, puckered lips, micrognathia, facial immobility, small nasal alae, ulnarly deviated ("windvane") fingers, and congenital contractures of the hips and knees including club feet and kyphoscoliosis. There are early feeding problems and failure to thrive (30 percent), and a few patients have had mental disability. Preventive management of whistling face syndrome should follow the recommendations of the arthrogryposis checklist with emphasis on evaluation of early nutrition and respiratory function. Some children have suffered aspiration and death (Gorlin et al., 1990, pp. 634–6), and anesthesia requires considerable expertise (Jones & Dolcourt, 1992; Mayhew, 1993). The improvement in joint function seen with many forms of arthrogryposis can be particularly evident in Freeman–Sheldon syndrome, so medical management should be aggressive and optimistic (Staheli et al., 1998). Seizures may also occur (Sackey et al., 1995).

Arthrogryposis syndromes

Terminology

Arthrogryposis multiplex congenita is a phenotype that has now been separated into many different syndromes. A conglomerate of signs and symptoms including deformity or fixation of the joints (limb contractures or ankylosis), dimpling over the joints, pterygia (webbing) across the joints, bony deformities (kyphoscoliosis) are seen in various arthrogryposis syndromes, and it may be difficult to classify individual patients (Hall, 1981; Jones, 1997, pp. 623–5; Staheli et al., 1998). Joint contractures and pulmonary hypoplasia may occur as a "fetal akinesia sequence" that is caused by fetal nerve or muscle dysfunction as well as maternal constraint (uterine anomaly, twin pregnancy).

Incidence, etiology, and differential diagnosis

The overall incidence of arthrogryposis is about 1 in 10,000 births (Hall, 1981), with some individual syndromes being quite rare (Table 18.1). As discussed above, any abnormality of the fetal genotype, the maternal metabolism, or the in utero environment that decreases fetal movement can produce congenital contractures. Severe fetal Werdnig–Hoffman disease or myopathy, maternal myasthenia gravis, and uterine constraints (twin pregnancy, bicornuate uterus) are all causes of arthrogryposis. Because several syndromes with arthrogryposis as a component exhibit autosomal recessive inheritance, the older, all-inclusive name "arthrogryposis multiplex congenita" was often described as an autosomal recessive disease. One of the more common forms of arthrogryposis (amyoplasia) is not genetic.

The differential diagnosis of children with congenital contractures is extensive, including many neuromuscular disorders in addition to the syndromes listed in Table 18.1. Chromosomal disorders (e.g., trisomy 18 that can be confused with Pena–Shokeir type I syndrome) and metabolic diseases (e.g., Zellweger syndrome with club feet) may include congenital contractures as a presenting symptom. Distinctive clinical findings include the "policeman's tip" positioning in amyoplasia, the pulmonary hypoplasia in Pena–Shokeir type I syndrome, the deeply set eyes in Pena–Shokeir type II syndrome, the puckered lips of Schwartz–Jampel or whistling face syndrome, and the webbing extending over the great toes in popliteal pterygium syndrome.

Diagnostic evaluation and medical counseling

A thorough physical examination is the cornerstone of diagnostic evaluation for the arthrogryposis syndromes. Webs, dimples, and positioning should be noted and the range of motion of each limb segment noted for future reference. Inspection for associated anomalies of the facies, eyes, mouth, trunk, and genitalia should then be conducted; children with a small thorax should be watched for evidence of respiratory insufficiency. Additional investigations may include cranial MRI scans in children with microcephaly, and a skeletal radiographic survey for the detection of osteopenia, fractures, cervical spine fusions, sacral fusions, etc. If there are minor anomalies of the craniofacies and limbs, then chromosomal studies should be performed. Ophthalmologic evaluations for cataracts, strabismus, or ptosis are important as a prelude to regular vision checks. Medical counseling will usually be optimistic unless there is severe pulmonary hypoplasia or evidence of microcephaly and facial dysmorphology. Many children with severe joint contractures make remarkable progress in motor rehabilitation.

Family and psychosocial counseling

Table 18.1 illustrates that syndromes with congenital contractures may be inherited as autosomal dominant or autosomal recessive diseases. If one includes severe presentations of neuropathies or myopathies, the X-linked recessive inheritance may also occur. The most likely inheritance mechanism will be autosomal recessive with a 25 percent recurrence risk, but amyoplasia (sporadic occurrence) or whistling face syndrome (autosomal dominant in some cases) may be associated with a minimal recurrence risk. Psychosocial counseling is needed for parents when severe developmental disabilities or major rehabilitative efforts are needed. Parent support groups are listed in the checklist, part 1.

Natural history and complications

Although many children with congenital contractures have an excellent prognosis, those with involvement of the central nervous system have increased morbidity and mortality (Hall, 1981). The complications of arthrogryposis mainly concern the bones and joints, but the syndromes listed in Table 18.1 illustrate numerous other problems that may occur. The arthrogryposis checklist, part 1, lists many of the more common complications of the arthrogryposis syndromes, including feeding and nutrition, ocular anomalies, high or cleft palate, micrognathia, hernias, kyphoscoliosis, limb contractures with or without webs, gastrointestinal anomalies, pulmonary hypoplasia and/or chronic pneumonitis, cardiac anomalies, urogenital anomalies, brain anomalies, and neurosensory deficits. After treatment of the contractures, later complications can include dental crowding, hernias, restrictive lung disease, degenerative arthritis, and motor disabilities.

Arthrogryposis syndromes preventive medical checklist

Once the initial assessment of cranial, skeletal, pulmonary, and urogenital development is completed, the clinician should initiate aggressive orthopedic and physical therapy to preserve muscle function and mobilize joints (Staheli et al., 1998).

Therapists must be cautioned to avoid forcing movement when there is ankylosis or osteopenia, and a skeletal radiographic survey is helpful to point out fragile areas. Ophthalmologic evaluations should be performed initially to document anomalies and serially to monitor vision. Feeding may be compromised by a high or cleft palate, by micrognathia, or by a small mouth with constricted lips; feeding evaluation and education are therefore essential. Observation of stool and urinary patterns is also important to rule out intestinal or genitourinary anomalies.

Later management (checklist, part 4) will consist of monitoring skeletal growth and symmetry, continued neurosensory testing including audiometric and ophthalmologic evaluations, orthopedic and physical medicine assessments to provide appliances or therapies for motor limitations, and dental evaluations to exclude tooth crowding or malocclusion (Staheli, 1998). Patients with neurologic symptoms may require school evaluations and family counseling appropriate for children with severe disabilities.

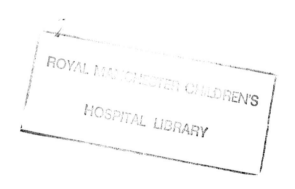

Preventive Management of Arthrogryposis syndromes

Clinical diagnosis: Pattern of manifestations including deformity or fixation of the joints (limb contractures or ankylosis), dimpling over the joints, pterygia (webbing) across the joints, and bony deformities (kyphoscoliosis, club feet). Abnormalities are mainly confined to the musculoskeletal system in disorders such as amyoplasia, but many syndromes include arthrogryposis within a broader spectrum of brain, heart, and kidney defects.

Incidence: Various disorders with an overall incidence of about 1 in 10,000 live births.

Laboratory diagnosis: No karyotypic or genetic mutations have been characterized; nerve or muscle biopsies are usually not definitive.

Genetics: Autosomal recessive inheritance applies for many disorders involving arthrogryposis, but amyoplasia (sporadic occurrence) or Freeman–Sheldon (autosomal dominant in some cases) may imply a minimal recurrence risk for normal parents having an affected child.

Key management issues: Aggressive orthopedic and physical therapy to preserve muscle function and mobilize joints, avoiding forced positioning in the presence of ankylosis or osteopenia; evaluation of feeding, stool, and urinary patterns to rule out anomalies; dental evaluations to exclude tooth crowding or malocclusion; monitoring of hearing, vision, growth, and skeletal development; early intervention and family support for patients with microcephaly and severe disabilities.

Growth Charts: The dependence of stature on the degree of limb deformity and its variation among syndromes precludes the use of specific charts; regular charts should be used to monitor head growth and weight gain.

Parent groups: National AVENUES: A National Support Group for Arthrogryposis Multiplex Congenita, P. O. Box 5192, Sonora CA, 95370, (209) 928-3688, avenues@sonnet.com, http://sonnet.com/avenues; CAST (Canadian Arthrogryposis Support Team), 365 Fiddler's Green Rd. S., Ancaster ON, Canada L9G 1X2, (905) 648-2007, cast@freenet.hamilton.ca

Basis for management recommendations: Multidisciplinary management outlined in detail by Staheli et al. (1998), complications below as documented by Hall (1981); Hall et al. (1983).

Summary of clinical concerns

General	Learning	Cognitive disability, learning differences for patients with microcephaly
	Growth	Failure to thrive, short stature
Facial	Face	Flat nasal bridge, hemangiomas, micrognathia
	Eye	Ptosis, microphthalmia, corneal opacities, strabismus
	Mouth	Oromotor dysfunction, dental crowding, high palate, microstomia
Surface	Neck/trunk	Torticollis, umbilical hernias, inguinal hernias
	Epidermal	Extensible skin
Skeletal	Cranial	Cranial asymmetry, craniosynostosis
	Axial	Scoliosis
	Limbs	Pterygia, contractures, ankyloses, degenerative arthritis
Internal	Digestive	Dysphagia, gastroschisis, intestinal atresias
	Pulmonary	Pulmonary hypoplasia, restrictive lung disease, respiratory obstruction
	Circulatory	Cardiac anomalies, cardiomyopathies
	Excretory	Renal anomalies, hydronephrosis, urinary tract infections
	Genital	Cryptorchidism, micropenis, labial hypoplasia
Neural	CNS	Brain anomalies, seizures
	Motor	Decreased movements, motor delays
	Sensory	Optic and otic nerve dysfunction, vision and hearing deficits
	Muscular	Amyoplasia, decreased muscle mass, decreased strength

Bold: frequency > 20%

Key references

Hall, J. (1981). *Pediatric Annals* 10:15–26
Hall, J. G., Reed, S. D. & Driscoll E. P. (1983). *American Journal of Medical Genetics* 15:571–8.
McCall, R. E. & Budden, J. (1992). *Orthopedics* 15:1417–22.
Staheli, L. T. et al. (1998). *Arthrogryposis. A Text Atlas.* Cambridge: Cambridge University Press.

Arthrogryposis syndromes

Preventive medical checklist (0–1yr)

Patient   **Birth Date** / /   **Number**

Pediatric	Screen	Evaluate		Refer/Counsel	
Neonatal / / *Newborn screen* ❑ *HB* ❑	Skeletal survey[3] ❑ Head MRI scan[3] ❑ Lung volume[3] ❑	Feeding Cranium, eyes Jaw, palate Spine, limbs Muscle mass	❑ ❑ ❑ ❑ ❑	Genetic evaluation Feeding specialist[3] Orthopedics Physical therapy Craniofacial surgery[3]	❑ ❑ ❑ ❑ ❑
1 month / /	Echocardiogram ❑	Feeding Heart Joint mobility	❑ ❑ ❑	Family support[4] Feeding specialist[3] Cardiology[3]	❑ ❑ ❑
2 months / / *HB[1]* ❑ *Hib* ❑ *DTaP, IPV* ❑ *RV* ❑	Hearing, vision[2] ❑	Feeding Heart, lungs Joint mobility Genitalia	❑ ❑ ❑ ❑	Early intervention[5] Developmental pediatrics[3] Genetic counseling	❑ ❑ ❑
4 months / / *HB[1]* ❑ *Hib* ❑ *DTaP/IPV* ❑ *RV* ❑	Hearing, vision[2] ❑	Feeding Heart, lungs Joint mobility Genitalia	❑ ❑ ❑ ❑	Early intervention[5] Feeding specialist[3]	❑ ❑
6 months / / *Hib* ❑ *IPV[1]* ❑ *DTaP* ❑ *RV* ❑	Hearing, vision[2] ❑	Feeding Heart, lungs Joint mobility Genitalia	❑ ❑ ❑ ❑	Family support[4] Feeding specialist[3] Orthopedics Physical therapy	❑ ❑ ❑ ❑
9 months / / *IPV[1]* ❑		Feeding Heart, lungs Joint mobility Genitalia	❑ ❑ ❑ ❑	Ophthalmology	❑
1 year / / *HB* ❑ *Hib[1]* ❑ *IPV[1]* ❑ *MMR[1]* ❑ *Var[1]* ❑	Hearing, vision[2] ❑	Feeding Heart, lungs Joint mobility Genitalia	❑ ❑ ❑ ❑	Family support[4] Early intervention[5] Genetics Orthopedics Physical therapy	❑ ❑ ❑ ❑ ❑

Clinical concerns for Arthrogryposis syndromes, ages 0–1 year

Craniosynostosis	Cardiac anomalies	Motor delays
Microphthalmia, cataracts	Pulmonary hypoplasia	Microcephaly, seizures
Strabismus	Joint contractures	Feeding problems
Trismus of jaw	Ankyloses, pterygia	Intestinal atresias

Guidelines for the neonatal period should be undertaken *at whatever age* the diagnosis is made; DTaP, acellular DTP; IPV, inactivated poliovirus (oral polio also used); RV, rotavirus; MMR, measles–mumps–rubella; Var, varicella; [1]alternative timing; [2]by practitioner; [3]as dictated by clinical findings; [4]parent group, family/sib, financial, and behavioral issues as discussed in the preface; [5]including developmental monitoring and motor/speech therapy.

Arthrogryposis syndromes

Preventive medical checklist (15m–6yrs)

Patient _____ **Birth Date** / / **Number** _____

Pediatric	Screen	Evaluate		Refer/Counsel	
15 months / / Hib[1] ☐ MMR[1] ☐ DTaP, IPV[1] ☐ Varicella[1] ☐		Feeding Heart, lungs Joint mobility Genitalia	☐ ☐ ☐ ☐	Family support[4] Early intervention[5] Orthopedics Physical therapy	☐ ☐ ☐ ☐
18 months / / DTaP, IPV[1] ☐ Varicella[1] ☐ Influenza[3] ☐				Cardiology[3] Ophthalmology	☐ ☐
2 years / / Influenza[3] ☐ Pneumovax[3] ☐ Dentist ☐	Hearing, vision[2] ☐	Feeding Heart, lungs Joint mobility Genitalia	☐ ☐ ☐ ☐	Family support[4] Developmental pediatrics[3] Genetics Orthopedics Physical therapy	☐ ☐ ☐ ☐ ☐
3 years / / Influenza[3] ☐ Pneumovax[3] ☐ Dentist ☐	Hearing, vision[2] ☐	Feeding Heart, lungs Joint mobility	☐ ☐ ☐	Family support[4] Preschool transition[5] Dentistry Orthopedics	☐ ☐ ☐ ☐
4 years / / Influenza[3] ☐ Pneumovax[3] ☐ Dentist ☐	Hearing, vision[2] ☐	Mobility Scoliosis	☐ ☐	Family support[4] Preschool program[5] Developmental pediatrics[3] Genetics Physical therapy	☐ ☐ ☐ ☐ ☐
5 years / / DTaP, IPV[1] ☐ MMR[1] ☐	Hearing, vision[2] ☐	Mobility Asymmetry Scoliosis	☐ ☐ ☐	School transition[5] Orthopedics Physical therapy	☐ ☐ ☐
6 years / / DTaP, IPV[1] ☐ MMR[1] ☐ Dentist ☐	Hearing, vision[2] ☐	Mobility Asymmetry Scoliosis	☐ ☐ ☐	Family support[4] Developmental pediatrics[3] Genetics Cardiology[3] Ophthalmology Orthopedics	☐ ☐ ☐ ☐ ☐ ☐

Clinical concerns for Arthrogryposis syndromes, ages 1–6 years

Craniosynostosis	Cardiac anomalies	Mental disability
Microphthalmia, cataracts	Pulmonary hypoplasia	Brain anomalies, seizures
Strabismus	Joint contractures	Feeding problems
Trismus of jaw	Synostoses, pterygia	Intestinal atresias

Guidelines for prior ages should be undertaken _at the time of diagnosis_; DTaP, acellular DTP; IPV, inactivated poliovirus (oral polio also used); MMR, measles–mumps–rubella; [1]alternative timing; [2]by practitioner; [3]as dictated by clinical findings; [4]parent group, family/sib, financial, and behavioral issues as discussed in the preface; [5]including developmental monitoring and motor/speech therapy.

Arthrogryposis syndromes

Preventive medical checklist (6+ yrs)

Patient		Birth Date / /	Number	

Pediatric	Screen	Evaluate		Refer/Counsel	
8 years / / *Dentist* ❏		Mobility Asymmetry Scoliosis	❏ ❏ ❏	School options Developmental pediatrics[3] Genetics Orthopedics	❏ ❏ ❏ ❏
10 years / / 	Hearing, vision[2] ❏	Mobility Asymmetry Scoliosis	❏ ❏ ❏	Ophthalmology[3] Cardiology[3]	❏ ❏
12 years / / *Td[1], MMR, Var* ❏ *CBC* ❏ *Dentist* ❏ *Scoliosis* ❏ *Cholesterol* ❏		Mobility Asymmetry Scoliosis	❏ ❏ ❏	Family support[4] School options Developmental pediatrics[3] Genetics Orthopedics	❏ ❏ ❏ ❏ ❏
14 years / / *CBC* ❏ *Dentist* ❏ *Cholesterol* ❏ *Breast CA* ❏ *Testicular CA* ❏	Hearing, vision[2] ❏	Mobility Asymmetry Scoliosis	❏ ❏ ❏	Cardiology[3] Ophthalmology[3]	❏ ❏
16 years / / *Td[1]* ❏ *CBC* ❏ *Cholesterol* ❏ *Sexual[5]* ❏ *Dentist* ❏		Mobility Asymmetry Scoliosis	❏ ❏ ❏	Vocational planning Developmental pediatrics[3] Genetics Orthopedics	❏ ❏ ❏ ❏
18 years / / *CBC* ❏ *Sexual[5]* ❏ *Cholesterol* ❏ *Scoliosis* ❏	Hearing, vision[2] ❏	Mobility Asymmetry Scoliosis	❏ ❏ ❏	Vocational planning Dentistry	❏ ❏
20 years[6] / / *CBC* ❏ *Sexual[5]* ❏ *Cholesterol* ❏ *Dentist* ❏	Hearing, vision[2] ❏	Mobility Asymmetry Scoliosis	❏ ❏ ❏	Family support[4] Cardiology[3] Ophthalmology[3] Orthopedics	❏ ❏ ❏ ❏

Clinical concerns for Arthrogryposis syndromes, ages 6+ years

Failure to thrive	Cardiac anomalies	Mental disability
Strabismus	Pulmonary hypoplasia	Brain anomalies, seizures
High palate	Joint contractures	Inguinal, umbilical hernias
Dental crowding	Asymmetry, scoliosis	Genital anomalies

Guidelines for prior ages should be undertaken *at the time of diagnosis*; Td, tetanus/diphtheria; MMR, measles–mumps–rubella; Var, varicella; [1]alternative timing; [2]by practitioner; [3]as dictated by clinical findings; [4]parent group, family/sib, financial, and behavioral issues as discussed in the preface; [5]birth control, STD screening if sexually active; [6]repeat every decade.

Part VIII

Management of neurodegenerative metabolic disorders

With several hundred diseases and an aggregate frequency of 1 in 600 births, a complete discussion of metabolic disorders is beyond the scope of this book. The classic reference of Scriver et al. (1995a) provides an encyclopedic and detailed description of inborn errors of metabolism. Selected here are several of the more common diseases that illustrate the role of generalists in the care of patients with metabolic disorders. Since the focus of this book is congenital malformations, emphasis is given to disorders that produce alterations in appearance and/or morphogenesis (Burton, 1998). From the standpoint of morphogenesis, these are metabolic dysplasias in the sense that they cause altered histiogenesis (see Chapter 1). Examples include the glycogen storage diseases, producing a "cherubic" facies and hepatomegaly; the mucopolysaccharidoses, producing a coarsened facies with dysostosis multiplex; and a variety of neuromuscular diseases in which severe hypotonia causes subtle facial alterations (bitemporal hollowing, down-turned corners of the mouth), single palmar creases, and contractures (e.g., club feet).

Most patients with inborn errors of metabolism will require consistent input from metabolic specialists for monitoring of injurious metabolites, dietary counseling, and prognostication. Ideally, the primary physician would coordinate general health care issues including growth, development, and school issues, leaving metabolic management to the specialist. In practice, the sweep of managed care may force many primary physicians to coordinate more of the dietary and metabolic management of patients with inborn errors of metabolism. Disorders that are unresponsive to dietary treatment, discussed in Chapter 19, are more similar to malformation syndromes in requiring chronic preventive management to realize an optimal quality of life. Despite their known or suspected metabolic etiology, these metabolic dysplasia syndromes are like other chronic disorders in needing informed primary care physicians to ensure optimal preventive care after the initial diagnostic evaluation.

19

Organellar and miscellaneous neurodegenerative disorders

Partitioning of the cell into organellar compartments offers the advantage and vulnerability of specialized function. Genetic mutations that alter the structure or targeting of organellar proteins may disrupt the entire organelle and produce multiple metabolic abnormalities. Examples of generalized organellar dysfunction include alterations of the mannose-6-phosphate targeting in lysosomes (e.g., I-cell disease), deletions of mitochondrial DNA (e.g., Kearns–Sayre syndrome), and mutations in peroxisomal membrane proteins (e.g., Zellweger syndrome). Other genetic mutations affect only one organellar protein, producing a more limited and specific phenotype (e.g., Fabry disease, Leber hereditary optic neuropathy, or adrenoleukodystrophy).

The dietary manipulations that are effective for the "small"-molecule disorders have limited use for organellar disorders. Deficiencies of lysosomal enzymes often lead to "storage" diseases, with the accumulation of "large" molecules that are internally synthesized and independent of dietary sources. Other lysosomal diseases, as well as disorders affecting the structure of mitochondria or peroxisomes, may involve an excess or deficiency of molecules within cellular compartments; these molecules are less accessible to manipulation by diet.

Many organellar disorders are progressive, involving a phase of normal development until the accumulation of metabolites interferes with organ function. Often several organs are affected, particularly the brain, eye, heart, liver, and skeleton. Most of the disorders exhibit insidious loss of previously acquired developmental milestones, followed by neurodegeneration and death. The age at which the deceleration of development occurs and the rate of progression vary widely. In a few diseases, and in some variants within a disease category, the nervous system is spared. Selected disorders affecting lysosomal, mitochondrial, or peroxisomal function are described in this chapter, with an emphasis on those causing syndromal disease. A miscellaneous category of metabolic dysplasias is also discussed, based on similarities in clinical presentation and natural history.

Lysosomal enzyme deficiencies

Lysosomes are one of several cytoplasmic organelles that form a network of protein transport between the plasma membrane and the Golgi apparatus (Sabatini & Adesnik, 1995). Endosomes from the Golgi may fuse with coated vesicles from the cell surface, acquire mannose-6-phosphate receptors that lead to the import of hydrolytic enzymes (multivesicular bodies), and shed these receptors to become a mature lysosome. External or internal cellular macromolecules can be transferred to the Golgi or to lysosomes via the multivesicular bodies, and those routed to mature lysosomes are degraded for the recycling of components. Deficiency of a single lysosomal hydrolase leads to abnormal accumulation of its substrate, causing lysosomal engorgement and disruption of other lysosomal hydrolases. Several types of macromolecules can then build up in susceptible organs. As outlined in this chapter, lysosomal enzyme deficiencies can be classified as lipidoses, mucolipidoses (oligosaccharidoses), or mucopolysaccharidoses according to the predominant type of macromolecule that is stored (Table 19.1).

Lysosomal diseases: Lipidoses and mucolipidoses (oligosaccharidoses)

The storage of lipid material is a common feature of several lysosomal enzyme deficiencies. Many, like Tay–Sachs disease, Sandhoff disease, Niemann–Pick disease, metachromatic leukodystrophy, G_{M2} gangliosidosis, or Krabbe disease, are predominantly neurodegenerative disorders that will not be discussed here. Preventive management of the neurolipidoses will involve regular neurologic, audiologic, and ophthalmologic evaluations that attend to neurosensory deficits, seizures, and progressive neurodevastation. Most neurolipidoses are lethal, autosomal recessive diseases requiring genetic counseling, extensive psychosocial support, physical/occupational therapy, and hospice services.

Other lipidoses affect many other structures besides the brain and eyes. Some of these involve the storage of both lipids and oligosaccharides, leading to a phenotype that resembles the mucopolysaccharidoses. These disorders have been called mucolipidoses or, because there is not a true "mucolipid" substance, oligosaccharidoses. Disorders of glycoprotein degradation including the mannosidoses, fucosidosis, and sialidoses could also be classified as oligosaccharidoses. Selected lipidoses and oligosaccharidoses are summarized in Table 19.1.

Disorders of glycoprotein degradation

Mannosidoses, fucosidosis, sialidoses, and aspartylglucosaminuria are autosomal recessive disorders caused by well-characterized enzyme deficiencies that allow prenatal diagnosis (Warner & O'Brien, 1983). Inspection of a blood smear for

Table 19.1 Selected lysosomal enzyme deficiencies

Disease or syndrome	Incidence (live births)	Deficient enzyme	Complications
Neurolipidoses			
Krabbe disease	1 in 200,000	Galactosyl-ceramidase	ND, blindness, deafness
Metachromatic leukodystrophy	1 in 50,000	Arylsulfatase A	ND, altered gait, incontinence, seizures, quadriparesis
Niemann–Pick diseases	1 in 40,000 (J)	Sphingomyelinase	ND, visceromegaly,
Tay–Sachs, Sandhoff disease (G$_{M2}$ gangliosidoses)	1 in 4000 (J) 1 in 100,000	Hexaminidase A,B	ND, cherry red spot
Other lipidoses			
Fabry disease	1 in 40,000	α-galactosidase	Angiokeratoma, band cataract, vascular disease, nerve pain, renal failure, hypohidrosis
Gaucher disease	1 in 1000 1 in 100,000	Glucocerebrosidase	ND (types 2,3), visceromegaly, bleeding, bone crises, joint disease, pulmonary disease
Oligosaccharidoses			
G$_{M1}$ gangliosidosis	~50 cases	β-Galactosidase	ND, Hurler-like, cherry red spots
I-cell disease	~50 cases	Phosphotransferase	ND, Hurler-like
Pseudo-Hurler syndrome	~50 cases	Phosphotransferase	ND, Hurler-like
Multiple sulfatase deficiency	~50 cases	Sulfatases	ND, Hurler-like, cherry red spot, ichthyosis
Mannosidosis	~50 cases	α-Mannosidase	ND, Hurler-like, seizures, cataracts
Mannosidosis	~50 cases	β-Mannosidase	ND, Hurler-like, hearing loss, infections
Fucosidosis	~100 cases	α-Fucosidase	ND, Hurler-like, angiokeratomas, hypohidrosis
Sialidosis	~50 cases	Sialidase	ND, Hurler-like, cherry red spot, angiokeratomas
Aspartylglucosaminuria	~100 cases	Aspartyl hydrolase	ND, Hurler-like, cataracts
Mucopolysaccharidoses			
Hurler syndrome (type IH)	1 in 100,000	α-Iduronidase	ND, coarse face and skin, viscous mucous, pectus, gibbus, dysostosis, visceromegaly
Scheie syndrome (type IS)	1 in 500,000	α-Iduronidase	
Hunter syndrome (type II)	1 in 65,000	Iduronate sulfatase	ND, Hurler-like

Table 19.1 (*cont.*)

Disease or syndrome	Incidence (live births)	Deficient enzyme	Complications
San Filippo syndrome (type III)	1 in 24,000	Heparan sulfatase	ND, Hurler-like (later onset)
Morquio syndrome (type IV)	1 in 40,000	β-Galactosidase	Dysostosis, short neck and trunk
Maroteaux–Lamy (type VI)	1 in 100,000	Arylsulfatase B	Hurler-like
Sly syndrome (type VII)	~20 cases	β-Glucuronidase	ND, Hurler-like

Notes:

J, Jewish population; ND, neurodegeneration.

vacuolated lymphocytes and urine screening for mannose, fucose, sialyl, or aspartylglucosamine oligosaccharides allow suspicion of the diagnoses, followed by demonstration of the appropriate enzyme deficiency in leukocytes (Cantz & Ullrich-Bott, 1990). Each of these diseases may be associated with a Hurler-like syndrome reminiscent of the mucopolysaccharidoses. Other clinical manifestations include moderate to severe mental retardation and seizures, cataracts and corneal opacities (α-mannosidosis, aspartylglucosaminuria), cherry red spots (sialidosis), hearing loss (β-mannosidosis), recurrent infections (β-mannosidosis), sweat abnormalities with hypohidrosis (fucosidosis), and angiokeratomas of the skin (fucosidosis, β-mannosidosis, sialidosis; Thomas & Beaudet, 1995). There are subtypes within these disorders that vary in their onset and progression. Adult survival is common in certain types of sialidosis and in aspartylglucosaminuria.

Preventive management should be similar to that outlined for the mucopolysaccharidoses, with focus on neurologic, ophthalmologic, and orthopedic evaluations (Warner & O'Brien, 1983; Thomas & Beaudet, 1995). Audiologic monitoring is particularly important for patients with mannosidosis and fucosidosis, and visual deterioration is noted in patients with sialidosis. Patients with aspartylglucosaminuria are susceptible to pulmonary infections and cardiac valvular disease in adulthood. The early intervention and psychosocial services emphasized for patients with mucopolysaccharidoses are certainly needed for severely affected patients with mannosidoses, fucosidosis, sialidoses, and aspartylglucosaminuria.

Fabry disease

Fabry disease was described in 1898 and initially named angiokeratoma corporis diffusum universale because of its characteristic skin lesions (Gorlin et al., 1990, pp.

129–31). It is an X-linked disorder caused by a deficiency of α-galactosidase, encoded by a locus in chromosome region Xq22. There is progressive deposition of glycolipids into the endothelium of blood vessels, accounting for most of the clinical manifestations. On the skin, glycolipid deposition produces dark-red to blue telangiectasias that cluster over the umbilicus, thorax, thighs, buttocks, and knees. There is also ectodermal dysplasia with sparse body and facial hair together with hypohidrosis. Blood vessel changes in many other organs produce retinal and conjunctival aneurysms with cloudiness of the cornea and a whitish band in the lens called "Fabry cataract" (Gorlin et al., 1990, pp. 129–32). Proteinuria with azotemia and renal failure, myocardial infarction, and cerebrovascular disease causes increased morbidity and mortality, with a mean survival of 41 years for untransplanted patients. Chronic pain from paresthesias begins in childhood, and these episodic crises of burning pain may drive patients to attempt suicide. Growth retardation, delayed puberty, abdominal pain, lymphedema of the limbs, and avascular necrosis of the femoral head are less common findings.

Preventive management for Fabry disease should include regular ophthalmologic evaluations, dermatologic monitoring of the skin lesions with possible cosmetic treatments, and periodic monitoring of blood pressure, renal functions, heart, and urinary sediment. Growth and development should be followed in early childhood, with possible referral for early intervention services if there are delays. Pain management is important, and clinicians should consider referring severely affected patients to pain specialists. Diphenylhydantoin and carbamazapine have been helpful in suppressing painful crises (Lockman et al., 1973). The α-galactosidase is a lysosomal enzyme that is taken up by deficient cells, so renal transplantation and enzyme therapies have had some success (Desnick et al., 1995).

Gaucher disease

Gaucher disease was described in 1882 based on a patient with massive splenomegaly (Beutler & Grabowski, 1995). Three types of the disease have been recognized, with types 2 and 3 being much rarer and having severe to moderate neurologic involvement. All three types are autosomal recessive, and involve accumulation of glucocerebroside due to deficiency of β-glucosidase. The incidence is about 1 in 1000 births for the Ashkenazic Jewish population and 1 in 100,000 in non-Jewish populations (Beutler & Grabowski, 1995).

Clinical manifestions of type 1 Gaucher disease include neurologic (spinal cord compression due to collapse of vertebrae), pulmonary (infiltrative disease with clubbing), gastroenterologic (hepatomegaly and occasional liver failure), hematologic (thrombocytopenia, splenic infarction or rupture), and skeletal (painful "bone crises," fractures) abnormalities (Beutler & Grabowski, 1995). Type 2 (acute neuronopathic) Gaucher disease may present as hydrops fetalis or infantile oculomotor abnormalities (e.g., strabismus). Severe neurologic features (hypertonia, choreo-athetosis, seizures) and visceromegaly are present during infancy, and death usually occurs by age 2 years. Type 3 Gaucher disease resembles type 2 in presenting with oculomotor changes and visceromegaly. The usual onset is between infancy and age 14 years, with survival to the third or fourth decade.

The diagnostic evaluation may include a bone marrow to demonstrate the foam-laden Gaucher cells, but should rest on the demonstration of β-glucosidase deficiency in leucocytes. DNA analysis for β-glucosidase gene mutations is also available, and is preferred when a mutation has been demonstrated in affected relatives.

Preventive management for Gaucher disease is outlined by Beutler & Grabowski (1995). After diagnosis, the first consideration is splenectomy for patients with massive splenomegaly or severe thrombocytopenia (platelet count less than 40,000). The need for penicillin prophylaxis of overwhelming infection may be mitigated by performing a partial splenectomy. With the advent of enzyme therapy, splenectomy is less commonly performed. Skeletal abnormalities may be severe, and periodic orthopedic evaluations should be performed. Patients should be counseled to avoid high-intensity exercise; swimming is a good choice for minimizing joint deterioration. Hip, knee, and shoulder joint replacements have been helpful in alleviating pain and restoring mobility, but surgeons should be experienced in dealing with bone thinning and pseudofractures. Phosphonates have shown anecdotal but not controlled benefits in treating bone disease.

Although the ability to target exogenous enzymes to lysosomes has made this category an attractive candidate for enzyme therapy, Gaucher disease is one of the few disorders where this has been achieved. Modified enzyme from human placenta (Ceredase or alglucerase) has been industrially produced and shown to improve hematologic and skeletal abnormalities in patients with Gaucher disease. Although the amounts of enzyme needed decline during the course of therapy, initial costs can be as high as $400,000 per year for an adult male (Figueroa et al., 1992). Furthermore, some manifestations (e.g., pulmonary disease) appear unaffected by enzyme therapy. A recombinant enzyme produced in bacteria (Cerezyme) has recently become available. Bone marrow transplant is also effective and expensive, but has the usual disadvantage of a 10–15 percent mortality rate.

G_{M1} gangliosidosis, I-cell disease, and pseudo–Hurler polydystrophy

Children with early and severe features of Hurler syndrome but with minimal urine mucopolysaccharide excretion were initially designated as having pseudo-Hurler syndrome. Since some children with these clinical features (e.g., those with G_{M1} gangliosidosis) had cherry red spots reminiscent of neurolipidosis, the term "mucolipidosis" was coined to designate the combined findings. Methods for detecting urine oligosaccharides by thin-layer chromatography replaced this name with the chemically accurate designation of oligosaccharidoses (Gorlin et al., 1990, pp. 117–28). The severe, aggregate manifestations of oligosaccharidoses relate in part to the many varieties of accumulated polysaccharides. Deficiency of a multi-substrate enzyme (β-galactosidase in G_{M1} gangliosidosis) or deficiency of multiple enzymes due to a disruption of the mannose-6-phosphate targeting system (I-cell disease, pseudo-Hurler polydystrophy) accounts for the accumulation of these complex oligosaccharides. Inclusions may be seen in leukocytes and fibroblasts, explaining the term "inclusion-cell disease." Multiple sulfatase deficiency also has a severe, multienzyme deficiency phenotype that combines features of lipidosis and mucopolysaccharidosis (see below).

G_{M1} gangliosidosis, I-cell disease, and pseudo-Hurler polydystrophy all have an onset of Hurlerlike features at birth or during infancy. A cherry red spot is often seen in G_{M1} gangliosidosis, with corneal clouding more common in I-cell disease and pseudo-Hurler polydystrophy (Gorlin et al., 1990, pp. 117–28). All can exhibit rapid progression of neurologic symptoms and Hurler-like somatic manifestations. As with other lysosomal storage disorders, there are milder clinical variants within these categories. Preventive management is essentially the same as detailed below for the mucopolysaccharidoses. An emphasis on preserving neurosensory, joint, and respiratory functions is important for patients with milder disease; survival is often limited to early childhood in the severe forms.

Multiple sulfatidosis

Most forms of sulfatide lipidosis (metachromatic leukodystrophies) cause neurode-generation and death without an unusual appearance. However, children with multi-ple sulfatase deficiency lack not only the arylsulfatases responsible for metachromatic leukodystrophy but also the mucopolysaccharide sulfatases that are deficient in dis-orders such as Hunter syndrome. These children have features resembling the muco-polysaccharidoses, and the disorder has been called Austin syndrome.

Clinical manifestations include a loss of milestones in the second year, with pro-gressive development of hearing loss, blindness, and seizures. Features of muco-polysaccharidosis may appear simultaneously with the neurologic deterioration, or may appear later. They include subtle coarse facies, visceromegaly, joint contrac-tures, pectus, and gibbus. Ichthyosis and cherry red spots may occur in multiple sulfatase deficiency as distinguishing features from the mucopolysaccharidoses. Preventive management should be as outlined for the mucopolysaccharidoses, with the additional provision of skin lotions for the treatment of ichthyosis. Some ameli-oration of symptoms has been produced by bone marrow transplantation, but the procedure has worsened the clinical course of patients who are already deteriorat-ing (Kolodny & Fluharty, 1995).

Lysosomal diseases: mucopolysaccharidoses

The mucopolysaccharidoses are a group of neurodegenerative disorders that exhibit somatic changes of the face and skeleton (Table 19.1). They are lysosomal storage diseases, caused by a deficiency of enzymes that sculpt complex chains of carbohydrate and protein (glycosaminoglycans). Glycosaminoglycans are a prominent component of the extracellular matrix, explaining the thickened secretions and subcutaneous tissues in children with mucopolysaccharidosis. The typical somatic changes embodied by Hurler syndrome are also seen in certain lipidoses or oligosaccharidoses (Table 19.1) distinguished from the mucopolysaccharidoses by their lower amounts of urinary glycosaminoglycans. The mucopolysaccharide-storage disorders offer a compelling strategy for enzyme or gene therapy that is derived from the classic experiments of Neufeld and colleagues (Neufeld & Muenzer, 1995): the deficient enzymes often contain a mannose-6-phosphate "tag" that targets them to lysosomes of the appropriate cells and allows a restoration of degradative function.

In contrast to neurolipidoses such as Tay–Sachs or Krabbe diseases, the mucopolysaccharide/oligosaccharide storage diseases develop a Hurler-like syndrome that extends beyond the neurodegeneration of the retina and brain (Table 19.1). At times that vary from birth to later adolescence, depending on the disease and/or severity, the patients develop insidious symptoms. These include coarsening of the facial features, thickening of the skin and hair, thickened secretions that cause chronic rhinorrea or communicating hydrocephalus, joint contractures, and skeletal deformities (Gorlin et al., 1990, pp. 99–117). The Hurler-like appearance becomes manifest during late fetal development in the infantile form of G_{M1} gangliosidosis, during early childhood in the Hurler and Hunter syndromes, and during adolescence in the milder forms of San Filippo or Maroteaux–Lamy syndromes (Table 19.1).

The degree of mental disability versus connective tissue or skeletal involvement varies among the different mucopolysaccharide storage disorders and among different patients with the same disorder. Patients with San Filippo syndrome have severe mental disability with milder somatic features, while those Morquio or Maroteaux–Lamy syndromes have normal mentality with severe somatic features. Despite these variations, a common set of strategies for diagnosis and preventive management are required for the mucopolysaccharidoses and oligosaccharidoses. The descriptions below are directed toward patients with mucopolysaccharidoses I (Hurler), II (Hunter), VI (Maroteaux–Lamy) and VII (Sly) syndromes, but can be modified for relevance to other conditions listed in Table 19.1. These modifications are outlined briefly in the sections devoted to complications and management.

Terminology

The mucopolysaccharidoses were first identified by the classical reports of Hurler and Hunter in the early 1900s (Spranger, 1987). Distinctive clinical manifestations and subsequent characterization of enzyme deficiencies led to the delineation of seven types, each bearing the eponym of its discoverer (Table 19.1). Scheie disease was initially designated as type V until it was realized that both Scheie and Hurler syndromes involve a deficiency of α-iduronidase. Although descriptive of their high content in mucus and their core polysaccharide chain, the substances designated as "mucopolysaccharides" are more properly termed "glycosaminoglycans." Many forms of glycosaminoglycans exist, and the relative proportions of keratan sulfate, dermatan sulfate, or heparan sulfate excreted in the urine can give preliminary insight into the type of mucopolysaccharidosis.

Incidence, etiology, and differential diagnosis

The incidence of disorders with the syndrome of coarse facies and dysostosis multiplex is estimated at 1 in 10,000–20,000 births, depending on the age of ascertainment. Individual disorders, exemplified by Hurler (1 in 100,000 births), Scheie (1 in 500,000 births), or Hunter (1 in 65,000 births) syndromes, are much more rare. The etiology of these disorders is a deficiency of lysosomal proteins that incorporate or degrade complex glycosaminoglycans within lysosomes. Specific enzyme deficiencies have been characterized for all of the clinically delineated mucopolysaccharide and oligosaccharide syndromes, and antibodies to the affected proteins have led to the cloning and characterization of the responsible genes. Following the rule for other enzymes involved in the same metabolic pathway or process, the genes responsible for mucopolysaccharide accumulation are distributed widely across the genome. All are autosomal recessive disorders, with the exception of Hunter syndrome, which is X-linked recessive. Proper biochemical and molecular diagnosis of affected children allows prenatal diagnosis in subsequent pregnancies.

The differential diagnosis is chiefly concerned with distinguishing among the members of the mucopolysaccharidosis/mucolipidosis category. Disorders with later onset of the characteristic facial and skeletal changes, such as San Filippo syndrome, may be confused with other causes of mental retardation and bony deformities. Chromosomal disorders and syndromes with contractures may be confused until the appropriate biochemical studies are performed.

Diagnostic evaluation and medical counseling

The presenting complaints of children with mucopolysaccharidoses will usually be developmental delay with or without unusual facial or skeletal findings. The more severe disorders may present with hydrops fetalis, infantile hydrocephalus, or even multiple fractures suggestive of osteogenesis imperfecta. For mildly stigmatized patients, an ophthalmologic examination for corneal clouding, skeletal radiographic survey for evidence of dysostosis, and a urine mucopolysaccharide screen are often obtained as evidence that the patient fits into the mucopolysaccharidosis category. Chromosomal studies may be considered for exclusion, and cranial imaging or liver biopsy may be obtained if there is macrocephaly or hepatosplenomegaly. It should be emphasized that random urine samples may give false negative results for mucopolysaccharides if they are too dilute, or false positive results if they are stored at room temperature and contaminated by bacteria. Nonspecific indicators of altered mucopolysaccharide metabolism, such as the measurement of radioactive sulfate accumulation in fibroblasts, may also give anomalous results. Patients with suggestive clinical findings should have serum, leukocyte, or fibroblast enzyme assays performed for the disorders in question; several academic centers offer panels of relevant leukocyte and serum assays. Serum levels of lysosomal enzymes are elevated in disorders such as mucolipidosis II (I-cell disease) where defective lysosomal transport allows the egress of multiple degradative enzymes.

Medical counseling must be tailored to the particular type of mucopolysaccharidosis or oligosaccharidosis. Many of these disorders are uniformly fatal, with the life span depending on complications and the dedication of the family to chronic care. Patients with G_{M1} gangliosidosis or I-cell disease will usually die in early childhood; those with Hurler or Hunter syndromes, in later childhood or adolescence. Complicating predictions are the varying phenotypes caused by similar enzyme deficiencies; the iduronidase deficiencies in Hurler and Scheie disease cause early death in the former disorder but allow a virtually normal life in the latter. Mild variants have also been described having the same iduronate sulfatase deficiency found in Hunter syndrome. In general, children with stigmata manifest in early childhood face a terminal illness with severe neurodevastation that renders them bedridden and dependent on gastrostomy feedings. Attention to the type of enzyme deficiency is also important, with the Morquio or Maroteaux–Lamy syndromes exhibiting normal intelligence despite severe somatic changes. Emphasis on minimizing pain and maximizing the quality of life is recommended, without attempting to predict the exact timing of disability and death.

Family and psychosocial counseling

Because all of the mucopolysaccharidoses and oligosaccharidoses are autosomal or X-linked recessive, a 25 percent recurrence risk can be predicted for subsequent children. In the X-linked Hunter syndrome, only males will have phenotypic expression unless carrier females experience deletion of their normal X chromosome locus due to chromosome rearrangement. Prenatal diagnosis is available through chorionic villus biopsy or amniocentesis, although overlap of heterozygote and affected homozygote enzyme levels have caused errors in some instances. In some of the disorders, common molecular mutations have been characterized that allow DNA diagnosis.

Psychosocial counseling is extremely important in the more severe mucopoly-saccharidoses because of the terrible burden of these diseases. Not only must parents learn that their apparently normal child will experience degeneration and death, but also they must witness the progressive coarsening and deformity of their child. Many patients also have severe behavioral changes that disrupt family life, with aggression, biting, hyperactivity, and inability to sleep. The large size and aggressiveness of some children warrant special measures for confinement, including a secured area to put the child and allow respite during selected family activities and sleep. Contacts with psychosocial and pastoral counseling services should be facilitated for all families with severely affected children, and parent support groups can be pivotal for family survival.

Natural history and complications

The majority of patients with mucopolysaccharidoses exhibit macrocephaly and early increase of growth until medical complications accumulate (mucopolysac-charidosis checklist, part 1). In Hurler syndrome, the accelerated growth falls off between one and two years of age, in Hunter syndrome, between three and six years (Gorlin et al., 1990, pp. 99–117). Behavioral changes often accompany the plateauing of development, with poor attention span, aggressive behavior, and temper tantrums. Hydrocephalus may be present. Chronic rhinorrhea and otitis are common, and the thick mucus together with a large tongue places patients at risk of airway obstruction or sleep apnea. Corneal clouding is prominent in the Hurler and Maroteaux–Lamy syndromes, but absent in Hurler syndrome. The skeletal changes include progressive contractures of the extremities and deformity of the chest and spine (pectus, gibbus, scoliosis). Inguinal and umbilical hernias as well as congenital hip dislocation may attest to the general affliction of connective tissue. Deformities of the thoracic cage, together with thickened alveolar secretions, often produce restrictive lung disease and interstitial pneumonitis (Gorlin et al., 1990, pp. 99–117). Odontoid hypoplasia and platyspondyly may cause cervical spinal cord compression, adding another source of unacknowledged pain or apnea (Brill et al., 1978).

As the disease progresses, the cardiac valves may become infiltrated and lead to congestive heart failure. Dental cysts and thin enamel may compromise oral hygiene and interfere with feeding, and infiltration of the intestine can produce chronic diarrhea. Joint fixations and neurosensory deficits lead to a withdrawn, bedridden patient with cardiorespiratory compromise. Pneumonias are a frequent cause of death. Distinctive findings among the mucopolysaccharidoses include more severe hearing loss in Hunter syndrome and the appearance of somatic features in later childhood or adolescence in Scheie syndrome. There are milder somatic features despite severe neurodegeneration in the four subtypes of San Filippo syndrome, thoracic dysplasia suggestive of a skeletal dysplasia in Morquio syndrome, and more severe cardiovascular infiltration in Maroteaux–Lamy syndrome. Hearing loss is prominent in both Morquio and Maroteaux–Lamy syndromes, and both usually have normal intellectual potential if not compromised by neurosensory deficits and medical problems. Sly syndrome exhibits striking variability, with some patients presenting as hydrops fetalis and others having only mild mental disability (Gorlin et al., 1990, pp. 99–117).

The mucopolysaccharidoses preventive medical checklist

If not part of the initial diagnostic evaluation, then a cranial MRI scan, ophthalmologic examination, audiologic assessment, and skeletal radiographic survey should be performed as soon as a specific enzymatic diagnosis is made (checklist, parts 2–4). Neurosensory evaluation is extremely important, and regular audiometric, and ophthalmologic evaluations are essential (Neufeld & Muenzer, 1995). Periodic examination of the skeleton is also important, with referral to orthopedics for the treatment of congenital hip dislocation, joint contractures, or scoliosis. Physical and occupational therapy are needed to maintain joint mobility, and these should be initiated through early intervention services. Radiologic evaluation of the cervical spine should be performed routinely, and patients with stridor, upper airway obstruction, gasping respirations, or apnea need sleep studies and otolaryngologic evaluation. Patients with Morquio syndrome are at particular risk for quadriparesis due to atlantoaxial instability. Hydrocephalus and cervical spinal cord compression may be sources of pain that the patient cannot describe, so a high index of suspicion is necessary with consideration of craniospinal MRI scans (Neufeld & Muenzer, 1995). Undetected pain, including discomfort from upper respiratory congestion and serous otitis, may exacerbate difficult behavior. Careful medical surveillance is an important adjunct to psychosocial and pastoral supports, which should be facilitated for all families.

Depending on the type of mucopolysaccharidosis, later changes in the cardiac valves, joints, and teeth may occur in midchildhood (Hurler syndrome) up to the third or fourth decade (Scheie syndrome). Regular cardiac and skeletal evaluations are needed, with good histories and range-of-motion examinations to detect joint problems such as carpal tunnel syndrome. Formal cardiology referral with echocardiography should be performed during the initial phase of disease progression as judged by somatic and skeletal features. Because corneal clouding and hearing loss may progress during adulthood in the Scheie, Morquio, and Maroteaux–Lamy syndromes, ophthalmologic and audiometric assessments should be performed throughout life. Bone marrow transplant has been tried in several types of muco-polysaccharide disease with promising results. Younger children with minimal brain and visceral dysfunction are the best candidates.

Mitochondrial disorders

Mitochondrial disorders encoded by nuclear DNA

Mitochondria contain a large complement of proteins that contribute to the two mitochondrial membranes and mediate import of peptides and other metabolites into the organelle (Soumalainen, 1997; Warner & Shapira, 1997). Mitochondria contain unique ribosomes and protein synthesis mechanisms, and serve in respiratory and oxidation pathways that supply energy for the cell (Robinson, 1995; Shofner & Wallace, 1995). Many mitochondrial proteins are encoded by nuclear DNA and imported into the organelle, exemplified by most components of the respiratory chain. Metabolic disorders caused by the alteration of nuclear-encoded mitochondrial proteins will exhibit Mendelian inheritance: usually autosomal recessive but occasionally X-linked recessive inheritance (Table 19.2). Other mitochondrial proteins are synthesized by the 16-kilobase mitochondrial genome, which is transmitted to embryonic cells in the maternal oocyte cytoplasm. Genetic disorders involving mitochondrial genome-encoded proteins often exhibit maternal inheritance, meaning that all offspring of affected mothers but no offspring of affected fathers exhibit the trait. In practice, the 1000 mitochondria in each cell may become heterogeneous in their genomic and/or protein structure, a phenomenon termed heteroplasmy. Clinical manifestations of mitochondrial genome-encoded disorders may thus change with time, representing the proportion of abnormal genomes within cells of susceptible tissues. Maternal inheritance may therefore be obscured by absent manifestations in mothers or offspring that have small proportions of abnormal mitochondria in the cells of susceptible tissues. Direct analysis of mitochondrial DNA is now available to distinguish between nuclear and mitochondrial-encoded disorders, and to measure the degree of heteroplasmy.

An underlying theme in the pathogenesis of mitochondrial DNA mutations is a diminished cellular energy supply. Any given mitochondrial DNA phenotype probably depends on the degree to which mitochondrial respiratory function is disrupted, the energy requirements of particular tissues and developmental stages, and the proportions of altered mitochondria. The most common manifestation of decreased energy supply is lactic acidemia. If the lactic acidemia is pronounced during the neonatal period, infants may have a slightly unusual facies. Other disorders with acidosis and severe hypotonia, such as glutaric acidemia type II, will have more extensive dysmorphology reminiscent of Zellweger syndrome (see below).

Table 19.2 Mitochondrial, peroxisomal, and miscellaneous metabolic dysplasias

Disease or syndrome	Incidence	Inheritance	Complications
Mitochondrial diseases caused by nuclear genes			
Glutaric acidemia II	~50 cases	AR	ND, acidosis, hypotonia, abnormal facies, demyelination, renal cysts, genital a.
Leigh disease, lactic acidemias	?	AR, XLR	ND, lactic acidosis, hypotonia, brain a., optic atrophy, ophthalmoplegia
Mitochondrial diseases caused by mitochondrial genes			
Kearn–Sayres disease	~300 cases	Maternal, AD, AR	Ptosis, ophthalmoplegia, retinitis, hearing loss, diabetes, hypoparathyroidism, myopathy, lactic acidosis
Peroxisomal diseases			
Adrenoleukodystrophy	1 in 50,000	XLR	ND, visual loss, adrenal insufficiency
Infantile Refsum disease	~50 cases	AR	ND, hypotonia, unusual facies, liver disease, hearing loss, retinitis, ichthyosis
Neonatal adrenoleukodystrophy	~200 cases	AR	ND, hypotonia, unusual facies, seizures, demyelination, brain a.
Zellweger syndrome	1 in 50,000	AR	ND, hypotonia, unusual facies, demyelination, brain a., liver disease, renal cysts, stippled epiphyses
Miscellaneous metabolic dysplasias			
Carbohydrate-deficient glycoprotein syndrome	~50 cases	AR	ND, liver disease, ataxia, retinitis, strabismus, abnormal fat, coagulopathy
Smith–Lemli–Opitz syndrome	~150 cases	AR	ND, hypotonia, abnormal facies, polydactyly, renal cysts, genital a.

Notes:

AR, autosomal recessive; XLR, X-linked recessive: ND, neurodegeneration; a., anomalies.

Glutaric acidemia Type II

Accumulation of glutaric acid, a five-carbon dicarboxylic acid, occurs in two very different disorders. Type I glutaric acidemia is a defect in lysine metabolism associated with macrocephaly, hypotonia, dystonia, and Reyelike episodes with vomiting, hepatomegaly, and encephalopathy (Goodman & Frerman, 1995). Death often occurs in the first decade. Type II glutaric acidemia is caused by an abnormality of the electron transfer flavoprotein (ETF) that is part of the mitochondrial respiratory chain (Frerman & Goodman, 1995). Similar disorders are caused by deficiencies of ETF or its dehydrogenase, and both exhibit autosomal recessive inheritance consistent with their encoding by the nuclear genome.

Clinical manifestations of glutaric acidemia type II are of three types: neonatal onset with malformations, neonatal onset without malformations, and onset in later childhood (Frerman & Goodman, 1995). Major and minor anomalies include macrocephaly, a large anterior fontanelle, high forehead, broad nasal root, telecanthus, rocker bottom feet, renal cysts, hypospadias, and chordee (Wilson et al., 1989). The neonatal presentation usually includes hypotonia and hepatomegaly associated with severe hypoglycemia and metabolic acidosis. Most patients with neonatal onset die in early infancy, often with hypertrophic cardiomyopathy. Later-onset patients have presented in early to later childhood with vomiting, hypoglycemia, and acidosis. The initial diagnostic evaluation should include: urine organic acid and ketone determination – potentially revealing glutaric, ethylmalonic, and adipic acids but no ketones; serum glucose, electrolyte, hepatic transaminase, and carnitine levels – potentially revealing hypoglycemia, acidosis, and liver disease; cranial MRI scan – potentially revealing demyelination; and abdominal CT scan – potentially showing renal cysts. A definitive diagnosis can be made by demonstrating deficiency of ETF or its dehydrogenase in cultured fibroblasts or liver.

Preventive management for glutaric acidemia II will be limited in neonatal onset patients, but should include chest radiography to monitor heart size, frequent electrolyte studies to monitor acidosis, and periodic urinalyses to monitor aminoaciduria and renal disease. Therapy with oral riboflavin (100 to 300 mg per day) and oral carnitine (100 mg per kilogram per day) have had some benefit in later-onset patients but not with neonates (Frerman & Goodman, 1995). A low fat and protein diet may also be helpful. Genetic and psychosocial counseling are important for parents, and later-onset patients should have early intervention services.

Leigh disease and lactic acidemias

Leigh disease, also known as subacute necrotizing encephalomyelopathy, is a phenotype that is produced by a variety of defects in the mitochondrial respiratory chain. The presentation has onset from early infancy to middle childhood, and includes hypotonia, developmental delay with regression, optic atrophy, strabismus, nystagmus, irregularities in breathing, muscle weakness, and lactic acidosis. Later neurologic symptoms may include ataxia and spasticity. The cranial MRI scan shows demyelination and/or hyperintense areas near the thalamus and basal ganglia. Occasional patients have retinitis or hypertrophic cardiomyopathy, and some have the ragged red fibers visualized on muscle biopsy specimens that are characteristic of mitochondrial disease (Shofner & Wallace, 1995).

The diagnosis of Leigh disease involves an analysis of respiratory chain components in muscle or leukocytes. Alterations in cytochrome c (respiratory complex

IV) are most common, but abnormalities of NADH dehydrogenase (respiratory complex I) or pyruvate dehydrogenase have also been reported. DNA analysis is the preferred diagnostic method, since several common mutations have been described (Shofner & Wallace, 1995). While most mutations causing Leigh disease have been in nuclear-encoded genes, a few examples with maternal inheritance have been demonstrated. It is important to realize that the phenotype is extremely variable and heterogeneous, overlapping with other mitochondrial diseases such as pigmentary retinopathy with degeneration or mitochondrial myopathy (Shofner & Wallace, 1995).

Also overlapping with the Leigh disease phenotype are numerous disorders of the mitochondrial respiratory chain that produce chronic lactic acidemia. The most common of this group is deficiency of the pyruvate dehydrogenase complex. Pyruvate dehydrogenase deficiency can cause severe neonatal lactic acidemia and death, more moderate lactic acidemia with severe developmental retardation, or intermittent lactic acidemia with ataxia after a carbohydrate load (Robinson, 1995). Clinical variability is probably related to the presence of multiple subunits in the pyruvate dehydrogenase complex, one of which is encoded on the X chromosome. Other causes include deficiency of enzymes in the glycolytic pathway (phosphenolpyruvate carboxykinase, pyruvate carboxylase). Lactic acidemias can exhibit autosomal recessive or X-linked recessive inheritance.

The initial diagnostic evaluation for children with Leigh disease or lactic acidemias should be performed in conjunction with metabolic disease specialists and include serum glucose, hepatic transaminase, electrolyte, lactate, and pyruvate levels. A high pyruvate and a high lactate (normal lactate/pyruvate ratio) would suggest defects in pyruvate dehydrogenase or other diseases such as glycogen-storage disease or defects in fatty acid oxidation. A high lactate/pyruvate ratio suggests a respiratory defect typical of Leigh disease and other mitochondrial disorders. A cranial MRI scan, ophthalmologic examination, and muscle biopsy should then reveal the typical basal ganglia demyelination, retinitis, or ragged red fibers of Leigh/respiratory chain disease, or demonstrate the more limited phenotype of lactic acidemia and neurodegeneration. Analysis for common mutations associated with Leigh disease or assay of pyruvate dehydrogenase and pyruvate carboxylase can then proceed as appropriate. The category of lactic acidemias is still expanding, and specific enzyme or DNA alterations may not be identified in many patients. Preventive management is limited to periodic neurologic and ophthalmologic evaluations, control of lactic acidosis, monitoring of growth and nutrition, and referral for early intervention services.

Several therapies have been tried for respiratory chain disorders and lactic acidemias, but disease heterogeneity has complicated the interpretation of results (Shofner & Wallace, 1995). A low-carbohydrate, ketogenic diet may be helpful for children with pyruvate dehydrogenase deficiency (Robinson, 1995). Dichloro-acetate at levels of 15 to 200 mg per kg per day often reduces lactate levels by 20 percent and has few side effects. Menadione (vitamin K_3) at 1.1–1.5 mg per kg per day and ascorbic acid at 50 mg per kg per day have been tried as electron donors to cytochrome c. Coenzyme Q (4.3 mg per kg per day), thiamine (100 mg per day), and riboflavin (300 mg per day as mentioned above) have also been tried (Shofner & Wallace, 1995). None of these treatments has produced a dramatic reversal of neurologic deterioration.

Mitochondrial disorders encoded by mitochondrial DNA

Mutations in the mitochondrial genome produce an overlapping group of disease findings that depend on the location and extent of altered DNA. Single nucleotide mutations may produce a limited phenotype such as Leber hereditary optic neuropathy (LHON) or maternally inherited sensorineural deafness (Shofner & Wallace, 1995). Large mitochondrial DNA deletions often affect several organ systems, exemplified by Kearns–Sayre syndrome. The findings in Kearns–Sayre syndrome are quite variable, and overlap with those of other mitochondrial DNA mutations. Among these are Pearson syndrome (bone marrow failure, pancreatic dysfunction with diabetes mellitus, ataxia, myopathy), diabetes mellitus with deafness, MERRF (mitochondrial encephalopathy with ragged red fibers), MELAS (mitochondrial encephalopathy with lactic acidemia and strokes), and myoneuro-gastrointestinal disorder (encephalopathy, diarrhea, malabsorption, weight loss, external ophthalmoplegia, and peripheral neuropathy – Shofner & Wallace, 1995).

Kearns–Sayre syndrome

Patients with Kearns–Sayre syndrome show manifestations before age 20 that include ophthalmoplegia, retinitis pigmentosa, generalized myopathy, and occasional cardiac conduction defects (Shofner & Wallace, 1995). If the onset of symptoms occurs after age 20, the patients are classified as having chronic progressive external ophthalmoplegia with or without other manifestations. Both diseases are associated with mitochondrial DNA deletions that occur during embryogenesis and increase their proportions with age, causing progressive disease. Another closely related condition is Pearson syndrome, with bone marrow failure, pancreatic insufficiency, and similar neurologic problems. Associated clinical manifestations in this spectrum of disorders include lactic acidemia, seizures, dementia, ataxia, optic atrophy, hearing loss, cardiac arrhythmias, diabetes mellitus, hypoparathyroidism, gastrointestinal dysmotility, renal failure with glomerulosclerosis, and neuropathies (Shofner & Wallace, 1995). Some patients have had renal tubular acidosis and others severe atrophy of the choroid and sclera which resembles choroidemia. Diagnosis is made by analysis of mitochondrial DNA for deletions and, more rarely, duplications. Preventive management for patients with Kearns–Sayre syndrome, chronic progressive external ophthalmoplegia, and overlapping conditions will include regular ophthalmologic, neurologic, and audiometric assessments; serum glucose, calcium, electrolyte, blood urea nitrogen, creatinine, and lactate monitoring; periodic electrocardiography; and, depending on the age of onset, referral for early intervention, special education, or job training services. Trial of coenzyme Q, vitamin K, and/or ascorbate therapy as mentioned above may be considered.

Peroxisomal diseases

Peroxisomes are single-membraned organelles that contain over 40 proteins, many with a prominent role in lipid metabolism. They were first observed by electron microscopy and called "microbodies," then named peroxisomes based on their content of catalase and peroxidases (Wilson et al., 1988). Clinical interest in peroxisomes was intensified when their absence from the liver of patients with Zellweger syndrome was discovered (Goldfischer et al., 1973). A spectrum of diseases was soon defined, each involving abnormal peroxisomal structure or deficiencies of peroxisomal enzymes. Several peroxisomal diseases are summarized in Table 19.2.

A major distinction among peroxisomal diseases is whether they cause severe disruption of peroxisome structure, with multiple enzyme deficiencies, or whether they involve deficiency of a single enzyme that is located within peroxisomes (Lazarow & Moser, 1985). Acatalasemia, X-linked adrenoleukodystrophy, and rhizomelic chondrodysplasia punctata are disorders that may be caused by deficiency of a single peroxisomal enzyme deficiency (catalase, ALDP protein, and dihydroxyacetone phosphate acyltransferase enzyme respectively), and their phenotypes (mouth ulcers, neurodegenerative disease, skeletal dysplasia) are strikingly different. Peroxisomal diseases that involve multiple enzyme deficiencies have overlapping clinical manifestations that often involve the central nervous system; many of these patients have a syndrome of hypotonia and facial features that is most dramatic in Zellweger syndrome (Wilson et al., 1988). Patients with multiple deficiencies of peroxisomal enzymes also have a common metabolic profile with elevated very-long-chain fatty acids, elevated pipecolic and phytanic acids, and deficient plasmalogens. In a few cases, these multiple-enzyme deficiency diseases have been shown to involve alterations in proteins within the peroxisomal membrane. It is therefore logical that mutations that disrupt the entire peroxisomal structure would cause a severe and multifaceted phenotype due to multiple enzymic deficiencies, while those that affect a single peroxisomal enzyme have a more limited and specific phenotype (Wilson et al., 1988; Lazarow & Moser, 1995).

Zellweger syndrome is the prototype for disorders involving multiple peroxisomal enzyme deficiencies. The following discussion is oriented toward patients with Zellweger syndrome, with modifications for similar but less severe disorders such as neonatal adrenoleukodystrophy or infantile Refsum syndrome.

Terminology

Bowen et al. (1964) reported the first patients with Zellweger syndrome, although two of their patients proved to have a separate disorder. The Refsum syndrome of ataxia, retinitis, and ichthyosis was described in 1946, and in 1974, severely affected patients with similar features were described as infantile Refsum syndrome (Wilson et al., 1988). The neurologic and adrenal changes of adrenoleukodystrophy, recognized initially as an X-linked disorder in 1923, were described as an autosomal recessive, neonatal variety in 1978. Grouping of these apparently separate diseases as a peroxisomal disease category was made possible when biochemical markers of peroxisome dysfunction were characterized: elevated very-long-chain fatty acids and deficient plasmalogens. Soon it was realized that patients presenting as Zellweger syndrome, neonatal adrenoleukodystrophy, or infantile Refsum syndrome had alterations in the metabolism of very-long-chain fatty acid and plasmalogens. Unlike adult adrenoleukodystrophy or Refsum syndrome, these early-onset disorders had similar phenotypes due to generalized peroxisomal dysfunction (Wilson et al., 1988).

As with other multifaceted disorders, observers have seized upon component manifestations of Zellweger syndrome and reported affected patients as having separate conditions. Some patients described as having "chondrodysplasia punctata," "hyperpipecolatemia," or infantile Refsum disease undoubtedly are part of the spectrum of Zellweger syndrome, and it will require further biochemical and molecular characterization to achieve a precise delineation of the generalized peroxisomal disease category (Wilson, 1986). Rhizomelic chondrodysplasia punctata is discussed in more detail in Chapter 11. Detection of reduced red cell plasmalogens is particularly useful in this condition.

Incidence, etiology, and differential diagnosis

Although population surveys have estimated incidences for Zellweger syndrome as low as 1 in 100,000 births (Danks et al., 1975), the aggregate incidence of generalized peroxisomal disorders is thought to be 1 in 25,000–50,000 births (Zellweger, 1987). The generalized peroxisomal disorders exhibit autosomal recessive inheritance, and selected patients with Zellweger syndrome have had mutations in the 70-kilodalton or 35-kilodalton peroxisomal membrane proteins (Lazarow & Moser, 1985). Alterations in very long chain fatty acid degradation, plasmalogen synthesis, or numerous other pathways presumably account for the effects on embryogenesis and neural development. There is little understanding of the pathogenesis of peroxisomal disorders, but the ability to increase peroxisome density by administering oral agents offers some promise for pre- and postnatal therapy.

The differential diagnosis includes many other disorders with hypotonia, neurologic dysfunction, and congenital contractures (Wilson et al., 1988). Congenital myopathies, disorders producing stippling of the epiphyses (chondrodysplasia punctatas), and even Down syndrome have been confused. It may be difficult to separate Zellweger syndrome from other generalized peroxisomal disorders because of the similar profile of enzymic deficiencies and metabolic alterations. Even the classical Zellweger phenotype is heterogeneous, since studies investigating the correction of cells in culture have suggested that mutations at 13 different genetic loci can cause this phenotype (Lazarow & Moser, 1995).

Diagnostic evaluation and medical counseling

Children with generalized peroxisomal disorders often come to medical attention because of infantile hypotonia, and frequently have cranial MRI scans that may show demyelination. Additional diagnostic findings include retinitis pigmentosa detected by ophthalmologic examination, stippled epiphyses detected by radiographic survey, and periportal fibrosis with iron storage on liver biopsy performed for hepatomegaly. The diagnosis is confirmed by a demonstration of altered metabolites, particularly the sensitive and specific assay for serum very-long-chain fatty acids developed by Moser and colleagues (Brown et al., 1982). Additional metabolic testing includes assay of erythrocyte plasmalogens and serum phytanic acid; leukocyte or fibroblast enzyme assay to demonstrate deficiencies of dihydroxyacetone phosphate acyltransferase (Wilson et al., 1986), phytanic oxidase, or sedimented catalase may also be employed (Lazarow & Moser, 1995). All of these measures are usually abnormal in patients with severe Zellweger syndrome, while more selective elevations of very-long-chain fatty acids (neonatal adrenoleukodystrophy) or phytanic acid (infantile Refsum disease) may point toward other disorders.

Most important for medical counseling is the age of presentation and the severity of neurologic features. Severely hypotonic neonates with brain anomalies by MRI have a severe prognosis, with likely death during infancy. It should be remembered that hepatic disease in Zellweger syndrome may be fulminant in the first few months and subside, so prognosis should be based on neurologic manifestations. Even milder patients with a Zellweger syndrome phenotype will have significant neurosensory deficits and mental disability. Parents should be prepared for a potentially lethal and handicapping disorder.

Family and psychosocial counseling

All of the generalized peroxisomal disorders are autosomal recessive, implying a 25 percent recurrence risk for future pregnancies. Prenatal diagnosis is reliable by measuring elevated metabolites or enzyme deficiencies in chorionic villi or amniocytes. Psychosocial and pastoral support appropriate for a potentially lethal disorder should be facilitated. Parent support groups are listed on the checklist for peroxisomal disorders, part 1.

Natural history and complications

The natural history of peroxisomal disorders varies from a turbulent and lethal neonatal course to a chronic debilitating condition with survival into adulthood. Patients with Zellweger syndrome have facial features that derive from the hypotonia and dysostosis. Patients with milder Zellweger syndrome, neonatal adrenoleukodystrophy, or infantile Refsum disease have similar but less dramatic craniofacial findings. The anterior fontanelle is large, the forehead is prominent, and there is a broad nasal root with down-turned corners of the mouth and micrognathia. Single palmar creases, a high palate, and club feet are residua of in utero hypotonia, and there may be Brushfield spots and epicanthal folds reminiscent of Down syndrome. Additional clinical manifestations include congenital heart defects, liver disease with hepatitis and cirrhosis, renal cysts, genital anomalies such as hypospadias and cryptorchidism, and intestinal anomalies (pyloric stenosis, malrotation). Patients with infantile Refsum syndrome are more likely to have ichthyosis.

The clinical course is dominated by neurologic abnormalities including seizures, sensorineural deafness, blindness, and severe mental disability. Neuropathologic analysis has been performed on 46 patients with Zellweger syndrome, showing pachymicrogyria (67 percent), heterotopias or migration defects (48 percent), gliosis (35 percent), demyelination (22 percent), and agenesis of the corpus callosum (20 percent) or olfactory lobes (7 percent; Wilson et al., 1986). Poor nutrition and failure to thrive are usual, with most patients requiring gastrostomy feedings. The high palate leads to dental crowding, and proteinuria or urinary tract abnormalities (horseshoe kidney, renal agenesis) may occur (checklist, part 1).

Generalized peroxisomal disorders preventive medical checklist

After or during the initial diagnostic evaluation, a cranial MRI or CT scan, skeletal survey, renal sonogram, auditory evoked response study, electroretinogram, and screening of liver functions should be performed (checklist, parts 2–4). Ophthalmologic and neurologic assessments will usually be indicated to evaluate lens opacities, retinal pigmentation, seizure activity, and hypotonia. Feeding and nutrition should be followed carefully, since many patients will require high-calorie formulas, and nasogastric or gastrostomy feedings. Coagulation profiles and precautions against bleeding may be required if there is liver disease, and some patients have had esophageal varices. Occasional patients have presented with hypothyroidism, so monitoring of thyroid, hearing, vision, and nutrition is important in early

childhood. Early intervention and psychosocial counseling appropriate for children with severe disabilities is appropriate.

Long-term survivors will need monitoring of developmental progress, hearing
and vision. Speech therapy and dental evaluations for tooth crowding are also
important. Periodic urinalyses are advised to evaluate aminoaciduria and potential
infections; children with abnormal genitalia should have urologic assessment and
monitoring during puberty. Adrenal function may be compromised in the peroxisomal disorders, so steroid supplementation may be considered during acute illnesses. A corticin stimulation test can be performed to confirm subtle adrenal
insufficiency. Cataracts and ichthyosis can be late complications, so regular skin
and eye examinations are needed (checklist, parts 2–4).

Dietary therapy has been attempted in the peroxisomal disorders by minimizing
dietary oleic acid and dairy products containing phytanic acid (Lazarow & Moser,
1995). Dietary supplementation of ether lipids produced increases in erythrocyte
plasmalogens, but no long-term clinical improvements (Wilson et al., 1986).

Miscellaneous metabolic disorders

Carbohydrate-deficient glycoprotein syndrome

A wide variety of signs and symptoms can occur in the carbohydrate-deficient glycoprotein syndrome, including mental disability, growth failure, ataxia, seizures,
strokes, strabismus, retinal degeneration, cardiomyopathy with pericardial effusions,
elevated hepatic enzymes, renal microcysts, and unusual distribution of body fat
(Jaeken & Carchon, 1993; Thomas & Beaudet, 1995). More than 150 patients have
been reported, and the inheritance is autosomal recessive. The initial symptoms are
often hypotonia and developmental delay, with peau d'orange appearance of the skin
and lipodystrophy being the most distinctive features. Multiple glycoproteins have
abnormal carbohydrate moieties, causing deficiencies of the coagulation proteins S
and C, antithrombin III, and factor IX, with abnormal transferrin being used as a
diagnostic marker from serum. There is as yet no mapping data or knowledge of the
gene responsible for carbohydrate-deficient glycoprotein syndrome.

Preventive management should consist of an initial diagnostic evaluation
including a cranial MRI scan, screening of serum coagulation factors as well as
transferrin, cardiologic evaluation to screen for cardiomyopathy or pericardial
effusion, and ophthalmologic evaluation to screen for strabismus or retinal
changes. Hematologic referral to consider anticoagulant therapy should be considered in patients with low levels of protein S, C, and antithrombin III; hyperreflexia,
ataxia, and muscle atrophy in children have been attributed to stroke-like episodes
(Thomas & Beaudet, 1995). Variants exist with mild mental disability, but most
families should be referred for early intervention and psychosocial services.

Smith–Lemli–Opitz syndrome

Many years after Smith et al. (1964) described the Smith–Lemli–Opitz syndrome of microcephaly, growth delay, and facial and genital abnormalities, a defect in cholesterol metabolism has been recognized in these patients (Opitz & De la Cruz, 1994). There are in addition more severe patients who may represent a type II form of the disorder. The original patients had a very distinctive phenotype with a low birth weight, microcephaly, a broad nasal root, micrognathia, genital anomalies including cryptorchidism and hypospadias, and syndactyly of toes 2 and 3. In the type II patients, the prenatal growth retardation and genital anomalies are more severe, with affected males having female external genitalia and sex reversal. Both disorders exhibit autosomal recessive inheritance and elevations of the metabolite 7-dehydrocholesterol, and it will require further research to know if they result from locus or allelic heterogeneity (Opitz & De la Cruz, 1994; Elias & Irons, 1995).

Other clinical manifestations of type I Smith–Lemli–Opitz syndrome include: ptosis (85 percent), strabismus (40 percent), anteverted nares (75 percent), brain abnormalities (seizures, agenesis of corpus callosum, hypoplasia of cerebellar vermis), postaxial polydactyly (25 percent), hypospadias (50 percent), cryptorchidism (50 percent), congenital heart lesions (septal defects, tetralogy of Fallot, aberrant subclavian artery – 20 percent), and renal anomalies (cystic or hypoplastic kidneys – 45 percent; Gorlin et al., 1990, pp. 890–5; Lin et al., 1997). The additional or more extreme features of type II Smith–Lemli–Opitz syndrome include hydrocephalus, congenital hip dislocation, genital ambiguity with internal testes and Mullerian duct remnants in some males, Hirschsprung disease, and cardiac defects or renal cysts in the majority of patients.

Preventive management for patients with the Smith–Lemli–Opitz syndromes will include a comprehensive initial evaluation to screen for anomalies of brain, heart, skeleton, urinary tract and internal genitalia. The timing of cranial, cardiac, skeletal, abdominal, and pelvic imaging studies should be coordinated with the severity of illness and probability of neonatal survival. Many patients, particularly with the type II Smith–Lemli–Opitz syndrome, have a lethal disorder that merits palliative management sufficient for diagnosis and genetic counseling. However, milder forms of the disorder have been described (Lowry & Yong, 1980), and occasional patients survive to adulthood. Blood for the measurement of elevated 7-dehydrocholesterol levels should be obtained in all suspect patients, since a positive result provides the option for prenatal diagnosis in subsequent pregnancies.

Early feeding and nutrition is important to monitor in infants with Smith–Lemli–Opitz syndrome because of hypotonia (50 percent of infants) or hypertonia (30 percent of older children). Pyloric stenosis in addition to gastrointestinal reflux and Hirschsprung disease is common, as are cleft palate (40 percent) or broad lateral palatine ridges that give the appearance of a high palate (60 percent). The debilitated condition and infectious susceptibility of these patients, together with palatal anomalies, make surveillance for upper respiratory infections/chronic otitis and regular audiologic assessments worthwhile. Early and regular ophthalmologic evaluations are needed for the strabismus and cataracts, along with neurologic monitoring if there is behavior suggestive of seizures or hypertonicity that interferes with feeding. Neonates with ambiguous genitalia require multidisciplinary assessment from urology, endocrinology, and genetics to determine sex assignment, and chromosomal studies will be indicated in most patients with Smith–Lemli–Opitz syndrome. Early intervention, preschool, rehabilitative, and psychosocial counseling services appropriate for patients with severe mental and physical disability should also be provided.

Preventive Management of Mucopolysaccharidosis

Clinical diagnosis: Variable, progressive pattern of manifestations that includes a coarse facial appearance, thickened skin and hair, chronic rhinorrhea, thickened gums, skeletal changes in the cranium, thorax and limbs, and mental deterioration. The progression is insidious with timing in early childhood for Hunter and Hurler syndromes, later childhood in Maroteaux–Lamy and San Filippo syndromes. Morquio syndrome resembles a skeletal dysplasia.

Incidence: Aggregate incidence for all types of 1 in 10,000–20,000 live births.

Laboratory diagnosis: Deficiency of specific lysosomal enzyme in leukocytes or fibroblasts.

Genetics: All types exhibit recessive inheritance with Hunter syndrome being X-linked recessive.

Key management issues: Cranial MRI, ophthalmology, audiology, skeletal survey at the time of diagnosis; monitoring of hearing, vision, respiratory status, and sleep, periodic examination for congenital hip dislocation, joint contractures, or scoliosis; radiographic evaluation for cervical spinal cord compression or hydrocephalus with irritability or respiratory problems, monitoring of the cardiac valves, joints, and teeth as the disease progresses.

Growth Charts: Early overgrowth, later short stature in most types, no specific charts are available.

Parent groups: National Mucopolysaccharidosis Society (MPS), 17 Kraemer St., Hicksville NY, 11801, (516) 931-6338, cohenzec@aol.com, http://www.members.aol.com/mpssociety/index.html.

Basis for management recommendations: Derived from the complications below as documented by Gorlin et al. (1990, pp. 99–117), Neufeld & Muenzer (1995). Clinical judgment should guide the use of imaging studies that require anesthesia, but the subtle manifestations of hydrocephalus or spinal cord compression should be realized.

Summary of clinical concerns

General	Learning	**Cognitive disability, neurodegeneration**
	Behavior	Poor attention span, outbursts, aggression
	Growth	Short stature
Facial	Face	Coarse appearance, chronic rhinitis
	Eye	Strabismus, corneal clouding, retinal degeneration
	Ear	**Chronic otitis**
	Nose	Chronic rhinorrea, thick mucus
	Mouth	Large tongue, dental cysts, thin enamel, sleep apnea
Surface	Neck/trunk	Short neck, umbilical hernia, inguinal hernias
	Epidermal	Hirsutism, coarse hair and skin
Skeletal	Cranial	Macrocephaly
	Axial	Platyspondyly, odontoid hypoplasia, and kyphoscoliosis (particularly in Morquio); spinal cord compression and cervical myelopathy (particularly in Maroteaux–Lamy)
	Limbs	Carpal tunnel syndrome, congenital hip dislocation, joint contractures
Internal	Digestive	Chronic diarrhea
	Pulmonary	Interstitial pneumonitis, airway obstruction
	Circulatory	Aortic insufficiency, cardiac valvular lesions, mitral valve prolapse
Neural	CNS	**Hydrocephalus**, headaches
	Sensory	Optic and otic nerve dysfunction, hearing and vision loss

Bold: frequency > 20%

Key references

Gorlin, R. J., Cohen, M. M., Jr. & Levin, L. S. (1990). *Syndromes of the Head and Neck*. New York: Oxford University Press.

Neufeld, E. F. & Muenzer, J. (1995). The mucopolysaccharidoses. In *The Metabolic and Molecular Bases of Inherited Disease*, 7th edn, ed. C. R. Scriver, A. L. Beaudet, W. S. Sly & D. Valle, pp. 2465–94. New York: McGraw-Hill, Inc.

The Mucopolysaccharidoses

Preventive medical checklist (0–1yr)

Patient   **Birth Date** / /   **Number**

Pediatric	Screen		Evaluate		Refer/Counsel	
Neonatal / / *Newborn screen* ❑ *HB* ❑	Head size Skeletal x-rays Enzyme assay	❑ ❑ ❑	Eyes Macroglossia Hip dislocation	❑ ❑ ❑	Genetic evaluation Careful anesthesia	❑ ❑
1 month / /	Head size	❑	Eyes Hydrocephalus Hip dislocation	❑ ❑ ❑	Family support[4]	❑
2 months / / *HB[1]* ❑ *Hib* ❑ *DTaP, IPV* ❑ *RV* ❑	Head size Hearing, vision[2]	❑ ❑	Eyes Hydrocephalus Hip dislocation	❑ ❑ ❑	Early intervention[5] Developmental pediatrics Genetic counseling	❑ ❑ ❑
4 months / / *HB[1]* ❑ *Hib* ❑ *DTaP/IPV* ❑ *RV* ❑	Head size Hearing, vision[2]	❑ ❑	Eyes Hydrocephalus Otitis	❑ ❑ ❑	Early intervention[5] ENT[3]	❑ ❑
6 months / / *Hib* ❑ *IPV[1]* ❑ *DTaP* ❑ *RV* ❑	Head size Hearing, vision[2]	❑ ❑	Eyes Hydrocephalus Otitis	❑ ❑ ❑	Family support[4]	❑
9 months / / *IPV[1]* ❑	Head size Audiology	❑ ❑	Eyes Hydrocephalus Otitis	❑ ❑ ❑	Ophthalmology[3] Careful anesthesia	❑ ❑
1 year / / *HB* ❑ *Hib[1]* ❑ *IPV[1]* ❑ *MMR[1]* ❑ *Var[1]* ❑	Head size Hearing, vision[2] Head CT scan[3] Cardiac echo	❑ ❑ ❑ ❑	Eyes Hydrocephalus Otitis	❑ ❑ ❑	Family support[4] Early intervention[5] Developmental pediatrics Genetics Cardiology	❑ ❑ ❑ ❑ ❑

Clinical concerns for the Mucopolysaccharidoses, ages 0–1 year

Hydrocephalus	Atlantoaxial instability	Developmental disability
Corneal clouding, glaucoma	Cardiac anomalies	Speech delay
Chronic otitis	Hip dislocation	Obstructive sleep apnea
Hearing loss	Kyphoscoliosis	Frequent infections

Guidelines for the neonatal period should be undertaken *at whatever age* the diagnosis is made; DTaP, acellular DTP; IPV, inactivated poliovirus (oral polio also used); RV, rotavirus; MMR, measles–mumps–rubella; Var, varicella; [1]alternative timing; [2]by practitioner; [3]as dictated by clinical findings – atlantoaxial instability (AAI) is a particular concern in the Morquio and Maroteaux–Lamy syndromes, hydrocephalus may be subtle; [4]parent group, family/sib, financial, and behavioral issues as discussed in the preface; [5]including developmental monitoring and motor/speech therapy.

The Mucopolysaccharidoses

Preventive medical checklist (15m–6yrs)

Patient		Birth Date / /	Number

Pediatric	Screen	Evaluate	Refer/Counsel
15 months / / *Hib[1]* ☐ *MMR[1]* ☐ *DTaP, OPV[1]* ☐ *Varicella[1]* ☐			Family support[4] ☐ Early intervention[5] ☐ Orthopedics[3] ☐ Physical medicine[3] ☐
18 months / / *DTaP, IPV[1]* ☐ *Varicella[1]* ☐ *Influenza[3]* ☐	Head size ☐	Hydrocephalus ☐ Otitis ☐ Sleep apnea ☐	Sleep study[3] ☐ Careful anesthesia ☐
2 years / / *Influenza[3]* ☐ *Pneumovax[3]* ☐ *Dentist* ☐	Head size ☐ Hearing, vision[2] ☐ Audiology ☐	Hydrocephalus ☐ AAI ☐ Sleep apnea ☐	Family support[4] ☐ Cardiology ☐ Genetics ☐ ENT[3] ☐ Ophthalmology[3] ☐
3 years / / *Influenza[3]* ☐ *Pneumovax[3]* ☐ *Dentist* ☐	Head size ☐ Hearing, vision[2] ☐ Audiology ☐ Head CT scan[3] ☐	Hydrocephalus ☐ AAI ☐ Sleep apnea ☐	Family support[4] ☐ Preschool transition[5] ☐ Cardiology ☐
4 years / / *Influenza[3]* ☐ *Pneumovax[3]* ☐ *Dentist* ☐	Head size ☐ Hearing, vision[2] ☐	Scoliosis ☐ AAI ☐	Family support[4] ☐ Preschool program[5] ☐ Developmental pediatrics[3] ☐ Genetics ☐ Ophthalmology[3] ☐
5 years / / *DTaP, IPV[1]* ☐ *MMR[1]* ☐	C-spine x-rays[4] ☐ Hearing, vision[2] ☐ Audiology ☐	Hydrocephalus ☐ Scoliosis ☐	School transition[5] ☐ Careful anesthesia ☐ Orthopedics[3] ☐ Physical medicine[3] ☐
6 years / / *DTaP, IPV[1]* ☐ *MMR[1]* ☐ *Dentist* ☐	Head size ☐ Hearing, vision[2] ☐ Head CT scan ☐	School progress ☐ Scoliosis ☐ AAI ☐ Sleep apnea ☐	Family support[4] ☐ Developmental pediatrics[3] ☐ Genetics ☐ Cardiology[3] ☐ Ophthalmology[3] ☐ ENT[3] ☐

Clinical concerns for the Mucopolysaccharidoses, ages 1–6 years

Hydrocephalus
Corneal clouding, glaucoma
Chronic otitis
Hearing loss

Atlantoaxial instability
Cardiac anomalies
Hip dislocation
Kyphoscoliosis

Developmental disability
Speech delay
Obstructive sleep apnea
Frequent infections

Guidelines for prior ages should be undertaken *at the time of diagnosis*; DTaP, acellular DTP; IPV, inactivated poliovirus (oral polio also used); MMR, measles–mumps–rubella; [1]alternative timing; [2]by practitioner; [3]as dictated by clinical findings – atlantoaxial instability (AAI) is a particular concern in the Morquio and Maroteaux–Lamy syndromes, hydrocephalus may be subtle; [4]parent group, family/sib, financial, and behavioral issues as discussed in the preface; [5]including developmental monitoring and motor/speech therapy.

The Mucopolysaccharidoses

Preventive medical checklist (6+ yrs)

Patient   **Birth Date** / /   **Number**

Pediatric	Screen	Evaluate		Refer/Counsel	
8 years / / *Dentist* ❏		Hydrocephalus Scoliosis	❏ ❏	School options Developmental pediatrics[3] Genetics Orthopedics[3]	❏ ❏ ❏ ❏
10 years / /	Head size ❏ Hearing, vision[2] ❏	School progress Scoliosis AAI	❏ ❏ ❏	Cardiology[3] Ophthalmology[3] ENT[3]	❏ ❏ ❏
12 years / / *Td[1], MMR, Var* ❏ *CBC* ❏ *Dentist* ❏ *Scoliosis* ❏ *Cholesterol* ❏	C-spine x-rays[3] ❏ Head CT scan[3] ❏	Hydrocephalus Sleep apnea Behavior	❏ ❏ ❏	Family support[4] School options Developmental pediatrics[3] Genetics Careful anesthesia	❏ ❏ ❏ ❏ ❏
14 years / / *CBC* ❏ *Dentist* ❏ *Cholesterol* ❏ *Breast CA* ❏ *Testicular CA* ❏	Hearing, vision[2] ❏	School progress Scoliosis AAI	❏ ❏ ❏	Cardiology[3] Ophthalmology[3]	❏ ❏
16 years / / *Td[1]* ❏ *CBC* ❏ *Cholesterol* ❏ *Sexual[5]* ❏ *Dentist* ❏	Head CT scan[3] ❏	Hydrocephalus Behavior	❏ ❏	Vocational planning Developmental pediatrics[3] Genetics Orthopedics[3]	❏ ❏ ❏ ❏
18 years / / *CBC* ❏ *Sexual[5]* ❏ *Cholesterol* ❏ *Scoliosis* ❏	Hearing, vision[2] ❏	School progress Hydrocephalus Behavior	❏ ❏ ❏	Vocational planning Genetics Careful anesthesia	❏ ❏ ❏
20 years[6] / / *CBC* ❏ *Sexual[5]* ❏ *Cholesterol* ❏ *Dentist* ❏	C-spine x-rays[3] ❏ Head CT scan[3] ❏ Hearing, vision[2] ❏	Hydrocephalus AAI Sleep apnea Behavior Work, residence	❏ ❏ ❏ ❏ ❏	Family support[4] Cardiology[3] Ophthalmology[3]	❏ ❏ ❏

Clinical concerns for the Mucopolysaccharidoses, ages 6+ years

Short stature	Atlantoaxial instability	Cognitive disability
Hydrocephalus	Cardiac valvular disease	Behavior problems
Corneal clouding, glaucoma	Kyphoscoliosis	Obstructive sleep apnea
Hearing, vision loss	Joint contractures	Frequent infections

Guidelines for prior ages should be undertaken *at the time of diagnosis*; Td, tetanus/diphtheria; MMR, measles–mumps–rubella; Var, varicella; [1]alternative timing; [2]by practitioner; [3]as dictated by clinical findings – atlantoaxial instability (AAI) is a particular concern in the Morquio and Maroteaux–Lamy syndromes, hydrocephalus may be subtle; [4]parent group, family/sib, financial, and behavioral issues as discussed in the preface; [5]birth control, STD screening if sexually active; [6]repeat every decade.

Preventive Management of Peroxisomal Disorders

Clinical diagnosis: Severe forms (i.e., Zellweger syndrome) exhibit a pattern of manifestations deriving from hypotonia and dysostosis, including large anterior fontanelle, bitemporal hollowing, down-turned corners of the mouth, single palmar creases, and club feet. Internal anomalies include brain heterotopias and demyelination, renal cysts, and liver disease. Milder forms (neonatal adrenoleukodystrophy, infantile Refsum disease) have mostly neurologic symptoms with atypical findings in chondrodysplasia punctata (ichthyosis, skeletal dysplasia) or infantile Refsum disease (ichthyosis).

Incidence: Aggregate incidence of 1 in 25,000–50,000 live births.

Laboratory diagnosis: Elevated serum, very long chain fatty or phytanic acids and decreased levels of red blood cell plasmalogens, mutations in genes for peroxisomal membrane proteins.

Genetics: Autosomal recessive inheritance with a 25 percent recurrence risk after one affected child (X-linked adrenoleukodystrophy is not a generalized peroxisomal disorder).

Key management issues: Monitoring of hearing, vision, skeletal development; periodic assessment of thyroid, adrenal, renal, and hepatic function, early intervention for motor and cognitive delays.

Growth Charts: Specific charts are not available.

Parent groups: United Leukodystrophy Foundation, 2304 Highland Drive, Sycamore IL, 60178, (800) 728-5483, ulf@ceet.niu.edu

Basis for management recommendations: Complications listed below as documented by Wilson et al. (1986), Lazarow & Moser (1995).

Summary of clinical concerns

General	Learning	**Cognitive disability** (100%)
	Growth	**Short stature, failure to thrive**
Facial	Face	**Prominent forehead** (94%), **broad nasal root** (69%)
	Eye	**Congenital cataracts** (71%), **hypoplastic optic disc** (36%), **retinitis pigmentosa** (38%)
	Mouth	**High palate** (82%), dental crowding
Surface	Epidermal	Ichthyosis
Skeletal	Cranial	**Large fontanelles** (94%)
	Axial	Scoliosis, asymmetry
	Limbs	**Stippled epiphyses** (69%), **club feet** (56%), camptodactyly (10%)
Internal	Digestive	**Hepatomegaly** (69%), liver iron storage, biliary dysgenesis, **hepatic cirrhosis** (61%), cholestasis
	Circulatory	Patent ductus arteriosus, cardiac septal defects
	Endocrine	**Adrenal hypoplasia** (86%), adrenal insufficiency
	Excretory	**Renal cortical cysts** (93%), aminoaciduria
	Genital	**Labial hypoplasia** (56%), **cryptorchidism** (75%)
Neural	CNS	**Migration defects** (22%) **seizures** (80%)
	Motor	**Hypotonia** (99%)
	Sensory	Optic and otic nerve dysfunction, vision loss, **hearing loss** (100%)

Most complications are for Zellweger syndrome; **bold**: frequency > 20%

Key references

Lazarow, P. B. & Moser, H. W. (1995). In *The Metabolic and Molecular Bases of Inherited Disease*, 7th edn, ed. C. R. Scriver et al. pp. 2287–2324. New York: McGraw-Hill, Inc.

Wilson, G. N. et al. (1986). *American Journal of Medical Genetics* 24:69–82.

Peroxisomal Disorders

Preventive medical checklist (0–1yr)

Patient		Birth Date / /		Number	

Pediatric	Screen		Evaluate		Refer/Counsel	
Neonatal / / *Newborn screen* ☐ *HB* ☐	Peroxisomal assays ☐ Skeletal x-rays ☐		Feeding ☐ Cataracts ☐ Club feet ☐		Genetic evaluation ☐ Ophthalmology ☐ Feeding specialist ☐ Developmental pediatrics ☐ Genetic counseling ☐	
1 month / /	LFTs ☐ Head MRI scan ☐ Renal sonogram ☐		Feeding ☐ Hepatomegaly ☐ Genitalia ☐		Family support[4] ☐ Cardiology ☐ Neurology ☐	
2 months / / *HB¹* ☐ *Hib* ☐ *DTaP, IPV* ☐ *RV* ☐	Growth ☐ Hearing, vision[2] ☐ LFTs ☐		Feeding ☐ Hepatomegaly ☐ Genitalia ☐		Early intervention[5] ☐ Developmental pediatrics ☐ Genetic counseling ☐	
4 months / / *HB¹* ☐ *Hib* ☐ *DTaP/IPV* ☐ *RV* ☐	Growth ☐ Hearing, vision[2] ☐ LFTs ☐		Feeding ☐ Hepatomegaly ☐		Early intervention[5] ☐ Genetics ☐ ENT ☐	
6 months / / *Hib* ☐ *IPV¹* ☐ *DTaP* ☐ *RV* ☐	Growth ☐ Hearing, vision[2] ☐ LFTs ☐		Feeding ☐ Hepatomegaly ☐		Family support[4] ☐	
9 months / / *IPV¹* ☐	Audiology ☐				Ophthalmology[3] ☐	
1 year / / *HB* ☐ *Hib¹* ☐ *IPV¹* ☐ *MMR¹* ☐ *Var¹* ☐	Hearing, vision[2] ☐ T4, TSH ☐ Urinalysis ☐		Feeding ☐ Hepatomegaly ☐		Family support[4] ☐ Early intervention[5] ☐ Developmental pediatrics ☐ Genetic counseling ☐ Neurology ☐	

Clinical concerns for Peroxisomal Disorders, ages 0–1 year

Large fontanelle	Cardiac anomalies	Developmental disability
Retinitis pigmentosa	Hepatic cirrhosis	Hypotonia
Cataracts	Club feet	Seizures
Hearing loss	Renal cortical cysts	Hypothyroidism

Guidelines for the neonatal period should be undertaken *at whatever age* the diagnosis is made; DTaP, acellular DTP; IPV, inactivated poliovirus (oral polio also used); RV, rotavirus; MMR, measles–mumps–rubella; Var, varicella; LFTs, liver function tests; [1]alternative timing; [2]by practitioner; [3]as dictated by clinical findings – asymmetry is common in patients with chondrodysplasia punctata; [4]parent group, family/sib, financial, and behavioral issues as discussed in the preface; [5]including developmental monitoring and motor/speech therapy.

Peroxisomal Disorders

Preventive medical checklist (15m–6yrs)

| Patient | | Birth Date / / | Number |

Pediatric	Screen	Evaluate	Refer/Counsel
15 months / / Hib[1] ☐ MMR[1] ☐ DTaP, IPV[1] ☐ Varicella[1] ☐			Family support[4] ☐ Early intervention[5] ☐
18 months / / DTaP, IPV[1] ☐ Varicella[1] ☐ Influenza[3] ☐	Growth ☐		
2 years / / Influenza[3] ☐ Pneumovax[3] ☐ Dentist ☐	Growth ☐		Developmental pediatrics ☐ Genetics ☐
3 years / / Influenza[3] ☐ Pneumovax[3] ☐ Dentist ☐	Hearing, vision[2] ☐ Audiology ☐ T4, TSH ☐ Adrenal function ☐	Feeding ☐ Hepatomegaly ☐	Family support[4] ☐ Preschool transition[5] ☐ Ophthalmology[3] ☐ Genetics ☐
4 years / / Influenza[3] ☐ Pneumovax[3] ☐ Dentist ☐	Hearing, vision[2] ☐ Urinalysis ☐	Eyes ☐ Skin ☐ Asymmetry ☐	Family support[4] ☐ Preschool program[5] ☐ Developmental pediatrics ☐ Genetics ☐ Ophthalmology ☐
5 years / / DTaP, IPV[1] ☐ MMR[1] ☐	Growth ☐ Hearing, vision[2] ☐ Audiology ☐ Urinalysis ☐	Eyes ☐ Skin ☐ Asymmetry ☐	School transition[5] ☐ Genetics ☐
6 years / / DTaP, IPV[1] ☐ MMR[1] ☐ Dentist ☐	Hearing, vision[2] ☐ Urinalysis ☐ Adrenal function ☐	School progress ☐ Eyes ☐ Skin ☐ Asymmetry ☐	Family support[5] ☐ Developmental pediatrics ☐ Genetics ☐ Cardiology[3] ☐ Ophthalmology[3] ☐ ENT[3] ☐

Clinical concerns for Peroxisomal Disorders, ages 1–6 years

Large fontanelle	Cardiac anomalies	Developmental disability
Retinitis pigmentosa	Hepatic cirrhosis	Hypotonia
Cataracts	Club feet	Seizures
Hearing loss	Renal cortical cysts	Hypothyroidism

Guidelines for prior ages should be undertaken *at the time of diagnosis*; DTaP, acellular DTP; IPV, inactivated poliovirus (oral polio also used); MMR, measles–mumps–rubella; [1]alternative timing; [2]by practitioner; [3]as dictated by clinical findings – asymmetry is common in patients with chondrodysplasia punctata; [4]parent group, family/sib, financial, and behavioral issues as discussed in the preface; [5]including developmental monitoring and motor/speech therapy.

Peroxisomal Disorders

Preventive medical checklist (6+ yrs)

Patient   **Birth Date** / /   **Number**

Pediatric	Screen	Evaluate	Refer/Counsel
8 years / / *Dentist* ❑	Growth ❑ Hearing, vision[2] ❑ Urinalysis ❑	Eyes ❑ Skin ❑ Asymmetry ❑	School options ❑ Developmental pediatrics ❑ Genetics ❑ Neurology[3] ❑
10 years / /	Hearing, vision[2] ❑ Urinalysis ❑	School progress ❑ Eyes ❑ Skin ❑ Asymmetry ❑	Ophthalmology[3] ❑ ENT[3] ❑
12 years / / *Td[1], MMR, Var* ❑ *CBC* ❑ *Dentist* ❑ *Scoliosis* ❑ *Cholesterol* ❑	Growth ❑ Hearing, vision[2] ❑ Urinalysis ❑ Adrenal function ❑	Eyes ❑ Skin ❑ Asymmetry ❑	Family support[5] ❑ School options ❑ Developmental pediatrics ❑ Genetics ❑ Cardiology[3] ❑
14 years / / *CBC* ❑ *Dentist* ❑ *Cholesterol* ❑ *Breast CA* ❑ *Testicular CA* ❑	Growth ❑ Hearing, vision[2] ❑ Urinalysis ❑	School progress ❑ Eyes ❑ Skin ❑ Asymmetry ❑	Genetics ❑ Neurology[3] ❑
16 years / / *Td[1]* ❑ *CBC* ❑ *Cholesterol* ❑ *Sexual[5]* ❑ *Dentist* ❑	Hearing, vision[2] ❑ Urinalysis ❑	Eyes ❑ Skin ❑ Asymmetry ❑	Vocational planning ❑ Developmental pediatrics ❑ Genetics ❑
18 years / / *CBC* ❑ *Sexual[5]* ❑ *Cholesterol* ❑ *Scoliosis* ❑	Hearing, vision[2] ❑ Urinalysis ❑	School progress ❑ Eyes ❑ Skin ❑ Asymmetry ❑	Vocational planning ❑ Genetics ❑ Neurology[3] ❑
20 years[6] / / *CBC* ❑ *Sexual[5]* ❑ *Cholesterol* ❑ *Dentist* ❑	Hearing, vision[2] ❑ Urinalysis, BP ❑ Adrenal function ❑	Eyes ❑ Skin ❑ Asymmetry ❑	Family support[5] ❑ Ophthalmology[3] ❑ Cardiology[3] ❑ Neurology[3] ❑

Clinical concerns for Peroxisomal Disorders, ages 6+ years

Retinitis pigmentosa	Cardiac anomalies	Cognitive disability
Cataracts	Hepatic cirrhosis	Seizures
Hearing loss	Renal cortical cysts	Adrenal insufficiency
Dental anomalies	Cryptorchidism	

Guidelines for prior ages should be undertaken *at the time of diagnosis*; Td, tetanus/diphtheria; MMR, measles–mumps–rubella; Var, varicella; [1]alternative timing; [2]by practitioner; [3]as dictated by clinical findings – asymmetry is common in patients with chondrodysplasia punctata; [4]parent group, family/sib, financial, and behavioral issues as discussed in the preface; [5]birth control, STD screening if sexually active; [6]repeat every decade.

20

Metabolic dysplasias susceptible to dietary treatment

The provision of dietary treatment is a powerful strategy for preventive management that is available for selected inborn errors of metabolism. Newborn screening programs allow recognition of certain of these disorders (e.g., phenylketonuria, galactosemia), while clinical acumen must be utilized for others (e.g., glycogen storage diseases).

An algorithm for approaching patients with suspected inborn errors of metabolism is presented in Chapter 1. The approach emphasizes the differences between abnormalities in "small" molecule metabolism (acute presentations with seizures, coma, hypoglycemia, acidosis, hyperammonemia, sepsis, or organ failure) and abnormalities in "large" molecule metabolism (facial changes, visceromegaly, or neurodegeneration). While there is overlap between these simplified categories, the "small" molecule disorders are often diagnosed by amino acid and organic acid screening, while the "large" molecule disorders are recognized by neurologic, ophthalmologic, and tissue biopsy studies. In this chapter, the "small" molecule diseases are represented by galactosemia and phenylketonuria, while the "large" molecule diseases are represented by the glycogen storage diseases.

The definitive diagnosis for any inborn error of metabolism is to characterize a primary defect in the responsible gene (by DNA diagnosis) or its protein product (by enzyme assay). Often the demonstration of abnormal metabolites in plasma, urine, or affected tissues allows categorization of the disease and guides selection of the gene or enzyme to be tested. Participation of a metabolic disease specialist in the initial diagnostic evaluation is strongly recommended for interpretation of complex laboratory results (e.g., urine organic acid profiles). After the diagnosis is confirmed, the primary physician assumes the more important role in management, either as a partner in ensuring dietary compliance or as a director of the preventive management program.

This chapter will discuss treatable metabolic diseases according to four categories – disorders of carbohydrate, amino acid, organic acid, and fatty acid metabolism. Among these disorders, only the glycogen storage diseases have sufficient population incidence and diversity of preventive measures to warrant presentation of a detailed checklist.

Table 20.1 Disorders of carbohydrate metabolism

Disease	Incidence (live births)	Deficient enzyme, locus	Clinical manifestations
Fructose-1,6-diphosphatase deficiency	Unknown	Fructose-1,6-diphosphatase	Hypoglycemia, lactic acidosis
Galactosemia, severe	1 in 50,000	GALT, 9p13, 4 kb gene, 11 exons, Q188R mutation in 70%	Neonatal liver disease, sepsis, later MR if untreated, ovarian failure with certain mutations
Galactosemia, mild	Unknown	Galactokinase 17q21	Cataracts
GSD type Ia (von Gierke)	1 in 100,000	G-6-Pase, 17p	Hypoglycemia, hyperuricemia, lactic acidemia, hepatomegaly
GSD type Ib	1 in 200,000	Abnormal microsomal transport G-6-Pase	Type Ia plus neutropenia
GSD type II (Pompe)	1 in 100,000	α-Glucosidase	Cardiac disease, early death
GSD types III and IV	1 in 100,000	Debrancher (1p21) or brancher (3p12) enzyme	Mild type Ia (III) or fatal cirrhosis (type IV)
GSD types VI and VIII	1 in 200,000	Phosphorylase kinase (unknown or Xp22)	Mild type Ia

Notes:
GSD, glycogen storage disease; GALT, galactose-1-phosphate uridyl transferase; G-6-P, glucose-6-phosphate; 9p17, band 17 on the short arm of chromosome 9.

Disorders of carbohydrate metabolism

The provision of glucose to cells is important for energy production in highly active tissues such as liver, skeletal muscle, and heart. Numerous steps in the provision of glucose to cells can be interrupted, including dietary intake, digestion into small molecules, absorption into the blood stream, conversion of other carbohydrates into glucose, maintenance of serum glucose levels, intake of glucose into cells, and storage of materials for gluconeogenesis during fasting. Hypoglycemia is the prototypic symptom of inborn errors of carbohydrate metabolism such as galactosemia or glycogen storage diseases (Table 20.1). Dietary deprivation, intestinal malabsorption, or inaccessibility of glucose to cells (e.g., diabetes mellitus) represent other alterations of carbohydrate metabolism that are better discussed in nutrition, gastroenterology, or endocrinology texts.

Galactosemia

The most common cause of galactosemia is deficiency of the enzyme galactose-1-phosphate uridyl transferase (GALT). The incidence ranges from 1 in 35,000 to 1 in 190,000 births, with an average figure of 1 in 62,000 births (Segal & Berry, 1995). The diagnosis is often suspected from clinical manifestations of vomiting, diarrhea, and jaundice after breast or formula feeding in the newborn period, and a urine clinitest will be positive for reducing substances (sugars such as glucose or galactose and other metabolites with aldehyde groups). In the 38 states with newborn screening programs, report of an elevated serum galactose should be returned within 1–2 weeks, but this may occur after serious complications have occurred. Timely collection of neonatal blood spots and follow-up of infants for feeding problems and jaundice may also challenge health care professionals in this era of early discharge from the nursery. A change to lactose-free formula should be instituted immediately once galactosemia is considered, until referral to metabolic specialists and assay of blood for GALT enzyme deficiency can confirm or exclude the diagnosis.

Clinical manifestations of galactosemia most commonly include cataracts, vomiting, diarrhea, and indirect hyperbilirubinemia in the neonatal period (Segal & Berry, 1995). The jaundice may occur after the usual physiologic elevation of bilirubin, and there may be associated hemolysis which masks the disease. Cataracts may be visible only on slit-lamp examination. Less commonly, infants are acutely ill with the lethargy, hypotonia, hepatic disease, and cerebral edema that will usually occur if lactose is not removed from the diet. There is predisposition to *E. coli* sepsis, and it is recommended that infants with *E. coli* infections be screened for GALT enzyme deficiency (Levy et al., 1977). Later manifestations include more chronic presentation in later infancy or childhood with failure to thrive, cataracts, hepatomegaly, and developmental delay. Even with dietary treatment, there is a significant incidence of speech problems (62 percent of sibs recognized and treated as newborns), decreased IQ, poor school performance, and psychological problems such as lack of motivation and withdrawal (Waggoner & Buist, 1993). Females may have streak or hypoplastic ovaries, hypergonadotropic hypogonadism (75 percent), amenorrhea, premature menarche, and infertility (Kaufman et al., 1986, 1987).

Preventive management of galactosemia begins with removal of breast milk or formula from the diet, followed by dietary counseling through experienced nutritionists at a metabolic disease center. Failure to remove lactose from the diet produces liver failure with cirrhosis, renal tubular dysfunction with aminoaciduria, cataracts, and death. Soybean formula (e.g., Isomil) or Nutramigen are recommended formulas, although the former has galactose-containing sugars such as raffinose and the latter is derived from cow's milk. The dangers of lactose in fruit and vegetables have been emphasized by some, but others feel that this lactose is not available for absorption and metabolism (Segal & Berry, 1995). Since galactose is not an essential nutrient, complete omission is the goal of dietary therapy. Assay of erythrocyte galactose-1-phosphate levels may be performed to monitor dietary compliance, but there is imperfect and controversial correlation between these levels and galactose intake (Segal & Berry, 1995). Milk avoidance should certainly be maintained throughout life, but other foods (e.g., cakes and bread) may be permitted in adolescence and adulthood. Better intellectual outcomes have been demonstrated in sibs having dietary restriction from birth as compared to their older sibs who required 7–400 days to make the diagnosis (Waggoner et al., 1990).

Because intellectual and ovarian dysfunction can occur even in well-controlled patients, developmental and speech assessments should be performed on children with galactosemia. Speech apraxias are particularly common, and older children have had cerebellar ataxias and tremors reminiscent of neurodegenerative disease. Since these changes may relate to kernicterus or other neonatal complications, galactosemics with turbulent neonatal histories should probably receive early intervention and preschool services. Monitoring of females for menstrual irregularities is also important, and pelvic sonography may be indicated when there is concern about puberty or fertility. Quarterly visits to the metabolic clinic are recommended for young children, with annual visits being sufficient for older and more stable patients.

Hereditary fructose intolerance and fructose 1,6-bisphosphatase deficiency

Hereditary fructose intolerance is a self-limiting disease that exerts its most severe effects during infancy (Gitzelmann et al., 1995). It is an autosomal recessive disorder that leads to deficiency of aldolase and acccumulation of fructose-1-phosphate in tissues. Infants and young children may present with severe vomiting, failure to thrive, hypoglycemia, jaundice, diarrhea, hepatic and renal disease (Pagliara et al., 1973). Reducing substances may be found in the urine, but definitive diagnosis may require a fructose challenge. Even small amounts of sucrose, fructose, or sorbitol may be lethal for some patients, although most survive and become normal when they are able to control their diet and avoid fructose-rich foods. Nutritional counseling is still needed once the diagnosis is suspected, since even the small amounts of fructose allowed by self-selection may cause hepatomegaly and growth failure. Monitoring of growth, development, and yearly assessment in the metabolic/nutrition clinic is appropriate preventive management for patients with hereditary fructose intolerance. Families and older patients should carry emergency treatment cards that emphasize the dangers of intravenous fluids containing sucrose, fructose, or sorbitol.

Fructose 1,6-bisphosphatase (FDPase) deficiency is a more severe disorder than hereditary fructose intolerance. More than 85 patients with this autosomal recessive disorder have been reported, and it can be diagnosed by assaying the cognate enzyme in liver. FDPase deficiency usually presents in the newborn period, with severe hypoglyemia, acidosis, hyperventilation, hypotonia and coma (Rallison et al., 1979). Unlike hereditary fructose intolerance, the patients rarely have hepatic or renal disease and there is no aversion to eating sweets or fruits containing fructose. Usually there are episodic attacks of inanition, vomiting, convulsions, hypoglycemia and acidosis before the diagnosis is recognized. These attacks are provoked by febrile illnesses and fasting. The clinical course is benign once fructose and sucrose are excluded from the diet, but high carbohydrate diet, frequent feeding, and treatment of intercurrent episodes with glucose and intravenous fluids may be required. Preventive management consists of nutritional counseling and early pediatric evaluation for intercurrent infections, watching for vomiting, diarrhea and acidosis. Families should be counseled regarding the danger of sucrose-containing intravenous fluids, and emergency treatment cards stipulating this prohibition should be carried by affected patients. For patients who are doing well, yearly visits to the metabolic clinic are sufficient.

Glycogen storage diseases

Terminology

Glycogen storage diseases are a group of genetic disorders that produce alterations in the amount or structure of glycogen. Since storage of glycogen occurs mainly in liver and muscle, the diseases were first classified based on the spectrum of hepatic and muscular disease. Type I glycogen storage disease was described as "hepatonephromegalia glycogenica" by von Gierke in 1929, and the disease is still known by that eponym (Chen & Burchell, 1995). Types III (Cori or Forbes disease), IV (Anderson disease) and VI (Hers disease) are also hepatic glycogenoses, while Type II (Pompe disease with cardiac manifestations) and Types V and VII (McArdle and Tarui diseases with muscle cramping) are muscle glycogenoses. Type II (Pompe) glycogen storage disease is a lysosomal storage disease that is quite different from other glycogenoses (Reuser et al., 1995).

Incidence, etiology, and differential diagnosis

The incidence of all types of glycogen storage diseases is about 1 in 20–25,000 births, with types I–IV accounting for over 90 percent of patients (Anonymous, 1993; Chen & Burchell, 1995). Most follow the general rule for metabolic diseases and exhibit autosomal recessive inheritance; the exceptions are the group of heterogenous disorders that comprise the X-linked recessive type VI category. Enzymes that regulate glucose/glycogen interconversion are responsible for the glycogen storage diseases, including type I (glucose-6-phosphatase), type II (lysosomal α-glucosidase), type III (debranching enzyme), type IV (branching enzyme), type V (muscle phosphorylase), type VI (phosphorylase and phosphorylase kinase), and type VII (phosphofructokinase). Differential diagnosis for the hepatic disorders will include other causes of hypoglycemia and acidosis: galactosemia, fructose bisphosphatase deficiency, fatty acid oxidation disorders or even infectious hepatitis may be considered until the typical metabolic profile and excess hepatic glycogen are demonstrated. Pompe disease can simulate endocardial fibroelastosis and other cardiomyopathies until the characteristic shortened P-R interval is demonstrated by electrocardiography. The muscle cramping of types V and VII can be confused with other disorders that interfere with muscle energy metabolism (i.e., hexokinase deficiency) until exercise testing, phosphorus magnetic resonance imaging, and muscle enzyme assays are employed.

Diagnostic evaluation and medical counseling

Although a variety of intravenous tolerance tests and associated imaging studies can be performed, the primary technique for diagnosis of glycogen storage diseases should involve biopsy of the appropriate organ followed by histologic and enzymatic study of the hepatic or muscle tissue. The exception is Pompe disease, where the abnormal lysosomal enzyme (α-glucosidase) is best assayed in fibroblasts grown from skin biopsy. The enzyme can be assayed in leukocytes prepared from whole blood, but α-glucosidase isozymes may contribute residual activities that are more difficult to interpret. Medical counseling can be optimistic for glycogen storage diseases other than types II and IV. Although patients with types I and III disease may have short stature and protuberant abdomens, improvements in management and natural amelioration after puberty allows normal adult function for many affected individuals. Emphasis on adherance to treatment regimens is important, since treatment is clearly related to the degree of short stature and adult complications. Families of patients with type II or type IV disease require psychosocial, pastoral, and hospice support appropriate for the early lethality of these disorders.

Family and psychosocial counseling

The recurrence risk for parents of children with glycogen storage disease will be 25 percent, with type VI families having the risk for affected sons rather than daughters. Carrier mothers do not have manifestations of type VI glycogen storage disease, so that enzyme assay of maternal tissues is required to determine if index patients with type VI disease represent new mutations. Molecular analysis may also be possible since genetic mapping studies have assigned the locus for type VI disease to chromosomal region Xp22, near the locus for the α-subunit of liver phosphorylase kinase (Chen & Burchell, 1995). Family counseling for patients with hepatic glycogenoses I and III should emphasize the importance of maintaining adequate carbohydrate supplies so that growth failure, abnormal body build, and medical complications can be minimized. Similar counseling regarding avoidance of high-intensity exercise should be given to patients with muscle glycogenoses types V and VII. Parent support groups are listed in the checklist, part 1.

Natural history and complications

The key derangement in patients with hepatic glycogenoses is the inability to mobilize hepatic glycogen into circulating glucose. Abnormal amounts or structures of glycogen accumulate and produce hepatomegaly, while the block in glucose liberation causes hypoglycemia, lactic acidosis, hyperuricemia, and hyperlipidemia. Lipids also accumulate in the liver and contribute to the hepatomegaly. The types of hepatic glycogenoses present variations on this theme of glycogen accumulation and glucose scarcity. In type I, shunting of glucose-6-phosphate through glycolysis causes increased lactate and acidosis. The lactate competes with renal urate excretion, and joins with increased nucleotide turnover to cause hyperuricemia. The exaggerated glycolysis also increases pools of NADH/NADPH and glycerol, favoring triglyceride synthesis and fatty liver. Types III and VI involve the same pathogenetic mechanisms as in type I, but to lesser degrees. In type IV, the accumulating glycogen is hepatotoxic and leads to early death from liver failure. The cause of toxicity is not known (Chen & Burchell, 1995).

As a result of these metabolic alterations, patients with hepatic glycogenoses exhibit early clinical manifestations of hypoglycemia, seizures and lactic acidosis (checklist, part 1). In later childhood, they may have short stature, cherubic or "doll-like" facies with increased adiposity, protuberant abdomen with hepatomegaly, and skin xanthomas. Ocular changes may include atrophy of the retinal pigment epithelium (Abe & Tamai, 1995). After puberty, which is often delayed, there is short stature, pancreatitis secondary to hyperlipidemia, gouty tophi and arthritis secondary to hyperuricemia, and renal disease with proteinuria, Fanconi syndrome, hypertension, hyperfiltration, or renal failure (Chen & Van Hove, 1995). Osteoporosis and pulmonary hypertension have also been reported, but increased atherosclerosis from hyperlipidemia has not been demonstrated. Most patients with type I glycogen storage disease develop hepatic adenomas in their second to third decade of life, and these are subject to hemorrhage or malignant transformation (Chen & Burchell, 1995). The hepatic adenomas and hepatocellular carcinomas may reflect increased amounts of long-chain, dicarboxylic fatty acids that are associated with peroxisome proliferators and liver cancers in rodents (Ockner et al., 1993).

Glycogenoses other than type I exhibit either milder or different clinical manifestations. Biochemical analysis of glucose-6-phosphatase compartmentalization in the cell has revealed a subtype of glycogen storage disease type I that has been designated type Ib. In addition to the clinical problems detailed above, these patients have neutropenia with recurrent bacterial infections, mouth ulcers, and intestinal lesions that present as inflammatory bowel disease (Wendel et al., 1993). Type III patients have more frequent cirrhosis, particularly if they are Japanese, and later onset muscular weakness and wasting. Type III patients may also develop arrythmias (Tada et al., 1995). Type VI patients may have growth delay, motor delay, mild hepatitis, hepatomegaly, and hyperlipidemia in childhood, but show improvement with age to become virtually asymptomatic in adulthood. The severe cirrhosis in type IV, the cardiomyopathy in type II, and the intermittent muscle cramping in types V and VII have already been mentioned as exceptions to the clinical manifestations summarized in the checklist, part 1.

Hepatic glycogen storage disease preventive medical checklist

The initial management concern in children with hepatic glycogenoses is to restore glucose homeostasis and prevent hypoglycemic seizures, lactic acidosis, hyperuricemia, and hyperlipidemia. Enzymic or DNA diagnosis is required to distinguish milder type III and VI patients who may not require therapy. Two dietary treatment methods are efficacious in preventing hypoglycemia and its secondary complications (Parker et al., 1993). The first involves placement of a nasogastric tube for administration of nocturnal glucose drip feedings. The rate is 8–10 mg per kg per minute in an infant and 5–7 mg per kg per minute in older children (Chen & Burchell, 1995). During the day, a high carbohydrate diet is administered to comprise a total load of 65–70 percent carbohydrate, 10–15 percent lipid, and 20–25 percent fat with about 33 percent of total intake administered as the nocturnal infusion. The first oral feeding must follow cessation of the infusion by no more than 30 minutes, and precautions to ensure pump and tube function are important since interruptions have been associated with sudden hypoglycemia and death. The second dietary treatment involves oral administration of uncooked cornstarch at 1.6 g per kg every 4 hours for infants younger than 2 years, changing to 1.75–2.5 g per kg every 6 hours. The cornstarch provides a slow-release form of glucose and is supplemented to provide a diet with similar composition to that mentioned for nocturnal infusion (Chen & Burchell, 1995).

Once dietary therapy is instituted, monitoring of growth and development, glucose levels, liver size, liver function tests, and tongue size is important. Patients with glycogen storage disease type Ib will require complete blood counts to monitor neutropenia, and inspection for mouth ulcers. Patients with type Ib disease who develop inflammatory bowel disease have been treated with colony-stimulating factors (Roe et al., 1992). Periodic assessments by an experienced dietician and metabolic specialist is recommended, and the option of liver transplantation should be considered in severe cases. Allopurinol should be given for children with hyperuricemia, maintaining the serum urate concentration below 6.4 mg per ml (Chen & Burchell, 1995). A bleeding time should be obtained prior to any surgery, and abnormal values corrected by intravenous glucose administration. In general, 10 percent dextrose solutions should be used for intravenous therapy rather than Ringer's lactate. Fructose and galactose should also be limited in the diet of type I patients since these sugars cannot be converted to glucose.

Management of older children with hepatic glycogen storage disease should include monitoring of glucose, liver function, uric acid, renal function, and liver size. The occurrence of hepatomas should be monitored by abdominal examination and periodic abdominal ultrasound, with periodic α-fetoprotein measurements to check for transformation to hepatocarcinoma. If there is poor growth, referral to endocrinology may be considered, and women should be counseled about worsening symptoms that occur with pregnancy. The presence of malignant hepatic tumors would constitute an immediate indication for liver transplant, and some patients have required renal transplant because of chronic renal failure (Chen & Van Hove, 1995; Rosh et al, 1995). Many patients with long-term dietary treatment are now reaching adulthood, and the outlook for normal stature and regression of hepatic adenomas seems good (Smit, 1993; Chen & Burchell, 1995).

Disorders of amino acid metabolism

Disorders of amino acid metabolism may be present acutely in the newborn period (hyperglycinemia, urea cycle disorders) or gradually with developmental delay and seizures (Table 20.2). The usual diagnostic procedures are a serum ammonia, plasma amino acids, and urine organic acids. Newborn screening is an important method for recognizing aminoacidopathies such as phenylketonuria, since dietary treatment can prevent mental retardation. Few of the amino acid disorders are associated with an abnormal facies or congenital malformations. Homocystinuria does involve an altered body habitus and is discussed in Chapter 16.

Phenylketonuria

Elevated plasma concentration of phenylalanine is associated with three categories of disease (Scriver et al., 1995b). The most frequent is classical phenylketonuria (PKU), due to deficiency of phenylalanine hydroxylase enzyme. Patients with PKU require diets low in phenylalanine to have normal mental development (Williamson et al., 1981). Milder deficiencies of phenylalanine hydroxylase produce hyperphenylalaninemia, a benign variant which rarely requires dietary treatment. A third category involves deficiency of biopterin, the cofactor for phenylalanine hydroxylase, and is more refractory to dietary management. Another disease occurs in infants of mothers with uncontrolled PKU during pregnancy; these infants have congenital anomalies and developmental delay reminiscent of fetal alcohol syndrome.

Table 20.2 Disorders of amino acid metabolism

Disease	Incidence (live births)	Deficient enzyme, locus	Clinical manifestations
Phenylketonuria	1 in 10,000	<1% PAH, 12q22, 90 kb gene with 13 exons, >100 diverse mutations	MD, mousy odor, seizures if untreated
Hyperphenylalaninemia	1 in 20,000	>1% PAH, 12q22, subset of mutations	None – benign phenotype
Hyperphenylalaninemia	1 in 1,000,000	Dihydropteridine reductase, 4p15, 730 bp open reading frame	Severe MD, seizures
Tyrosinemia type I	Unknown	Fumarylacetoacetate hydrolase, 15q23	Liver disease, cirrhosis
Oculocutaneous albinism	1 in 30,000	Tyrosinase, 11q14	Pale skin, eyes, sun sensitivity, nystagmus
Alkaptonuria	1 in 100,000	Homogentisic acid oxidase, 3q2	Dark urine, pigmented cartilage, arthritis
Homocystinuria	1 in 350,000	Cystathionine-β-synthase deficiency, 21q21	Marfanoid habitus, vascular thromboses
Maple syrup urine disease	1 in 180,000	Branched chain keto-acid dehydrogenase subunits, 1p31, 6p21, 7q31, 19q13	MD, ketoacidosis; lactic acidosis with E3 subunit deficiency

PKU, like hyperphenylalaninemia and the biopterin deficiencies, is an autosomal recessive disorder. The incidence of PKU is 1 in 10,000 births in Caucasian populations, while hyperphenylalaninemia is 4- or 5-fold lower and the biopterin deficiences 100-fold lower. Children with PKU are often lightly pigmented, presumably because of tyrosine deficiency (tyrosine is the product of phenylalanine hydroxylase) and decreased melanin synthesis. Developmental delay, seizures, scleroderma-like changes, and skin rashes may occur. Demyelination of the brain may be demonstrated on cranial MRI scan if dietary control is inadequate. Untreated patients with PKU will have severe mental retardation, while adolescents terminating treatment may have depression, distractibility, anxiety, and agoraphobia (Scriver et al., 1995b).

Preventive management for PKU begins with accurate diagnosis. Health care providers must be vigilant to ensure that newborn screening is performed in an era of early neonatal discharge. Elevated phenylalanine in blood spots is often reported within 10–14 days and a repeat sample is requested. Children with confirmed elevations should be referred to a metabolic disease center for quantitative blood phenylalanine and tyrosine determinations and biopterin testing. Once the diagnosis of PKU is confirmed, forceful medical and dietary counseling of the parents is essential to ensure compliance with a diet low in phenylalanine. Parents should also be cautioned about aspartame, the artifical sweetener that contains phenylalanine. Genetic counseling regarding the 25 percent recurrence risk and the feasibility of prenatal diagnosis by DNA analysis should be mentioned. Some patients, particularly those with biopterin deficiencies, have some mental disability despite good dietary compliance.

After the initial diagnostic evaluation and counseling, management consists of monitoring of nutrition and development. Many states have guidelines for management of children with PKU. Follow-up is best coordinated with a metabolic center and a nutritionist knowledgable about phenylalanine-free foods and formulae. Parents should be encouraged to compile three-day diet records when the child is 6 months, 1 year, 2 years, and 3 years old to assess knowledge and compliance. Most programs recommend monitoring of blood phenylalanine and tyrosine levels ate least every 6 months and more often if compliance is in question. A variety of child behavior and developmental testing should also be performed. Termination of the diet has been tried at age 6 years, but most centers recommend lifelong restriction (Koch et al., 1982; Scriver et al., 1995b). Teenagers are often aware of decreased concentration and school abilities when their intake of phenylalanine increases. Women with PKU must be counseled regarding the risks of pregnancy, since they must have good dietary control before and during the embryonic period. Many of these women have difficulty resuming a stringent diet, particularly when they have mental disability. Infants born to poorly controlled mothers may have microcephaly, growth failure, congenital heart disease, ocular and orthopedic anomalies. Preventive management of these infants can utilize the checklist for fetal alcohol syndrome that is presented in Chapter 5.

Maple syrup urine disease

Maple syrup urine disease involves accumulation of branched chain amino and organic acids, producing acidosis and neurologic symptoms (Chuang & Shih, 1995). It is an autosomal recessive disorder with a frequency of about 1 in 185,000 births. The primary defects involve alteration of the branched chain α-keto acid dehydrogenase, a complex of at least 5 proteins and a thiamine cofactor. In the most severe variety, neonates become lethargic at age 4–7 days, then progress to hypotonia, dystonic posturing, ketosis, and acidosis. Subtle dysmorphic features may accompany acidosis in patients with maple syrup urine disease, pyruvate dehydrogenase deficiency, and related disorders. Seizures, coma, and a bulging fontanelle and a maple syrup odor may be noted. The diagnosis is made by blood amino acid and urine organic acid profiles, which show the branched chain amino acids and keto acids (valine, leucine, isoleucine). Several milder forms of the disease have been described and discriminated by molecular analysis; one of these responds to thiamine.

Preventive management relies on a sufficiently early diagnosis to avoid severe neurologic lesions. The initial diagnosis and dietary counseling is best made at a metabolic center, where the specialized testing and dietary management is available (Goodman et al., 1969). Once the diagnosis is suspected, thiamine at 50–300 mg per day should be given for at least 3 weeks (Chuang & Shih, 1995). Special formulas lacking in branched chain amino acids should be administered, and blood branched chain amino acid levels followed weekly for 6 months. Once the levels are stable, determinations can occur at 6–12 month intervals, but regular evaluations for skin and mouth lesions should occur. Intercurrent infections and/or dehydration can be lethal to these patients, and parents should be warned to contact their physician early for symptoms of illness, loss of appetite, or behavioral changes. Exchange transfusion and parenteral nutrition may be required during acute episodes (Chuang & Shih, 1995). Many patients sustain some neurologic damage, so early intervention and other services appropriate for children with disabilities are needed (Kaplan et al., 1991).

Disorders of organic and fatty acid metabolism

The prominent symptom of organic acidemias is metabolic acidosis. In disorders of fatty acid oxidation, acute decompensation may occur after a normal early childhood, often related to fasting and an intercurrent illness. Several organic acidemias and fatty acid oxidation disorders are accompanied by hypoglycemia and absence of the usual ketones (Table 20.3). More than eight disorders of fatty acid oxidation have been described, epitomized by medium chain coenzyme A dehydrogenase deficiency. Affected patients have episodic hypoglycemia, acidosis, and carnitine deficiency, sometimes with cardiomyopathy and skeletal myopathy. They do not have an unusual appearance or congenital malformations. Disorders of fatty acid oxidation are important to recognize, since they can often be treated with low fat diets, frequent feeding, and carnitine supplementation.

While organic acidemias often exhibit demyelination, seizures, and other neurologic problems, they also are not typically associated with dysmorphology. An exception is biotinidase or multiple carboxylase deficiency, where patients may have ocular problems, deafness and alopecia.

Biotinidase and holocarboxylase synthetase deficiencies

Biotin is a vitamin cofactor for several carboxylase enzymes including propionyl coenzyme A carboxylase and pyruvate carboxylase. These mitochondrial carboxylases are important for fatty acid synthesis and amino acid catabolism, and their

Table 20.3 Organic acidemias and fatty acid oxidation disorders

Disease	Incidence (live births)	Deficient enzyme, locus	Clinical manifestations
Propionic acidemia	Unknown	Propionyl-CoA carboxylase subunits, 3q13, 13q22	MD, acidosis, hypoglycemia, hyperammonemia, neutropenia
Methylmalonic acidemia	1 in 20,000	Methylmalonyl-CoA mutase, 6p12	Same as propionic
Methylmalonic acidemia plus homocystinuria	Unknown	Methylcobalamin (vit. B12) synthesis	MD, milder acidosis, neutropenia
Multiple carboxylase deficiency	1 in 25,000	Biotinidase	Sparse hair, rashes, acidosis, anion gap
Multiple carboxylase deficiency	Unknown	Holocarboxylase synthetase deficiency	Sparse hair, rashes, acidosis, anion gap
LCHAD deficiency	Unknown	Long chain hydroxyacyl CoA dehydrogenase	Liver disease, cardiomyopathy
MCAD deficiency	1 in 20,000	Medium chain acyl-CoA dehydrogenase, 1p31	Nonketotic hypoglycemia, acidosis, sudden death
SCAD deficiency	Unknown	Short chain acyl-CoA dehydrogenase	MD, lethargy, vomiting, hypotonia

combined deficiency produces elevations of lactate, propionate, ammonia, alanine, and ketone bodies (Wolf & Heard, 1991). Biotin is chemically attached to these carboxylases (biotinylation), and must be recycled through action of the enzyme biotinidase. Defective biotinylation (holocarboxylase synthetase deficiency) or defective biotin recycling (biotinidase deficiency) are two disorders that produce similar clinical results: organic aciduria, acidosis, variable neurologic problems, skin rashes, and alopecia. These disorders are important to recognize because they can be partially or completely cured by administration of biotin (Wolf, 1995).

Holocarboxylase synthetase deficiency has been described in less than 20 patients, producing lactic acidosis, ketosis, organic aciduria including propionic and lactic acids, hyperammonemia, skin rashes, poor feeding, lethargy, seizures, ataxia, and hair loss. More than 100 patients have been described with biotinidase deficiency, a later-onset disorder with similar clinical symptoms (Wolf & Heard, 1991). Children with either disorder have increased susceptibility to bacterial and fungal infections, and patients have died with disseminated sepsis before treatment can be given. Most children with holocarboxylase synthetase deficiency present before 3 months, while that age is the median age of presentation for patients with biotinidase deficiency.

The initial diagnostic evaluation for children with biotin deficiencies should include urine organic acids, blood amino acids, blood ammonia, glucose, electrolytes, neurology, and ophthalmology examinations. The definitive diagnosis is established by enzyme assay of component carboxylases and biotinidase in serum, leukocytes, or fibroblasts. Preventive management for disorders of biotin metabolism begins with administration of 60–80 mg per day of oral biotin when the diagnosis is suspected (Wolf, 1995). Biotin therapy is curative if begun before severe infection or neurologic devastation. Prenatal diagnosis is also available for these autosomal recessive disorders, and administration of 10 mg per day of oral biotin to mothers during the last trimester, followed by treatment of the infant, has resulted in normal children with demonstrable enzyme deficiencies. It is not clear if prenatal in addition to postnatal therapy is necessary for these normal outcomes. Once treatment is begun, the child should have regular assessments of hearing, vision, and development. Audiometry and ophthalmology evaluations are particularly important, since hearing loss and optic atrophy respond more slowly to therapy (Wolf, 1995). Feeding and nutrition should also be carefully monitored in early childhood. Baseline neurologic and dermatologic examinations may be useful to detect motor weakness, ataxia, and rashes that may persist despite successful biotin therapy. Early intervention services should be considered in children with prominent neurologic symptoms or developmental delays; speech problems have been recognized in less than 10 percent of treated patients with biotinidase deficiency (Wolf & Heard, 1991; Wolf, 1995).

Preventive Management of Glycogen Storage Diseases

Clinical diagnosis: Pattern of manifestations including short stature, cherubic face, prominent abdomen with enlarged liver, and liver disease with recurrent hypoglycemia, hypercholesterolemia, hyperuricemia, and acidosis. Type I is the classic hepatic disease with type Ib having neutropenia; types III and VI are milder versions of type I while type IV has lethal cirrhosis; type II lethal cardiac, and types V, VII skeletal muscle disease.

Laboratory diagnosis: Liver biopsy to document glycogen storage, specific enzyme assays in liver biopsy tissue.

Genetics: Autosomal recessive with a 25% recurrence risk after the first affected child; type VIII is X-linked recessive.

Key management issues: Dietary therapy with complex carbohydrates coordinated by a metabolic disease center, monitoring of growth, development, glucose levels, liver size, liver function tests, and tongue size; assessment of blood counts and inspection for mouth ulcers in type Ib; allopurinol therapy for hyperuricemia; screening for hepatic tumors by abdominal examination, periodic abdominal ultrasound, and α-fetoprotein measurements; bleeding times prior to surgery; endocrine referrals for poor growth; options for liver transplantation in severe cases; counseling women about worsening disease during pregnancy.

Growth Charts: Short stature is common, but no specific charts are available.

Parent groups: National Association for Glycogen Storage Diseases, P. O. Box 896,Durant IA, 52747, (319) 785-6038.

Basis for management recommendations: Derived from the complications as documented by Chen & Burchell (1995).

Summary of clinical concerns

General	Behavior	Rebellious because of abnormal appearance, short stature
	Growth	**Short stature**
	Tumors	**Hepatic adenomas** (decades 2–3), hepatocarcinoma
Facial	Eye	Retinal lesions (hyperlipidemia)
	Mouth	Oral ulcers (type Ib)
Surface	Neck/trunk	**Protuberant abdomen**
	Epidermal	Skin xanthomas
Skeletal	Limbs	Gouty arthritis (postpubertal), osteoporosis
Internal	Digestive	**Hepatomegaly**, intermittent diarrhea, pancreatitis, inflammatory bowel disease (type Ib), lethal cirrhosis (Type IV)
	Circulatory	Pulmonary hypertension and congestive heart failure (type I), cardiomyopathy (types II, III)
	Endocrine	Delayed puberty, normal fertility
	RES	Easy bruising, epistaxis, prolonged bleeding time (impaired platelet adhesion due to hypoglycemia), neutropenia in type Ib
	Excretory	Enlarged kidneys; proteinuria, glomerular disease, renal failure in adulthood
Neural	CNS	Seizures (hypoglycemia), hypotonia (type IV)
	Muscular	Muscle atrophy, myopathy (types IV, V, VII), cramps (types V, VII)

Bold: frequency > 20%

Key references

Chen, Y. T. & Burchell, A. (1995). In *The Metabolic and Molecular Bases of Inherited Disease*, 7th edn, ed. C. R. Scriver et al. New York: McGraw-Hill, Inc.

Rosh, J. R. et al. (1995). *Journal of Pediatric Gastroenterology & Nutrition* 20:225–8.

Glycogen Storage Diseases I, III–IV

Preventive medical checklist (0–1yr)

Patient   **Birth Date** / /   **Number**

Pediatric	Screen	Evaluate	Refer/Counsel
Neonatal / / *Newborn screen* ❑ *HB* ❑	Glucose, LFTs ❑ CBC ❑ Bleeding time (before surgery) ❑	Feeding ❑ Abdominal exam ❑ Macroglossia ❑	Parent group ❑ Dietician ❑ Genetic evaluation ❑
1 month / /	Glucose, LFTs ❑	Feeding ❑ Abdominal exam ❑	Family support[4] ❑ Dietician ❑
2 months / / *HB[1]* ❑ *Hib* ❑ *DTaP, IPV* ❑ *RV* ❑	Glucose, LFTs ❑	Feeding ❑ Abdominal exam ❑ Macroglossia ❑	Genetic counseling ❑ Dietician ❑
4 months / / *HB[1]* ❑ *Hib* ❑ *DTaP/IPV* ❑ *RV* ❑	Glucose, LFTs ❑	Feeding ❑ Abdominal exam ❑	Dietician ❑
6 months / / *Hib* ❑ *IPV[1]* ❑ *DTaP* ❑ *RV* ❑	Glucose, LFTs ❑ CBC ❑ Hearing[3] ❑	Feeding ❑ Abdominal exam ❑ Macroglossia ❑ Otitis, sinusitis[5] ❑	Family support[4] ❑
9 months / / *IPV[1]* ❑	ABR[3] ❑	Feeding ❑ Abdominal exam ❑	
1 year / / *HB* ❑ *Hib[1]* ❑ *IPV[1]* ❑ *MMR[1]* ❑ *Var[1]* ❑	Glucose, LFTs ❑ Abdominal U/S[3] ❑ Serum AFP ❑ Bleeding time (before surgery) ❑	Feeding ❑ Abdominal exam ❑	Family support[4] ❑ Genetics ❑ Dietician ❑ Liver transplant[3] ❑

Clinical concerns for Glycogen Storage Diseases, ages 0–1 year

Hypoglycemia, seizures	Hepatomegaly	Epistaxis
Hyperlipidemia	Hepatic adenomas	Prolonged bleeding time
Hyperuricemia	Lumbar lordosis	Proteinuria
Sinusitis, otitis[5]	Neutropenia, infections[5]	Obesity

Guidelines for the neonatal period should be undertaken *at whatever age* the diagnosis is made; DTaP, acellular DTP; IPV, inactivated poliovirus (oral polio also used); RV, rotavirus; MMR, measles–mumps–rubella; Var, varicella; LFTs, liver function studies; CBC, complete blood count; U/S, ultrasound, [1]alternative timing; [2]by practitioner; [3]as dictated by clinical findings; [4]parent group, family/sib, financial, and behavioral issues as discussed in the preface; [5]for those with glycogen storage disease Ib.

Glycogen Storage Diseases I, III–IV

Preventive medical checklist (15m–6yrs)

Patient   **Birth Date** / /   **Number**

Pediatric	Screen		Evaluate		Refer/Counsel	
15 months / / *Hib*[1] ❑ *MMR*[1] ❑ *DTaP, IPV*[1] ❑ *Varicella*[1] ❑			Feeding Abdominal exam	❑ ❑	Family support[4] Dietician	❑ ❑
18 months / / *DTaP, IPV*[1] ❑ *Varicella*[1] ❑ *Influenza*[3] ❑	Glucose, LFTs	❑	Feeding Abdominal exam	❑ ❑	Dietician	❑
2 years / / *Influenza*[3] ❑ *Pneumovax*[3] ❑ *Dentist* ❑	Glucose, LFTs Audiology[3] Urinalysis	❑ ❑ ❑	Feeding Abdominal exam Otitis, sinusitis[5]	❑ ❑ ❑	Genetics Dietician	❑ ❑
3 years / / *Influenza*[3] ❑ *Pneumovax*[3] ❑ *Dentist* ❑	Glucose, LFTs Audiology[3] Abdominal U/S[3]	❑ ❑ ❑	Feeding Abdominal exam Otitis, sinusitis[5]	❑ ❑ ❑	Family support[4] Dietician	❑ ❑
4 years / / *Influenza*[3] ❑ *Pneumovax*[3] ❑ *Dentist* ❑	Glucose, LFTs CBC Bleeding time Urinalysis, BP	❑ ❑ ❑ ❑	Abdominal exam	❑	Genetics Dietician	❑ ❑
5 years / / *DTaP, IPV*[1] ❑ *MMR*[1] ❑	Glucose, LFTs CBC Bleeding time Urinalysis, BP	❑ ❑ ❑ ❑	Abdominal exam	❑	Dietician	❑
6 years / / *DTaP, IPV*[1] ❑ *MMR*[1] ❑ *Dentist* ❑	Glucose, LFTs Serum AFP Abdominal U/S Urinalysis, BP	❑ ❑ ❑ ❑	Abdominal exam	❑	Family support[4] Genetics Dietician Endocrinology[3] Liver transplant[3]	❑ ❑ ❑ ❑ ❑

Clinical concerns for Glycogen Storage Diseases, ages 1–6 years

Hypoglycemia, seizures	Hepatomegaly	Epistaxis
Hyperlipidemia	Hepatic adenomas	Prolonged bleeding time
Hyperuricemia	Lumbar lordosis	Proteinuria
Sinusitis, otitis[5]	Neutropenia, infections[5]	Obesity

Guidelines for prior ages should be undertaken *at the time of diagnosis*; DTaP, acellular DTP; IPV, inactivated poliovirus (oral polio also used); MMR, measles–mumps–rubella; LFTs, liver function studies; CBC, complete blood count; U/S, ultrasound, AFP, α-fetoprotein; [1]alternative timing; [2]by practitioner; [3]as dictated by clinical findings; [4]parent group, family/sib, financial, and behavioral issues as discussed in the preface; [5]for those with glycogen storage disease Ib.

Glycogen Storage Diseases I, III–IV

Preventive medical checklist (6+ yrs)

Patient   **Birth Date**   /   /   **Number**

Pediatric	Screen		Evaluate		Refer/Counsel	
8 years / / *Dentist* ☐	Glucose, LFTs CBC, bleed time Urinalysis, BP	☐ ☐ ☐	Abdominal exam	☐	Genetics Dietician Endocrinology[3]	☐ ☐ ☐
10 years / /	Glucose, LFTs Urinalysis, BP Serum AFP Abdominal U/S	☐ ☐ ☐ ☐	Abdominal exam	☐	Dietician Endocrinology[3]	☐ ☐
12 years / / *Td[1], MMR, Var* ☐ *CBC* ☐ *Dentist* ☐ *Scoliosis* ☐ *Cholesterol* ☐	Glucose, LFTs Urinalysis, BP CBC Bleeding time	☐ ☐ ☐ ☐	Abdominal exam	☐	Family support[4] Genetics Dietician Endocrinology[3]	☐ ☐ ☐ ☐
14 years / / *CBC* ☐ *Dentist* ☐ *Cholesterol* ☐ *Breast CA* ☐ *Testicular CA* ☐	Glucose, LFTs Urinalysis, BP Serum AFP Abdominal U/S	☐ ☐ ☐ ☐	Abdominal exam	☐	Dietician	☐
16 years / / *Td[1]* ☐ *CBC* ☐ *Cholesterol* ☐ *Sexual[5]* ☐ *Dentist* ☐	Glucose, LFTs Urinalysis, BP CBC Bleeding time	☐ ☐ ☐ ☐	Abdominal exam	☐	Genetics Dietician	☐ ☐
18 years / / *CBC* ☐ *Sexual[5]* ☐ *Cholesterol* ☐ *Scoliosis* ☐	Glucose, LFTs Urinalysis, BP Serum AFP Abdominal U/S	☐ ☐ ☐ ☐	Abdominal exam	☐	Dietician Dentistry	☐ ☐
20 years[6] / / *CBC* ☐ *Sexual[5]* ☐ *Cholesterol* ☐ *Dentist* ☐	Growth Hearing, vision[2] Abdominal U/S CBC Bleeding time	☐ ☐ ☐ ☐ ☐	Glucose, LFTs Urinalysis, BP Serum AFP Abdominal exam	☐ ☐ ☐ ☐	Liver transplant[3]	☐

Clinical concerns for Glycogen Storage Diseases, ages 6+ years

Hypoglycemia, seizures	Short stature	Osteoporosis
Hyperlipidemia	Obesity	Epistaxis
Hyperuricemia	Hepatomegaly	Prolonged bleeding time
Lactic acidosis	Hepatic adenomas, cancers	Proteinuria, renal failure

Guidelines for prior ages should be undertaken *at the time of diagnosis*; Td, tetanus/diphtheria; MMR, measles–mumps–rubella; Var, varicella; LFTs, liver function studies; CBC, complete blood count; U/S, ultrasound, AFP, α-fetoprotein; [1]alternative timing; [2]by practitioner; [3]as dictated by clinical findings; [4]parent group, family/sib, financial, and behavioral issues as discussed in the preface; [5]birth control, STD screening if sexually active; [6]repeat every decade.

References

Aase, J. M. (1992). Dysmorphologic diagnosis for the pediatric practitioner. *Pediatric Clinics of North America* 39:135–56.

Abe, T. & Tamai, M. (1995). Ocular changes of glycogen storage disease type I. *Ophthalmologica* 209:92–5.

Abel, E. L. (1988). Fetal alcohol syndrome in families. *Neurotoxicology and Teratology* 10:1–2.

Abel, E. L. (1995). An update on incidence of FAS: FAS is not an equal opportunity birth defect. *Neurotoxicology and Teratology* 17:437–43.

Abel, E. L. & Sokol, R. J. (1987). Incidence of fetal alcohol syndrome and economic impact of FAS-related anomalies. *Drug and Alcohol Dependence* 19:51–70.

Ackerman, J., Chau, V. & Gilbert-Barness, E. (1996). Pathological case of the month. Congenital muscular torticollis. *Archives of Pediatric and Adolescent Medicine* 150:1101–2.

Adams, J., Vorhees, C. V. & Middaugh, L. D. (1990). Developmental neurotoxicology of anticonvulsants: Human and animal evidence on phenytoin. *Neurotoxicology and Teratology* 12:203–14.

Ades, L. C., Waltham, R. D., Chiodo, A. A. & Bateman, J. F. (1995). Myocardial infarction resulting from coronary artery dissection in an adolescent with Ehlers-Danlos syndrome type IV due to a type III collagen mutation. *British Heart Journal* 74:112–16.

Admiraal, R. J. & Huygen, P. L. (1997). Vestibular areflexia as a cause of delayed motor skill development in children with the CHARGE association. *International Journal of Pediatric Otorhinolaryngology* 39:205–22.

Adra, A., Cordero, D., Mejides, A., Yasin, S., Salman, F. & O'Sullivan, M. J. (1994). Caudal regression syndrome: etiopathogenesis, prenatal diagnosis, and perinatal management. *Obstetrical and Gynecological Survey* 49:508–16.

Agency for Health Care Policy and Research (1993). *Clinical Practice Guideline Development.* Washington, DC: Government Printing Office. AHCPR #93–0023.

Agha, A. & Hashimoto, K. (1995). Multiple lentigines (Leopard) syndrome with Chiari I malformation. *Journal of Dermatology* 22:520–3.

Ainsworth, S. R. & Aulicino, P. L. (1993). A survey of patients with Ehlers–Danlos syndrome. *Clinical Orthopaedics and Related Research* 286:250–6.

Akbarnia, B. A., Gabriel, K. R., Beckman, E. & Chalk, D. (1992). Prevalence of scoliosis in neurofibromatosis. *Spine* 17:S244–8.

Alagille, D., Estrada, A., Hadchouel, M., Gautier, M., Odievre, M. & Dommergues. J. P. (1987).

Syndromic paucity of interlobular bile ducts (Alagille syndrome or arteriohepatic dysplasia): review of 80 cases. *Journal of Pediatrics* 110:195–200.

Albanese, A. & Stanhope, R. (1993). Growth and metabolic data following growth hormone treatment of children with intrauterine growth retardation. *Hormone Research* 39:8–12.

Allanson, J. E. (1987). Noonan syndrome. *Journal of Medical Genetics* 24:9–13.

Allanson, J. E. (1989). Time and natural history: The changing face. *Journal of Craniofacial Genetics and Developmental Biology* 9:21–8.

Allanson, J. E. & Cole, T. R. (1996). Sotos syndrome: evolution of facial phenotype subjective and objective assessment. *American Journal of Medical Genetics* 65:13–20.

Allanson, J. E. & Hall, J. G. (1986). Obstetric and gynecologic problems in women with chondrodystrophies. *Obstetrics and Gynecology* 67:74–8.

Allanson, J. E., Hennekam, R. C. & Ireland, M. (1997). De Lange syndrome: subjective and objective comparison of the classical and mild phenotypes. *Journal of Medical Genetics* 34:645–50.

Allingham-Hawkins, D. J. & Tomkins, D. J. (1995). Heterogeneity in Roberts syndrome. *American Journal of Medical Genetics* 55:188–94.

American Cleft Palate-Craniofacial Association (1993). Parameters for evaluation and treatment of patients with cleft lip/palate or other craniofacial anomalies. *The Cleft Palate-Craniofacial Journal* 30:S1–S8.

Amman, A. J., Wara, D. W., Cowan, M. J., Barrett, D. J. & Stiehm, E. R. (1982). The DiGeorge syndrome and the fetal alcohol syndrome. *American Journal of Diseases of Children* 136:906–8.

Anderson, P. J., Hall, C., Evans, R. D., Harkness, W. J., Hayward, R. D. & Jones, B. M. (1997). The cervical spine in Crouzon syndrome. *Spine* 22:402–5.

Angelman, H. (1961). Syndrome of coloboma with multiple congenital abnormalities in infancy. *British Medical Journal* 1:1212–14.

Anonymous. (1985). Case history of a child with Williams syndrome. *Pediatrics* 75:962–8.

Anonymous. (1993). Identification and characterization of the tuberous sclerosis gene on chromosome 16. The European Chromosome 16 Tuberous Sclerosis Consortium. *Cell* 75:1305–15.

Anonymous. (1993). Glycogen storage disease type I. Proceedings of a workshop. *European Journal of Pediatrics* 152 (Suppl. 1):S1–S88.

Anonymous. (1996). Positional cloning of a gene involved in the pathogenesis of Treacher Collins syndrome. The Treacher Collins Syndrome Collaborative Group. *Nature Genetics* 12:130–6.

Antley, R. & Bixler, D. (1975). Trapezoidocephaly, midfacial hypoplasia, and cartilage abnormalities with multiple synostosis and skeletal fractures. *Birth Defects* 11:397–401.

Apajasalo, M., Sintonen, H., Rautonen, J. & Kaitila, I. (1998). Health-related quality of life of patients with genetic skeletal dysplasias. *European Journal of Pediatrics* 157:114–21.

Applegate, K. E. & Sargent, S. K. (1995). Spontaneous colonic ischemia in a patient with Riley–Day syndrome. *Pediatric Radiology* 25:12–13.

Arbour, L., Rosenblatt, B., Clow, C. & Wilson, G. N. (1988). Post-operative dystonia in a female patient with homocystinuria. *Journal of Pediatrics* 113:863–4.

Argenta, L. C., David, L. R., Wilson, J. A. & Bell, W. O. (1996). An increase in infant cranial deformity with supine sleeping position. *Journal of Craniofacial Surgery* 7:5–11.

Assadi, F. K. (1990). Renal tubular dysfunction in fetal alcohol syndrome. *Pediatric Nephrology* 4:48–51.

Astley, S. J. & Clarren, S. K. (1995). A fetal alcohol syndrome screening tool. *Alcoholism Clinical and Experimental Research* 19:1565–71.

Attanasio, A., James, D., Reinhardt, R. & Rekers-Mombarg, L. (1995). Final height and long-term outcome after growth hormone therapy in Turner syndrome: results of a German multicenter trial. *Hormone Research* 43:147–9.

Auerbach, A. D. & Verlander, P. C. (1997). Disorders of DNA replication and repair. *Current Opinions in Pediatrics* 9:600–16.

Axelrod, F. B. & Pearson, J. (1984). Congenital sensory neuropathies: Diagnostic distinction from familial dysautonomia. *American Journal of Diseases of Children* 138:947–9.

Axelrod, F. B., Porges, R. F. & Sein, M. E. (1987). Neonatal recognition of familial dysautonomia. *Journal of Pediatrics* 110:946–8.

Ayers, G. (1994). Statistical profile of special education in the United States. *Teaching Exceptional Children* 26 (suppl. 3): 3–4.

Azcona, C., Albanese, A., Bareille, P. & Stanhope, R. (1998). Growth hormone treatment in growth hormone-sufficient and -insufficient children with intrauterine growth retardation/Russell-Silver syndrome. *Hormone Research* 50:22–7.

Baba, H., Maezawa, Y., Furusawa, N., Chen, Q., Imura, S. & Tomita, K. (1995). The cervical spine in the Klippel–Feil syndrome. A report of 57 cases. *International Orthopedics* 19:204–8.

Bachrach, S. J., Walter, R. S. & Trzcinski, K. (1998). Use of glycopyrrolate and other anticholinergic medications for sialorrhea in children with cerebral palsy. *Clinical Pediatrics* 37:485–90.

Balling, R., Mutter, G., Gruss, P. & Kessel, M. (1989). Craniofacial abnormalities induced by ectopic expression of the homeobox gene Hox-1.1. *Cell* 58:337–47.

Bannayan, G. A. (1971). Lipomatosis, angiomatosis and macroencephaly: A previously undescribed congenital syndrome. *Archives of Pathology* 92:1–5.

Bantz, E. W. (1984). Valproic acid and congenital malformation. *Clinical Pediatrics* 23:332–33.

Baraitser, M., Winter, R. M. & Brett, E. M. (1983). Greig cephalosyndactyly: Report of 13 affected individuals in three families. *Clinical Genetics* 24:257–65.

Bardach, J., Morris, H. L., Olin, W. H., Gray, S. D., Jones, D. L., Kelly, K. M., Shaw, W. C. & Semb, G. (1992). Results of multidisciplinary management of bilateral cleft lip and palate at the Iowa Cleft Palate Center. *Plastic and Reconstructive Surgery* 89:419–32.

Barnicoat, A. (1997). Screening for fragile X syndrome: a model for genetic disorders? *British Medical Journal* 315:1174–5.

Bartolucci, G. & Younger, J. (1994). Tentative classification of neuropsychiatric disturbances in Prader–Willi syndrome. *Journal of Intellectual Disability Research* 38:621–9.

Batshaw, M. L. (1994). *The Child with Developmental Disabilities*. Philadelphia: W.B. Saunders.

Baty, B. J., Blackburn, B. L. & Carey, J. C. (1994a). Natural history of trisomy 18 and trisomy 13: I. Growth, physical assessment, medical histories, survival and recurrence risk. *American Journal of Medical Genetics* 49:175–88.

Baty, B. J., Jorde, L. B., Blackburn, B. L. & Carey, J. C. (1994b). Natural history of trisomy 18 and trisomy 13: II. Psychomotor development. *American Journal of Medical Genetics* 49:189–94.

Bauer, S. (1994). Urologic care of the child with spina bifida. *Spina Bifida Spotlight*, July:1–4.

Baumgardner, T. L., Reiss, A. L., Freund, L. S. & Abrams, M. T. (1995). Specification of the neuro-behavioral phenotype in males with fragile X syndrome. *Pediatrics* 95:744–52.

Bawle, E. & Quigg, M. H. (1992). Ectopia lentis and aortic root dilatation in congenital contractural arachnodactyly. *American Journal of Medical Genetics* 42:19–21.

Beazley, D. M. & Egerman R. S. (1998). Toxoplasmosis. *Seminars in Perinatology* 22:332–8.

Bebb, G. G., Grannis, F. W., Jr., Paz, I. B., Slovak, M. L. & Chilcote, R. (1998). Mediastinal germ cell tumor in a child with precocious puberty and Klinefelter syndrome. *Annals of Thoracic Surgery* 66:547–8.

Bebin, E. M., Kelly, P. J. & Gomez, M. R. (1993). Surgical treatment for epilepsy in cerebral tuberous sclerosis. *Epilepsia* 34:651–7.

Belkengren, R. & Sapala, S. (1998). Pediatric management problems. Plagiocephaly. *Pediatric Nursing* 24:82–5.

Bellus, G. A., McIntosh, I., Smith, E. A., Aylsworth, A. S., Kaitila, I., Horton, W. A., Greenhaw, G. A., Hecht, J. T. & Francomano, C. A. (1995). A recurrent mutation in the tyrosine kinase domain of fibroblast growth factor receptor 3 causes hypochondroplasia. *Nature Genetics* 10:357–9.

Bembi, B., Parma, A., Bottega, M., Ceschel, S., Zanatta, M., Martini, C. & Ciana, G. (1997). Intravenous pamidronate treatment in osteogenesis imperfecta. *Journal of Pediatrics* 131:622–5.

Bender, B. G., Linden, M. G. & Robinson, A. (1993). Neuropsychiatric impairment in 42 adolescents with sex chromosome abnormalities. *American Journal of Medical Genetics* 48:169–73.

Ben-Neriah, Z., Yagel, S. & Ariel, I. (1995). Renal anomalies in Marden–Walker syndrome: a clue for prenatal diagnosis. *American Journal of Medical Genetics* 57:417–19.

Berde, C., Willis, D. C. & Sandberg E. C. (1983). Pregnancy in women with pseudoxanthoma elasticum. *Obstetrics and Gynecology Survey* 38:339–44.

Berry, G.T. & Bennett, M. J. (1998): A focused approach to diagnosing inborn errors of metabolism. *Contemporary Pediatrics* 15:79–102.

Beuren, A. J., Apitz, J. & Harmjanz, D. (1962). Supravalvular aortic stenosis in association with mental retardation and certain facial appearance. *Circulation* 26:1235–40.

Beutler, E. & Grabowski, G. A. (1995). Gaucher disease. In *The Metabolic and Molecular Bases of Inherited Disease*, 7th edn, ed. C. R. Scriver, A. L. Beaudet, W. S. Sly & D. Valle, pp. 2641–70. New York: McGraw-Hill, Inc.

Bhargava, S. A., Putnam, P. E., Kocoshis, S. A., Rowe, M. & Hanchett, J. M. (1996). Rectal bleeding in Prader–Willi syndrome. *Pediatrics* 97:265–7.

Biehl, R. F. (1996). Legislative mandates. In *Developmental Disabilities in Infancy and Childhood*, ed. A. J. Capute & P. J. Accardo, pp. 513–24. Baltimore: Paul H. Brookes.

Binder, H., Conway, A., Hason, S., Gerber, L. H., Marini, J., Berry, R. & Weintrob, J. (1993). Comprehensive rehabilitation of the child with osteogenesis imperfecta. *American Journal of Medical Genetics* 45:265–9.

Bird, H., Collins, A. L., Oley, C. & Lindsay, S. (1995). Crossover analysis in a British family suggests that Coffin–Lowry syndrome maps to a 3.4-cM interval in Xp22. *American Journal of Medical Genetics* 59:512–16.

Blair, S. N., Kohl III, H. W. Barlow, C. E., Paffenbarger, R. S., Jr., Gibbons, L. W. & Macera, C. A

(1995). Changes in physical fitness and all-cause mortality. *Journal of the American Medical Association* 273:1093–8.

Blake, K. D., Davenport, S. L., Hall, B. D., Hefner, M. A., Pagon, R. A., Williams, M. S., Lin, A. E. & Graham, J. M., Jr. (1998). CHARGE association: an update and review for the primary pediatrician. *Clinical Pediatrics* 37:159–73.

Blake, K., Kirk, J. M. & Ur E. (1993). Growth in CHARGE association. *Archives of Disease in Childhood* 68:508–9.

Blake, K.D., Russell-Eggitt, I.M., Morgan, D.W., Ratcliffe, J.M. & Wyse R.K.H. (1990). Who's in charge? Multidisciplinary management of patients with CHARGE association. *Archives of Disease in Childhood* 65:217–23.

Blasco, P. A. & Stansbury, J. C. (1996). Glycopyrrolate treatment of chronic drooling. *Archives of Pediatric and Adolescent Medicine* 150:932–5.

Blythe, W. R., Logan, T. C., Holmes, D. K. & Drake, A. F. (1996). Fibromatosis colli: a common cause of neonatal torticollis. *American Family Physician* 54:1965–7.

Bogdanovic, R., Komar, P., Cvoric, A., Nikolic, V., Sinotic, M., Zdravkovic, D., Ognjanovic, M. & Abinun, M. (1994). Focal glomerular sclerosis and nephrotic syndrome in spondyloepiphyseal dysplasia. *Nephron* 66:219–24.

Boj, J. R., von Arx, J. D., Cortada, M., Jimenez, A. & Golobart, J. (1993). Dentures for a 3-year-old with ectodermal dysplasia. *American Journal of Dentistry* 6:165–7.

Bomalaski, M. D., Teague, J. L. & Brooks, B. (1995). The long-term impact of urological management on the quality of life of children with spina bifida. *Journal of Urology* 154:778–81.

Bonthron, D. T., Macgregor, D. F. & Barr, D. G. (1993). Nager acrofacial dysostosis: minor familial manifestations supporting dominant inheritance. *Clinical Genetics* 43:127–31.

Bos, A. P., Broers C. J. M., Hazebroek, F. W. J., van Hemel, J. O., Tibboel, D., Wesby-van Sway, E. & Molenaar, J. C. (1992). Avoidance of emergency surgery in newborn infants with trisomy 18. *Lancet* 339:913–17.

Boschert, S. (1995). Many objections to new fetal alcohol guidelines. *Pediatric News* November 11.

Botto, L. D., Khoury, M. J., Mastroiacovo, P., Castilla, E. E., Moore, C. A., Skjaerven, R., Mutchinick, O. M., Borman, B., Cocchi, G., Czeizel, A. E., Goujard, J., Irgens, L. M., Lancaster, P. A., Martinez-Frias, M. L., Merlob, P., Ruusinen, A., Stoll, C. & Sumiyoshi, Y. (1997). The spectrum of congenital anomalies of the VATER association: an international study. *American Journal of Medical Genetics* 71:8–15.

Botvin, G. J., Baker, E., Dusenbury, L., Botvin, E. B. & Diaz, T. (1995). Long-term follow-up results of a randomized drug abuse prevention trial in a middle-class population. *Journal of the American Medical Association* 273: 1106–12.

Bowen, P., Lee, C. S. H., Zellweger, H. & Lindenberg, R. (1964). A familial syndrome of multiple congenital defects. *Bulletin of Johns Hopkins* 114:402–14.

Bowling, B. S. & Chandna, A. (1994). Superior lacrimal canalicular atresia and nasolacrimal duct obstruction in the CHARGE association. *Journal of Pediatric Ophthalmology and Strabismus* 31:336–7.

Boyle, C., Decouflé, P. & Yeargin-Allsopp, M. (1994). Prevalence and health impact of developmental disabilities in US children. *Pediatrics* 93:399–403.

Brent, R. L. (1988). Improving the quality of expert witness testimony. *Pediatrics* 82:511–13.

Brent, R. L. (1995). Bendectin: review of the medical literature of a comprehensively studied human nonteratogen and the most prevalent tortogen-litogen. *Reproductive Toxicology* 9:337–49.

Briault, S., Hill, R., Shrimpton, A., Zhu, D., Till, M., Ronce, N., Margaritte-Jeannin, P., Baraitser, M., Middleton-Price, H., Malcolm S., Thompson, E., Hoo, J., Wilson, G., Romano, C., Guichet, A., Pembrey, M., Fontes, M., Poustka, A. & Moraine, C. (1997). A gene for FG syndrome maps in the Xq12–q21.31 region. *American Journal of Medical Genetics* 73:87–90.

Brill, C. B., Rose, J. S., Godmilow, L., Sklower, S., Willner, J. & Hirschhorn, K. (1978). Spastic quadriparesis due to C1–C2 subluxation in Hurler syndrome. *Journal of Pediatrics* 92:441–3.

Brisigotti, M., Fabbretti, G., Pesce, F., Gatti, R., Cohen, A., Parenti, G. & Callea, F. (1993). Congenital bilateral juvenile granulosa cell tumor of the ovary in leprechaunism: a case report. *Pediatric Pathology* 13:549–58.

Briskin, H. & Liptak G. S. (1995). Helping families with children with developmental disabilities. *Pediatric Annals* 24:262–6.

Brook-Carter, P. T., Peral, B., Ward, C. J., Thompson, P. J., Hughes, M., Maheshwar, M., Nellist, M., Gamble, V., Harris, P. C. & Sampson, J. R. (1994). Deletion of the TSC2 and PKD1 genes associated with severe infantile polycystic kidney disease – a contiguous gene syndrome. *Nature Genetics* 8:328–32.

Brown, D. M., Vandenburgh, K., Kimura, A.E., Weingeist, T. A., Sheffield, V.C. & Stone, E. M. (1995). Novel frameshift mutations in the procollagen 2 gene (COL2A1) associated with Stickler syndrome (hereditary arthro-ophthalmopathy). *Human Molecular Genetics* 4:141–2.

Brown, F.R. III, McAdams, A. J., Cummins, J. W., Konkol, R., Singh, I., Moser, A. B. & Moser, H. W. (1982). Cerebro-hepato-renal (Zellweger) syndrome and neonatal adrenoleukodystrophy: Similarities in phenotype and accumulation of very long chain fatty acids. *Johns Hopkins Medical Journal* 151:344–61.

Brueton, L. A., Chotai, K. A. van Herwerden, L., Schinzel, A. & Winter, R. M. (1992). The acrocallosal syndrome and Greig syndrome are not allelic disorders. *Journal of Medical Genetics* 29:635–7.

Brumsen, C., Hamdy, N. A. & Papapoulos, S. E. (1997). Long-term effects of bisphosphonates on the growing skeleton. Studies of young patients with severe osteoporosis. *Medicine* 76:266–83.

Bruni, O., Cortesis, F., Giannotti, F. & Curatolo, P. (1995). Sleep disorders in tuberous sclerosis: a polysomnographic study. *Brain and Development* 17:52–6.

Brunt, P. W. & McKusick, V. A. (1970). Familial dysautonomia: a report of genetic and clinical studies, with a review of the literature. *Medicine* 49:343–74.

Bryden, D. C., Remington, S. A. & Mason, C. (1995). Treacher Collins syndrome and difficult intubation. *British Journal of Hospital Medicine* 53:419.

Bucciarelli, R. L. & Eitzman, D. V. (1988). Baby Doe: Where do we stand now. *Contemporary Pediatrics* January:116–28.

Buehler, B. A., Dellmont, D., van Waes, M. & Finnell, R. H. (1990). Prenatal determination of risk for the fetal hydantoin syndrome. *New England Journal of Medicine* 322:1567–72.

Bühler, E. M. & Malik, N. J. (1984). The tricho-rhino-phalangeal syndrome(s): Chromosome 8 deletion. Is there a shortest region of overlap between reported cases? TRP I and TRP II syndromes: Are they separate entities? *American Journal of Medical Genetics* 19:113–19.

Burch, M., Sharland, M., Shinebourne, E., Smith, G., Patton, M. & McKenna, W. (1993). Cardiologic abnormalities in Noonan syndrome: Phenotypic diagnosis and echocardiographic assessment of 118 patients. *Journal of the American College of Cardiology* 22:1189–92.

Burd, L. & Martsolf, J. T. (1989). Fetal alcohol syndrome: Diagnosis and syndromal variability. *Physiology and Behavior* 46:39–43.

Burd, L., Vesely, B., Martsolf, J. & Korbeshian, J. (1990). Prevalence study of Prader–Willi syndrome in North Dakota. *American Journal of Medical Genetics* 37:97–9.

Burn, J. (1986). Syndrome of the month: Williams syndrome. *Journal of Medical Genetics* 23:389–395.

Burn, J., Camm, J., Davies, M. J., Peltonen, L., Schwartz, P. J. & Watkins, H. (1997). The phenotype/genotype relation and the current status of genetic screening in hypertrophic cardiomyopathy, Marfan syndrome, and the long QT syndrome. *Heart* 78:110–16.

Burton, B. K. (1998). Inborn errors of metabolism in infancy: a guide to diagnosis. *Pediatrics* 102:E69.

Butler, M. G. & Meaney, F. J. (1991). Standards for selected anthropometric measurements in Prader–Willi syndrome. *Pediatrics* 88:853–60.

Butler, M. G. & Wadlington, W. B. (1987). Robinow syndrome: report of two patients and review of literature. *Clinical Genetics* 31:77–85.

Butler, M. G., Brunschwig, A., Miller, L. K. & Hagerman, R. J. (1992). Standards for selected anthropometric measurements in males with the fragile X syndrome. *Pediatrics* 89:1059–62.

Byers, P. H. (1994). Ehlers–Danlos syndrome: recent advances and current understanding of the clinical and genetic heterogeneity. *Journal of Investigative Dermatology* 103 (suppl. 5):47S-52S.

Cabana, M. D., Capone, G., Fritz, A. & Berkovitz, G. (1997). Nutritional rickets in a child with Down syndrome. *Clinical Pediatrics* 36:235–7.

Canadian Task Force on the Periodic Health Examination. (1994). *The Canadian Guide to Clinical Preventive Health Care.* Ottawa, Ontario: Canada Communication Group Publishing.

Cantz, M. & Ullrich-Bott, B. (1990). Disorders of glycoprotein degradation. *Journal of Inherited Metabolic Disease* 13:523–6.

Capute, A. & Accardo, P. (1996). Cerebral palsy: the spectrum of motor dysfunction. In *Developmental Disabilities in Infancy and Childhood*, 2nd edn, vol. 2, ed. A. Capute & P. Accardo, pp. 81–94. Baltimore: Paul Brookes.

Capute, A. J. (1998). On the treatment of cerebral palsy: the outcome of 177 patients, 74 totally untreated, by Richmond Paine, MD (*Pediatrics*,1962;29:605–616). *Pediatrics* 102:233–4.

Carden, S. M., Boissy, R. E., Schoettker, P. J. & Good, W. V. (1998). Albinism: modern molecular diagnosis. *British Journal of Ophthalmology* 82:189–95.

Carey, J. (1992). Health supervision and anticipatory guidance for children with genetic disorders (including specific recommendations for trisomy 21, trisomy 18, and neurofibromatosis). *Pediatric Clinics of North America* 39:25–53.

Carey, J. C. (1998). Neurofibromatosis–Noonan syndrome. *American Journal of Medical Genetics* 75:263–4.

Carlson, W. E., Vaughan, C. L., Damiano, D. L. & Abel, M. F. (1997). Orthotic management of gait in spastic diplegia. *American Journal of Physical Medicine and Rehabilitation* 76:219–25.

Carolino, J., Perez, J. A. & Popa, A. (1998). Osteopetrosis. *American Family Medicine* 57:1293–6.

Carpenter, P. K. (1994). Prader–Willi syndrome in old age. *Journal of Intellectual Disability Research* 38:529–31.

Cassidy, S. B. (1987). Prader–Willi syndrome. Characteristics management and etiology. *Alabama Journal of Medical Sciences* 24:169–75.

Cassidy, S. B., Pagon, R. A., Pepin, M. & Blumhagen, J. D. (1983). Family studies in tuberous sclerosis. Evaluation of apparently unaffected parents. *Journal of the American Medical Association* 249:1302–4.

Cassidy, S. B., Blonder, O., Courtney, V. W., Ratzan, S. K. & Carey, D. E. (1986). Russell–Silver syndrome and hypopituitarism. Patient report and literature review. *American Journal of Diseases of Children* 140:155–9.

Cassidy, S. B. & Schwartz, S. (1998). Prader–Willi and Angelman syndromes. Disorders of genomic imprinting. *Medicine* 77:140–51.

Centers for Disease Control (1992). Spina bifida incidence at birth – United States, 1983–1990. *Morbidity and Mortality Weekly Report* 41:497–500.

Centers for Disease Control (1995). Health insurance coverage and receipt of preventive health services – United States, 1993. *Journal of the American Medical Association* 273:1083–4.

Centers for Disease Control (1995). Update: trends in fetal alcohol syndrome – United States, 1979–1993. *Journal of the American Medical Association* 273:1406.

Centers for Disease Control (1997a). Alcohol consumption among pregnant and childbearing-aged women – United States, 1991 and 1995. *Morbidity and Mortality Weekly Report* 46:346–50.

Centers for Disease Control (1997b). Rubella and congenital rubella syndrome – United States, 1994–1997. *Morbidity and Mortality Weekly Report* 16:350–4.

Centers for Disease Control (1997c). Surveillance for fetal alcohol syndrome using multiple sources – Atlanta, Georgia, 1981–1989. *Morbidity and Mortality Weekly Report* 46:1118–20.

Cerniglia, F. R., Jr. (1997). Frankie's story – spina bifida from the parents' perspective [editorial]. *Journal of Urology* 158:1291.

Charnas, L. R. & Marini, J. C. (1993). Communicating hydrocephalus, basilar invagination, and other neurologic features in osteogenesis imperfecta. *Neurology* 43:2603–8.

Charney, E. B. (1990). Myelomeningocele. In *Pediatric Primary Care: A Problem-Oriented Approach*, ed. M. W. Schwartz, p. 663. Chicago: Mosby-Year Book.

Charrow, J., Listernick, R. & Ward, K. (1993). Autosomal dominant multiple café-au-lait spots and neurofibromatosis-1: evidence of non-linkage. *American Journal of Medical Genetics* 45:606–8.

Chen, A., Francis, M., Ni, L., Cremers, C. W., Kimberling, W. J., Sato, Y., Phelps, P. D., Bellman, S. C., Wagner, M. J. & Pembrey, M. (1995). Phenotypic manifestations of the branchio-oto-renal syndrome. *American Journal of Medical Genetics* 58:365–70.

Chen, E., Johnson, J. P., Cox, V. A. & Golabi, M. (1993). Simpson–Golabi–Behmel syndrome: congenital diaphragmatic hernia and radiologic findings in two patients and follow-up of a previously reported case. *American Journal of Medical Genetics* 46:574–8.

Chen, Y. T. & Burchell, A. (1995). Glycogen storage diseases. In *The Metabolic and Molecular Bases of Inherited Disease,* 7th edn, ed. C. R. Scriver, A. L. Beaudet, W. S. Sly & D. Valle, pp. 935–65. New York: McGraw-Hill, Inc.

Chen, Y. T. & Van Hove, J. L. (1995). Renal involvement in type I glycogen storage disease. *Advances in Nephrology from the Necker Hospital* 24:357–65.

Cheney, C. & Ramsdel, J. (1987). Effect of medical records' checklists on implementation of periodic health measures. *American Journal of Medicine* 83:129–36.

Cheng, T. L., Perrin, E. C., DeWitt, T. G. & O'Connor, K. G. (1996). Use of checklists in pediatric practice. *Archives of Pediatric and Adolescent Medicine* 150:768–9.

Chestnut, R., James H. E. & Jones, K. L. (1992). The Vater association and spinal dysraphia. *Pediatric Neurosurgery* 18:144–8.

Chevenix-Trench, G., Wicking, C., Berkman, J., Sharpe, H., Hockey, A., Haan, E., Oley, C., Ravine, D., Turner, A. & Goldgar, D. (1993). Further localization of the gene for nevoid basal cell carcinoma syndrome (NBCSS) in 15 Australian families: linkage and loss of heterozygosity. *American Journal of Human Genetics* 53:760–7.

Chi-Lum, B. I. (1995). Putting more prevention into medical training. *Journal of the American Medical Association* 273:1402–3.

Chitayat, D., Hodgkinson, K. A., Chen, M. F., Haber, G. D., Nakishima, S. & Sando, I. (1992). Branchio-oto-renal syndrome: further delineation of an underdiagnosed syndrome. *American Journal of Medical Genetics* 43:970–5.

Chuang, D. T. & Shih, V. E. (1995). Disorders of branched chain amino acid and keto acid metabolism. In *The Metabolic and Molecular Bases of Inherited Disease*, 7th edn, ed. C. R. Scriver, A. L. Beaudet, W. S. Sly & D. Valle, pp. 1239–77. New York: McGraw-Hill, Inc.

Chudley, A. E. & Hagerman, R. J. (1987). Fragile X syndrome. *Journal of Pediatrics* 110:821–31.

Church, M. W. & Gerkin, K. P. (1988). Hearing disorders in children with fetal alcohol syndrome: Findings from case reports. *Pediatrics* 82:147–54.

Church, M. W. & Kaltenbach, J. A. (1997). Hearing, speech, language, and vestibular disorders in the fetal alcohol syndrome: a literature review. *Alcoholism Clinical & Experimental Research* 21:495–512.

Clark, A. N. G. & Zuha, M. S. (1977). Klinefelter syndrome in the aged. *Age and Ageing* 6:118–22.

Clark, J. R., Smith, L. J., Kendall, B. E., Tasker R. C. & Wilkerson, K. A. (1995). Unexpected brainstem compression following routine surgery in a child with oto-palato-digital syndrome. *Anaesthesia* 50:641–3.

Clarke, D. J. (1993). Prader–Willi syndrome and psychoses. *British Journal of Psychiatry* 163:680–4.

Cluzel, P., Pierot, L., Leung, A., Gaston, A., Kieffer, E. & Chiras, J. (1994). Vertebral arteriovenous fistulae in neurofibromatosis: report of two cases and review of the literature. *Neuroradiology* 36:321–5.

Coberly, S., Lammer, E. & Alashari, M. (1996). Retinoic acid embryopathy: case report and review of literature. *Pediatric Pathology & Laboratory Medicine* 16:823–36.

Coffin, G. S. & Siris, E. (1970). Mental retardation with absent fifth fingernail and terminal phalanx. *American Journal of Diseases of Children* 119:433–9.

Cohen, M. M., Jr. (1971). Variability versus "incidental findings" in the first and second branchial arch syndrome: Unilateral variants with anophthalmia. *Birth Defects* 7:103–8.

Cohen, M. M., Jr. (1975). An etiologic and nosologic overview of craniosynostosis syndromes. *Birth Defects* 11:137–89.

Cohen, M. M., Jr. (1979). Craniosynostosis and syndromes with craniosynostosis: Incidence, genetics, penetrance, variability and new syndrome updating. *Birth Defects* 15:85–9.

Cohen, M. M., Jr. (1987). The elephant man did not have neurofibromatosis. *Proceedings of the Greenwood Genetics Center* 6:187–92.

Cohen, M. M., Jr. (1991). Hallermann–Streiff syndrome: A review. *American Journal of Medical Genetics* 41:488–99.

Cohen, M. M., Jr. (1993). Pfeiffer syndrome update, clinical subtypes, and guidelines for differential diagnosis. *American Journal of Medical Genetics* 45:300–7.

Cohen, M. M., Jr. (1995). Craniosynostoses: Phenotypic/molecular correlations. *American Journal of Medical Genetics* 56:334–9.

Cohen, M. M., Jr., Hall, B. D., Smith, D. W., Graham, C. B. & Lampert. K. J. (1973). A new syndrome with hypotonia, obesity, mental deficiency, and facial, oral, ocular and limb anomalies. *Journal of Pediatrics* 83:280–4.

Cohen, M. M., Jr. & Hayden, P. W. (1979). A new recognized hamartomatous syndrome. *Birth Defects* 15(5B):291–6.

Cohen, M. M., Jr. & Kreiborg, S. (1992). Upper and lower airway obstruction in the Apert syndrome. *American Journal of Medical Genetics* 44:90–3.

Cohen, M. M., Jr. & Kreiborg, S. (1993). Growth pattern in Apert syndrome. *American Journal of Medical Genetics* 47:617–23.

Cohen, P. R. (1994). Incontinentia pigmenti: clinicopathologic characteristics and differential diagnosis. *Cutis* 54:161–6.

Cohen, W. I. (1992). Down syndrome preventive medical check list. *Down Syndrome Papers and Abstracts for Professionals* 15:1–7.

Cole, D. E. (1993). Psychosocial aspects of osteogenesis imperfecta: an update. *American Journal of Medical Genetics* 45:207–11.

Cole, T. R. & Hughes, H. E. (1990). Sotos syndrome. *Journal of Medical Genetics* 27:571–6.

Cole, T. R. & Hughes, H. E. (1994). Sotos syndrome: a study of the diagnostic criteria and natural history. *Journal of Medical Genetics* 31:20–32.

Committee on Genetics, American Academy of Pediatrics. (1994). Health supervision for children with Down syndrome. *Pediatrics* 93:855–9.

Committee on Genetics, American Academy of Pediatrics. (1995a). Health supervision for children with achondroplasia. *Pediatrics* 95:443–51.

Committee on Genetics, American Academy of Pediatrics. (1995b). Health supervision for children with neurofibromatosis. *Pediatrics* 96:368–71.

Committee on Genetics, American Academy of Pediatrics. (1995c). Health supervision for children with Turner syndrome. *Pediatrics* 96:1166–73.

Committee on Genetics, American Academy of Pediatrics. (1996a). Health supervision for children with fragile X syndrome. *Pediatrics* 98:297–300.

Committee on Genetics, American Academy of Pediatrics. (1996b). Health supervision for children with Marfan syndrome. *Pediatrics* 98:818–21.

Committee on Sports Medicine and Fitness, American Academy of Pediatrics. (1995). Atlantoaxial instability in Down syndrome: Subject review. *Pediatrics* 96:151–4.

Conley, M. E., Beckwith, J. B., Mancer, J. F. K. & Tenckhoff, L. (1979). The spectrum of DiGeorge syndrome. *Journal of Pediatrics* 94:883–90.

Cooley, W. C. (1994a). The ecology of support for caregiving families. *Journal of Behavioral and Developmental Pediatrics* 15:117–19.

Cooley, W. C. (1994b). Changing care in private practice: Management of chronic conditions in the primary care setting. In *Ross Roundtable on Management of Chronic Illness and Disability in the Primary Care Setting*, pp. 69–86. Washington, DC.

Cooley, W. C. (1994c). Pediatric training and family-centered care. In *Families, Physicians, and Children with Special Health Care Needs: Collaborative Medical Education Models*, ed. R. Darling & M. Peter, pp. 109–22. Southport, CT: Greenwood Press.

Cooley, W. C. & Graham, J. M., Jr. (1991). Down syndrome – an update and review for the primary pediatrician. *Clinical Pediatrics* 30:233–53.

Cooley, W., Rawnsley, E., Melkonian, G., Moses, C., McCann, D., Virgin, B., Couglan, J. & Moeschler, J. (1990). Autosomal dominant familial spastic paraplegia: report of a large New England family. *Clinical Genetics* 38:57–68.

Cooper, S. (1987). The fetal alcohol syndrome. *Journal of Child Psychology and Psychiatry and Allied Disciplines* 28:223–7.

Coppes, M. J., Sohl, H., Teshima, I. E., Mutiranga, A., Ledbetter, D. H. & Weksberg, R. (1993). Wilms tumor in a patient with Prader–Willi syndrome. *Journal of Pediatrics* 122:730–3.

Cordero, L. & Landon, M. B. (1993). Infant of the diabetic mother. *Clinics in Perinatology* 20:635–47.

Corsello, G., Giuffre, M., Carcione, A., Cuzto, M. L., Piccione, M. & Ziino, O. (1996). Lymphoproliferative disorders in Sotos syndrome: observation of two cases. *American Journal of Medical Genetics* 64:588–93.

Coselli, J. S., LeMaire, S. A. & Buket, S. (1995). Marfan syndrome: the variability and outcome of operative management. *Journal of Vascular Surgery* 21:432–43.

Costa, T., Scriver, C. R. & Childs, B. (1985). The effect of Mendelian disease on human health: a measurement. *American Journal of Medical Genetics* 21:231–42.

Cotton, J. L. & Williams, R. G. (1995). Noonan syndrome and neuroblastoma. *Archives of Pediatric and Adolescent Medicine* 149:1280–1.

Couriel, J. M., Bisset, R., Miller, R., Thomas, A. & Clarke, M. (1993). Assessment of feeding problems in neurodevelopmental handicap: a team approach. *Archives of Disease in Childhood* 69:609–13.

Crabbe, L. S., Bensky, A. S., Hornstein, L. & Schwartz, D. C. (1993). Cardiovascular abnormalities in children with fragile X syndrome. *Pediatrics* 91:714–15.

Crockard, H. A. & Stevens, J. M. (1995). Craniovertebral junction anomalies in inherited disorders: part of the syndrome or caused by the disorder? *European Journal of Pediatrics* 154:504–12.

Crocker, A. C. (1989). The spectrum of medical care for developmental disabilities. In *Developmental Disabilities: Delivery of Medical Care for Children and Adults*, ed. I. L Rubin & A. C. Crocker. Philadelphia: Lea and Febiger.

Cronk, C., Crocker, A. C., Pueschel, S. M., Shea, A. M., Zackai, E., Pickens, G. & Reed, R. B. (1988). Growth charts for children with Down syndrome: 1 month to 18 years of age. *Pediatrics* 81:102–110.

Crow, Y. J., Zuberi, S. M., McWilliam, R., Tolmie, J. L., Hollman, A., Pohl, K. & Stephenson, J. B. (1998). "Cataplexy" and muscle ultrasound abnormalities in Coffin–Lowry syndrome. *Journal of Medical Genetics* 35:94–8.

Crowe, A. V., Kearnes, D. B. & Mitchell, D. B. (1989). Tracheal stenosis in Larsen's syndrome. *Archives of Otolaryngology* 115:626.

Crowe, F. W., Schull, J. & Neel, J. V. (1956). *A Clinical, Pathological and Genetic Study of Multiple Neurofibromatosis.* Springfield IL: Charles C. Thomas.

Cruickshank, W. (1976). The problem and its scope (cerebral palsy). In *Cerebral Palsy: a Developmental Disability* 3rd edn, ed. W. Cruickshank, pp. 1–28. Syracuse: Syracuse University Press.

Cull, C. & Wyke, M. (1984). Memory function of children with spina bifida and shunted hydrocephalus. *Developmental Medicine and Child Neurology,* 26:177–83.

Cuneo, B. F., Driscoll, D. A., Gidding, S. S. & Langman, C. B. (1997). Evolution of latent hypoparathyroidism in familial 22q11 deletion syndrome. *American Journal of Medical Genetics* 69:50–5.

Cuneo, B. F., Langman, C. B., Ilbawi, M. N., Ramakrishnan, V., Cutilletta, A. & Driscoll, D. A. (1996). Latent hypoparathyroidism in children with conotruncal cardiac defects. *Circulation* 93:1702–8.

Cunningham, C. C., Morgan, P. A. & McGucken, R. B. (1984). Down syndrome: is dissatisfaction with disclosure of diagnosis inevitable? *Developmental Medicine and Child Neurology* 26:33–9.

Cunningham, M. L. & Jerome, J. T. (1997). Linear growth characteristics of children with cleft lip and palate. *Journal of Pediatrics* 131:707–11.

Curfs, L. M., Wiegers, G., Sommers, A. M., Borghgraef, J. R. M. & Fryns, J. P. (1991). Strengths and weaknesses in the cognitive profile of youngsters with Prader–Willi syndrome. *Clinical Genetics* 40:430–4.

Curry, C. J. R., Magenis, R. E., Brown, M., Lanman, J. T., Jr., Tsai, J., O'Lague, P., Goodfellow, P., Mohandas, T., Bergner, E. A. & Shapiro, L. J. (1984). Inherited chondrodysplasia punctata due to a deletion of the terminal short arm of an X chromosome. *New England Journal of Medicine* 311:1010–15.

D'Angelo, V. A., Ceddia, A. M., Zelante, L. & Florio, F. P. (1998). Multiple intracranial aneurysms in a patient with Seckel syndrome. *Childs Nervous System* 14:82–4.

Danks, D. M., Tippet, P., Adams, C. & Campbell, P. (1975). Cerebro-hepato-renal syndrome of Zellweger. A report of eight cases with comments on the incidence, the liver lesion, and a fault in pipecolic acid metabolism. *Journal of Pediatrics* 86:382–7.

David, A., Mercier, J. & Verloes, A. (1996). Child with manifestations of Nager acrofacial dysostosis, and the MURCS, VACTERL, and pulmonary agenesis associations: complex defect of blastogenesis? *American Journal of Medical Genetics* 62:1–5.

David, K. M., Copp, A. J., Stevens, J. M., Hayward, R. D. & Crockard, H. A. (1996). Split cervical spinal cord with Klippel–Feil syndrome: seven cases. *Brain* 119:1859–72.

Davies, D. R., Armstrong, J. G., Thakker, N., Horner, K., Guy, S. P., Clancy, T., Sloan, P., Blair, V., Dodd, C., Warnes, T. W., Harris, R. & Evans, D. G. R. (1995). Severe Gardner syndrome in familes with mutations restricted to a specific region of the APC gene. *American Journal of Human Genetics* 57:1151–8.

Davies, P. S., Evans, S., Broomhead, S., Clough, H., Day, J. M., Laidlaw, A. & Barnes, N. D. (1998). Effect of growth hormone on height, weight, and body composition in Prader–Willi syndrome. *Archives of Disease in Childhood* 78:474–6.

Davit-Spraul, A., Pourci, M. L., Atger, V., Cambillau, M., Hadchouel, M., Moatti, N. & Legrand, A. (1996). Abnormal lipoprotein pattern in patients with Alagille syndrome depends on icterus severity. *Gastroenterology* 111:1023–32.

De Grouchy, J. & Turleau, C. (1984). *Clinical Atlas of Human Chromosomes*. New York: John Wiley & Sons, Inc.

De Haan, M., van der Kamp, J. J., Briet, E. & Dubbeldam. J. (1988). Noonan syndrome: partial factor XI deficiency. *American Journal of Medical Genetics* 29:277–82.

De Moerlooze, L. & Dickson, C. (1997). Skeletal disorders associated with fibroblast growth factor receptor mutations. *Current Opinions in Genetics and Development* 7:378–85.

De Paepe, A., Devereux, R. B., Dietz, H. C., Hennekam, R. C. & Pyeritz, R. E. (1996). Revised diagnostic criteria for the Marfan syndrome. *American Journal of Medical Genetics* 62:417–26.

DeBaun, M. R., Siegel, M. J. & Choyke, P. L. (1998). Nephromegaly in infancy and early childhood: a risk factor for Wilms tumor in Beckwith–Wiedemann syndrome. *Journal of Pediatrics* 132:401–4.

DeBaun, M. R. & Tucker, M. A. (1998). Risk of cancer during the first four years of life in children from The Beckwith–Wiedemann Syndrome Registry. *Journal of Pediatrics* 132:398–400.

Delatycki, M. & Gardner, R. J. (1997). Three cases of trisomy 13 mosaicism and a review of the literature. *Clinical Genetics* 51:403–7.

DeLuca, P. A. (1996). The musculoskeletal management of children with cerebral palsy. *Pediatric Clinics of North America* 43:1135–50.

DeLuke, D. M., Marchand, A., Robles, E. C. & Fox, P. (1997). Facial growth and the need for orthognathic surgery after cleft palate repair: literature review and report of 28 cases. *Journal of Oral and Maxillofacial Surgery* 55:694–7.

Desnick, R. J., Ioannou, Y. A. & Eng, C. M. (1995). α-galactosidase A deficiency: Fabry disease. In *The Metabolic and Molecular Bases of Inherited Disease*, 7th edn, ed. C. R. Scriver, A. L. Beaudet, W. S. Sly & D. Valle, pp. 2741–84. New York: McGraw-Hill, Inc.

Devriendt, K., Swillen, A. & Fryns, J. P. (1998). Deletion in chromosome region 22q11 in a child with CHARGE association. *Clinical Genetics* 53:408–10.

Devriendt, K., Thienen, M. N., Swillen, A. & Fryns, J. P. (1996). Cerebellar hypoplasia in a patient with velo-cardio-facial syndrome. *Developmental Medicine and Child Neurology* 38:949–53.

Dhillon, R., Reddy, T. D. & Redington, A. (1998). Acquired coarctation of the aorta in William's syndrome. *Heart* 80:205–6.

Dhooge, I., Lemmerling, M., Lagache, M., Standaert, L., Govaert, P. & Mortier, G. (1998). Otological manifestations of CHARGE association. *Annals of Otology, Rhinology and Laryngology* 107:935–41.

DiGeorge, A. M. (1965). Discussions on a new concept of the cellular base of immunology. *Journal of Pediatrics* 67:907.

Digilio, M. C., Giannotti, A., Marino, B., Guadagni, A. M., Orzalesi, M. & Dallapiccola, B. (1997). Radial aplasia and chromosome 22q11 deletion. *Journal of Medical Genetics* 34:942–4.

Dise, J. E. & Lohr, M. E. (1998). Examination of deficits in conceptual reasoning abilities associated with spina bifida. *American Journal of Physical Medicine and Rehabilitation* 77:247–51.

Dixon, M. J. (1995). Treacher Collins syndrome. *Journal of Medical Genetics* 32:806–8.

Dixon, M. J. (1998). Treacher Collins syndrome: from linkage to prenatal testing. *Journal of Laryngology and Otology* 112:705–9.

Dobyns, W. (1987). Developmental aspects of lissencephaly and the lissencephaly syndromes. *Birth Defects: Original Article Series* 23:225–41.

Dobyns, W. B., Kirkpatrick, J. B., Hittner, H. M., Roberts, R. M. & Kretzer, F. C. (1985). Syndromes with lissencephaly II. Walker–Warburg and cerebro-oculo-muscular syndromes and a new syndrome with type II lissencephaly. *American Journal of Medical Genetics* 22:157–95.

Dobyns, W. B., Pagon, R. A., Armstrong, D., Curry, C. J. R., Greenberg, F., Grix, A., Holmes L. B., Laxova, R., Michels, V. V., Robinow, M. & Zimmerman, R. L (1989). Diagnostic criteria for Walker–Warburg syndrome. *American Journal of Medical Genetics* 32:195–210.

Dobyns, W. B., Reiner, O., Carrozzo, R. & Ledbetter, D. H. (1993). Lissencephaly. A human brain malformation associated with deletion of the LIS1 gene located at chromosome 17p13. *Journal of the American Medical Association* 270:2838–42.

Dodge, N. N. & Dobyns, W.B. (1995). Agenesis of the corpus callosum and Dandy–Walker malformation associated with hemimegalencephaly in the sebaceous nevus syndrome. *American Journal of Medical Genetics* 56:147–50.

Donnenfeld, A. E., Packer, R. J., Zackai, E. H., Chee, C. M., Sellinger, B. & Emanuel, B. S. (1989). Clinical, cytogenetic, and pedigree findings in 18 cases of Aicardi syndrome. *American Journal of Medical Genetics* 32:461–7.

Duerbeck, N. B. (1997). Fetal alcohol syndrome. *Comprehensive Therapy* 23:179–83.

Dunbar, J. D., Sussman, M. D. & Aiona, M. D. (1995). Hip pathology in the trichorhinophalangeal syndrome. *Journal of Pediatric Orthopedics* 15:381–5.

Duncan, P. A., Shapiro, L. R. & Klein, R. M. (1991). Sacrococcygeal dysgenesis association. *American Journal of Medical Genetics* 41:153–61.

Dunkley, C. J. & Dearlove, O. R. (1996). Delayed recovery from anaesthesia in Rubinstein–Taybi syndrome. *Paediatric Anaesthesia* 6:245–6.

Dunn, I. J. & Palmer, P. E. (1998). Toxoplasmosis. *Seminars in Roentgenology* 33:81–5.

Dutheil, P., Vabres, P. Cayla, M. C. & Enjolras, O. (1995). Incontinential pigmenti: late sequelae & genotypic diagnosis: a three-generation study of four patients. *Pediatric Dermatology* 12:107–11.

DuVall, G. A. & Walden, D. T. (1996). Adenocarcinoma of the esophagus complicating Cornelia de Lange syndrome. *Journal of Clinical Gastroenterology* 22:131–3.

Dworkin, P. H. (1989). British and American recommendations for developmental monitoring: the role of surveillance. *Pediatrics* 84:1000–10.

Ebara, S., Anwar, M. M., Okawa, A., Kajiura, I., Hiroshima, K. & Ono, K. (1996). The cervical spine in athetoid cerebral palsy. A radiological study of 180 patients. *Journal of Bone and Joint Surgery, Britain* 78:613–19.

Eberle, A. J. (1993). Congenital hypothyroidism presenting as apparent spondyloepiphyseal dysplasia. *American Journal of Medical Genetics* 47:464–7.

Edwards, J. H., Harnden, D. G. Cameron, A. H., Crosse, V. M. & Wolff. O. H. (1960). A new trisomic syndrome. *Lancet* 1:787–90.

Einhorn, T. A. & Kaplan, F. S. (1994). Traumatic fractures of heterotopic bone in patients who have fibrodysplasia ossificans progressiva. A report of 2 cases. *Clinical Orthopaedics and Related Research* 308:173–7.

Elder, D. E., Minutillo, C. & Pemberton, P. J. (1995). Neonatal herpes simplex infection: keys to early diagnosis. *Journal of Paediatric and Child Health* 31:307–11.

Elia, M., Di Lello, R., Romano, C. & Schepis, C. (1995). A case of FG syndrome with gingival hyperplasia and keloids. *Pediatric Dermatology* 12:387–9.

Elias, E. R. & Irons, M. (1995) Abnormal cholesterol metabolism in Smith–Lemli–Opitz syndrome. *Current Opinions in Pediatrics* 7:710–14.

Elkayam, U., Ostrzega, E., Shotan, A. & Mehra, A. (1995). Cardiovascular problems in pregnant women with the Marfan syndrome. *Annals of Internal Medicine* 123:117–22.

Elliott, A. M., Chen, M. F., Azouz, E. M. & Teebi, A. S. (1995). Developmental anomalies suggestive of the human homologue of the mouse mutant disorganization. *American Journal of Medical Genetics* 55:240–3.

Elliott, F., Bayly, M. R., Cole, T., Temple, I. K. & Maher, E. R. (1994). Clinical features and natural history of Beckwith–Wiedemann syndrome: presentation of 74 new cases. *Clinical Genetics* 46:168–74.

Elsawi, M. M., Pryor, J. P., Klufio, G., Barnes, C. & Patton. M. A. (1994). Genital tract function in men with Noonan syndrome. *Journal of Medical Genetics* 31:468–70.

Emery, A. E. H. & Rimoin, D. (1990). Nature and incidence of genetic disease. In *Principles and Practice of Medical Genetics,* 2nd edn, ed. A. E. H. Emery & D. L. Rimoin, pp. 3–6. Edinburgh: Churchill Livingstone.

Engin, C., Yavuz, S. S. & Sahin, F. I. (1997). Congenital muscular torticollis: is heredity a possible factor in a family with five torticollis patients in three generations? *Plastic and Reconstructive Surgery* 99:1147–50.

Ensink, R. J., Marres, H. A., Brunner, H. G. & Cremers, C. W. (1996). Hearing loss in the Saethre–Chotzen syndrome. *Journal of Laryngology and Otology* 110:952–7.

Epps, R. E., Pittelkow, M. R. & Su, W. P. (1995). TORCH syndrome. *Seminars in Dermatology* 14:179–86.

Epstein, C. J. (1995). Down syndrome (trisomy 21). In *The Metabolic and Molecular Bases of Inherited Disease,* 7th edn, ed. C. R. Scriver, A. L. Beaudet, W. S. Sly & D. Valle. pp. 749–94. New York: McGraw-Hill, Inc.

Escobar, V., Bixler, D., Gleiser, S., Weaver, D. D. & Gibbs, T. (1978). Multiple pterygium syndrome. *American Journal of Diseases of Children* 132:609–11.

Evans, J. A., Vitez, M. & Czeizel, A.(1993). On the biologic nature of associations: Evidence from a study of radial ray deficiencies and associated malformations. *Birth Defects:Original Article Series* 29:63–81.

Evans, M. (1995). Peutz–Jeghers syndrome. *Canadian Journal of Surgery* 38:209.

Ewart, A. K., Morris, C. A., Atkinson, D., Jin, W., Sternes, K., Spallone, P., Stock, A. D., Leppert,

M. & Keating, M. T. (1993a). Hemizygosity at the elastin locus in a developmental disorder, Williams syndrome. *Nature Genetics* 5:11–16.

Ewart, A. K., Morris, C. A., Ensing, G. J., Loker, J., Moore, C., Leppert, M. & Keating. M. (1993b). A human vascular disorder, supravalvular aortic stenosis, maps to chromosome 7. *Proceedings of the National Academy of Sciences, USA* 90:3226–30.

Fahmy, J., Kaminsky, C. K. & Parisi, M. T. (1998). Perlman syndrome: a case report emphasizing its similarity to and distinction from Beckwith–Wiedemann and prune-belly syndromes. *Pediatric Radiology* 28:179–82.

Famy, C., Streissguth, A. P. & Unis, A. S. (1998). Mental illness in adults with fetal alcohol syndrome or fetal alcohol effects. *American Journal of Psychiatry* 155:552–4.

Fariello, R. G., Chun, R. W. M., Doro, J. M., Buncic, M. R. & Prichard, J. S. (1977). EEG recognition of Aicardi's syndrome. *Archives of Neurology* 34:563–6.

Feremback, D. (1963). Frequency of spina bifida occulta in prehistoric human skeletons. *Nature* 199:100.

Fernandez-Palazzi, F., McLaren, A. T. & Slowie, D. F. (1992). Report on a case of Hutchinson–Gilford progeria, with special reference to orthopedic problems. *European Journal of Surgery* 2:378–82.

Field, M. J., ed. (1994). *Setting Priorities for Clinical Practice Guidelines*. Washington, DC: National Academy Press.

Figueroa, M. L., Rosenbloom, B. E., Kay, A. C., Garver, P., Thuerston, D. W, Koziol, J. A., Gelbart, T. & Beutler, E. (1992). A less costly regimen of alglucerase to treat Gaucher's disease. *New England Journal of Medicine* 327:1632–9.

Finegan, J. K., Cole, T. R., Kingwell, E., Smith, M. L., Smith, M. & Sitarenios, G. (1994). Language and behavior in children with Sotos syndrome. *Journal of the American Academy of Child and Adolescent Psychiatry* 33:1307–15.

Finelli, L., Crayne, E. M. & Spitalny, K. C. (1998). Treatment of infants with reactive syphilis serology, New Jersey: 1992 to 1996. *Pediatrics* 102:27.

Finkbohner, R., Johnston, D., Crawford, E. S., Coselli, J. & Milewicz, D. M. (1995). Marfan syndrome. Long-term survival and complications after aortic aneurysm repair. *Circulation* 91:728–33.

Finnell, R. H. & Chernoff, G. F. (1984). Variable patterns of malformations in the mouse fetal hydantoin syndrome. *American Journal of Medical Genetics* 19:463–71.

Fisch, G. S. (1993). What is associated with the fragile X syndrome. *American Journal of Medical Genetics* 48:112–21.

Fisher, E. & Scambler, P. (1994). Human haploinsufficiency – one for sorrow, two for joy. *Nature Genetics* 7:5–7.

Fletcher, J., Bohan, T., Brandt, M., Brookshire, B., Beaver, S., Francis, D., Davidson, K., Thompson, N. & Miner, M. (1992). Cerebral white matter and cognition in hydrocephalic children. *Archives of Neurology* 49:818–24.

Fletcher, J. M., McCauley, S. R., Brandt, M. E., Bohan, T. P., Kramer, L. A., Francis, D. J., Thorstad, K. & Brookshire, B. L. (1996). Regional brain tissue composition in children with hydrocephalus. Relationships with cognitive development. *Archives of Neurology* 53:549–57.

Fowler, K. B., Stagno, S., Pass, R. F., Britt, W. J., Boll, T. J. & Alford, C. A. (1992). The outcome of congenital cytomegalovirus infection in relation to maternal antibody status. *New England Journal of Medicine* 326:663–7.

Frame, P. S., Berg. A. O. & Woolf, S. (1997). U.S. Preventive Services Task Force: highlights of the 1996 report. *American Family Physician* 55:567–76, 581–2.

Franceschetti, A. & Klein, D. (1949). Mandibulofacial dysostosis: New hereditary syndrome. *Acta Ophthalmologica* 27:143–224.

Francke, U., Harper, J. F., Darras, B. T., Cowan, J. M., McCabe E. R. B., Kohlschütter, A. A. & Seltzer, W. K. (1987). Congenital adrenal hypoplasia, myopathy, and glycerol kinase deficiency: molecular genetic evidence for deletions. *American Journal of Human Genetics* 40:212–27.

Franco, B., Meroni, G., Parenti, G., Levilliers, J., Bernard, L., Gebbia, M., Cox, L., Maroteaux, P., Sheffield, L. & Rappold, G. A. (1995). A cluster of sulfatase genes, mutations in chondrodysplasia punctata, and insights into the mechanism of warfarin. *Cell* 81:15–25.

Fraser, C. R. (1962). Our genetic "load." A review of some aspects of genetical variation. *Annals of Human Genetics* 25:387–415.

Frawley, P. A., Broughton, N. S. & Menelaus, M. B. (1996). Anterior release for fixed flexion deformity of the hip in spina bifida. *Journal of Bone and Joint Surgery, Britain* 78:299–302.

Freed, G. L., Clark, S. J., Konrad, T. R. & Pathman, D. E. (1996). Variation in patient charges for vaccines and well-child care. *Archives of Pediatric and Adolescent Medicine* 150:421–6.

Freed, M. D., Moodie, D. S., Driscoll, D. J. & Bricker, J. T. (1997). Health supervision for children with Turner syndrome. *Pediatrics* 99:146.

Frerman, F. E. & Goodman, S.I. (1995). Nuclear-encoded defects of the mitochondrial respiratory chain, including glutaric acidemia type II. In *The Metabolic and Molecular Bases of Inherited Disease*, 7th edn, ed. C. R. Scriver, A. L. Beaudet, W. S. Sly & D. Valle, pp. 1611–29. New York: McGraw-Hill, Inc.

Freud, S. (1897). Attempts at classification of various types of infantile cerebral paralysis. In *Infantile Cerebral Paralysis*, pp. 230–60. Coral Gables, FL: University of Miami Press.

Freund, L. S., Reiss, A. L. & Abrams, M. T. (1993). Psychiatric disorders associated with fragile X in the young female. *Pediatrics* 91:321–9.

Frias, J. L., Feldman, A. H., Rosenbloom, A. L., Finkelstein, S. N., Hoyt, W. F. & Hall, B. D. (1978). Normal intelligence in two children with Carpenter syndrome. *American Journal of Medical Genetics* 2:191–9.

Friedman, J. M. (1990). A practical approach to dysmorphology. *Pediatric Annals* 19:95–101.

Fries, M. H., Kuller, J. A. & Norton, M. E. (1993). Facial features of infants exposed prenatally to cocaine. *Teratology* 48:413–20.

Froster, U. G. & Baird, P. A. (1993). Amniotic band sequence and limb defects: data from a population-based study. *American Journal of Medical Genetics* 46:497–500.

Fryburg, J. S., Pelegano, J. P., Bennett, M. J. & Bebin, E. M. (1994). Long-chain-3-hydroxy-coenzyme-A-dehydrogenase (L-CHAD) deficiency in a patient with Bannayan–Riley–Ruvalcaba syndrome. *American Journal of Medical Genetics* 52:97–102.

Fryer, A., Smith, C., Rosenbloom, L. & Cole, T. (1997). Autosomal dominant inheritance of Weaver syndrome. *Journal of Medical Genetics* 34:418–19.

Fryns, J. P. (1979). A new lethal syndrome with cloudy cornea, diaphragmatic defects, and distal limb deformities. *Human Genetics* 50:65–70.

Fryns, J. P. (1992). Aarskog syndrome: The changing phenotype with age. *American Journal of Medical Genetics* 43:420–7.

Fryns, J. P. (1997). Progressive hydrocephalus in Noonan syndrome *Clinical Dysmorphology* 6:379.

Fryns, J. P. & Descheemaeker, M. J. (1995). Aarskog syndrome: severe neurological deficit with spastic hemiplegia resulting from perinatal cerebrovascular accidents in two non-related males. *Clinical Genetics* 48:54–5.

Fryns, J. P. & Smeets, E. (1998). "Cataplexy" in Coffin–Lowry syndrome. *Journal of Medical Genetics* 35:702.

Gabbe, S. G. (1977). Congenital malformations in infants of diabetic mothers. *Obstetrical and Gynecological Survey* 32:125–30.

Gabriel, R. & McComb, J. (1985). Malformations of the central nervous system. In *Textbook of Child Neurology*, 3rd edn, ed. J. Menkes, pp. 189–270. Philadelphia: Lea and Febiger.

Galan, E. & Kousseff, B. G. (1995). Peripheral neuropathy in Ehlers–Danlos syndrome. *Pediatric Neurology* 12:242–5.

Ganel, A. & Horoszowski, H. (1996). Limb lengthening in children with achondroplasia. Differences based on gender. *Clinical Orthopedics* 332:179–83.

Ganesan, V. & Kirkham, F. J. (1997). Noonan syndrome and moyamoya. *Pediatric Neurology* 16:256–8.

Garcia, C. R., Torriani, F. J. & Freeman, W. R. (1998). Cidofovir in the treatment of cytomegalo-virus (CMV) retinitis. *Ocular Immunology and Inflammation* 6:195–203.

Garro, A.J., Gordon, B. H. J. & Lieber, C. S. (1992). Alcohol abuse: Carcinogenic effects and fetal alcohol syndrome. In *Medical and Nutritional Complications of Alcoholism*, ed. C. S. Lieber, pp. 459–93. New York: Plenum Publishing Corporation.

Garty, B. Z., Daliot, D., Kauli, R., Arie, R., Grosman, J., Nitzan, M. & Danon, Y. L. (1994). Hearing impairment in idiopathic hypoparathyroidism and pseudohypoparathyroidism. *Israel Journal of Medical Sciences* 30:587–91.

Garvey, P., Elovitz, M. & Landsberger, E. J. (1998). Aortic dissection and myocardial infarction in a pregnant patient with Turner syndrome. *Obstetrics and Gynecology* 91:864.

Gaston, H. (1996). Patients with hydrocephalus should have regular eye checks. *British Medical Journal* 312:57.

Gath, A. & Gumley, D. (1984). Down syndrome and the family: follow-up of children first seen in infancy. *Developmental Medicine and Child Neurology* 26:500–8.

Gellis, S. & Feingold, M. (1973). Schwartz–Jampel syndrome. *American Journal of Diseases of Children* 126:339–40.

George, C. D., Patton, M. A., El Sawi, M., Sharland, M. & Adam, E. J. (1993). Abdominal ultra-sound in Noonan syndrome: a study of 44 patients. *Pediatric Radiology* 23:316–18.

Geralis, E. (ed.) (1991). *Children With Cerebral Palsy – a Parents' Guide*. Baltimore: Woodbine Press.

German, J. (1993). Bloom syndrome: a mendelian prototype of somatic mutational disease. *Medicine* 72:393–406.

German, J. & Passarge, E. (1989). Bloom's syndrome. XII. Report from the registry for 1987. *Clinical Genetics* 35:57–69.

German, J., Roe, A. M., Leppert, M. F. & Ellis, N. A. (1994). Bloom syndrome: an analysis of consanguinous families assigns the locus mutated to chromosome band 15q26.1. *Proceedings of the National Academy of Sciences, USA* 91:6669–73.

Gerritsen, E. J., Vossen, J. M., Fasth, A., Friedrich, W., Morgan, G., Padmos, A., Vellodi, A., Porras, O., O'Meara, A. & Porta, F. (1994). Bone marrow transplantation for autosomal recessive osteopetrosis. A report from the Working Party on Inborn Errors of the European Bone Marrow Transplantation Group. *Journal of Pediatrics* 125:896–902.

Gerszten, P. C., Albright, A. L. & Johnstone, G. F. (1998). Intrathecal baclofen infusion and subsequent orthopedic surgery inpatients with spastic cerebral palsy. *Journal of Neurosurgery* 88:1009–13.

Ghosh, A. K. & O'Bryan, T. (1995). Ehlers–Danlos syndrome with reflux nephropathy. *Nephron* 70:266.

Giangreco, C. A., Steele, M. W., Aston, C. E., Cummins, J. H. & Wenger, S. L. (1996). A simplified six-item checklist for screening for fragile X syndrome in the pediatric population. *Journal of Pediatrics* 129:611–14.

Gill, T. M. & Feinstein, A. R. (1994). A critical appraisal of the quality of quality of life measurements. *Journal of the American Medical Association* 272:619–26.

Gitzelmann, R., Steinmann, B. & Van der Berghe, G. (1995). Disorders of fructose metabolism. In *The Metabolic and Molecular Bases of Inherited Disease*, 7th edn, ed. C. R. Scriver, A. L. Beaudet, W. S. Sly & D. Valle, pp. 905–34. New York: McGraw-Hill, Inc.

Glascoe, F. P. & Dworkin, P. H. (1995). The role of parents in the detection of developmental and behavioral problems. *Pediatrics* 95:829–36.

Glascoe, F. P., Martin, E. D. & Humphrey, S. (1990). A comparative review of developmental screening tests. *Pediatrics* 86:547–54.

Glass, L., Shapiro, I., Hodge, S. E., Bergstrom, L. & Rimoin, D. L. (1981). Audiologic findings of patients with achondroplasia. *International Journal of Pediatric Otorhinolaryngology* 3:129–35.

Glover, T. W., Verga, V., Rafael, J., Barcroft, C. & Gorski, J. L. (1993). Translocation breakpoint in Aarskog syndrome maps to Xp11.21 between ALAS2 and DXS323. *Human Molecular Genetics* 2:1717–18.

Gluck, G. S. & Mawn, S. V. (1992). The Klippel–Feil syndrome: Implications for naval service. *Military Medicine* 157:318–22.

Goens, M. B., Campbell, D. & Wiggins, J. W. (1992). Spontaneous chylothorax in Noonan syndrome. Treatment with prednisone. *American Journal of Diseases of Children* 146:1453–6.

Goldberg, R., Motzkin, B., Marion, R., Scambler, P. J & Shprintzen, R. J. (1993). Velo–Cardio–Facial Syndrome: A review of 120 patients. *American Journal of Medical Genetics* 45:313–19.

Golden, G. (1979). Neural tube defects. *Pediatrics in Review* 1:187–9.

Golden, J. A., Nielsen, G. P., Pober, B. R. & Hyman, B. T. (1995). The neuropathology of Williams syndrome. *Archives of Neurology* 52:209–12.

Goldenhar, M. (1952). Associations malformatives de l'oeil et de l'oreille, en particulier le syndrome dermöide epibulbaire-appendices auriculaires-fistula auris congenita et ses relations avec la dysostose mandibulo-faciale. *Journale de Génétique Humaine* 1:243–82.

Goldfischer, S., Moore, C. L., Johnson, A. B., Spiro, A. J., Valsamis, M. P., Wisniewski, H. K., Ritch, R. H., Norton, W. T., Rapin, I. & Gartner L. M. (1973). Peroxisomal and mitochondrial defects in the cerebro-hepato-renal syndrome of Zellweger. *Science* 182:62–4.

Goldson, E. & Hagerman, R. J. (1993). Fragile X syndrome and failure to thrive. *American Journal of Diseases of Children* 147:605–7.

Goldstein, N. A., Armfield, D. R., Kingsley, L. A., Borland, L. M., Allen, G. C. & Post, J. C. (1998). Postoperative complications after tonsillectomy and adenoidectomy in children with Down syndrome. *Archives of Otolaryngology – Head and Neck Surgery* 124:171–6.

Gooch, J. L. & Sandell, T. V. (1996). Botulinum toxin for spasticity and athetosis in children with cerebral palsy. *Archives of Physical Medicine and Rehabilitation* 77:508–11.

Goodban, M. T. (1993). Survey of speech and language skills with prognostic indicators in 116 patients with Cornelia de Lange syndrome. *American Journal of Medical Genetics* 47:1059–63.

Goodman, S. I. & Frerman, F. E. (1995). Organic acidemias due to defects in lysine oxidation: 2-ketoadipic acidemia and glutaric acidemia. In *The Metabolic and Molecular Bases of Inherited Disease*, 7th edn, ed. C. R. Scriver, A. L. Beaudet, W. S. Sly & D. Valle, pp. 1451–60. New York: McGraw-Hill, Inc.

Goodman, S. I., Pollak, S., Miles, B. & O'Brien, D. (1969). The treatment of maple syrup urine disease. *Journal of Pediatrics* 75:485–8.

Gorlin, R. J. (1987). Nevoid basal cell carcinoma syndrome. *Medicine* 66:96–113.

Gorlin, R. J., Anderson, R. C. & Moller, J. H. (1971). Multiple lentigines syndrome revisited. *Birth Defects* 7:110–15.

Gorlin, R. J., Cohen, M. M., Jr., Condon, L. M. & Burke, B. A. (1992). Bannayan–Riley–Ruvalcaba syndrome. *American Journal of Medical Genetics* 44:307–14.

Gorlin, R. J., Cohen, M. M., Jr. & Levin L. S. (1990). *Syndromes of the Head and Neck.* New York: Oxford University Press.

Gorlin, R. J., Sedano, H. O. & Cervenka, J. (1968). Popliteal pterygium syndrome: a syndrome comprising cleft lip-palate, popliteal, and intercrural pterygia, digital, and genital anomalies. *Pediatrics* 41:503–9.

Gorry, M. C., Preston, R. A.. White, G. J., Zhang, Y., Singhal, V. K., Losken, H. W., Parker, M. G., Nwokoro, N. A., Post, J. C. & Ehrlich, G. D. (1995). Crouzon syndrome. Mutations in two spliceoforms of FGFR2 and a common point mutation shared with Jackson–Weiss syndrome. *Human Molecular Genetics* 4:1387–90.

Gorski, J. L. & Burright, E. N. (1993). The molecular genetics of incontinentia pigmenti. *Seminars in Dermatology* 12:255–65.

Gosain, A. K., Conley, S. F., Marks, S. & Larson, D. L. (1996a). Submucous cleft palate: diagnostic methods and outcomes of surgical treatment. *Plastic and Reconstructive Surgery* 97:1497–509.

Gosain, A. K., McCarthy, J. G. & Pinto, R. S. (1994). Cervicovertebral anomalies and basilar impression in Goldenhar syndrome. *Plastic and Reconstructive Surgery* 93:498–506.

Gosain, A. K., McCarthy, J. G. & Wisoff, J. H. (1996b). Morbidity associated with increased intracranial pressure in Apert and Pfeiffer syndromes: the need for long-term evaluation. *Plastic and Reconstructive Surgery* 97:292–301.

Gould, S. J. (1981). *The Mismeasure of Man.* New York: W.W. Norton & Company, Inc.

Grabb, W. C. (1965). The first and second branchial arch syndrome. *Plastic and Reconstructive Surgery* 36:485–508.

Graham, J. M., Jr., Hanson, J. W., Darby, B. L., Barr, H. M. & Streissguth, A. P. (1988). Independent dysmorphology evaluations at birth and 4 years of age for children exposed to various amounts of alcohol *in utero*. *Pediatrics* 81:772–8.

Graham, J. M., Jr., Morse, R. P., Rachenmacher, S., Lin, A., Hall, B. D., MacLeod, P. J. & Pyeritz, R. E. (1989). Infantile Marfan syndrome. *Proceedings of the Greenwood Genetics Center* 8:213–14.

Grahame, R. & Pyeritz, R. E. (1995). The Marfan syndrome: joint and skin manifestations are prevalent and correlated. *British Journal of Rheumatology* 34:126–31.

Grebe, T.A., Rimsza, M. E., Richter, S. F., Hansen, R. C. & Hoyme, H. E. (1993). Further delineation of the epidermal nevus syndrome: two cases with new findings and literature review. *American Journal of Medical Genetics* 47:24–30.

Green, A. J., Johnson, P. H. & Yates, J. R. (1994). The tuberous sclerosis gene on chromosome 9q34 acts as a growth suppressor. *Human Molecular Genetics* 10:1833–4.

Green, M., ed. (1994). *Bright Futures. Guidelines for Health Supervision of Infants, Children, and Adolescents*. Arlington VA: National Center for Education in Maternal and Child Health.

Greenberg, F. (1990). Williams syndrome professional symposium. *American Journal of Medical Genetics* supplement 6:85–8.

Greenberg, F. (1993). DiGeorge syndrome: an historical review of clinical and cytogenetics features. *Journal of Medical Genetics* 30:803–6.

Greenberg, F., Guzzetta, V., Montes de Oca-Luna, R., Magenis, R. E., Smith, A. C. M., Richter, S. F., Kondo, I., Dobyns, W. B., Patel, P. I. & Lupski, J. R. (1991). Molecular analysis of Smith–Magenis syndrome: a possible contiguous-gene syndrome associated with del(17)(p11.2). *American Journal of Human Genetics* 49:1207–18.

Greenberg, F., Lewis, R. A., Potocki, L., Glaze, D., Parke, J., Killian, J., Murphy, M. A., Williamson, D., Brown, F., Dutton, R., McCluggage, C., Friedman, E., Sulek, M. & Lupski, J. R. (1996). Multi-disciplinary clinical study of Smith–Magenis syndrome (deletion 17p11.2). *American Journal of Medical Genetics* 62:247–54.

Greenberg, F., Stein, F., Gresik, M. V., Finegold, M. J., Carpenter, R. J., Riccardi, V. M. & Beaudet, A. L. (1986). The Perlman familial nephroblastomatosis syndrome. *American Journal of Medical Genetics* 24:101–10.

Greenhaw, G. A., Hebert, A., Duke-Woodside, M. E., Butler, I. J., Hecht, J. T., Cleaver, J. E., Thomas, G. H. & Horton, W. A. (1992). Xeroderma pigmentosum and Cockayne syndrome: overlapping clinical and biochemical phenotypes. *American Journal of Human Genetics* 50:677–9.

Greenswag, L. R. (1987). Adults with Prader–Willi syndrome. *Developmental Medicine and Child Neurology* 29:145–52.

Griebel, M., Oakes, W. & Worley, G. (1991). The Chiari malformation associated with myelomeningocele. In *Comprehensive Management of Spina Bifida*, ed. H. Rekate, pp. 67–92. Boca Raton, FL: CRC Press.

Gross, A. J. (1996). Response to growth hormone in children with chondrodysplasia. *Journal of Pediatrics* 128:S14–S17.

Grundy, R. G., Pritchard, J., Baraitser, M., Risdon, A. & Robards, M. (1992). Perlman and Wiedemann–Beckwith syndromes: two distinct conditions associated with Wilms tumor. *European Journal of Pediatrics* 151:895–8.

Grunebaum, M., Kornreich, L., Horev, G. & Ziv, N. (1996). Tracheomegaly in Brachmann–de Lange syndrome. *Pediatric Radiology* 26:184–7.

Guerina, N. G. (1994): Congenital infection with *Toxoplasma gondii*. *Pediatric Annals* 23:138–51.

Guille, J. T., Miller, A., Bowen, J. R., Forlin, E. & Caro, P. A. (1995). The natural history of Klippel–Feil syndrome: clinical, roentgenographic, and magnetic resonance imaging findings at adulthood. *Journal of Pediatric Orthopedics* 15:617–26.

Guion-Almeida, M. L., Richieri-Costa, A., Saavedra, D. & Cohen, M. M., Jr. (1996). Frontonasal dysplasia: analysis of 21 cases and literature review. *International Journal of Oral and Maxillofacial Surgery* 25:91–7.

Gunay-Aygun, M., Cassidy, S. B. & Nicholls, R. D. (1997). Prader–Willi and other syndromes associated with obesity and mental retardation. *Behavioral Genetics* 27:307–24.

Gupte, G., Mahajan, P. Shreenivas, V. K., Kher, A. & Bharucha, B. A. (1992). Wildervanck syndrome (cervico-oculo-acoustic syndrome). *Journal of Postgraduate Medicine* 38:180–2.

Hacker, S. M., Ramos-Caro, F. A., Beers, B. B. & Flowers, F. P. (1993). Juvenile pseudoxanthoma elasticum: recognition and management. *Pediatric Dermatology* 10:19–25.

Haeusler, G., Frisch, H., Schmitt, K., Blumel, P., Plochl, E., Zachman, M. & Waldhor, T. (1995). Treatment of patients with Ullrich–Turner syndrome with conventional doses of growth hormone and the combination with testosterone or oxandrolone: effect on growth, IGF-1, and IGFBP-3 concentrations. *European Journal of Pediatrics* 154:437–44.

Hagerman, R. J. (1997). Fragile X syndrome. Molecular and clinical insights and treatment issues. *Western Journal of Medicine* 166:129–37.

Hagerman, R. J., Jackson, C., Amiri, K., Silverman, A. C., O'Connor, R. & Sobesky, W. (1992). Girls with fragile X syndrome: physical and neurocognitive status and outcome. *Pediatrics* 89:395–400.

Hakonarson, H., Moskovitz, J., Daigle, K. L., Cassidy, S. B. & Cloutier, M. M. (1995). Pulmonary function abnormalities in Prader–Willi syndrome. *Journal of Pediatrics* 126:565–70.

Hall, B. D. (1971). Aglossia-adactylia. *Birth Defects* 7:233–6.

Hall, B. D. (1979). Choanal atresia and associated multiple anomalies. *Journal of Pediatrics* 95:395–8.

Hall, B. D., de Lorimier, A. & Foster, L. H. (1983). A new syndrome of hemangiomatous branchial clefts, lip pseudoclefts, and abnormal facial appearance. *American Journal of Medical Genetics* 14:135–8.

Hall, J. G. (1976). Embryopathy associated with oral anticoagulant therapy. *Birth Defects* 12:33–7.

Hall, J. (1981). An approach to congenital contractures (arthrogryposis). *Pediatric Annals* 10:15–26.

Hall, J. (1986). Analysis of Pena–Shokeir phenotype. *American Journal of Medical Genetics* 25:99–117.

Hall, J. G. (1988). Somatic mosaicism: Observations related to clinical genetics. *American Journal of Human Genetics* 43:355–63.

Hall, J. G. (1990). Genomic imprinting: Review and relevance to human diseases. *American Journal of Human Genetics* 46:857–53.

Hall, J. G. (1993). CATCH 22. *Journal of Medical Genetics* 30:801–2.

Hall, J. (1997). Arthrogryposis multiplex congenita: etiology, genetics, classification, diagnostic approach, and general aspects *Journal of Pediatric Orthopedics* 6:159–66.

Hall, J. G. & Gilchrist, D. M. (1990). Turner syndrome and its variants. *Pediatric Clinics of North America* 37:1421–40.

Hall, J. G., Reed, S. D. & Driscoll E. P. (1983a). Part I. Amyoplasia: A common sporadic condition with congenital contractures. *American Journal of Medical Genetics* 15:571–90.

Hall, J. G., Reed, S. D., McGillivray, B. C., Herrmann, J., Partington, M. W., Schinzel, A., Shapiro, J. & Weaver, D. D. (1983b). Part II. Amyoplasia: twinning in amyoplasia – A specific type of arthrogryposis with an apparent excess of discordantly affected identical twins. *American Journal of Medical Genetics* 15:591–8.

Hall, J. G., Reed, S. D. & Greene, G. (1982a). The distal arthrogryposes: Delineation of new entities, review, and nosologic discussion. *American Journal of Medical Genetics* 11:185–239.

Hall, J. G., Sybert, V. P., Williamson, R. A., Fisher, N. L. & Reed, S. D. (1982b). Turner's syndrome. *Western Journal of Medicine* 137:32–44.

Hall, J. W. III & Denneny, J. C. (1993). Audiologic and otolaryngologic findings in progeria: case report. *Journal of the Academy of Audiology* 4:116–21.

Hall, J. W. III, Prentice, C. H., Smiley, G. & Werkhaven, J. (1995). Auditory dysfunction in selected syndromes and patterns of malformations: review and case findings. *Journal of the American Academy of Audiology* 6:80–92.

Hammadeh, M. Y., Dutta, S. N., Cornaby, A. J. & Morgan, R. J. (1995). Congenital urological anomalies in Sotos syndrome. *British Journal of Urology* 76:133–5.

Hanshaw, J. B. (1994). Congenital cytomegalovirus infection. *Pediatric Annals* 23:124–8.

Hanson, J. W. (1986). Teratogen update: Fetal hydantoin effects. *Teratology* 33:349–53.

Hanson, J. W. & Smith, D. W. (1975a). The fetal hydantoin syndrome. *Journal of Pediatrics* 87:285–90.

Hanson, J. W. & Smith. D. W. (1975b). Teratogenicity of anticoagulants. *Journal of Pediatrics* 87:838–45.

Hanson, J. W., Jones, K. L. & Smith, D. W. (1976). Fetal alcohol syndrome. Experience with 41 patients. *Journal of the American Medical Association* 235:1458–60.

Happle, R. (1979). X-linked dominant chondrodysplasia punctata. *Human Genetics* 53:65–73.

Happle, R. (1995). Epidermal nevus syndromes. *Seminars in Dermatology* 14:111–21.

Harris, J., Robert, E. & Kallen, B. (1997). Epidemiology of choanal atresia with special reference to the CHARGE association. *Pediatrics* 99:363–7.

Harris, S. (1984). Predictive value of the movement assessment of infants. *Journal of Developmental and Behavioral Pediatrics* 5:336.

Hartsfield, J. K., Jr., Hall, B. D., Grix, A. W., Kousseff, B. G., Salazar, J. F. & Haufe, S. M. (1993). Pleiotropy in Coffin–Lowry syndrome: sensorineural hearing deficit and premature tooth loss as early manifestations. *American Journal of Medical Genetics* 45:552–7.

Harvey, A. S., Leaper, P. M. & Bankier, A. (1991). CHARGE association: Clinical manifestations and developmental outcome. *American Journal of Medical Genetics* 39:48–55.

Hayashi, M., Sakamoto, K., Kurata, K., Nagata, J., Satoh, J. & Morimatsu, Y. (1996). Septo-optic dysplasia with cerebellar hypoplasia in Cornelia de Lange syndrome. *Acta Neuropathologica (Berlin)* 92:625–30.

Hayashi, N., Valdes-Dapena, M. & Green, W. R. (1998). CHARGE association: histopathological report of two cases and a review. *Journal of Pediatric Ophthalmology & Strabismus* 35:100–6.

Hecht, F. & Beals, R. K. (1972). "New" syndrome of congenital contractural arachnodactyly originally described by Marfan in 1896. *Pediatrics* 49:574.

Hellstrom, A., Jansson, C., Boguszewski, M., Olegard, R., Lagreid, L. & Albertsson-Wikland, K. (1996). Growth hormone status in six children with fetal alcohol syndrome. *Acta Paediatrica* 85:1456–62.

Hendrix, J. D., Jr. & Greer, K. E. (1996). Rubinstein–Taybi syndrome with multiple flamboyant keloids. *Cutis* 57:346–8.

Hennekam, R. C. M., Tilanus, M., Hamel, B. C. J., Voshart-van Heeren, H. Mariman, E. C. M., van Beersum, S. E. C., van den Boogaard, M. J. & Breuning, M. H. (1993). Deletion at chromosome 16p13.3 as a cause of Rubinstein–Taybi syndrome: Clinical aspects. *American Journal of Human Genetics* 52:255–62.

Hennessy, C. H., Moriarty, D. G., Zack, M. M., Scherr, P. A. & Brackbill, R. (1994). Measuring health-related quality of life for public health surveillance. *Public Health Reports* 109:665–72.

Henning, K. A., Li, L., Iyer, N., McDaniel, L. D., Reagan, M. S., Legerski R., Schultz, R. A., Stefanini, M., Lehmann, A. R., Mayne, L.V. & Friedberg, E. C. (1995). The Cockayne syndrome group A gene encodes a WD repeat protein that interacts with CSB protein and a subunit of RNA polymerase II, TFIIH. *Cell* 82:1–20.

Henry, I., Puesch, A., Riesewijk, A., Ahnie, L., Mannens, M., Beldjord, C., Bitoun, P., Tournade, M., Landrieu, P. & Junien, C. (1993). Somatic mosaicism for partial paternal isodisomy in Wiedemann–Beckwith syndrome: a post-fertilization event. *European Journal of Human Genetics* 1:19–29.

Henthorn, P. S. & Whyte, M. P. (1992). Missense mutations of the tissue-nonspecific alkaline phosphatase gene in hypophosphatasia. *Clinical Chemistry* 38:2501–5.

Herman, G. E., Greenberg, F. & Ledbetter D. H. (1988). Multiple congenital anomaly/mental retardation (MCA/MR) syndrome with Goldenhar complex due to a terminal del(22q). *American Journal of Medical Genetics* 29:909–15.

Herman, T. E. & Siegel, M. J. (1997). Special imaging casebook. Trisomy 13 and occult dysraphism with tethered cord. *Journal of Perinatology* 17:172–4.

Hermann, J. & Opitz, J. M. (1977). The SC phocomelia and the Roberts syndrome: Nosologic aspects. *European Journal of Pediatrics* 125:117–34.

Herman-Staab, B. (1994). Screening, management, and appropriate referral for pediatric behavior problems. *Nurse Practitioner* 19:40–49.

Hersh, J. H. (1989). Toluene embryopathy: Two new cases. *Journal of Medical Genetics* 26:333–7.

Hersh, J. H., Cole, T. R., Bloom, A. S., Bertolone, S. J. & Hughes, H. E. (1992). Risk of malignancy in Sotos syndrome. *Journal of Pediatrics* 120:572–4.

Hertle, R. W., Ziylan, S. & Katowitz, J. A. (1993). Ophthalmic features and visual prognosis in the Treacher Collins syndrome. *British Journal of Ophthalmology* 77:642–5.

Higashi, K. & Matsuki, C. (1994). Coffin–Lowry syndrome with sensorineural deafness and labyrinthine anomaly. *Journal of Laryngology and Otology.* 108:147–8.

Hill, R. M., Hegemier, S. & Tennyson, L. M. (1989). The fetal alcohol syndrome: A multihandicapped child. *Neurotoxicology* 10:585–96.

Hirata, K., Triposkiadis, F., Sparks, E., Bowen, J., Boudoulas, H. & Wooley. C. F. (1992). The Marfan syndrome: cardiovascular physical findings and diagnostic correlates. *American Heart Journal* 123:743–52.

Hoar, D. I., Field, L. L., Beards, F., Hoganson, G., Rollnick, B. & Hoo, J. J. (1992). Tentative assignment of gene for oto-palato-digital syndrome to distal Xq (Xq26–q28). *American Journal of Medical Genetics* 42:170–2.

Hockey, A., Bower, C., Goldblatt, J. & Knowles, S. (1996). Fetal valproate embryopathy in twins: genetic modification of the response to a teratogen. *Birth Defects Original Article Series* 30:401–5.

Hodgkins, P., Lees, M., Lawson, J., Reardon, W., Leitch, J., Thorogood, P., Winter, R. M. & Taylor, D. S. (1998). Optic disc anomalies and frontonasal dysplasia. *British Journal of Ophthalmology* 82:290–3.

Hoffenberg, E. J., Narkewicz, M. R., Sondheimer, J. M., Smith, D. J., Silverman, A. & Sokol, R. J. (1995). Outcome of syndromic paucity of interlobular bile ducts (Alagille syndrome) with onset of cholestasis in infancy. *Journal of Pediatrics* 127:220–4.

Hofman, K. J., Harris, E. L., Bryan R. N. & Denckla, M. B. (1994). Neurofibromatosis type 1: the cognitive phenotype. *Journal of Pediatrics* 124:A1–S8.

Holden, K. R., Jabs, E. W. & Sponseller, P. D. (1992). Roberts/pseudothalidomide syndrome and normal intelligence: approaches to diagnosis and management. *Developmental Medicine and Child Neurology* 34:534–9.

Holder, S. E., Winter, R. M., Kamath, S. & Scambler, P. J. (1993). Velocardiofacial syndrome in a mother and daughter: variability of the clinical phenotype. *Journal of Medical Genetics* 30:825–7.

Holl, R. W., Kunze, D., Etzrodt, H., Teller, W. & Heinze, E. (1994). Turner syndrome: final height, glucose tolerance, bone density and psychosocial status in 25 adult patients. *European Journal of Pediatrics* 153:11–16.

Hollier, L. M. & Cox, S. M. (1998). Syphilis. *Seminars in Perinatology* 22:323–31.

Holm, V. A., Cassidy, S. B., Butler, M. G., Hanchett, J. M., Greenswag L. R., Whitman, B. Y. & Greenberg, F. (1993). Prader–Willi syndrome: Consensus diagnostic criteria. *Pediatrics* 91:398–402.

Holmes, J. M. & Coates, C. M. (1994). Assessment of visual acuity in children with trisomy 18. *Ophthalmic Genetics* 15:115–20.

Holtzman, N. A. (1988). Recombinant DNA technology, genetic tests, and public policy. *American Journal of Human Genetics* 42:623–45.

Holtzman, N. A. (1989). *Proceed with Caution: The Use of Recombinant DNA Testing For Genetic Testing*. Baltimore: Johns Hopkins University Press.

Hook, E. B. & Lindsjö, A. (1978). Down syndrome in live births by single year maternal age interval in a Swedish study: Comparison with results from a New York State study. *American Journal of Human Genetics* 30:19–27.

Hordnes, K. (1994). Ehlers–Danlos syndrome and delivery. *Acta Obstetrica et Gynecologica Scandinavica* 73:671–3.

Horton, W. A. (1996). One gene, three chondrodysplasias: Déja vu. *Genes, Growth and Hormones* 12:14.

Horton, W. A., Rotter, J. I., Rimoin, D. L., Scott, C. I. & Hall, J.G. (1978) Standard growth curves for achondroplasia. *Journal of Pediatrics* 93:435–8.

Horwitz, S. M., Leaf, P. J., Leventhal, J. M., Forsyth, B. & Speechley, K. N. (1992). Identification and management of psychosocial and developmental problems in community-based, primary care pediatric practices. *Pediatrics* 89:480–5.

Hoyme, H. E., Procopio, F., Crooks, W., Feingold, M. & Jones, K. L. (1987). The incidence of neoplasia in children with isolated congenital hemihypertrophy. *Proceedings of the Greenwood Genetics Center* 6:126.

Hsueh, W. A., Hsu, T. H. & Federman, D. D. (1978). Endocrine features of Klinefelter's syndrome. *Medicine* 57:447–61.

Hu, P. Y., Ernst, A. R., Sly, W. S., Venta, P. J., Skaggs, L. A. & Tashian. R. E. (1994). Carbonic anhydrase II deficiency: single base pair deletion in exon 7 is the predominant mutation in Caribbean Hispanic patients. *American Journal of Human Genetics* 54:602–8.

Huang, M. H., Gruss, J. S., Clarren, S. K., Mouradian, W. E., Cunningham, M. L., Roberts, T. S., Loeser, J. D. & Cornell, C. J. (1996). The differential diagnosis of posterior plagiocephaly: true lambdoid synostosis versus positional molding. *Plastic and Reconstructive Surgery* 98:765–74.

Huang, M. H., Mouradian, W. E., Cohen, S. R. & Gruss, J. S. (1998). The differential diagnosis of abnormal head shapes: separating craniosynostosis from positional deformities and normal variants. *Cleft Palate and Craniofacial Journal* 35:204–11.

Humphreys, R. (1986). Tethering: theories of development and pathophysiology. In *Spina Bifida: A Multidisciplinary Approach,* ed. R. McLaurin, pp. 215–20. New York: Praeger.

Hunt, A. (1993). Development, behaviour and seizures in 300 cases of tuberous sclerosis. *Journal of Intellectual Disability Research* 37:41–51.

Hyman, S. L. (1996). A transdisciplinary approach to self-injurious behavior. In *Developmental Disabilities in Infancy and Childhood*, ed. A. J Capute & P. J. Accardo, pp. 317–36. Baltimore: Paul H. Brookes.

Ichinose, M., Tojo, K., Nakamura, K., Matsuda, H., Tokudome, G., Ohta, M., Sakai, S. & Sakai, O. (1996). Williams syndrome associated with chronic renal failure and various endocrinological abnormalities. *Internal Medicine* 35:482–8.

Ilan, Y., Eid, A., Rivkind, A. I., Weiss, D., Dubin, Z. & Yatsiv, S. (1993). Gastrointestinal involvement in homocystinuria. *Journal of Gastroenterology and Hepatology* 8:60–2.

Ingram, T. (1984). A historical review of the definition and classification of the cerebral palsies. In *The Epidemiology of the Cerebral Palsies*, ed. F. Stanley & E. Alberman, pp. 1–11, Philadelphia: J. B. Lippincott.

Ioan, D. M., Popa, M. & Fryns, J. P. (1993). An unclassifiable type of spondylo-peripheral epiphyseal dysplasia associated with 21 trisomy. *Genetic Counseling* 4:59–62.

Iosub, S., Fuchs, M., Bingol, N. & Gromisch, D. S. (1981). Fetal alcohol syndrome revisited. *Pediatrics* 68:475–9.

Iskandar, B. J., McLaughlin, C., Mapstone, T. B., Grabb, P. A. & Oakes, W. J. (1998). Pitfalls in the diagnosis of ventricular shunt dysfunction: radiology reports and ventricular size. *Pediatrics* 101:1031–6.

Izquierdo, N. J., Traboulsi, E. I., Enger, C. & Maumenee, I. H. (1994). Strabismus in the Marfan syndrome. *American Journal of Ophthalmology* 117:632–5.

Jackson, C. E., Weiss, L. Reynolds, W. A., Forman, T. F. & Peterson, J. A. (1976). Craniosynostosis, mid-facial hypoplasia, and foot abnormalities: An autosomal dominant phenotype in a large Amish kindred. *Journal of Pediatrics* 88:963–8.

Jackson, G. (1996). Checklists will help us stay SHARP [editorial]. *British Journal of Clinical Practice* 50:235–6.

Jackson, I. T., Bauer, B., Saleh, J., Sullivan, C. & Argenta, L. C. (1989). A significant feature of Nager's syndrome: Palatal agenesis. *Plastic and Reconstructive Surgery* 84:219–26.

Jackson, L., Kline, A. D., Barr, M. A. & Koch, S. (1993). De Lange syndrome. A clinical review of 310 individuals. *American Journal of Medical Genetics* 47:940–6.

Jackson, P. (1990). Primary care needs of children with hydrocephalus. *Journal of Pediatric Health Care* 4: 59–71.

Jacobs, I. N., Gray, R. F. & Todd, N. W. (1996). Upper airway obstruction in children with Down syndrome. *Archives of Otolaryngology – Head and Neck Surgery* 122:945–50.

Jacobs, R. F. (1998). Neonatal herpes simplex virus infections. *Seminars in Perinatology* 22:64–71.

Jaeken, J. & Carchon, H. (1993.) The carbohydrate-deficient glycoprotein syndromes: Recent developments. *International Journal of Pediatrics* 88:60–5.

Jahrsdoerfer, R. A. & Jacobson, J. T. (1995). Treacher Collins syndrome: otologic and auditory managment. *Journal of the American Academy of Audiology* 6:93–102.

James, H. (1992). Hydrocephalus in infancy and childhood. *American Family Physician* 45:733–42.

Janniger, C. K. & Schwartz, R. A. (1993). Tuberous sclerosis: recent advances for the clinician. *Cutis* 51:167–74.

Jarrold, C., Baddeley, A. D. & Hewes, A. K. (1998). Verbal and nonverbal abilities in the Williams syndrome phenotype: evidence for diverging developmental trajectories. *Journal of Child Psychology and Psychiatry* 39:511–23.

Jenkins, R. R. & Saxena, S. B. (1995). Keeping adolescents healthy. *Contemporary Pediatrics* 12:76–89.

Jeret, J., Serur, D., Wisniewski, K. & Lubin, R. (1987). Clinicopathological findings associated with agenesis of the corpus callosum. *Brain and Development* 9:255–64.

Jessop, D. J. & Stein, R. E. K. (1995). Consistent but not the same. Effect of method on chronic condition rates. *Archives of Pediatric and Adolescent Medicine* 149:1105–10.

Johns, M. B., Hovell, M. F., Drastal, C. A., Lamke, C. & Patrick, K. (1992). Promoting prevention services in primary care: a controlled trial. *American Journal of Preventive Medicine* 8:135–45.

Johnson, A., Palomaki, G. & Haddow, J. (1990). Maternal serum alpha-fetoprotein levels in pregnancies among black and white women with fetal open spina bifida: a United States collaborative study. *American Journal of Obstetrics and Gynecology* 67:1–16.

Johnson, J. P., Golabi, M., Norton, M. E., Rosenblatt, R. M., Feldman, G. M., Yang, S. P., Hall, B. D., Fries, M. H. & Carey, J. C. (1998). Costello syndrome: phenotype, natural history, differential diagnosis, and possible cause. *Journal of Pediatrics* 133:441–8.

Johnson, M. C., Strauss, A. W., Dowton, S. B., Spray, T. L., Huddleston, C. B., Wood, M. K., Slaugh, R. A. & Watson, M. S. (1995). Deletion within chromosome 22 is common in patients with absent pulmonary valve syndrome. *American Journal of Cardiology* 76:66–9.

Johnston, L. B. & Borzyskowski, M. (1998). Bladder dysfunction and neurological disability at presentation inclosed spina bifida. *Archives of Disease in Childhood* 79:33–8.

Jones, B. M., Hayward, R., Evans, R. & Britto, J. (1997). Occipital plagiocephaly: an epidemic of craniosynostosis? *British Medical Journal* 315:693–4.

Jones, K. L. (1990). Williams syndrome: An historical perspective of its evolution, natural history, and etiology. *American Journal of Medical Genetics* supplement 6:89–96.

Jones, K. L. (1997). *Smith's Recognizable Patterns of Human Malformation,* 5th edn. Philadelphia: W.B. Saunders.

Jones, K. L. & Smith. D. W. (1975a). The fetal alcohol syndrome. *Teratology* 12:1–10.

Jones, K. L. & Smith, D. W. (1975b). The Williams elfin facies syndrome. A new perspective. *Journal of Pediatrics* 86:718–23.

Jones, K. L., Smith, D. W., Ulleland, C. N. & Streissguth, A. P. (1973). Pattern of malformation in offspring of chronic alcoholic mothers. *Lancet* 1:1267–71.

Jones, M. R., de Sa, L. C. & Good, W. V. (1993). Atypical iris colobomata and Pfeiffer syndrome. *Journal of Pediatric Ophthalmology and Strabismus* 30:266–7.

Jones, R. & Dolcourt, J. L. (1992). Muscle rigidity following halothane anesthesia in two patients with Freeman–Sheldon syndrome. *Anesthesiology* 77:599–600.

Jorde, L. B., Carey, J. C. & White, R. L. (1994). *Medical Genetics.* St. Louis: Mosby.

Kalter, H. & Warkany, J. (1983). Congenital malformations. Etiologic factors and their role in prevention. *New England Journal of Medicine* 308:424–31.

Kane, A. A., Mitchell, L. E., Craven, K. P. & Marsh, J. L. (1996). Observations on a recent increase in plagiocephaly without synostosis. *Pediatrics* 97:877–85.

Kaplan, L. C. (1989). The CHARGE association: Choanal atresia and multiple congenital anomalies. *Otolaryngology Clinics* 22:661–72.

Kaplan, P., Levison, M. & Kaplan, B. S. (1995). Cerebral artery stenoses in Williams syndrome cause strokes in childhood. *Journal of Pediatrics* 126:943–5.

Kaplan, P., Mazur, A., Field, M., Berlin, J. A., Berry, G. T., Heidenreich, R., Yudkoff, M. & Segal, S. (1991). Intellectual outcome in children with maple syrup urine disease. *Journal of Pediatrics* 119:46–50.

Karasick, D., Schweitzer, M. E. & Vaccaro, A. R. (1998). The traumatized cervical spine in Klippel–Feil syndrome: imaging features. *American Journal of Roentgenology* 170:85–8.

Kaufman, F. R., Donnell, G. N. & Lobo, R. A. (1987). Ovarian androgen secretion in patients with galactosemia and premature ovarian failure. *Fertility and Sterility* 47:1033–4.

Kaufman, F. R., Donnell, G. N., Roe, T. F. & Kogut, M. D. (1986). Hypergonadotropic hypogonadism in female patients with galactosemia. *New England Journal of Medicine* 305:464–7.

Kawai, M., Yorifuji, T., Yamanaka, C., Sasaki, H., Momoi, T. & Furusho, K. (1997). A case of Robinow syndrome accompanied by partial growth hormone insufficiency treated with growth hormone. *Hormone Research* 48:41–3.

Kaye, L. D., Rothner, A. D., Beauchamp, G. R., Meyers, S. M. & Estes, M. L. (1992). Ocular findings associated with neurofibromatosis-2. *Ophthalmology* 99:1424–9.

Keeney, G., Gebarski, S. S. & Brunberg, J. A. (1992). CT of severe inner ear anomalies, including aplasia, in a case of Wildervanck syndrome. *American Journal of Neuroradiology* 13:201–2.

Kemp, B., Hauptmann, S., Schroder, W., Amo-Takyi, B., Leeners, B. & Rath, W. (1995).

Dysgerminoma of the ovary in a patient with triple-X syndrome. *International Journal of Gynaecology and Obstetrics* 50:51–3.

Kennedy, P. T. & McAuley, D. J. (1998). Association of posterior fossa dermoid cyst and Klippel–Feil syndrome. *American Journal of Neuroradiology* 19:195.

Khakoo, A., Thomas, R., Trompeter, R., Duffy, P., Price, R. & Pope, F. M. (1997). Congenital cutis laxa and lysyl oxidase deficiency. *Clinical Genetics* 51:109–14.

Khoury, M. J., Cordero, J. F., Greenberg, F., James, L. M. & Erickson, J. D. (1983). A population study of the VACTERL association: evidence for its etiologic heterogeneity. *Pediatrics* 71:815–20.

Kiel, E. A., Frias, J. L. & Victorica, B. E. (1983). Cardiovascular malformations in the Larsen syndrome. *Pediatrics* 71:942–6.

King, R. A., Hearing, V. J., Creel, D. J. & Oetting, W. S. (1995). Albinism. In *The Metabolic and Molecular Bases of Inherited Disease*, 7th edn, ed. C. R. Scriver, A. L. Beaudet, W. S. Sly & D. Valle, pp. 4353–92. New York: McGraw-Hill, Inc.

Kinsman, S. (1996). Childhood-acquired hydrocephalus. In *Developmental Disabilities in Infancy and Childhood*, 2nd edn, ed. A. Capute & P. Accardo, Vol. 2, pp. 189–97. Baltimore: Paul Brookes.

Kinzler, K. W. & Vogelstein, B. (1992). The colorectal cancer gene hunt: Current findings. *Hospital Practice* November:51–58.

Kirkpatrick, J.A., Wagner, M.L. & Pilling, G.P. (1983). A complex of anomalies associated with tracheoesophageal fistula and esophageal atresia. *American Journal of Roentgenology* 95:208–13.

Kirschner, B. S. & Pachman, L. M. (1976). IgA deficiency and recurrent pneumonia in the Schwartz–Jampel syndrome. *Journal of Pediatrics* 88:1060–1.

Kline, A. D., Barr, M. & Jackson L. G. (1993a). Growth manifestations in the Brachmann–de Lange syndrome. *American Journal of Medical Genetics* 47:1042–9.

Kline, A. D., Stanley, C., Belevich, J., Brodsky, K., Barr, M. & Jackson, L. (1993b). Developmental data on individuals with the Brachmann–de Lange syndrome. *American Journal of Medical Genetics* 48:1053–8.

Knoll, J. H. M., Nicholls, R. D., Magenis, R. E., Graham, J. M., Jr., Lalande, M. & Latt, S. A. (1989). Angelman and Prader–Willi syndromes share a common chromosome 15 deletion but differ in parental origin of the deletion. *American Journal of Medical Genetics* 32:285–90.

Koch, H., Grzonka, M. & Koch, J. (1992). Popliteal pterygium syndrome with special consideration of the cleft malformation: case report. *Cleft Palate-Craniofacial Journal* 29:80–4.

Koch, R., Azen, C. G., Friedman, E. G. & Williamson, M. L. (1982). Preliminary report on the effects of diet discontinuation in PKU. *Journal of Pediatrics* 100:870–5.

Koenekoop, R. K., Rosenbaum, K. N. & Traboulsi, E. I. (1995). Ocular findings in a family with Sotos syndrome (cerebral gigantism). *American Journal of Ophthalmology* 119:657–8.

Kohl, S. (1997). Neonatal herpes simplex virus infection. *Clinical Perinatology* 24:129–50.

Kohlmeier, L., Gasner, C. & Marcus, R. (1993). Bone mineral status of women with Marfan syndrome. *American Journal of Medicine* 95:568–72.

Kolodny, E. H. & Fluharty, A. L. (1995). Metachromatic leukodystrophy and multiple sulfatase deficiency: Sulfatide lipidosis. In *The Metabolic and Molecular Bases of Inherited Disease*, 7th edn, ed. C. R. Scriver, A. L. Beaudet, W. S. Sly & D. Valle, pp. 2693–2739. New York: McGraw-Hill, Inc.

Konkol, R. J. (1994). Is there a cocaine baby syndrome? *Journal of Child Neurology* 9:225–6.

Kosztolanyi, G. (1997). Leprechaunism/Donohue syndrome/insulin receptor gene mutations: a syndrome delineation story from clinicopathological description to molecular understanding. *European Journal of Pediatrics* 156:253–7.

Kottke, T. E., Brekke, M. L. & Solberg, L. I. (1993). Making 'time' for preventive services. *Mayo Clinic Proceedings* 68:785–91.

Kousseff, B. G., Newkirk, P. & Root, A. W. (1994). Brachmann–de Lange syndrome. 1994 update. *Archives of Pediatrics and Adolescent Medicine* 148:749–55.

Kozma, C. (1996). Autosomal dominant inheritance of Brachmann–de Lange syndrome. *American Journal of Medical Genetics* 66:445–8.

Kraemer, K. H., Levy, D. D., Parris, C. N., Gozukara, E. M., Moriwaki, S., Adelberg, S. & Seidman, M. M. (1994). Xeroderma pigmentosum and related disorders: examining the linkage between defective DNA repair and cancer. *Journal of Investigative Dermatology* 103 (suppl 5):96S–101S.

Kreiborg, S., Barr, M., Jr. & Cohen, M. M., Jr. (1992). Cervical spine in the Apert syndrome. *American Journal of Medical Genetics* 43:704–8.

Kuban, K. C. K. & Leviton, A. (1994). Cerebral palsy. *New England Journal of Medicine* 330:188–195.

Kumar, P. (1996). Cleft lip and amniotic bands. *British Journal of Plastic Surgery* 49:74–5.

Kumar, S., Kimberling, W. J., Connolly, C. J., Tinley, S., Marres, H. A. & Cremers, C.W. (1994). Refining the region of branchio-oto-renal syndrome and defining the flanking markers on chromosome 8q by genetic mapping. *American Journal of Human Genetics* 55:1188–94.

Kurnit, D. M., Steele, M. W., Pinsky, L. & Dibbins, A. (1978). Autosomal dominant transmission of a syndrome of anal, ear, renal, and radial congenital malformations. *Journal of Pediatrics* 93:270–3.

Kuroki, Y., Suzuki, Y., Chyo, H., Hata, A. & Matsui, I. (1981). A new malformation syndrome of long palpebral fissures, large ears, depressed nasal tip, and skeletal anomalies associated with postnatal dwarfism and mental retardation. *Journal of Pediatrics* 99:570–3.

Kwittken, P. L., Sweinberg, S. K., Campbell, D. E. & Pawlowski, N. A. (1995). Latex hypersensitivity in children: clinical presentation and detection of latex-specific immunoglobulin E. *Pediatrics* 95:693–9.

Lammer, E. J. (1985). Retinoic acid embryopathy. *New England Journal of Medicine* 313:837–41.

Larsen, J. H., Schottstaedt, E. R. & Bost, F. C. (1950). Multiple congenital dislocations associated with characteristic facial abnormality. *Journal of Pediatrics* 37:574–81.

Lazarow, P. B. & Moser, H. W. (1995.) Disorders of peroxisome biogenesis. In *The Metabolic and Molecular Bases of Inherited Disease*, 7th edn, ed. C. R. Scriver, A. L. Beaudet, W. S. Sly & D. Valle, pp. 2287–2324. New York: McGraw-Hill, Inc.

Lee, B., Thirunavukkarasu, K., Zhou, L., Pastore, L., Baldini, A., Hecht, J., Geoffroy, V., Ducy, P. & Karsenty, G. (1997). Missense mutations abolishing DNA binding of the osteoblast-specific transcription factor OSF2/CBFA1 in cleidocranial dysplasia. *Nature Genetics* 16:307–10.

Lee, D., Lanza, J. & Har-El, G. (1996). Waardenburg syndrome. *Otolaryngology – Head and Neck Surgery* 114:166–7.

Lee, J. H., Gamble, J. G., Moore, R. E. & Rinsky, L. A. (1995). Gastrointestinal problems in patients who have type III osteogenesis imperfecta. *Journal of Bone and Joint Surgery* 77:1352–6.

Lee, J. J., Imrie, M. & Taylor, V. (1994). Anaesthesia and tuberous sclerosis. *British Journal of Anaesthesia* 73:421–5.

Lee, J., Nunn, J. & Wright, C. (1996). Height and weight achievement in cleft lip and palate. *Archives of Disease in Childhood* 76:70–2.

Lee, N. B., Kelly, L. & Sharland, M. (1992). Ocular manifestations of Noonan syndrome. *Eye* 6:328–34.

Leger, R. & Meeropol, E. (1992). Children at risk: latex allergy and spina bifida. *Journal of Pediatric Nursing* 7:373–6.

LeHeup, B. P., Masutti, J. P., Droulle, P. & Tisserand, J. (1995). The Antley–Bixler syndrome: report of two familial cases with severe renal and anal anomalies. *European Journal of Pediatrics* 154:130–3.

Leicher-Düber, A., Schumacher, R. & Spranger, J. (1990). Stippled epiphyses in fetal alcohol syndrome. *Pediatric Radiology* 20:369–70.

Leitch, R. J. & Winter, R. M. (1996). Midline craniofacial defects and morning glory disc anomaly. A distinct clinical entity. *Acta Ophthalmologica Scandinavica* (Suppl. 219):16–19.

Lemoine, P., Haurrousseau, M., Borteyru, J. P. & Menuet, J. C. (1968). Les enfants de parents alkooliques. Anomalies observées: À propos de 127 cases. *Ouest Medicine* 21:476–82.

Leonetti, J. P. (1995). The diagnosis and management of acoustic neuromas: Contemporary practice guidelines. *Comprehensive Therapy* 21:68–73.

Lepage, C., Noreau, L. & Bernard, P. M. (1998). Association between characteristics of locomotion and accomplishment of life habits in children with cerebral palsy. *Physical Therapy* 78:458–69.

Leppig, K. A., Viskochil, D., Neil, S., Rubenstein, A., Johnson, V. P., Zhu, X. L., Brothman, A. R. & Stephens, K. (1996). The detection of contiguous gene deletions at the neurofibromatosis 1 locus with fluorescence *in situ* hybridization. *Cytogenetics and Cell Genetics* 72:95–8.

Lesch, M. & Nyhan, W. L. (1964). A familial disorder of uric acid metabolism and central nervous system dysfunction. *American Journal of Medicine* 36:561–70.

Leung, A. K. C. (1985). Wiedemann–Beckwith syndrome and hypothyroidism. *European Journal of Pediatrics* 144:295.

Leung, A. K. & Robson, W. L. (1992). Association of preauricular sinuses and renal anomalies. *Urology* 40:259–61.

Levin, A. V., Seidman, D. J., Nelson, L. B. & Jackson, L. G. (1990). Ophthalmologic findings in the Cornelia de Lange syndrome. *Journal of Pediatric Ophthalmology and Strabismus* 27:94–102.

Levine, B., Skope, L. & Parker, R. (1991). Cherubism in a patient with Noonan syndrome. *Journal of Oral and Maxillofacial Surgery* 49:1014–18.

Levine, E. A., Ronan, S. G., Shirali, S. S. & Gupta, T. K. (1992). Malignant melanoma in a child with oculocutaneous albinism. *Journal of Surgical Oncology* 51:138–142.

Levy, H. L., Sepe, S. J., Shih, V. E, Vawter, F. G. & Klein, J. O. (1977). Sepsis due to *Escherichia coli* in neonates with galactosemia. *New England Journal of Medicine* 297:823–5.

Levy, P. A. (1998). Amniotic bands. *Pediatric Reviews* 19:249–55.

Lewis, C. E. (1988). Disease prevention and health promotion practices of primary care physicians in the United States. *American Journal of Preventive Medicine* 4 (suppl.):9–16.

Lewis, D. P., Van Dyke, D. C., Stumbo, P. J. & Berg, M. J. (1998). Drug and environmental factors associated with adverse pregnancy outcomes. Part I: Antiepileptic drugs, contraceptives, smoking, and folate. *Annals of Pharmacotherapy* 32:802–17.

Lichtig, C., Ludatscher, R. M., Mandel, H. & Gershoni-Baruch, R. (1993). Muscle involvement in the Walker–Warburg syndrome. Clinicopathologic features of four cases. *American Journal of Clinical Pathology* 100:493–6.

Lidang Jensen, M., Rix, M., Schroder, H. D., Teglbjaerg, P. S. & Ebbesen, F. (1995). Fetal akinesia-hypokinesia deformation sequence (FADS) in 2 siblings with myotonic dystrophy. *Clinical Neuropathology* 14:105–8.

Limbird, T. J. (1989). Slipped capital femoral epiphysis associated with Russell–Silver syndrome. *Southern Medical Journal* 82:902–4.

Lin, A. E., Ardinger, H. H., Ardinger, R. H., Jr., Cunniff, C. & Kelley, R. I. (1997). Cardiovascular malformations in Smith–Lemli–Opitz syndrome. *American Journal of Medical Genetics* 68:270–8.

Linden, M. G., Bender, B. G. & Robinson, A. (1995). Sex chromosome tetrasomy and pentasomy. *Pediatrics* 96:672–82.

Lindsay, E. A., Goldberg, R., Jurecic, V., Morrow, B., Carlson, C., Kucherlapati, R. S., Shprintzen, R. J. & Baldini, A. (1995). Velo-cardio-facial syndrome: frequency and extent of 22q11 deletions. *American Journal of Medical Genetics* 57:514–22.

Lipkin, P. H. (1991). Epidemiology of the developmental disabilities. In *Developmental Disabilities in Infancy and Childhood,* ed. A. J. Capute & P. J. Accardo, pp. 43–67. Baltimore: Paul H. Brookes.

Lipson, A. H., Yuille, D., Angel, M., Thompson, P. G., Vandervoord, J. G. & Beckenham, E. J. (1991). Velocardiofacial (Shprintzen) syndrome: an important syndrome for the dysmorphologist to recognize. *Journal of Medical Genetics* 28:596–604.

Liptak, G., Bloss, J., Briskin, H., Campbell, J., Hebert, E. & Revell, G. (1988). The management of children with spinal dysraphism. *Journal of Child Neurology* 3:3–20.

Liptak, G. S. & Revell, G. M. (1989). Community physician's role in the case management of children with chronic illness. *Pediatrics* 84:465–71.

Little, B. B., Snell, L.M., Rosenfeld, C. R., Gilstrap, L.C. III & Gant, N. F. (1990). Failure to recognize fetal alcohol syndrome in newborn infants. *American Journal of Diseases of Children* 144:1142–6.

Little, B. B., Wilson, G. N. & Jackson, G. (1996). Is there a cocaine syndrome? Dysmorphic and anthropometric assessment of infants exposed to cocaine. *Teratology* 54:145–9.

Little, W. (1862). On the influence of abnormal parturition, difficult labour, premature birth, and asphyxia neonatorum on the mental and physical condition of the child, especially in relation to deformities. *Transactions of the Obstetrical Society of London* 3:293–344.

Liu, X., Newton, V. & Read, A. (1995). Hearing loss and pigmentary disturbances in Waardenburg syndrome with reference to WS type II. *Journal of Laryngology and Otology* 109:96–100.

Lockman, L. A., Hunninghake, D. B., Krivit, W. & Desnick, R. J. (1973.) Relief of pain of Fabry's disease by diphenylhydantoin. *Neurology* 23:871–5.

Lomas, F. E., Dahlstrom, J. E. & Ford, J. H. (1998). VACTERL with hydrocephalus: family with X-linked VACTERL-H. *American Journal of Medical Genetics* 76:74–8.

Lonnqvist, L., Child, A., Kainulainen, K., Davidson, R., Puhakka, L. & Peltonen, L. (1994). A novel mutation of the fibrillin gene causing ectopia lentis. *Genomics* 19:573–6.

Lopez-Rangel, E., Maurice, M., McGillivaray, B. & Friedman. J. M. (1992). Williams syndrome in adults. *American Journal of Medical Genetics* 44:720–9.

Lopponen, T., Saukkonen, A. L., Serlo, W., Lanning, P. & Knip, M. (1995). Slow prepubertal linear growth but early pubertal growth spurt in patients with shunted hydrocephalus. *Pediatrics* 95:917–23.

Lopponen, T., Saukkonen, A. L., Serlo, W., Tapanainen, P., Ruokonen, A. & Knip, M. (1996). Accelerated pubertal development in patients with shunted hydrocephalus. *Archives of Disease in Childhood* 74:490–6.

Lowry, R. B. & Yong, S. L. (1980). Borderline normal intelligence in the Smith-Lemli-Opitz (RSH) syndrome. *American Journal of Medical Genetics* 5:137–143.

Lu, C. & Ridker, P. M. (1994). Echocardiographic diagnosis of congenital absence of the pericardium in a patient with VATER association defects. *Clinical Cardiology* 17:503–4.

Lubinsky, M. (1986). Current concepts: VATER and other associations: Historical perspectives and modern interpretations. *American Journal of Medical Genetics* (suppl. 2):9–16.

Lubinsky, M. & Moeschler, J. (1986). Different clusters within the VATER association distinguished through cardiac defects. *Dysmorphology and Clinical Genetics* 1:80–2.

Lubs, H. A., Chiurazzi, P., Arena, J. F., Schwartz, C., Tanebjaerg, L. & Neri, G. (1996). XLMR genes: Update 1996. *American Journal of Medical Genetics* 64:147–57.

Lumley, M. A., Jordan, M., Rubenstein, R., Tsipouras, P. & Evans, M. I. (1994). Psychosocial functioning in the Ehlers–Danlos syndrome. *American Journal of Medical Genetics* 53:149–52.

Lurie, I. W. & Ferencz, C. (1997). VACTERL-hydrocephaly, DK-phocomelia, and cerebro-cardioradio-reno-rectal community. *American Journal of Medical Genetics* 70:144–9.

Luzuriaga, K. & Sullivan, J. L. (1994). Pathogenesis of vertical HIV infection: implications for intervention and management. *Pediatric Annals* 23:159–66.

Lynch, H. T., Lynch, J., Conway, T., Watson, P., Feunteun, J., Lenoir, G., Narod, S. & Fitzgibbons, R., Jr. (1994). Hereditary breast cancer and family cancer syndromes. *World Journal of Surgery* 18:21–31.

Lyon, A. J., Preece, M. A. & Grant, D. B. (1985). Growth curve for girls with Turner syndrome. *Archives of Disease in Childhood* 60:932–6.

MacCollin, M., Mohney, T., Trofatter, J., Wertelecki, W., Ramesh, V. & Gusella, J. (1993). DNA diagnosis of neurofibromatosis 2. Altered coding sequence of the *merlin* tumor suppressor in an extended pedigree. *Journal of the American Medical Association* 270:2316–20.

MacDonald, I. & Dearlove, O. R. (1995). Anaesthesia and Robinow syndrome. *Anaesthesia* 50:1097.

MacDonald, M. R., Kolodziej, P., Schaefer, G. B. & Olney, A. H. (1997). Stickler syndrome. *Ear Nose and Throat Journal* 76:706–9.

Macias, V. R., Day, D. W., King, T. E. & Wilson, G. N. (1992). Clasped-thumb mental retardation (MASA) syndrome: Confirmation of linkage to Xq28. *American Journal of Medical Genetics* 43:408–14.

Madigan, W. P., Wertz, D., Cockerham, G. C. & Thach, A. B. (1994). Retinal detachment in osteogenesis imperfecta. *Journal of Pediatric Ophthalmology and Strabismus* 31:268–9.

Maiman, L. A., Becker, M. H., Liptak, G. S., Nazarian, L. F. & Rounds, K. A. (1988). Improving pediatricians' compliance-enhancing practices: a randomized trial. *American Journal of Diseases of Children* 142:773–9.

Maino, D. M., Kofman, J., Flynn, M. F. & Lai, L. (1994). Ocular manifestations of Sotos syndrome. *Journal of the American Optometry Association* 65:339–46.

Majnemer, A. (1998). Benefits of early intervention for children with developmental disabilities. *Seminars in Pediatric Neurology* 5:62–9.

Makitie, O. & Kaitila, I. (1997) Growth in diastrophic dysplasia. *Journal of Pediatrics* 130:641–6.

Makitie, O., Sulisalo, T., de la Chapelle, A. & Kaitila, I. (1995). Cartilage-hair hypoplasia. *Journal of Medical Genetics* 32:39–43.

Mandoki, M. W. & Sumner, G. S. (1991). Klinefelter syndrome: The need for early identification and treatment. *Clinical Pediatrics* 30:161–4.

Manfredi, R., Zucchini, A., Azzaroli, L. & Manfredi, G. (1993). Pseudohypoparathyroidism associated with idiopathic growth hormone deficiency. Role of treatment with biosynthetic growth hormone. *Journal of Endocrinologic Investigation* 16:709–13.

Mapstone, C. L., Weaver, D. D. & Yu, P.-L. (1986). Analysis of growth in the VATER association. *American Journal of Diseases of Children* 140:386–90.

Marcus, C. L. (1996). Images in clinical medicine. Periodic breathing in an infant with hydrocephalus. *New England Journal of Medicine* 334:1577.

Marcus, J. C. (1987). Neurologic findings in the fetal alcohol syndrome. *Neuropediatrics* 18:158–60.

Marden, P. M. & Walker, W. A. (1966). A new generalized connective tissue dysplasia: Association with multiple congenital anomalies. *American Journal of Diseases of Children* 112:225–8.

Marge, M. (1984). The prevention of communication disorders. *American Speech–Language–Hearing Association* 26:29–33.

Marini, J. C. & Gerber, N. R. (1997). Osteogenesis imperfecta. Rehabilitation and prospects for gene therapy. *Journal of the American Medical Association* 277:746–50.

Marini, J.C., Bordenick, S., Heavner, G., Rose, S. & Chrousos, G. P. (1993). Evaluation of growth hormone axis and responsiveness to growth stimulation of short children with osteogenesis imperfecta. *American Journal of Medical Genetics* 45:261–4.

Markert, M. L., Majure, M., Harville, T. O., Hulka, G. & Oldham, K. (1997). Severe laryngomalacia and bronchomalacia in DiGeorge syndrome and CHARGE association. *Pediatric Pulmonology* 24:364–9.

Maródi, L., Rigó, G. & Káposzta, R. (1994). Picture of the month (Alagille syndrome). *Archives of Pediatrics and Adolescent Medicine* 148:287–8.

Maron, B. J., Moller, J. H., Seidman, C. E., Vincent, G. M., Dietz, H. C., Moss, A. J., Sondheimer, H. M., Pyeritz, R. E., McGee, G. & Epstein, A. E. (1998). Impact of laboratory molecular diagnosis on contemporary diagnostic criteria for genetically transmitted cardiovascular diseases: hypertrophic cardiomyopathy, long-QT syndrome, and Marfan syndrome. A statement for healthcare professionals from the Councils on Clinical Cardiology, Cardiovascular Disease in the Young, and Basic Science, American Heart Association. *Circulation* 98:1460–71.

Marres, H. A., Cremers, C. W., Marres, E. H. & Huygen, P. L. (1995). Ear surgery in Treacher Collins syndrome. *Annals of Otology, Rhinology, and Laryngology* 104:31–41.

Martin, A., State, M., Koenig, K., Schultz, R., Dykens, E. M., Cassidy, S. B. & Leckman, J. F. (1998). Prader–Willi syndrome. *American Journal of Psychiatry* 155:1265–73.

Martin, J. P. & Bell, J. (1943). A pedigree of mental defect showing sex-linkage. *Journal of Neurology and Psychiatry* 6:154–7.

Martínez-Frías, M. L. (1994). Epidemiologic analysis of outcomes of pregnancy in diabetic mothers: Identification of the most characteristic and most frequent congenital anomalies. *American Journal of Medical Genetics* 51:108–113.

Martinez-Lage, J. F., Garcia Santos, J. M., Poza, M., Puche, A., Casas, C. & Costa, T. R. (1995). Neurosurgical management of Walker–Warburg syndrome. *Childs Nervous System* 11:145–53.

Martinez-Perez, D., Vander Woude, D. L., Barnes, P. D., Scott, R. M. & Mulliken, J. B. (1996). Jugular foraminal stenosis in Crouzon syndrome. *Pediatric Neurosurgery* 25:252–5.

Massey, J. Y. & Roy, F. H. (1973). Ocular manifestations of the happy puppet syndrome. *Journal of Pediatric Ophthalmology* 10:282–4.

Matsubara, S., Yoshino, M. & Takamori, T. (1994). Benign neurogenic amyotrophy in Klinefelter's syndrome. *Journal of Neurology, Neurosurgery and Psychiatry* 57:640–2.

Mattson, S. N., Riley, E. P., Gramling, L., Delis, D. C. & Jones, K. L. (1997). Heavy prenatal alcohol exposure with or without features of fetal alcohol syndrome leads to IQ deficits. *Journal of Pediatrics* 131:718–21.

Mayfield, J. (1991). Comprehensive orthopedic management in myelomeningocele. In *Comprehensive Management of Spina Bifida*, ed. H. Rekate, pp.113–63. Boca Raton, FL: CRC Press.

Mayhew, J. F. (1993). Anesthesia for children with Freeman–Sheldon syndrome. *Anesthesiology* 78:408.

Mazzanti, L., Cacciari, E., Bergamaschi, R., Tassinari, D., Magnani, C., Perri, A., Scarano, E. & Pluchinotta, V. (1997). Pelvic ultrasonography in patients with Turner syndrome: age-related findings in different karyotypes. *Journal of Pediatrics* 131:135–40.

Mazzocco, M. M. (1998). A process approach to describing mathematics difficulties in girls with Turner syndrome. *Pediatrics* 102:492–6.

McAlister, W. H. (1998). Invited commentary: posterior deformational plagiocephaly. *Pediatric Radiology* 28:727–8.

McAllion, S. J. & Paterson, C. R. (1996). Causes of death in osteogenesis imperfecta. *Journal of Clinical Pathology* 49:627–30.

McCall, R. E. & Budden, J. (1992). Treatment of multiple pterygium syndrome. *Orthopedics* 15:1417–22.

McCauley, E., Ross, J. L., Kushner, H. & Cutler, G., Jr. (1995). Self-esteem and behavior in girls with Turner syndrome. *Journal of Developmental and Behavioral Pediatrics* 16:82–8.

McClone, D., Czyzewski, D., Raimondi, A. & Sommers, R. (1982). Central nervous system infections as a limiting factor in the intelligence of children with myelomeningocele. *Pediatrics* 70:338–42.

McCool, M. & Weaver, D. D. (1994). Branchio-oculo-facial syndrome: broadening the spectrum. *American Journal of Medical Genetics* 49:414–21.

McCowan, L. M. & Becroft, D. M. (1994). Beckwith–Wiedemann syndrome, placental abnormalities, and gestational proteinuric hypertension. *Obstetrics and Gynecology* 83:813–17.

McDonald-McGinn, D. A., Driscoll, L., Bason, L., Christensen, K. M., Zavod, W., Clark, B. J., Emanuel, B. S. & Zackai, E. H. (1995). Autosomal dominant Opitz syndrome secondary to a 22q11.2 deletion. *American Journal of Human Genetics* 57 (suppl): A20.

McFarlin, B. L. & Bottoms, S. F. (1996). Maternal syphilis: the next pregnancy. *American Journal of Perinatology* 13:513–18.

McGaughran, J. M., Gaunt, L., Dore, J., Petrij, F., Dauwerse, H. G. & Donnai, D. (1996). Rubinstein–Taybi syndrome with deletions of FISH probe RT1 at16p13.3: two UK patients. *Journal of Medical Genetics* 33:82–3.

McGinnis, J. M. & Lee, P. R. (1995). *Healthy People 2000* at mid-decade. *Journal of the American Medical Association* 273:1123–9.

McKusick, V. A. (1994). *Mendelian Inheritance in Man. Catalogs of Human Genes and Genetic Disorders,* 11th edn. Baltimore: Johns Hopkins University Press. (Also available online at www.ncbi.nlm.nih.gov/omim/).

McMaster, M. J. (1994). Spinal deformity in Ehlers–Danlos syndrome. Five patients treated by spinal fusion. *Journal of Bone and Joint Surgery* 76:773–7.

McNeal, D., Hawtrey, C., Wolraich, M. & Mapel, J. (1983). Symptomatic neurogenic bladder in a cerebral palsied population. *Developmental Medicine and Child Neurology* 25:612–16.

Mehlman, C. T., Rubinstein, J. H. & Roy, D. R. (1998). Instability of the patellofemoral joint in Rubinstein–Taybi syndrome. *Journal of Pediatric Orthopedics* 18:508–11.

Mehta, A. V. & Ambalavanan, S. K. (1997). Occurrence of congenital heart disease in children with Brachmann–de Lange syndrome. *American Journal of Medical Genetics* 71:434–5.

Mehta, D. I., Hill, I. D., Singer-Granick, C., Balloch, Z. & Blecker, U. (1995). Primary sclerosing cholangitis and multiple autoimmune disorders in a patient with Down syndrome. *Clinical Pediatrics* 34:502–5.

Meinecke, P. & Rodewald, A. (1989). Kabuki make-up syndrome in a caucasian. *Dysmorphology and Clinical Genetics* 3:103–7.

Meisels, S. J. (1989). Can developmental screening tests identify children who are developmentally at risk? *Pediatrics* 83:578–85.

Meldon, S., Brady, W. & Young, J. S. (1996). Presentation of Ehlers–Danlos syndrome: iliac artery pseudoaneurysm rupture. *Annals of Emergency Medicine* 28:231–4.

Melnick, M., Bixler, D., Nance, W. E., Silk, K. & Yune, H. (1976). Familial branchio-oto-renal dysplasia: A new addition to the branchial arch syndromes. *Clinical Genetics* 9:25–34.

Menard, R. M., Delaire, J. & Schendel, S. A. (1995). Treatment of the craniofacial complications of Beckwith–Wiedemann syndrome. *Plastic and Reconstructive Surgery* 96:27–33.

Mendez, H. M. M. & Opitz, J. M. (1985). Noonan syndrome: a review. *American Journal of Medical Genetics* 21:493–506.

Menezes, A. V., MacGregor, D. L. & Buncic, J. R. (1994). Aicardi syndrome: natural history and possible predictors of severity. *Pediatric Neurology* 11:313–18.

Meyerson, M. D. & Nisbet, J. B. (1987). Nager syndrome: An update of speech and hearing characteristics. *Cleft Palate Journal* 24:142–51.

Milani-Comparetti, A. & Gidoni, E. 1976. Routine developmental examination in normal and retarded infants. *Developmental Medicine and Child Neurology* 9:631.

Milerad, J., Larson, O., Hagberg, C. & Ideberg, M. (1997). Associated malformations in infants with cleft lip and palate: a prospective, population-based study. *Pediatrics* 100:180–6.

Miller, F. & Bachrach, S. J. (1995). *Cerebral Palsy: A Complete Guide for Caregiving*. Baltimore: Johns Hopkins University Press.

Miller, M. T., Epstein, R. J., Sugar, J., Pinchoff, B. S., Sugar, A., Gammon, J. A., Mittelman, D., Dennis, R. F. & Israel, J. (1984). Anterior segment anomalies associated with the fetal alcohol syndrome. *Journal of Pediatric Ophthalmology and Strabismus* 21:8–18.

Miller, R. W. & Rubinstein, J. H. (1995). Tumors in Rubinstein–Taybi syndrome. *American Journal of Medical Genetics* 56:112–15.

Millman, B., Gibson, W. S. & Foster, W. P. (1995). Branchio-oto-renal syndrome. *Archives of Otolaryngology – Head and Neck Surgery* 121:922–5.

Mills, J. L., Baker, L. & Goldman, A. S. (1979). Malformations in infants of diabetic mothers occur before the seventh gestational week. Implications for treatment. *Diabetes* 28:292–3.

Mitchell, J. A., Giangiacomo, J., Hefner, M. A., Thelin, J. W. & Pickens, J. M. (1985). Dominant CHARGE association. *Ophthalmology and Pediatric Genetics* 6:31–5.

Mizuguchi, M., Takashima, S., Kakita, A., Yamada, M. & Ikeda, K. (1995). Lissencephaly gene product. Localization in the central nervous system and loss of immunoreactivity in Miller–Dieker syndrome. *American Journal of Pathology* 147:1142–51.

Moessinger, A. C. (1983). Fetal akinesia deformation sequence: An animal model. *Pediatrics* 72:857–63.

Molnar, G. E. (1979). Cerebral palsy: prognosis and how to judge it. *Pediatric Annals* 8:596–605.

Moore, G. E. (1995). Molecular approaches to the study of human craniofacial dysmorphologies. *International Review of Cytology* 158:215–17.

Moore, M. H. (1993). Upper airway obstruction in the syndromal craniosynostoses. *British Journal of Plastic Surgery* 46:355–62.

Moore, M. H., Cantrell, S. B., Trott, J. A. & David, D. J. (1995a). Pfeiffer syndrome: a clinical review. *Cleft Palate-Craniofacial Journal* 32:62–70.

Moore, M. H., Guzman-Stein, G., Proudman, T. W., Abbot, A. H., Weatherway, D. J. & David, D. J. (1994). Mandibular lengthening by distraction for airway obstruction in Treacher Collins syndrome. *Journal of Craniofacial Surgery* 5:22–25.

Moore, M. H., Lodge, M. L. & Clark, B. E. (1995b). Spinal anomalies in Pfeiffer syndrome. *Cleft Palate-Craniofacial Journal* 32:251–4.

Morgan, D., Bailey, M., Phelps, P., Bellman, S., Grace, A. & Wyse, R. (1993). Ear-Nose-Throat abnormalities in the CHARGE association. *Archives of Otolaryngology – Head and Neck Surgery* 119:49–54.

Moriyama, Y., Nishida, T., Toyohira, H., Saigenji, H., Shimokawa, S., Taira, A. & Kuriwaki, K. (1995). Acute aortic dissection in a patient with osteogenesis imperfectae. *Annals of Thoracic Surgery* 60:1397–9.

Morris, C. A., Demsey, S. A., Leonard, C. O., Dilts, C. & Blackburn. B. (1988). Growth data for Williams syndrome patients, collected with the assistance of the Williams Syndrome National Association. In *Growth References: Third Trimester to Adulthood*, ed. Saul, R. A., Seaver, L. H.,

Sweet, K. M., Geer, J. S., Phelan, M. C. & Mills, C. M., pp. 128–32. Greenville SC: Keys Printing.

Morris, C. A., Leonard, C. O., Dilts, C. & Demsey, S. A. (1990). Adults with Williams syndrome. *American Journal of Medical Genetics* 6:102–7.

Morrison, P. J., Mulholland, H. C., Craig, B. G. & Nevin, N. C. (1992). Cardiovascular abnormalities in the oculo-auriculo-vertebral spectrum (Goldenhar syndrome). *American Journal of Medical Genetics* 44:425–8.

Mostofsky, S. H., Mazzocco, M. M., Aakalu, G., Warsofsky, I. S., Denckla, M. B. & Reiss, A. L. (1998). Decreased cerebellar posterior vermis size in fragile X syndrome: correlation with neurocognitive performance. *Neurology* 50:121–30.

Moulis, H., Garsten, J. J., Marano, A. R. & Elser, J. M. (1992). Tuberous sclerosis complex: Review of the gastrointestinal manifestations and report of an unusual case. *American Journal of Gastroenterology* 87:914–18.

Msall, M. E. (1996). Functional assessment in neurodevelopmental disabilities. In *Developmental Disabilities in Infancy and Childhood,* ed. A. J. Capute & P. J. Accardo, pp. 371–92. Baltimore: Paul H. Brookes.

Msall, M. E., Reese, M. S., DiGaudio, K., Griswold, K., Granger, C. V. & Cooke, R. E. (1990). Symptomatic atlantoaxial instability associated with medical and rehabilitative procedures in children with Down syndrome. *Pediatrics* 85:447–9.

Msall, M. E., DiGaudio, K. M. & Malone, A. F. (1991). Health, developmental, and psychosocial aspects of Down Syndrome. *Infants and Young Children* 4:35–45.

Msall, M. E., DiGaudio, K., Duffy, L. C., LaForest, S., Braun, S. & Granger, C. V. (1994a). WeeFIM. Normative sample of an instrument for tracking functional independence in children. *Clinical Pediatrics* July:431–8.

Msall, M. E., DiGaudio, K., Rogers, B. T., LaForest, S., Ctanzaro, N. L., Campbell, J., Wilczenski, F. & Duffy, L. C. (1994b). The functional independence measure for children (WeeFIM). *Clinical Pediatrics* July:421–30.

Mudd, S. H., Skovby, F. Levy, H. L., Pettigrew, R. D., Wilcken, B., Pyeritz, R. E., Andria, G., Boers, G. H. J., Bromberg, I. L., Cerone, R., Fowler, B., Groebe, H., Schmidt, H. & Schweitzer, L. (1985). The natural history of homocystinuria due to cystathionine-β-synthase deficiency. *American Journal of Human Genetics* 37:1–31.

Mueller, R. F., Pagon, R. A., Pepin, M. G., Haas, J. E., Kawabori, I., Stevenson, J. G., Stephan, M. J., Blumhagen, J. D. & Christie, D.L. (1984). Arteriohepatic dysplasia: phenotypic features and family studies. *Clinical Genetics* 25:323–31.

Mulinare, J., Cordero, J. F., Erickson, J. D. & Berry, R. J. (1988). Periconceptional use of multivitamins and the occurrence of neural tube defects. *Journal of the American Medical Association* 260:3141–5.

Munro, G. (1986). Epidemiology and the extent of mental retardation. *Psychiatric Clinics of North America* 9:591–602.

Murovic, J. A., Posnick, J. C., Drake, J. M., Humphreys, R. P., Hoffman, H. J. & Hendricks, E. B. (1993). Hydrocephalus in Apert syndrome: a retrospective review. *Pediatric Neurosurgery* 19:151–5.

Nadel, A., Green, J. & Holmes, L. (1990). Absence of need for amniocentesis in patients with elevated levels of maternal serum alpha-feto-protein and normal ultrasonographic examinations. *New England Journal of Medicine* 323:557–61.

Naeye, R. L., Peters, E. C., Bartholomew, M. & Landis, J. R. (1989). Origins of cerebral palsy. *American Journal of Diseases of Children* 143:1154–61.

Nance, M. A., Neglia, J. P., Talwar, D. & Berry, S. A. (1990). Neuroblastoma in a patient with Sotos' syndrome. *Journal of Medical Genetics* 27:130–2.

Nanson, J. L. & Hiscock, M. (1990). Attention deficits in children exposed to alcohol prenatally. *Alcoholism Clinical and Experimental Research* 14:656–61.

Narvaez, J., Narvaez, J. A., Majos, C., Clavaguera, M. T. & Alegre-Sancho, J. J. (1996). Subarachnoid haemorrhage secondary to ruptured cerebral aneurysm in a patient with osteogenesis imperfecta. *British Journal of Rheumatology* 35:1332–3.

National Institutes of Health (NIH). (1988). Consensus Development Conference Statement: Neurofibromatosis. *Neurofibromatosis* 1:172–8.

National Institutes of Health (NIH) Consensus Development Conference Consensus Statement (1991). December 11–13, 9(4):1–24. Acoustic Neuroma.

Neff, J. M. & Anderson, G. (1995). Protecting children with chronic illness in a competitive marketplace. *Journal of the American Medical Association* 274:1866–9.

Nellhaus, G. (1986). Head circumference from birth to eighteen years. *Pediatrics* 41:106–14.

Nelson, K. & Ellenberg, J. (1986). Antecedents of cerebral palsy: multivariate analysis of risk. *New England Journal of Medicine* 315:81–6.

Neufeld, E. F. & Muenzer, J. (1995). The mucopolysaccharidoses. In *The Metabolic and Molecular Bases of Inherited Disease*, 7th edn, ed. C. R. Scriver, A. L. Beaudet, W. S. Sly & D. Valle, pp. 2465–94. New York: McGraw-Hill, Inc.

Nevin, N. C., Silvestri, J., Kernohan, D. C. & Hutchinson, W. M. (1994). Oral-facial-digital syndrome with retinal abnormalities: OFDS type IX. A further case report. *American Journal of Medical Genetics* 51:228–31.

Nguyen, P. N. & Sullivan, P. K. (1993). Issues and controversies in the management of cleft palate. *Clinics in Plastic Surgery* 20:671–82.

Nickerson, E., Greenberg, F., Keating, M. T., McCaskill, C. & Shaffer, L. G. (1995). Deletions of the elastin gene at 7q11.23 occur in ~90 percent of patients with Williams syndrome. *American Journal of Human Genetics* 56:1156–61.

Nielsen, J., Pelsen, B. & Sørenson, K. (1988). Follow-up of 30 Klinefelter males treated with testosterone. *Clinical Genetics* 33:262–9.

Nigam, A. & Samuel, P. R. (1994). Hyperacusis and Williams syndrome. *Journal of Laryngology and Otology* 108:494–6.

Niikawa, N., Matsuura, N., Fukushima, Y., Ohsawa, T. & Kajii, T. (1981). Kabuki make-up syndrome: A syndrome of mental retardation, unusual facies, large and protruding ears, and postnatal growth deficiency. *Journal of Pediatrics* 99:565–9.

Niki, H., Staheli, L. T. & Mosca, V. S. (1997). Management of clubfoot deformity in amyoplasia. *Journal of Pediatric Orthopedics* 17:803–7.

Nitahara, J., Dozor, A. J., Schroeder, S. A. & Rifkinson-Mann, S. (1996). Apnea as a presenting sign of hydrocephalus. *Pediatrics* 97:587–9.

Noonan, J. A. (1997). Health supervision for children with Turner syndrome. *Pediatrics* 99:146–7.

Noonan, J. A. & Ehmke, D. A. (1963). Associated noncardiac malformations in children with congenital heart disease. *Journal of Pediatrics* 63:468–70.

North, K. N., Fulton, A. B. & Whiteman, D. A. (1995a). Identical twins with Cohen syndrome. *American Journal of Medical Genetics* 58:54–8.

North, K. N., Whiteman, D. A., Pepin, M. G. & Byers, P. H. (1995b). Cerebrovascular complications in Ehlers–Danlos syndrome type IV. *Annals of Neurology* 38:960–4.

Nowak, K. C. & Weider, D. J. (1998). Pediatric nocturnal enuresis secondary to airway obstruction from cleft palate repair. *Clinical Pediatrics* 37:653–7.

Nowicki, M. J. & Peterson, R. B. (1998). Dubowitz syndrome and achalasia: two rare conditions in a child. *Clinical Pediatrics* 37:197–200.

Nuss, R. & Manco-Johnson, M. (1995). Hemostasis in Ehlers–Danlos syndrome. Patient report and literature. *Clinical Pediatrics* 34:552–5.

Oakes, W. J. (1992). The natural history of patients with the Sturge–Weber syndrome. *Pediatric Neurosurgery* 18:287–90.

Ockner, R. K., Kaikaus, R. M. & Bass, N. M. (1993). Fatty-acid metabolism and the pathogenesis of hepatocellular carcinoma: review and hypothesis. *Hepatology* 18:669–76.

Ohlsson, R., Nystrom, A., Pfeifer-Ohlsson, S., Tohönen, V., Hedborg, F., Schofield, P., Flam, F. & Ekstrom, T. J (1993). IGF2 is parentally imprinted during human embryogenesis and in the Beckwith–Wiedemann syndrome. *Nature Genetics* 4:94–7.

Okada, K., Iida, K., Sakusabe, N., Saitoh, H., Abe, E. & Sato, K. (1994). Pseudo-hypoparathyroidism-associated spinal stenosis. *Spine* 19:1186–9.

Oley, C. A., Baraitser, M. & Grant, D. B. (1988). A reappraisal of the CHARGE association. *Journal of Medical Genetics* 25:147–56.

Olitsky, S. E., Sadler, L. S. & Reynolds, J. D. (1997). Subnormal binocular vision in the Williams syndrome. *Journal of Pediatric Ophthalmology and Strabismus* 34:58–60.

Olney, A. H. & Kolodziej, P. (1998). Velocardiofacial syndrome (Shprintzen syndrome, chromosome 22q11 deletion syndrome). *Ear Nose and Throat Journal* 77:460–1.

Olson, A. & Cooley, W. (1996). The role of medical professionals in supporting child self-competence. In *Making Our Way: Building Self-Competence Among Youth With Disabilities*, ed. L. Powers & G. Singer, pp. 134–9. Baltimore: Paul Brookes.

Opitz, J. M. (1985). Editorial comment: The Brachmann–de Lange syndrome. *American Journal of Medical Genetics* 22:89–102.

Opitz, J. M. (1987). Editorial comment: G syndrome (hypertelorism with esophageal abnormality and hypospadias, or hypospadias-dysphagia, or "Opitz-Frias" or "Opitz-G" syndrome – perspective in 1987 and bibliography. *American Journal of Medical Genetics* 28:275–85.

Opitz, J. M. (1993). Blastogenesis, normal and abnormal. In *Proceedings of the Second International Workshop on Fetal Genetic Pathology*, ed. J. M. Opitz & N. W. Paul, pp. 3–37. New York: Wiley–Liss.

Opitz, J. M. (1994). Brachmann–de Lange syndrome. A continuing enigma. *Archives of Pediatrics and Adolescent Medicine* 148:1206–7.

Opitz, J. M. & De la Cruz, F. (1994). Cholesterol metabolism in the RSH/Smith–Lemli–Opitz syndrome: summary of an NICHD conference. *American Journal of Medical Genetics* 50:326–38.

Opitz, J. M. & Wilson, G. N. (1996). Causes and pathogenesis of birth defects. In *Potter's Pathology of the Fetus and Infant,* ed. E. Gilbert-Barness, pp. 44–64. Philadelphia: Mosby Year Book.

Opitz, J. M., Richieri-Costa, A., Aase, J. M. & Benke, P.J. (1988). FG syndrome update 1988. Note of 5 new patients and bibiliography. *American Journal of Medical Genetics* 30:309–28.

Orioli, I. M., Castilla, E. E. & Barbosa-Neto, J. G. (1986). The birth prevalence rates for the skeletal dysplasias. *Journal of Medical Genetics* 23:328–32.

Orlow, S. J. (1997). Albinism: an update. *Seminars in Cutaneous Medicine and Surgery* 16:24–9.

Orr, D. J., Slaney, S., Ashworth, G. J. & Poole, M. D. (1997). Craniofrontonasal dysplasia. *British Journal of Plastic Surgery* 50:153–61.

Overall, J. C., Jr. (1994). Herpes simplex virus infection of the fetus and newborn. *Pediatric Annals* 23:131–6.

Ozbey, H., Ozbey, N. & Tunnessen, W. W., Jr. (1998). Picture of the month. Leprechaunism. *Archives of Pediatric and Adolescent Medicine* 152:1031–2.

Paavola, P., Salonen, R., Weissenbach, J. & Peltonen, L. (1995). The locus for Meckel syndrome with multiple congenital anomalies maps to chromosome 17q21–q24. *Nature Genetics* 11:213–15.

Pagliara, A. S., Karl, I. E., Hammond, M. & Kipnis, D. M (1973). Hypoglycemia in infancy and childhood. Parts I and II. *Journal of Pediatrics* 82:365–79; 558–77.

Pagon, R. A., Chandler, J. W., Collie, W. R., Clarren, S. K., Moon, J., Minkin, S. A. & Hall, J. G. (1978). Hydrocephalus, agyria, retinal dysplasia, encephalocele (HARD E) syndrome: an autosomal recessive condition. *Birth Defects* 14:233–41.

Pagon, R. A., Graham, J. M., Jr., Zonana, J. & Yong, S.-L. (1981). Coloboma, congenital heart disease, and choanal atresia with multiple anomalies: CHARGE association. *Journal of Pediatrics* 99:223–7.

Palfrey, J. S., Singer, J. D., Walker, D. K. & Butler, J. A. (1987). Early identification of children's special needs: a study of five metropolitan communities. *Journal of Pediatrics* 111:651–9.

Palmer, F. & Hoon, A. (1995). Cerebral palsy. In *Developmental and Behavioral Pediatrics,* ed. S. Parker & B. Zuckerman, pp. 88–94. Boston: Little, Brown, and Co.

Paris, J. J., Weiss, A. H. & Soifer, S. (1992). Ethical issues in the use of life-prolonging interventions for an infant with trisomy 18. *Journal of Perinatology* 12:366–8.

Park, S. K., Chang, S. H., Cho, S. B., Baek, H. S. & Lee, D. Y. (1994). Cockayne syndrome: a case with hyperinsulinemia and growth hormone deficiency. *Journal of Korean Medical Science* 9:74–7.

Park, W. J., Meyers, G. A., Li, X., Theda, C., Day, D., Orlow, S .J., Jones, M.C. & Jabs, E. W. (1995). Novel FGFR2 mutations in Crouzon and Jackson–Weiss syndromes show allelic heterogeneity and phenotypic variability. *Human Molecular Genetics* 4:1229–33.

Parker, P. H., Ballew, M. & Greene, H. L. (1993). Nutritional management of glycogen storage disease. *Annual Review of Nutrition* 13:83–109.

Pasteris, N. G., Buckler, J., Cadle, A. B. & Gorski, J. L. (1997). Genomic organization of the faciogenital dysplasia (FGD1; Aarskog syndrome) gene. *Genomics* 43:390–4.

Patau, K., Smith, D. W., Therman, E., Inhorn, S. L. & Wagner, H. P. (1960). Multiple congenital anomaly caused by an extra autosome. *Lancet* 1:790–3.

Paterson, C. R., Ogston, S. A. & Henry, R. M. (1996). Life expectancy in osteogenesis imperfecta. *British Medical Journal* 312:351.

Patton, M. A. (1988). Russell–Silver syndrome. *Journal of Medical Genetics* 25:557–60.

Pauli, R. M. (1988). Mechanism of bone and cartilage maldevelopment in the Warfarin embryopathy. *Pathology and Immunopathology Research* 7:107–13.

Pauli, R. M., Scott, C. I., Wassman, E. R., Gilbert, E. F., Leavitt, L. A., Hoeve, J. V., Hall, J. G., Partington, M. W., Jones, K. L., Sommer, A., Feldman, W., Langer, L. O., Rimoin, D. L., Hecht, J. T. & Lebovitz, R. (1984). Apnea and sudden unexpected death in infants with achondroplasia. *Journal of Pediatrics* 104:342–8.

Pauli, R. M., Horton, V. K., Glinski, L. P. & Reiser, C. A. (1995). Prospective assessment of risks for cervicomedullary-junction compression in infants with achondroplasia. *American Journal of Human Genetics* 56:732–44.

Pavlidis, K., McCauley, E. & Sybert, V. P. (1995). Psychosocial and sexual functioning in women with Turner syndrome. *Clinical Genetics* 47:85–9.

Pedersen, J. F. & Mølsted-Pedersen, L. (1979). Early growth retardation in diabetic pregnancy. *British Medical Journal* 1:18–19.

Pena, S. D. J. & Shokeir, M. H. K. (1974). Syndrome of camptodactyly, multiple ankyloses, facial anomalies, and pulmonary hypoplasia: a lethal condition. *Journal of Pediatrics* 85:373–5.

Pena, S. D. J. & Shokeir, M. H. K. (1976). Syndrome of camptodactyly, multiple ankyloses, facial anomalies, and pulmonary hypoplasia – further delineation and evidence for autosomal recessive inheritance. *Birth Defects* 12:201–8.

Pereyo, N. G., Lugo-Janer, G. J. & Sanchez, J. L. (1993). Atrophic macules in an infant. Goltz syndrome (focal dermal hypoplasia [FDH] syndrome). *Archives of Dermatology* 129:897–900.

Perlman, M., Levin, M. & Wittels, B. (1973). Renal hamartomas, nephroblastomatosis, and fetal gigantism. *Journal of Pediatrics* 83:414–18.

Perrot, L. J. & Mrak, R. E. (1993). Cardiac involvement in a child with unsuspected pseudoxanthoma elasticum. *Pediatric Pathology* 13:273–9.

Pfeiffer, R. A. (1969). Associated deformities of the head and hands. *Birth Defects* 5:18–34.

Pharoah, P. O., Cooke, T., Johnson, M. A., King, R. & Mutch, L. (1998). Epidemiology of cerebral palsy in England and Scotland, 1984–9. *Archives of Disease in Childhood (Fetal and Neonatal Edition)* 79:F21–5.

Phelan, M. C., Rogers, R. C., Clarkson, K. B., Bowyer, F. P., Levine, M. A., Estabrooks, L. L., Severson, M. C. & Dobyns, W. B. (1995). Albright hereditary osteodystrophy and del(2)(q37.3) in four unrelated individuals. *American Journal of Medical Genetics* 58:1–7.

Phillips, E. (1998). Toxoplasmosis. *Canadian Family Physician* 44:1823–5.

Pierga, J. Y., Giacchetti, S., Vilain, E., Extra, J. M., Brice, P., Espie, M., Maragi, J. A., Fellous, M. & Marty, M. (1994). Dysgerminoma in a pure 45,X Turner syndrome: report of a case and review of the literature. *Gynecologic Oncology* 55:459–64.

Pilia, G., Hughes-Benzie, R. M., MacKenzie, A., Baybayan, P., Chen, E. Y.. Huber, R., Neri, G., Cao, A., Forabosco, A. & Schlessinger. D. (1996). Mutations in GPC3, a glypican gene, cause the Simpson–Golabi–Behmel overgrowth syndrome. *Nature Genetics* 12:241–7.

Pillay, T., Winship, W. S. & Ramdial, P. K. (1998). Pigmentary abnormalities in trisomy of chromosome 13. *Clinical Dysmorphology* 7:191–4.

Pinar, H., Carpenter, M. W., Abuelo, D. & Singer, D. B. (1994). Fryns syndrome: a new definition. *Pediatric Pathology* 14:467–78.

Piombo, M., Rosanda, C., Pasino, M., Marasini, M., Cerruti, P. & Comelli, A. (1993). Acute lymphoblastic leukemia in Noonan syndrome: report of two cases. *Medical and Pediatric Oncology* 21:454–5.

Piussan, C., Mathieu, M., Berquin, P. & Fryns, J. P. (1996). Fragile X mutation and FG syndrome-like phenotype. *American Journal of Medical Genetics* 64:395–8.

Pizio, H. F., Scott, M. H. & Richard, J. M. (1994). Tortuosity of the retinal vessels in Aarskog syndrome (faciogenital dysplasia). *Ophthalmic Genetics* 15:37–40.

Pizzutillo, P. D., Woods, M., Nicholson, L. & MacEwen, G. D. (1994). Risk factors in Klippel–Feil syndrome. *Spine* 19:2110–16.

Plissart, L., Borghgraef, M. & Fryns, J. P. (1996). Temperament in Williams syndrome. *Genetic Counseling* 7:41–6.

Plomp, A. S., De Die-Smulders, C. E., Meinecke, P., Ypma-Verhulst, J. M., Lissone, D. A. & Fryns, J. P. (1995). Coffin–Lowry syndrome: clinical aspects at different ages and symptoms in female carriers. *Genetic Counseling* 6:259–68.

Plotnick, L., Attie, K. M., Blethen, S. L. & Sy, J. P. (1998). Growth hormone treatment of girls with Turner syndrome: the National Cooperative Growth Study experience. *Pediatrics* 102:479–81.

Pober, B. R., Lacro, R. V., Rice C., Mandell, V. & Teele, R. L. (1993). Renal findings in 40 individuals with Williams syndrome. *American Journal of Medical Genetics* 46:271–4.

Poddevin, F., Delobel, B., Courreges, P. & Bayart, M. (1995). Antley–Bixler syndrome: case report and review of the literature. *Genetic Counseling* 6:241–6.

Pollack, I. F., Losken, H. W. & Fasick, P. (1997). Diagnosis and management of posterior plagiocephaly. *Pediatrics* 99:180–5.

Pollard, R. C. & Beasley, J. M. (1996). Anaesthesia for patients with trisomy 13 (Patau's syndrome). *Paediatric Anaesthesia* 6:151–3.

Pope, F. M., Komorowska, A., Lee, K. W. Speight, P., Zorawska, H., Ranta, H., Coonar, H. S. & MacKenzie, J. L. (1992). Ehlers–Danlos syndrome type I with novel dental features. *Journal of Oral Pathology and Medicine* 21:418–21.

Porter, M. E., Gardner, H. A., DeFeudis, P. & Endler. N. S. (1988). Verbal deficits in Klinefelter (XXY) adults living in the community. *Clinical Genetics* 33:246–53.

Posnick, J. C. (1996). Unilateral coronal synostosis (anterior plagiocephaly): current clinical perspectives. *Annals of Plastic Surgery* 36:430–47.

Posnick, J. C. (1997) Treacher Collins syndrome: perspectives in evaluation and treatment. *Journal of Oral and Maxillofacial Surgery* 55:1120–33.

Posnick, J. C. & Tompson, B. (1995). Cleft-orthognathic surgery: complications and long-term results. *Plastic and Reconstructive Surgery* 96:255–66.

Poswillo, D. (1973). The pathogenesis of the first and second branchial arch syndrome. *Oral Surgery, Oral Medicine, Oral Pathology* 35:302–29.

Prader, A., Labhart, A. & Willi, H. (1956). Ein Syndrom von Adipositas, Kleinwuchs, Kryptorchismus und Oligophrenie nach myotonieartigem Zustand in Neugeborenenalter. *Schweiz Medicine Woschenschrift* 86:1260–1.

Preis, S., Raymaekers-Buntinx, I. & Majewski, F. (1995). Acrofacial dysostosis of unknown type: nosology of the acrofacial dysostoses. *American Journal of Medical Genetics* 56:155–60.

Prockop, D. J. & Kivirikko, K. I. (1995). Collagens: molecular biology, diseases, and potentials for therapy. *Annual Review of Biochemisty* 64:403–34.

Pron, G., Galloway, C., Armstrong, D. & Posnick, J. (1993). Ear malformation and hearing loss in patients with Treacher Collins syndrome. *Cleft Palate–Craniofacial Journal* 30:97–103.

Ptacek, L. J., Opitz, J. M., Smith, D. W., Gerritsen, T. & Waisman, H. A. (1963). The Cornelia de Lange syndrome. *Journal of Pediatrics* 63:1000–20.

Pueschel, S. M., ed. (1978). *Down syndrome. Growing and learning.* Kansas City: Sheed Andrews & McMeel, Inc.

Pueschel, S. M. (1998). Should children with Down syndrome be screened for atlantoaxial instability? *Archives of Pediatric and Adolescent Medicine* 152:123–5.

Pueschel, S. M. & Pueschel, J. K., ed. (1992). *Biomedical Concerns in Persons with Down Syndrome.* Baltimore: Paul H. Brookes.

Pujol, R. M., Casanova, J. M., Perez, M., Matias-Guiu, X., Planaguma, M. & de Moragas, J. M. (1992). Focal dermal hypoplasia (Goltz syndrome): report of two cases with minor cutaneous and extracutaneous manifestations. *Pediatric Dermatology* 9:112–16.

Putnam, E. A., Zhang, H., Ramirez F. & Milewicz, D. M. (1995). Fibrillin-2 (FBN2) mutations result in the Marfan-like disorder, congenital contractural arachnodactyly. *Nature Genetics* 11:456–8.

Pyeritz, R. E. (1981). Maternal and fetal complications of pregnancy in the Marfan syndrome. *American Journal of Medicine* 71:784–90.

Pyeritz, R. E. (1993). Marfan syndrome. In *Connective Tissue and its Heritable Disorders,* ed. P.M. Royce & B. Steinmann, Ch. 14. New York: Wiley–Liss.

Pyeritz, R. E. & McKusick, V. A. (1979). The Marfan syndrome: Diagnosis and management. *New England Journal of Medicine* 300:772–6.

Pyeritz, R. E., Murphy, E. A., Lin, S. J. & Rosell, E. M. (1985). Growth and anthropometrics in the Marfan syndrome. In *Endocrine Genetics and the Genetics of Growth,* ed. C. J. Papadatos, C. S. Bartsocas, pp. 355–66. New York: Alan R. Liss.

Qazi, Q., Masakawa, A., Milman, D., McGann, B., Chua, A. & Haller, J. (1979). Renal anomalies in fetal alcohol syndrome. *Pediatrics* 63:886.

Qiu, W. W., Yin, S. S. & Stucker, F. J. (1998). Audiologic manifestations of Noonan syndrome. *Otolaryngology – Head and Neck Surgery* 118:319–23.

Quan, L. & Smith, D.W. (1973). The VATER association, Vertebral defects, Anal atresia, T-E fistula with esophageal atresia, Radial and Renal dysplasia: A spectrum of associated defects. *Journal of Pediatrics* 82:104–7.

Qureshi, I. L. & Khan, N. U. (1996). Experience with frontonasal dysplasia of varying severity. *Journal of Pediatric Surgery* 31:885–9.

Raffin, T. A. (1991). Withholding and withdrawing life support. *Hospital Practice* March:133–55.

Rallison, M. L., Meikle, A. W. & Zigrang, W. D. (1979). Hypoglycemia and lactic acidosis associated with fructose-1,6-diphosphatase deficiency. *Journal of Pediatrics* 94:933–6.

Rappo, P. D. (1997). Health supervision for children with Turner syndrome. *Pediatrics* 99:146.

Rauen, K. ed. (1990). *Guidelines for Spina Bifida Health Care Services Throughout Life.* Washington, DC: Spina Bifida Association of America.

Ray, S. & Rubin, A. P. (1994). Anaesthesia in a child with Schwartz–Jampel syndrome. *Anaesthesia* 49:600–2.

Read, A. P. & Newton, V. E. (1997). Waardenburg syndrome. *Journal of Medical Genetics* 34:656–65.

Reardon, W. & Winter, R. M. (1994). Saethre–Chotzen syndrome. *Journal of Medical Genetics* 31:393–6.

Rebsdorf Pederson, E., Hartvigsen, A., Fischer Hansen, B., Toftgaard, C., Konstantin-Hansen, K. & Bullow, S. (1994). Managment of Peutz–Jeghers syndrome. Experience with patients from the Danish Polyposis Register. *International Journal of Colorectal Disease* 9:177–9.

Redl, G. (1998). Massive pyramidal tract signs after endotracheal intubation: a case report of spondyloepiphyseal dysplasia congenita. *Anesthesiology* 89:1262–4.

Reece, E. A., Hmko, C. J., Wu, Y.-K. & Wiznitzer, A. (1993). Metabolic fuel mixtures and diabetic embryopathy. *Clinics in Perinatology* 20:517–32.

Reilly, S., Skuse, D. & Poblete, X. (1996). Prevalence of feeding problems and oral motor dysfunction in children with cerebral palsy: a community survey. *Journal of Pediatrics* 129:877–82.

Reiser, C. A., Pauli, R. M. & Hall, J. G. (1984). Achondroplasia: Unexpected familial recurrence. *American Journal of Medical Genetics* 19:245–50.

Reiss, A. L., Hagerman, R. J., Vinogradov, S., Abrams, M. & King, R. J. (1988). Psychiatric disability in female carriers of the fragile X syndrome. *Archives of General Psychiatry* 45:25–30.

Rekate, H. L. (1998). Occipital plagiocephaly: a critical review of the literature. *Journal of Neurosurgery* 89:24–30.

Reuser, A. J., Kroos, M. A., Hermans, M. M., Bijvoet, A. G., Verbeet, M. P., Van Diggelman, O. P., Kleijer, W. J. & Van der Ploeg, A. T. (1995). Glycogenosis type II (acid maltase deficiency). *Muscle and Nerve* 3:S61–S69.

Riccardi, V. M. (1981). von Recklinghausen neurofibromatosis. *New England Journal of Medicine* 305:1617–26.

Riela, A. R., Thomas, I. T., Gonzalez, A. R. & Ifft, R. D. (1995). Fryns syndrome: neurologic findings in a survivor. *Journal of Child Neurology* 10:110–13.

Riley, H. D. & Smith, W. R. (1960). Macrocephaly, pseudopapilledema and multiple hemangiomas. *Pediatrics* 26:293–300.

Rimell, F. L., Shapiro, A. M., Shoemaker, D. L. & Kenna, M. A. (1995). Head and neck manifestations of Beckwith–Wiedemann syndrome. *Otolaryngology – Head and Neck Surgery* 113:262–5.

Rittler, M., Paz, J. E. & Castilla, E. E. (1996). VACTERL association, epidemiologic definition and delineation. *American Journal of Medical Genetics* 63:529–36.

Rizzu, P., Overhauser, J., Jackson, L. G. & Baldini, A. (1995). Brachmann–de Lange syndrome: Toward the positional cloning of a locus at 3q27. *American Journal of Human Genetics* 57:A334.

Roach, E. S. & Delgado, M. R. (1995). Tuberous sclerosis. *Dermatologic Clinics* 13:151–61.

Roach, E. S., Gomez, M. R. & Northrup, H. (1998). Tuberous sclerosis complex consensus conference: Revised clinical diagnostic criteria. *Journal of Child Neurology* 13:624–8.

Roach, E. S., Smith, M., Huttenlocher, P., Bhat, M., Alcorn, D. & Hawley, L. (1992). Diagnostic criteria: tuberous sclerosis complex. *Journal of Child Neurology* 7:221–4.

Robertson, S., Tsang, B. & Aftimos, S. (1997). Cerebral infarction in Noonan syndrome. *American Journal of Medical Genetics* 71:111–14.

Robinson, B. H. (1995). Lactic acidemia (disorders of pyruvate carboxylase, pyruvate dehydrogenase). In *The Metabolic and Molecular Bases of Inherited Disease,* 7th edn, ed. C. R. Scriver, A. L. Beaudet, W. S. Sly & D. Valle, pp. 1479–99. New York: McGraw-Hill, Inc.

Robinson, G. C., Conry, J. L. & Conry, R. F. (1987). Clinical profile and prevalence of fetal alcohol syndrome in an isolated community in British Columbia. *Canadian Medical Association Journal* 137:203–7.

Robinson, L. K., James, H. E., Mubarak, S. J., Allen, E. J. & Jones, K. L. (1985). Carpenter syndrome: Natural history and clinical spectrum. *American Journal of Medical Genetics* 20:461–9.

Robson, A. K., Blanshard, J. D., Jones, K., Albery, E. H., Smith, I. M. & Maw, A. R. (1992). A conservative approach to management of otitis media with effusion in cleft palate children. *Journal of Laryngology and Otology* 106:788–92.

Roddi, R., Jansen, M. A., Vaandrager, J. M. & van der Meulen, J. C. (1995). Plagiocephaly – new classification and clinical study of a series of 100 patients. *Journal of Craniomaxillofacial Surgery* 23:347–54.

Roe, T. F., Coates, T. D., Thomas, D. W., Miller, J. H. & Gilsanz, V. (1992). Treatment of chronic inflammatory bowel disease in glycogen storage disease type Ib with colony-stimulating factors. *New England Journal of Medicine* 326:1666–9.

Roge, C., Cooper, M. & Tarnoff, H. (1997). Health supervision for children with Turner syndrome. *Pediatrics* 99:145–6.

Rohrich, R. J., Rowsell, A. R., Johns, D. F., Drury, M. A., Grieg, G., Watson, D. J., Godfrey, A. M. & Poole, M. D. (1996). Timing of hard palatal closure: a critical long-term analysis. *Plastic and Reconstructive Surgery* 98:236–46.

Rollnick, B. R., Kaye, C. I., Nagatoshi, K., Hauck, W. & Martin, A. O. (1987). Oculoauriculovertebral dysplasia and variants: Phenotypic characteristics of 294 patients. *American Journal of Medical Genetics* 26:361–75.

Romano, A. A., Blethen, S. L., Dana, K. & Noto, R. A. (1996). Growth hormone treatment in Noonan syndrome: the National Cooperative Growth Study experience. *Journal of Pediatrics* 128:S18–21.

Root, S. & Carey, J. C. (1994). Survival in trisomy 18. *American Journal of Medical Genetics* 49:170–4.

Rose, C. S., King, A. A., Summers, D., Palmer, R., Yang, S., Wilkie, A. O., Reardon, W., Malcolm, S. & Winter, R. M. (1994). Localization of the genetic locus for Saethre–Chotzen syndrome to a 6 cM region of chromosome 7 using four cases with apparently balanced translocations at 7p12.2. *Human Molecular Genetics* 3:1405–8.

Rose, G. (1992). *The Strategy of Preventive Medicine.* Oxford: Oxford University Press.

Rosenbloom, L. (1995). Diagnosis and management of cerebral palsy. *Archives of Disease in Childhood* 72:350–4.

Rosenfield, R. L., Perovic, N., Devine, N., Mauras, N., Moshang, T., Root, A. W. & Sy, J. P. (1998). Optimizing estrogen replacement treatment in Turner syndrome. *Pediatrics* 102:486–8.

Rosh, J. R., Collins, J., Groisman, G. M., Schwersenz, A. H., Schwartz, M. Miller, C. M. & LeLeiko, N. S. (1995). Management of hepatic adenoma in glycogen storage disease Ia. *Journal of Pediatric Gastroenterology and Nutrition* 20:225–8.

Ross, D. A., Witzel, M. A., Armstrong, D. C. & Thomson, H. G. (1996). Is pharyngoplasty a risk in velocardiofacial syndrome? An assessment of medially displaced carotid arteries. *Plastic and Reconstructive Surgery* 98:1182–90.

Ross, J. L., Feuillan, P., Long, L. M., Kowal, K., Kushner, H. & Cutler, G. B., Jr. (1995). Lipid abnormalities in Turner syndrome. *Journal of Pediatrics* 126:242–5.

Ross, J. L., Roeltgen, D., Feuillan, P., Kushner, H. & Cutler, G. B., Jr. (1998). Effects of estrogen on nonverbal processing speed and motor function in girls with Turner's syndrome. *Journal of Clinical Endocrinology and Metabolism* 83:3198–204.

Rossbach, H. C., Sutcliffe, M. J., Haag, M. M., Grana, N. H., Rossi, A. R. & Barbosa, J. L. (1996). Fanconi anemia in brothers initially diagnosed with VACTERL association with hydrocephalus, and subsequently with Baller–Gerold syndrome. *American Journal of Medical Genetics* 61:65–7.

Rossig, C., Wasser, S. & Oppermann, P. (1994). Audiologic manifestations in fetal alcohol syndrome assessed by brainstem auditory-evoked potentials. *Neuropediatrics* 25:245–9.

Rossiter, B. J. F. & Caskey, C. T. (1995). Hypoxanthine-guanine phosphoribosyltransferase deficiency: Lesch–Nyhan syndrome and gout. In *The Metabolic and Molecular Bases of Inherited Disease,* 7th edn, ed. C. R. Scriver, A. L. Beaudet, W. S. Sly & D. Valle, pp. 1679–1706. New York: McGraw-Hill, Inc.

Rossiter, E. J. (1993). The use of developmental screening and assessment instruments by paediatricians in Australia. *Journal of Paediatrics and Child Health* 29:357–9.

Rossiter, J. P., Repke, J. T., Morales, A. J., Murphy, E. A. & Pyeritz, R. E. (1995). A prospective longitudinal evaluation of pregnancy in the Marfan syndrome. *American Journal of Obstetrics and Gynecology* 173:1599–1606.

Rossmiller, D. R. & Pasic, T. R. (1994). Hearing loss in Townes–Brocks syndrome. *Otolaryngology – Head and Neck Surgery* 111:175–80.

Rouvreau, P., Glorion, C., Langlais, J., Noury, H. & Pouliquen, J. C. (1998). Assessment and neurologic involvement of patients with cervical spine congenital synostosis as in Klippel–Feil syndrome: study of 19 cases. *Journal of Pediatric Orthopedics B* 7:179–85.

Rowley, P. T. (1969). Familial hearing loss associated with branchial fistulas. *Pediatrics* 44:978–85.

Roy, M.-S., Milot, J. A., Polomeno, R. C. & Barsoum-Homsy, M. (1992). Ocular findings and visual evoked potential response in the Prader–Willi syndrome. *Canadian Journal of Ophthalmology* 307–11.

Rubenstein, L. K. & Vitsky, P. L. (1988). Dental management of patients with Russell–Silver syndrome. *Journal of Pedidontics* 12:215–19.

Rubin, K. (1998). Turner syndrome and osteoporosis: mechanisms and prognosis. *Pediatrics* 102:481–5.

Rubin, L. L. & Crocker, A. C. (1989). *Developmental Disabilities. Delivery of Medical Care for Children and Adults.* Philadephia: Lea & Febiger.

Russell, L. J., Weaver D. D. & Bull, M. J. (1981). The axial mesodermal dysplasia spectrum. *Pediatrics* 67:176–82.

Rutter, S. C. & Cole, T. R. (1991). Psychological characteristics of Sotos syndrome. *Developmental Medicine and Child Neurology* 33:898–902.

Ruvalcaba, R. H. A., Myhre, S. & Smith, D. W. (1980). Sotos syndrome with intestinal polyposis and pigmentary changes of the genitalia. *Clinical Genetics* 18:413–18.

Ryken, T. C. & Menezes, A. H. (1994). Cervicomedullary compression in achondroplasia. *Journal of Neurosurgery* 81:43–8.

Saal, H. M., Samango-Sprouse, C. A., Rodnan, L. A., Rosenbaum, K. N. & Custer, D. A. (1993). Brachmann–de Lange syndrome with normal IQ. *American Journal of Medical Genetics* 47:995–8.

Sabatini, D. D. & Adesnik, M. B. (1995). The biogenesis of membranes and organelles. In *The Metabolic and Molecular Bases of Inherited Disease,* 7th edn, ed. C. R. Scriver, A. L. Beaudet, W. S. Sly & D. Valle, pp. 459–553. New York: McGraw-Hill, Inc.

Sabry, M. A. & Farag, T. I. (1996). Hand anomalies in fetal-hydantoin syndrome: from nail/pha-langealhypoplasia to unilateral acheiria. *American Journal of Medical Genetics* 62:410–12.

Sackey, A., Coulter, B., Fryer, A. & Van Velzen, D. (1995). Epilepsy in the Freeman Sheldon syndrome. *Journal of Child Neurology* 10:335–7.

Sadler, L.S., Robinson, L.K. & Msall, M. E. (1995). Diabetic embryopathy: possible pathogenesis. *American Journal of Medical Genetics,* 55:363–6.

Sadove, A. M. (1996). Positional plagiocephaly [editorial]. *Journal of Craniofacial Surgery* 7:3.

Saldino, R. M., Steinbach H. L. & Epstein, C. J. (1972). Familial acrocephalosyndactyly (Pfeiffer syndrome). *American Journal of Roentgenology* 116:609–22.

Salim, M. A., Alpert, B. S., Ward, J. C. & Pyeritz, R. E. (1994). Effect of beta-adrenergic blockade on aortic root rate of dilation in the Marfan syndrome. *American Journal of Cardiology* 74:629–33.

Salle, J. L., de Fraga, J. C., Wojciechowski, M. & Antunes, C. R. (1992). Congenital rupture of the scrotum: an unusual complication of meconium peritonitis. *Journal of Urology* 148:1242–3.

Salonen, R. (1984). The Meckel syndrome: clinicopathologic findings in 67 patients. *American Journal of Medical Genetics* 18:671–89.

Sardor, G.G., Smith, D. F. & MacLeod, P. W. (1981). Cardiac malformations in the fetal alcohol syndrome. *Journal of Pediatrics* 98:771–3.

Sarwark, J. F. (1996). Spina bifida. *Pediatric Clinics of North America* 43:1151–8.

Sarwark, J. F. & Kramer, A. (1998). Pediatric spinal deformity. *Current Opinion in Pediatrics* 10:82–6.

Sataloff, R. T., Spiegel, J. R., Hawkshaw, M., Epstein, M. M. & Jackson, L. (1990). Cornelia de Lange syndrome. Otolaryngologic manifestations. *Archives of Otolaryngology – Head and Neck Surgery* 116:1044–6.

Saudubray, J.-M. & Charpentier, C. (1995). Clinical phenotypes. Diagnosis/algorithms. In *The Metabolic and Molecular Bases of Inherited Disease,* 7th edn, ed. C. R. Scriver, A. L. Beaudet, W. S. Sly & D. Valle, pp. 327–400. New York: McGraw-Hill, Inc.

Saul, R. A., Harden, K. J., Stevenson, R. E., Wilkes, G., Hannig, V. L., Simensen, R. J., Strickland, A. L. & Taylor, H. A. (1983). Clinical features in fragile X syndrome. *Proceedings of the Greenwood Genetics Center* 2:58–67.

Saul, R. A., Seaver, L. H., Sweet, K. M., Geer, J. S., Phelan, M. C. & Mills, C. M. (1998). *Growth References: Third Trimester to Adulthood*, pp. 128–32. Greenville SC: Keys Printing.

Saul, R. A. & Stevenson, R. E. (1986). Are Bannayan and Ruvalcaba–Myhre–Smith syndrome discrete entities? *Proceedings of the Greenwood Genetics Center* 5:3–7.

Sawin, P. D. & Menezes, A. H. (1997). Basilar invagination in osteogenesis imperfecta and related osteochondrodysplasias: medical and surgical management. *Journal of Neurosurgery* 86:950–60.

Say, B. (1975). Misuse of acronyms and the VATER association. *Journal of Pediatrics* 86:315.

Say, B. & Gerald, P. S. (1968). A new polydactyly, imperforate anus, vertebral anomalies syndrome. *Lancet* 1:688–9.

Schaefer, G. B., Bodensteiner, J. B., Buehler, B. A., Lin, A. & Cole, T. R. (1997). The neuroimaging findings in Sotos syndrome. *American Journal of Medical Genetics* 68:462–5.

Schaffer, S. J. & Campbell, J. R. (1994). The new CDC and AAP lead poisoning prevention recommendations: consensus versus controversy. *Pediatric Annals* 23:592–9.

Schardein, J. L. (1985). *Chemically Induced Birth Defects*. New York: Marcel Dekker, Inc.

Schepis, C., Failla, P., Siragusa, M. & Romano, C. (1994). Skin picking: the best cutaneous feature in the recognition of Prader–Willi syndrome. *International Journal of Dermatology* 33:866–7.

Schinzel, A. (1979). Postaxial polydactyly, hallux duplication, absence of the corpus callosum, macroencephaly and severe mental retardation: A new syndrome? *Helvetia Pediatrica Acta* 34:141–6.

Schinzel, A. (1984). *Catalogue of Unbalanced Chromosome Aberrations in Man*. Berlin: de Gruyter.

Schlictemeier, T. L., Tomlinson, G. E., Kamen, B. A., Waber, L. J. & Wilson, G. N. (1994). Multiple coagulation defects and the Cohen syndrome. *Clinical Genetics* 45:212–16.

Schmickel, R. D. (1986). Contiguous gene syndromes. A component of recognizable syndromes. *Journal of Pediatrics* 1909:231–41.

Schneider, M. B., Dittmar, S. & Boxer, R. A. (1993). Anterior sacral meningocele presenting as a pelvic/abdominal mass in a patient with Marfan syndrome. *Journal of Adolescent Health* 14:325–8.

Schotland, H. M, Eldridge, R., Somer, S. S. & Malawar, M. (1992). Neurofibromatosis-1 and osseous fibrous dysplasia in a family. *American Journal of Medical Genetics* 43:815–22.

Schrander-Stumpel, C., de Die-Smulders, C., de Krom, M., Schyns-Fleuran, S., Hamel, B., Jaeken, D. & Fryns, J. P. (1993). Marden–Walker syndrome: case report, literature review, and nosologic discussion. *Clinical Genetics* 43:303–8.

Schrander-Stumpel, C., Gerver, W. J., Meyer, H., Engelen, J., Mulder, H. & Fryns. J. P. (1994). Prader–Willi-like phenotype in fragile X syndrome. *Clinical Genetics* 45:175–80.

Schrander-Stumpel, C., Howeler, C., Jones, M., Sommer, A., Stevens, C., Tinschert, S., Israel, J. & Fryns, J. P. (1995). Spectrum of X-linked hydrocephalus (HSAS), MASA syndrome, and complicated spastic paraplegia (SPG1): Clinical review with six additional families. *American Journal of Medical Genetics* 57:107–16.

Schrander-Stumpel, C., Meinecke, P., Wilson, G., Gillessen-Kaesbach, G., Tinschert, S., Konig, R., Philip, N., Rizzo, R., Schrander, J., Pfeiffer, L., Maat-Kievit, A., van der Burgt, I., van Essen, T., Latta, E., Hillig, U., Verloes, A., Journel, H. & Fryns, J. P. (1994). The Kabuki

(Niikawa–Kuroki) syndrome: further delineation of the phenotype in 29 non-Japanese patients. *European Journal of Pediatrics* 153:438–45.

Schwartz, I. D. & Root, A. W. (1991). The Klinefelter syndrome of testicular dysgenesis. *Endocrinology and Metabolism Clinics of North America* 20:153–63.

Schwartz, I. D., Schwartz, K. J., Kousseff, B. G., Bercu, B. B. & Root, A. W. (1990). Endocrinopathies in Cornelia de Lange syndrome. *Journal of Pediatrics* 117:920–3.

Schwartz, M. F., Esterly, N. B., Fretzin, D. F., Pergament, E. & Rozenfeld, I. H. (1977). Hypomelanosis of Ito (incontinentia pigmenti achromians): A neurocutaneous syndrome. *Journal of Pediatrics* 90:236–40.

Schwartz, O. & Jampel, R. S. (1962). Congenital blepharophimosis associated with a unique generalized myopathy. *Archives of Ophthalmology* 68:52–7.

Scott, C. S., Neighbor, W. E. & Brock, D. M. (1992). Physicians' attitudes toward preventive care services: a seven-year prospective cohort study. *American Journal of Preventive Medicine* 8:241–8.

Scriver, C. R., Beaudet, A. L., Sly, W. S. & Valle, D., ed. (1995a). *The Metabolic and Molecular Bases of Inherited Disease*, 7th edn. New York: McGraw-Hill, Inc.

Scriver, C. R., Kaufman, S., Eisensmith, R. C. & Woo, S. L. C. (1995b). The hyperphenylalaninemias. In *The Metabolic and Molecular Bases of Inherited Disease*, 7th edn, ed. C. R. Scriver, A. L. Beaudet, W. S. Sly & D. Valle, pp. 1015–76. New York: McGraw-Hill, Inc.

Scrutton, D. & Baird, G. (1997). Surveillance measures of the hips of children with bilateral cerebral palsy. *Archives of Disease in Childhood* 76:381–4.

Seckel, H. P. G. (1960). *Bird-headed Dwarfs*, p. 241 Springfield IL: Charles C. Thomas.

Seegmiller, J. E., Rosenbloom, F. M. & Kelley, W. N. (1967). Enzyme defect associated with a sex-linked human neurological disorder and excessive purine synthesis. *Science* 155:1682–4.

Segal, S. & Berry, G.T. (1995). Disorders of galactose metabolism. In *The Metabolic and Molecular Bases of Inherited Disease*, 7th edn, ed. C. R. Scriver, A. L. Beaudet, W. S. Sly & D. Valle, pp. 967–1000. New York: McGraw-Hill, Inc.

Seller, M. (1994). Risks in spina bifida. *Developmental Medicine and Child Neurology* 36:1021–5.

Sells, J. M., Jaffe, K. M. & Hall, J. G. (1996). Amyoplasia, the most common type of arthrogryposis: the potential for good outcome. *Pediatrics* 97:225–31.

Seppala, M. T., Haltia, M. J., Sankila, R. J., Jaaskelainen, J. E. & Heiskanen, O. (1995). Long-term outcome after removal of spinal neurofibroma. *Journal of Neurosurgery* 82:572–7.

Serville, F., Lacombe, D., Saura, R., Billeaud, C. & Sergent, M. P. (1993). Townes–Brocks syndrome in an infant with translocation t(5;16). *Genetic Counseling* 4:109–12.

Sethi, R., Schwartz, R. A. & Janniger, C. K. (1996). Oculocutaneous albinism. *Cutis* 57:397–401.

Shah, P. B., Zasloff, M. A., Drummond, D. & Kaplan, F.S. (1994). Spinal deformity in patients who have fibrodysplasia ossificans progressiva. *Journal of Bone and Joint Surgery* 76:1442–50.

Shah, U. K., Ohlms, L. A., Neault, M. W., Willson, K. D., McGuirt, W. F., Jr., Hobbs, N., Jones, D. T., McGill, T. J. & Healy, G. B. (1998). Otologic management in children with the CHARGE association. *International Journal of Pediatric Otorhinolaryngology* 44:139–47.

Shanley, S., Ratcliffe, J., Hockey, A., Haan, E., Oley, C., Ravine, D., Martin, N., Wicking, C. & Chenevix-Trench, G. (1994). Nevoid basal cell carcinoma syndrome: review of 118 affected individuals. *American Journal of Medical Genetics* 50:282–90.

Shanske, A. & Marion, R. (1998). Central nervous system anomalies in Seckel syndrome: report of a new family and review of the literature. *American Journal of Medical Genetics* 77:250.

Shapira, H., Friedman, E., Mouallem, M. & Farfel, Z. (1996). Familial Albright's hereditary osteodystrophy with hypoparathyroidism: normal structural Gs alpha gene. *Journal of Clinical Endocrinology and Metabolism* 81:1660–2.

Shapiro, B. J. (1983). Down syndrome – a disorder of homeostasis. *American Journal of Medical Genetics* 14:241–69.

Sharland, M., Burch, M., McKenna, W. M. & Paton, M. A. (1992). A clinical study of Noonan syndrome. *Archives of Disease in Childhood* 67:178–183.

Sharland, M., Morgan, M., Smith, G., Burch, M. & Patton, M. A. (1993). Genetic counselling in Noonan syndrome. *American Journal of Medical Genetics* 45:437–40.

Shashi, V., Clark, P., Rogol, A. D. & Wilson, W. G. (1995). Absent pituitary gland in two brothers with an oral-facial-digital syndrome resembling OFDS II and VI: a new type of OFDS? *American Journal of Medical Genetics* 57:22–6.

Shaw, N. J. (1997). Bisphosphonates in osteogenesis imperfecta. *Archives of Disease in Childhood* 77:92–3.

Sheldon, S. H. (1998). Obstructive sleep apnea and growth in children with cleft palate. *Journal of Pediatrics* 132:1078–9.

Shepard, T. H. (1992). *Catalog of Teratogenic Agents*, 5th edn., Baltimore: Johns Hopkins University Press.

Shofner, J. M. & Wallace, D. C. (1995). Oxidative phosphorylation diseases. In *The Metabolic and Molecular Bases of Inherited Disease*, 7th edn, ed. C. R. Scriver, A. L. Beaudet, W. S. Sly & D. Valle, pp. 1535–1609. New York: McGraw-Hill, Inc.

Shohat, M., Flaum, E., Cobb, S. R., Lachman, R., Rubin, C., Ash, C. & Rimoin, D. L. (1993). Hearing loss and temporal bone structure in achrondroplasia. *American Journal of Medical Genetics* 45:548–51.

Shohat, M., Tick, D., Barakat, S., Bu, X., Melmed, S. & Rimoin, D. L. (1996). Short-term recombinant human growth hormone treatment increases growth rate in achondroplasia. *Journal of Clinical Endocrinology and Metabolism* 81:4033–7.

Shprintzen, R. J., Goldberg, R. B., Lewin, M. L., Sidoti, E. J., Berkman, M. D., Argamaso, R. V. & Young, D. (1978). A new syndrome involving cleft palate, cardiac anomalies, typical facies, and learning disabilities: velo-cardio-facial syndrome. *Cleft Palate Journal* 15:56–62.

Shprintzen, R. J. & Singer, L. (1992). Upper airway obstruction and the Robin sequence. *International Anesthesiology Clinics* 30:109–14.

Shurtleff, D. (1986). Selection process for infants. In *Myelodysplasias and Exotrophies: Significance, Prevention, and Treatment*, ed. D. Shurtleff, pp. 89–115. Orlando, Florida: Grune and Stratton.

Shurtleff, D., Lemire, R. & Warkany, J. (1986). Embryology, etiology, and epidemiology. In *Myelodysplasias and Exotrophies: Significance, Prevention, and Treatment*, ed. D. Shurtleff, pp. 39–64. Orlando, Florida: Grune and Stratton.

Siebert, J. W., Anson, G. & Longmaker, M. T. (1996). Microsurgical correction of facial asymmtery in 60 consecutive cases. *Plastic and Reconstructive Surgery* 97:354–63.

Siegel, P. T., Clopper, R. & Stabler, B. (1998). The psychological consequences of Turner syndrome and review of the National Cooperative Growth Study psychological substudy. *Pediatrics* 102:488–91.

Sigaudy, S. (1998). Costello syndrome. *Journal of Medical Genetics* 35:238–40.

Sillence, D. O., Senn, A. & Danks, D. M. (1979). Genetic heterogeneity in osteogenesis imperfecta. *Journal of Medical Genetics* 16:101–16.

Silverman, D. I., Burton, K. J., Gray, J., Bosner, M. S., Kouchoukos, N. T., Roman, M. J., Boxer, M., Devereux, R. B. & Tsipouras, P. (1995). Life expectancy in the Marfan syndrome. *American Journal of Cardiology* 75:157–60.

Simonian, P. T. & Staheli, L. T. (1995). Periarticular fractures after manipulation for knee contractures in children. *Journal of Pediatric Orthopedics* 15:288–91.

Singer, G. H. S. (1991). *The evolution of models of family adaptation to disability.* Unpublished manuscript. Hood Center for Family. Dartmouth Medical School. Lebanon, NH.

Singer, G. H. S. & Irvin, L. K. (1991). Supporting families of persons with severe disabilities: emerging findings, practices, and questions. In *Critical Issues in the Lives of People With Severe Disabilities*, ed. L. H. Meyer, C. A. Peck & L. Brown, pp. 271–312. Baltimore: Paul Brookes.

Sirotnak, J., Brodsky, L. & Pizzuto, M. (1995). Airway obstruction in the Crouzon syndrome: case report and review of the literature. *International Journal of Pediatric Otorhinolaryngology* 31:235–46.

Sison, C. G., Ostrea, E. M., Jr., Reyes, M. P. & Salari, V. (1997). The resurgence of congenital syphilis: a cocaine-related problem. *Journal of Pediatrics* 130:289–92.

Skovby, F. (1993). The homocystinurias. In *Connective Tissue and its Heritable Disorders*, ed. P. M. Royce & B. Steinmann, Ch. 15. New York: Wiley–Liss.

Sloan, T. B. & Kaye. C. I. (1991). Rumination risk of aspiration of gastric contents in the Prader–Willi syndrome. *Anesthesia and Analgesia* 73:492–5.

Smit, G. P. (1993). The long-term outcome of patients with glycogen storage disease type Ia. *European Journal of Pediatrics* 152 (Suppl. 1):S52–S55.

Smith, A. C., Dykens, E. & Greenberg, F. (1998a). Behavioral phenotype of Smith–Magenis syndrome (del 17p11.2). *American Journal of Medical Genetics* 81:179–85.

Smith, A. C., Dykens, E. & Greenberg, F. (1998b). Sleep disturbance in Smith–Magenis syndrome (del 17 p11.2). *American Journal of Medical Genetics* 81:186–91.

Smith, D. W., Lemli, L. & Opitz, J. M. (1964). A newly recognized syndrome of multiple congenital anomalies. *Journal of Pediatrics* 64:210–17.

Smullen, S., Willcox, T., Wetmore, R. & Zackai, E. (1994). Otologic manifestations of neurofibromatosis. *Laryngoscope* 104:663–5.

Smyth, C. M. & Bremner, W. J. (1998). Klinefelter syndrome. *Archives of Internal Medicine* 158:1309–14.

Snider, R. L. (1994). Unusual presentation of a third ventricular cyst in a patient with basal cell nevus syndrome. *Pediatric Dermatology* 11:323–6.

Soekarman, D., Cobben, J., Vogels, M. A., Spauwen, P. H. & Fryns, J. P. (1995). Variable expression of the popliteal pterygium in two 3-generation families. *Clinical Genetics* 47:169–74.

Soekarman, D. & Fryns, J. P. (1994). Corpus callosum agenesis in Coffin–Lowry syndrome. *Genetic Counseling* 5:77–80.

Solomon, L. M. & Esterly, N. B. (1975). Epidermal and other congenital organoid nevi. *Current Problems in Pediatrics* 6:3–56.

Soper, R., Chaloupka, J. C., Fayad, P. B., Greally, J. M., Shaywitz, B. A., Awad, I. A. & Pober, B. R. (1995). Ischemic stroke and intracranial multifocal cerebral arteriopathy in Williams syndrome. *Journal of Pediatrics* 126:945–8.

Sørensen, K. (1992). Physical and mental development of adolescent males with Klinefelter syndrome. *Hormone Research* 37(suppl. 3):55–61.

Sørenson, K. & Nielsen, J. (1977). Twenty psychotic males with Klinefelter's syndrome. *Acta Psychiatrica Scandinavica* 56:249–55.

Sorge, G., Polizzi, A., Ruggieri, M., Smilari, P. & Mauceri, L. (1996). Early fatal course in three brothers with FG syndrome. *Clinical Pediatrics* 35:365–7.

Sotos, J. F., Dodge, P. R., Muirhead, D., Crawford, J. D. & Talbot, N. B. (1964). Cerebral gigantism in childhood. *New England Journal of Medicine* 271:109–16.

Soyer, A. D. & McConnell, J. R. (1995). Progressive scoliosis in Dubowitz syndrome. *Spine* 20:2335–7.

Spahis, J. (1994). Sleepless nights. Obstructive sleep apnea in the pediatric patient. *Pediatric Nursing* 20:469–72.

Sperli, D., Concolino, D. Barbato, C. Strisciuglio, P. & Andria, G. (1993). Long survival of a patient with Marshall–Smith syndrome without respiratory complications. *Journal of Medical Genetics* 30:877–9.

Sperling, M. A. & Menon, R. K. (1997). Infant of the diabetic mother. *Current Therapy in Endocrinology and Metabolism* 6:405–9.

Spigelman, A. D., Arese, P. & Phillips, R. K. (1995). Polyposis: the Peutz–Jeghers syndrome. *British Journal of Surgery* 82:1311–14.

Spina Bifida Association of America (1994). *Preventing Secondary Conditions Associated with Spina Bifida or Cerebral Palsy*. Crystal City VA: Spina Bifida Association of America.

Sporik, R., Dinwiddie, R. & Wallis, C. (1997). Lung involvement in the multisystem syndrome CHARGE association. *European Respiratory Journal* 10:1354–5.

Spranger, J. (1987). Mini review: Inborn errors of complex carbohydrate metabolism. *American Journal of Medical Genetics* 28:489–99.

Spranger, J. W., Opitz, J. M. & Bidder, V. (1971). Heterogeneity of chondrodysplasia punctata. *Human Genetics* 11:190–212.

Spranger, J., Benirschke, K., Hall, J. G., Lenz, W., Lowry, R. B., Opitz, J. M., Pinsky, L., Schwarzacher, H. G. & Smith, D. W. (1982). Errors of morphogenesis: Concepts and terms. Recommendations of an international working group. *Journal of Pediatrics* 100:160–7.

Spranger, J., Winterpacht, A. & Zabel, B. (1994). The type II collagenopathies: a spectrum of chondrodysplasias. *European Journal of Pediatrics* 153:56–65.

Spritz, R. A. (1997). Piebaldism, Waardenburg syndrome, and related disorders of melanocyte development. *Seminars in Cutaneous Medicine and Surgery* 16:15–23.

Srivastava, V. K. (1995). Wound healing in trophic ulcers in spina bifida patients. *Journal of Neurosurgery* 82:40–3.

Staheli, L. T., Hall, J. G., Jaffe, K. M. & Paholke, D. O. (1998). *Arthrogryposis: A Text Atlas*. Cambridge: Cambridge University Press.

Staley, L.W., Hull, C. E., Mazzocco, M. M., Thibodeau, S. N., Snow, K., Wilson, V. L., Taylor, A., McGavran, L., Weiner, D., Riddle, J., O'Connor, R. & Hagerman, R. J. (1993). Molecular-clinical correlations in children and adults with fragile X syndrome. *American Journal of Diseases of Children* 147:723–6.

Stankovic, B., Krstic, V. Stankov, B., Jojic, L. Nagulic, M. & Artiko, G. (1994). Jackson–Weiss syndrome registered in four successive generations. The facies of Crouzon's syndrome with foot abnormalities. *Documenta Ophthalmologica* 85:281–6.

Stanley, C. S., Thelin, J. W. & Miles, J. H. (1988). Mixed hearing loss in Larsen syndrome. *Clinical Genetics* 33:395–8.

Staples, A. J., Sutherland, G. R., Haan, E. A. & Clisby, S. (1991). Epidemiology of Down syndrome in South Australia, 1960–89. *American Journal of Human Genetics*, 49:1014–24.

Stark, M., Assum, G. & Krone, W. (1995). Single-cell PCR performed with neurofibroma Schwann cells reveals the presence of both alleles of the neurofibromatosis type 1 (NF1) gene. *Human Genetics* 96:619–23.

Stein, D. J., Keating, J., Zar, H. J. & Hollander, E. (1994). A survey of the phenomenology and pharmacotherapy of compulsive and impulsive-aggressive symptoms in Prader–Willi syndrome. *Journal of Neuropsychiatry and Clinical Neurosciences* 6:23–9.

Steinberger, D., Mulligan, J. B. & Muller, U. (1995). Predisposition for cysteine substitutions in the immunoglobulin-like chain of FGFR2 in Crouzon syndrome. *Human Genetics* 96:113–15.

Steinbok, P. (1995). Dysraphic lesions of the cervical spinal cord. *Neurosurgery Clinics of North America* 6:367–76.

Steinlin, M. I., Nadal, D., Eich, G. F., Martin, E. & Boltshauser, E. J. (1996). Late intrauterine cytomegalovirus infection: clinical and neuroimaging findings. *Pediatric Neurology* 15:249–53.

Steinmann, B., Royce, P. M. & Superti-Furga, A. (1993). The Ehlers–Danlos syndrome. In *Connective Tissue and its Heritable Disorders,* ed. P. M. Royce & B. Steinmann, Ch. 11. New York: Wiley–Liss.

Stephan, M. J., Hall, B. D., Smith, D. W. & Cohen, M. M., Jr. (1975). Macrocephaly in association with unusual cutaneous angiomatosis. *Journal of Pediatrics* 87:353–9.

Stevens, C. A. & Bhakta, M. G. (1995). Cardiac abnormalities in the Rubinstein–Taybi syndrome. *American Journal of Medical Genetics* 59:346–8.

Stevens, C. A., Hennekam, R. C. M. & Blackburn, B. L. (1990). Growth in the Rubinstein–Taybi syndrome. *American Journal of Medical Genetics* suppl. 6:51–5.

Stevens, C. A., McClanahan, C., Steck, A., Shiel, F. O. & Carey, J. C. (1994). Pulmonary hypoplasia in the Fraser cryptophthalmos syndrome. *American Journal of Medical Genetics* 52:427–31.

Stevenson, R. D. (1995). Use of segmental measures to estimate stature in children with cerebral palsy. *Archives of Pediatric and Adolescent Medicine* 149:658–62.

Stevenson, R. E. (1993). The environmental basis of human anomalies. In *Human Malformations and Related Anomalies,* ed. R. E. Stevenson, J. G. Hall & R. M. Goodman, pp. 137–68. New York: Oxford University Press.

Stevenson, R. E., Hall, J. G. & Goodman, R. M., ed. (1993). *Human Malformations and Related Anomalies.* New York: Oxford University Press.

Stiehm, E. R. (1995). Now is the time for routine voluntary HIV testing of pregnant women. *Archives of Pediatric and Adolescent Medicine* 149:484–5.

Strange, P. R. & Lang, P. G., Jr. (1992). Long-term management of basal cell nevus syndrome with topical tretinoin and 5-fluorouracil. *Journal of the American Academy of Dermatology* 27:842–5.

Stratton, R. F., Young, R. S., Heiman, H. S. & Carter, J. M. (1993). Fryns syndrome. *American Journal of Medical Genetics* 45:562–4.

Stray-Gunderson, K. (1986). *Babies with Down Syndrome: A New Parents guide.* Kensington, MD: Woodbine House.

Streissguth, A. P., Aase, J. M., Clarren, S. K., Randels, S. P., LaDue, R. A. & Smith, D. F. (1991). Fetal alcohol syndrome in adolescents and adults. *Journal of the American Medical Association* 265:1961–7.

Streissguth, A. P., Bookstein, F. L., Barr, H. M., Press, S. & Sampson, P. D. (1998). A fetal alcohol behavioral scale. *Alcoholism, Clinical & Experimental Research* 22:325–33.

Strömland, K. (1987). Ocular involvement in the fetal alcohol syndrome. *Survey of Ophthalmology* 31:277–84.

Suevo, D. M. (1997). The infant of the diabetic mother. *Neonatal Network* 16:25–33.

Sujansky, E. & Conradi, S. (1995). Outcome of Sturge–Weber syndrome in 52 adults. *American Journal of Medical Genetics* 57:35–45.

Sulik, K. K., Johnston, M. C. & Webb, M. A. (1981). Fetal alcohol syndrome: Embryogenesis in a mouse model. *Science* 214:936–8.

Summers, J. A., Behr, S. K. & Turnbull, A. P. (1989). Positive adaptation and coping strengths of families who have children with disabilities. In *Support for Caregiving Families*, ed. G. H. S. Singer & L. K. Irvin, pp. 27–40. Baltimore: Paul Brookes.

Suomalainen, A. (1997). Mitochondrial DNA and disease. *Annals of Medicine* 29:235–46.

Suresh, D. (1991). Posterior spinal fusion in Sotos' syndrome. *British Journal of Anaesthesia* 66:728–32.

Sybert, V. P. (1990). Mosaicism in Turner syndrome. *Growth Genetics and Hormones* 6:4–8.

Sybert, V. P. (1994). Hypomelanosis of Ito: a description, not a diagnosis. *Journal of Investigative Dermatology* 103 (suppl 5):141S–143S.

Tada, H., Kurita, T., Ohe, T., Shimomura, K., Ishihara, T., Yamada, Y. & Osawa, N. (1995). Glycogen storage disease type III associated with ventricular tachycardia. *American Heart Journal* 130:911–12.

Tanaka, K., Sato, A., Naito, T., Kuramochi, K., Itabashi, H. & Takemura, Y. (1992). Noonan syndrome presenting growth hormone neurosecretory dysfunction. *Internal Medicine* 31:908–11.

Tanboga, I., Pince, S. & Duzdar, L. D. (1992). Dental management of a child with EEC syndrome. *International Journal of Paediatric Dentistry* 2:99–103.

Tasker, R. C., Dundas, I., Laverty, A., Fletcher, M., Lane, R. & Stocks, J. (1998). Distinct patterns of respiratory difficulty in young children with achondroplasia: a clinical, sleep, and lung function study. *Archives of Disease in Childhood* 79:99–108.

Tassabehji, M., Newton, V. E., Liu, X. Z., Brady, A., Donnai, D., Krajewska-Walasek, M., Murday, V., Norman, A., Obersztyn, E. & Reardon, W. (1995). The mutational spectrum in Waardenburg syndrome. *Human Molecular Genetics* 4:2131–7.

Tassabehji, M., Strachan, T., Sharland, M., Colley, A., Donnai, D., Harris, R. & Thakker, N. (1993). Tandem duplication within a neurofibromatosis type 1 (NF1) gene exon in a family with features of Watson syndrome and Noonan syndrome. *American Journal of Human Genetics* 53:90–5.

Tavormina, P. L., Shiang, R., Thompson, L. M.. Zhu, Y. Z., Wilkin, D. J., Lachman, R. S., Wilcox, W. R.. Rimoin, D. L., Cohn, D. H. & Wasmuth, J. J. (1995). Thanatophoric dysplasia (types I and II) caused by distinct mutations in fibroblast growth factor receptor 3. *Nature Genetics* 9:321–8.

Taybi, H. (1962). Generalized skeletal dysplasia with multiple anomalies. *American Journal of Roentgenology, Radium Therapy, and Nuclear Medicine* 88:450–6.

Taylor, A. I. (1968). Autosomal trisomy syndromes: a detailed study of 27 cases of Edwards' syndrome and 27 cases of Patau's syndrome. *Journal of Medical Genetics* 5:227–52.

Taylor, A. K., Safanda, J. F., Fall, M. Z., Quince, C., Lang, K. A., Hull, C. E. Carpenter, I., Staley, L. W. & Hagerman, R. J. (1994). Molecular predictors of cognitive involvement in female carriers of fragile X syndrome. *Journal of the American Medical Association* 271:507–14.

Taylor, G. A. & Madsen, J. R. (1996). Neonatal hydrocephalus: hemodynamic response to fontanelle compression – correlation with intracranial pressure and need for shunt placement. *Radiology* 201:685–9.

Teebi, A. S., Rucquoi, J. K. & Meyn, M. S. (1993). Aarskog syndrome: report of a family with review and discussion of nosology. *American Journal of Medical Genetics* 46:501–9.

Tekkok, I. H. (1996). Syringomyelia as a complication of Goldenhar syndrome. *Childs Nervous System* 12:291.

Tellier, A. L., Lyonnet, S., Cormier-Daire, V., de Lonlay, P., Abadie, V., Baumann C., Bonneau, D., Labrune, P., Lacombe, D., Le Merrer M., Nivelon, A,. Philip, N., Briard, M. L. & Munnich, A. (1996). Increased paternal age in CHARGE association. *Clinical Genetics* 50:548–50.

Temtamy, S. A. (1966). Carpenter's syndrome: Acrocephalopolysyndactyly. An autosomal recessive syndrome. *Journal of Pediatrics* 69:111–20.

Thomas, G. H. & Beaudet, A. L. (1995). Disorders of glycoprotein degradation and structure: α-mannosidosis, β-mannosidosis, fucosidosis, sialidosis, aspartylglucosaminuria, and carbohydrate-deficient glycoprotein syndrome. In *The Metabolic and Molecular Bases of Inherited Disease*, 7th edn, ed. C. R. Scriver, A. L. Beaudet, W. S. Sly & D. Valle, pp. 2529–63. New York: McGraw-Hill, Inc.

Thomas, I. T., Frias, J. L., Cantu, E. S., Lafer, C. Z.. Flannery, D. B. & Graham, J. G., Jr. (1989). Association of pigmentary anomalies with chromosomal and genetic mosaicism and chimerism. *American Journal of Human Genetics* 45:193–205.

Thomas, I. T., Frias, J. L., Felix, V., Sanchez de Leon, L., Hernandez, R. A. & Jones, M. C. (1986). Isolated and syndromic crypophthalmos. *American Journal of Medical Genetics* 25:85–98.

Thomas, P. K. (1992). Autonomic involvement in the inherited neuropathies. *Clinical Autonomic Research* 2:51–6.

Thompson, R. S., Taplin, S. H., McAfee, T. A., Mandelson, M. T. & Smith, A. E. (1995). Primary and secondary prevention services in clinical practice. *Journal of the American Medical Association* 271:1130–5.

Thyen, U., Aksu, F., Bartsch, O. & Herb, E. (1992). Acrocallosal syndrome: association with cystic malformation of the brain and neurodevelopmental aspects. *Neuropediatrics* 23:292–6.

Tinker, A., Uren, N. & Schofield, J. (1989). Severe pulmonary hypertension in Ullrich–Noonan syndrome. *British Heart Journal* 62:74–7.

Topaloglu, H., Serdaroglu, A., Okan, M., Guceyener, K. & Topcu, M. (1993). Improvement of myotonia with carbamazepine in three cases with the Schwartz–Jampel syndrome. *Neuropediatrics* 24:232–4.

Townes, P. L. & Brocks, E. R. (1972). Hereditary syndrome of imperforate anus with hand, foot, and ear anomalies. *Journal of Pediatrics* 81:321–6.

Treacher Collins, E. (1960). Cases with symmetrical congenital notches in the outer part of each lid and defective development of the malar bones. *Transactions of the Ophthalmological Society, UK* 20:190–2.

Trifiletti, R. R., Incorporata, G., Polizzi, A., Cocuzza, M. D., Bolan, E. A. & Parano, E. (1995). Aicardi syndrome with multiple tumors; a case report with literature review. *Brain and Development* 17:283–5.

Trivier, E., De Cesare, D., Jacquot, S., Pannetier, S., Zackai, E., Young, I., Mandel, J. L., Sassone-Corsi P. & Hanauer, A. (1997). Mutations in the kinase Rsk-2 associated with Coffin–Lowry syndrome. *Nature* 384:567–70.

Trousdale, R. T. (1998). Fetal hydantoin syndrome: an unusual cause of hip dysplasia. *Orthopedics* 21:210–12.

Tsang, V. T., Pawade, A., Karl, T. R. & Mee, R. B. (1994). Surgical management of Marfan syndrome in children. *Journal of Cardiac Surgery* 9:50–4.

Tsao, C. Y. & Westman, J. A. (1997). Infantile spasms in two children with Williams syndrome. *American Journal of Medical Genetics* 71:54–6.

Tsao, C. Y., Sommer, A. & Hamoudi, A. B. (1993). Aicardi syndrome, metastatic angiosarcoma of the leg, and scalp lipoma. *American Journal of Medical Genetics* 45:594–6.

Tsuchiya, K., Forsythe, M., Robin, N. H. & Tunnessen, W. W., Jr. (1998). Picture of the month. Fragile X syndrome. *Archives of Pediatric and Adolescent Medicine* 152:89–90.

Tsukahara, M. & Opitz, J. M. (1996). Dubowitz syndrome: review of 141 cases including 36 previously unreported patients. *American Journal of Medical Genetics* 63:277–89.

Tsusaki, B. & Mayhew, J. F. (1998). Anaesthetic implications of Cornelia de Lange syndrome. *Paediatric Anaesthesia* 8:181.

Turk, J. (1995). Fragile X syndrome. *Archives of Disease in Childhood* 72:3–5.

Turken, A., Balci, S., Senocak, M. E. & Hicsonmez, A. (1996). A large inguinal hernia with undescended testes and micropenis in Robinow syndrome. *Clinical Dysmorphology* 5:175–8.

Turner, G., Robinson, H., Wake, S., Laing, S. & Partington, M. (1997). Case finding for the fragile X syndrome and its consequences. *British Medical Journal* 315:1223–4.

Tyrala, E. E. (1996). The infant of the diabetic mother. *Obstetrics and Gynecology Clinics of North America* 23:221–41.

U. S. Department of Health and Human Services. (1987). *Surgeon General's Report on Children with Special Health Care Needs*. DHHS Publication #HRS/D/MC87–2. Rockville, MD.

U. S. Public Health Service. (1991). *Healthy People 2000: National Health Promotion and Disease Prevention Objectives*. Washington, DC: U.S. Government Printing Office, PHS 91–50212.

U. S. Public Health Service. (1994). *Put Prevention Into Practice Education and Action Kit*. Washington, DC: U.S. Government Printing Office. #017–001–00492–8.

Udwin, O. & Yule, W. (1991). A cognitive and behavioral phenotype in Williams syndrome. *Journal of Clinical and Experimental Neuropsychology* 13:232–44.

Udwin, O., Howlin, P., Davies, M. & Mannion, E. (1998). Community care for adults with

Williams syndrome: how families cope and the availability of support networks. *Journal of Intellectual and Disability Research* 42:238–45.

Uitto, J., Fazio, M. J. & Christiano, A. M. (1993). Cutis laxa and premature aging syndromes. In *Connective Tissue and its Heritable Disorders*, ed. P.M. Royce & B. Steinmann, Ch. 14. New York: Wiley–Liss.

Unuvar, E., Oguz, F., Sahin, K., Nayir, A., Ozbey, H. & Sidal, M. (1998). Coexistence of VATER association and recurrent urolithiasis: a case report. *Pediatric Nephrology* 12:141–3.

Usowicz, A.G., Golabi, M. & Curry, C. (1986). Upper airway obstruction in infants with fetal alcohol syndrome. *American Journal of Diseases of Children* 140:1039–41.

Van Den Berg, D. J. & Francke, U. (1993). Roberts syndrome: a review of 100 cases and a new rating system for severity. *American Journal of Medical Genetics* 47:1104–23.

Van Hove, J. L., Spiridigliozzi, G. A., Heinz, R., McConkie-Rosell, A., Iofolla, A. K. & Kahler, S. G. (1995). Fryns syndrome survivors and neurologic outcome. *American Journal of Medical Genetics* 39:334–40.

Van Lie Peters, E. M., Aronson, D. C. Everts, V. & Dooren, L. J. (1993). Failure of calcitriol treatment in a patient with malignant osteopetrosis. *European Journal of Pediatrics* 152:818–21.

Vari, R., Puca, A. & Meglio, M. (1996). Cleidocranial dysplasia and syringomyelia. Case report. *Journal of Neurosurgical Science* 40:125–8.

Vaughan, W. B., Sanders, D. W., Grosfeld, J. L., Plumley, D. A., Rescorla, F. J., Scherer, L. R. III, West, K. W. & Breitfeld, P. P. (1995). Favorable outcome in children with Beckwith–Wiedemann syndrome and intraabdominal malignant tumors. *Journal of Pediatric Surgery* 30:1042–4.

Vellman, R. A. (1990). *Meeting the Needs of People with Disabilities. A Guide for Librarians, Educators and Other Service Professionals*. Pheonix, AZ: Oryx Press.

Verkh, Z., Russell, M. & Miller, C. A. (1995). Osteogenesis imperfecta type II: microvascular changes in the CNS. *Clinical Neuropathology* 14:154–8.

Viljoen, D. (1994). Congenital contractural arachnodactyly (Beals syndrome). *Journal of Medical Genetics* 31:640–3.

Vits, L., van Camp, G., Coucke, P., Wilson, G., Schrander-Stumpel, C., Lyonnet, S., Munnich, A., Schwartz, C. E. & Willems, P. J. (1994). MASA syndrome is allelic to X-linked hydrocephalus at the L1CAM locus. *Nature Genetics* 7:108–13.

Volpe, E. P. (1986). Is Down syndrome a modern disease? *Perspectives in Biology and Medicine* 29:423–36.

Vortkamp, A., Gessler, M. & Grzeschik, K.-H. (1991). GLI3 zinc-finger gene interrupted by translocations in Greig syndrome families. *Nature* 352:539–40.

Waber, L. (1990). Inborn errors of metabolism. *Pediatric Annals* 19:105–18.

Waggoner, D. D., Buist, N. R. & Donnell, G. N. (1990). Long-term prognosis in galactosemia: results of a survey of 350 cases. *Journal of Inborn Errors of Metabolism* 13:802–8.

Wagner, A. (1997). Distinguishing vesicular and pustular disorders in the neonate. *Current Opinions in Pediatrics* 9:396–405.

Wainwright, H., Bowen, R. & Radcliffe, M. (1995). Lipoma of corpus callosum associated with dysraphic lesions and trisomy 13. *American Journal of Medical Genetics* 57:10–13.

Warner, R. H. & Rosett, H. L. (1975). The effects of drinking on offspring. An historical survey of the American and British literature. *Journal of Studies on Alcohol* 36:1395–1420.

Warner, T. G. & O'Brien J. S. (1983). Genetic defects in glycoprotein metabolism. *Annual Review of Genetics* 17:395–441.

Warner, T. T. & Schapira, A. H. (1997). Genetic counselling in mitochondrial diseases. *Current Opinions in Neurology* 10:408–12.

Warren, S. T. & Nelson, D. L. (1994). Advances in molecular analysis of fragile X syndrome. *Journal of the American Medical Association* 271:536–42.

Washington, K., Rourk, M. H., Jr., McDonagh, D. & Oldham, K. T. (1993). Inflammatory cloacogenic polyp in a child: part of the spectrum of solitary rectal ulcer syndrome. *Pediatric Pathology* 13:409–14.

Watanabe, H., Umeda, M., Seki, T. & Ishikawa, I. (1993). Clinical and laboratory studies of severe periodontal disease in an adolescent associated with hypophosphatasia. A case report. *Journal of Periodontology* 64:174–80.

Waterhouse, W. J., Enzenauer, R. W. & Martyak, A. P. (1993). Successful strabismus surgery in a child with Moebius syndrome. *Annals of Ophthalmology* 25:292–4.

Waters, K. A., Everett, F., Sillence, D., Fagan, E. & Sullivan, C. E. (1993). Breathing abnormalities in sleep I achondroplasia. *Archives of Disease in Childhood* 69:191–6.

Watt-Morse, M. L., Laifer, S. A. & Hill, L. M. (1995). The natural history of fetal cytomegalovirus infection as assessed by serial ultrasound and fetal blood sampling: a case report. *Prenatal Diagnosis* 15:567–70.

Weaver, D. D., Graham, C. B., Thomas, I. T. & Smith, D. W. (1974). A new overgrowth syndrome with accelerated skeletal maturation, unusual facies, and camptodactyly. *Journal of Pediatrics* 84:547–52.

Weaver, D. D., Mapstone, C. L. & P.-L. Yu. (1986). The VATER association: Analysis of 46 patients. *American Journal of Diseases of Children* 140:225–9.

Webster, W. S. (1998). Teratogen update: congenital rubella. *Teratology* 58:13–23.

Weinhouse, E., Riggs, T. W. & Aughton, D. J. (1995). Isolated bicuspid aortic valve in a newborn with Down syndrome. *Clinical Pediatrics* 34:116–17.

Weissgold, D. J., Maguire, A. M., Kalin, N. S. & Hertle, R. W. (1995). Persistent hyperplastic primary vitreous in association with Aicardi syndrome. *Journal of Pediatric Ophthalmology and Strabismus* 32:52–4.

Weksberg, R. & Squire, J. A. (1996). Molecular biology of Beckwith–Wiedemann syndrome. *Medical and Pediatric Oncology* 27:462–9.

Weller, T. H. (1971). The cytomegaloviruses: ubiquitous agents with protean clinical manifestations. *New England Journal of Medicine* 285:203–14.

Wendel, U., Schroten, H., Burdach, S. & Wahn, V. (1993). Glycogen storage disease type Ib: infectious complications and measures for prevention. *European Journal of Pediatrics* 152 (Suppl. 1):S49–S51.

Weng, E. Y., Mortier, G. R & Graham, J. M., Jr. (1995). Beckwith–Wiedemann syndrome. An update and review for the primary pediatrician. *Clinical Pediatrics* 34:317–32.

Wertheimer, E., Lu, S. P., Backeljauw, P. F., Davenport, M. L. & Taylor, S. I. (1993). Homozygous deletion of the human insulin receptor gene results in leprechaunism. *Nature Genetics* 5:71–3.

Westaby, S. (1995). Management of aortic dissection. *Current Opinion in Cardiology* 10:505–10.

Wheeler, A. H. (1997). Therapeutic uses of botulinum toxin. *American Family Physician* 55:541–5.

White, C. C., Koplan, J. P. & Orenstein W. A. (1985). Benefits, risks and costs of immmunization for measles, mumps and rubella. *American Journal of Public Health* 75:739–44.

Wight, J. N., Jr. & Salem, D. (1995). Sudden cardiac death and the "athlete's heart." *Archives of Internal Medicine* 155:1473–80.

Wildervanck, L. S. (1962). Hereditary malformations of the ear in three generations. *Acta Oto-Laryngologia* 54:533–60.

Wilkie, A. O. & Wall, S. A. (1996). Craniosynostosis: novel insights into pathogenesis and treatment. *Current Opinions in Neurology* 9:146–52.

Wilkin, D., Hallam, L. & Doggett, M.-A. (1993). *Measures of Need and Outcome for Primary Health Care*. Oxford: Oxford University Press.

Williams, C. A. & Frias, J. L. (1982). The Angelman (happy puppet) syndrome. *American Journal of Medical Genetics* 11:453–60.

Williams, C. J., Smith, R. A., Ball, R. J. & Wilkinson, H. (1997). Hypercalcaemia in osteogenesis imperfecta treated with pamidronate. *Archives of Disease in Childhood* 76:169–70.

Williams, C. R., O'Flynn, E., Clarke, N. M. & Morris, R. J. (1996). Torticollis secondary to ocular pathology. *Journal of Bone and Joint Surgery, Britain* 78:620–4.

Williams, D. W. III & Elster, A. D. (1992). Cranial CT and MR in the Klippel–Trenauney–Weber syndrome. *American Journal of Neuroradiology* 13:291–4.

Williams, J. C. P., Barratt-Boyes, B. G. & Lowe, J. B. (1961). Supravalvular aortic stenosis. *Circulation* 24:1311–18.

Williams, M. S., Josephson, K. D. & Wargowski, D. S. (1993). Marden–Walker syndrome: a case report and critical review of the literature. *Clinical Dysmorphology* 2:211–19.

Williams, M. S., Rooney B. L., Williams, J., Josephson, K. & Pauli. R. (1994). Investigation of thermoregulatory characteristics in patients with Prader–Willi syndrome. *American Journal of Medical Genetics* 49:302–7.

Williamson, M. L., Koch, R., Azen, C. & Chang, C. (1981). Correlates of intelligence test results in treated phenylketonuria children. *Pediatrics* 68:161–7.

Wills, K. (1993). Neuropsychological functioning in children with spina bifida and/or hydrocephalus. *Journal of Clinical Child Psychology* 22:247–65.

Wills, K., Holmbeck, G., Dillon, K. & McClone, D. (1990). Intelligence and achievement in children with myelomeningocele. *Journal of Pediatric Psychology* 15:161–76.

Wilmshurst, S., Ward, K., Adams, J. E., Langton, C. M. & Mughal, M. Z. (1996). Mobility status and bone density in cerebral palsy. *Archives of Disease in Childhood* 75:164–5.

Wilson, D. I., Burn, J., Scambler, P. & Goodship. J. (1993). DiGeorge syndrome: part of CATCH 22. *Journal of Medical Genetics* 30:852–6.

Wilson, G. N. (1983). Cranial defects in the Goldenhar syndrome. *American Journal of Medical Genetics* 14:435–43.

Wilson, G. N. (1986). What is Zellweger syndrome? *Journal of Pediatrics* 109:398.

Wilson, G. N. (1988). Heterochrony and human malformation. *American Journal of Medical Genetics* 29:311–21.

Wilson, G. N. (1990). Office approach to the genetics patient. *Pediatric Annals* 19:79–91.

Wilson, G. N. (1992). Genomics of human dysmorphogenesis. *American Journal of Medical Genetics* 42:187–96.

Wilson, G. N. (1998). Thirteen cases of Niikawa–Kuroki syndrome: report and review with emphasis on medical complications and preventive management. *American Journal of Medical Genetics* 79:112–20.

Wilson, G. N., Holmes, R. D., Custer, J., Lipkowitz, J. L., Stover, J., Datta, N. & Hajra. A. (1986). Zellweger syndrome: Diagnostic assays, syndrome delineation, and potential therapy. *American Journal of Medical Genetics* 24:69–82.

Wilson, G. N., Holmes, R. D. & Hajra, A. K. (1988). Peroxisomal disorders: Clinical commentary and future prospects. *American Journal of Medical Genetics* 30:771–92.

Wilson, G. N., de Chadarévian, J.-P. Kaplan, P. Loehr J.P., Frerman F.E. & Goodman. S.I. (1989). Glutaric aciduria type II: Review of the phenotype and report of an unusual glomerulopathy. *American Journal of Medical Genetics* 32:395–401.

Wilson, G. N., Richards, C. S., Katz, K. & Brookshire, G. S. (1992). Nonspecific X-linked mental retardation with aphasia exhibiting genetic linkage to chromosomal region Xp11. *Journal of Medical Genetics* 29:629–34.

Wilson, L. C., Oude, M. E., Luttikhuis, P., Clayton, P. T., Fraser, W.D. & Tremblath, R. C. (1994). Parental origin of Gs alpha gene mutations in Albright's hereditary osteodystrophy. *Journal of Medical Genetics* 31:835–9.

Wilson, M. E. H. (1995). Assumptions, prevention, and the need for research. *Archives of Pediatric and Adolescent Medicine* 149:356.

Winter, R. M. (1986). Dubowitz syndrome. *Journal of Medical Genetics* 23:11–13.

Winter, R. M., Baraister, M., Laurence, K. M., Donnai, D. & Hall, C. M. (1983). The Weissenbacher–Zweymüller, Stickler, and Marshall syndromes: Further evidence for their identity. *American Journal of Medical Genetics* 16:189–200.

Witlin, A. G., Olson, G. L., Gogola, J. & Hankins, G. D. (1998). Disseminated neonatal herpes infection. *Obstetrics and Gynecology* 92:721.

Witt, D. R., Hoyme, H. E., Zonana, J., Manchester, D. K., Fryns, J. P., Stevenson, J. G., Curry, C. J. & Hall, J. G. (1987). Lymphedema in Noonan syndrome: clues to pathogenesis and prenatal diagnosis and review of the literature. *American Journal of Medical Genetics* 27:841–56.

Witt, D. R., Keena, B. A., Hall, J. G. & Allanson, J. E. (1986). Growth curves for height in Noonan syndrome. *Clinical Genetics* 30:150–3.

Witt, D. R., McGillivaray, B. C., Allanson, J. E., Hughes, H. E., Hathaway, W. E., Zipursky, A. & Hall. J. G. (1988). Bleeding diathesis in Noonan syndrome: a common association. *American Journal of Medical Genetics* 31:305–17.

Witt, P. D. & Marsh, J. L. (1997). Advances in assessing outcome of surgical repair of cleft lip and cleft palate. *Plastic and Reconstructive Surgery* 100:1907–17.

Witt, P. D., March, J. L. Marty-Grames, L., Muntz, H. R. & Gay, W. D. (1995). Management of the hypodynamic velopharynx. *Cleft Palate–Craniofacial Journal* 32:179–87.

Witt, P. D., Myckatyn, T., Marsh, J. L., Grames, L. M. & Dowton, S. B. (1997). Need for velopharyngeal management following palatoplasty: an outcome analysis of syndromic and nonsyndromic patients with Robin sequence. *Plastic and Reconstructive Surgery* 99:1522–9.

Woldorf, J. W. & Johnson, K. (1994). Gross motor development of a 7-year-old girl with trisomy 18. *Clinical Pediatrics* 33:120–2.

Wolf, B. (1995). Disorders of biotin metabolism. In *The Metabolic and Molecular Bases of*

Inherited Disease, 7th edn, ed. C. R. Scriver, A. L. Beaudet, W. S. Sly & D. Valle, pp. 3151–77. New York: McGraw-Hill, Inc.

Wolf, B. & Heard, G. S. (1991). Biotinidase deficiency. *Advances in Pediatrics* 38:1–22.

Wolkstein, M. A., Atkin, A. K., Willner, J. P. & Mindel, J. S. (1983). Diffuse choroidal atrophy and Klinefelter syndrome. *Acta Ophthalmolgica* 61:313–21.

Wong, B. J. & Hashisaki, G. T. (1996). Treatment of Bloom syndrome patients: guidelines and report of a case. *Otolaryngology – Head and Neck Surgery* 114:295–8.

Wong, R. S., Follis, F. M., Shively, B. K. & Wernly, J. A. (1995). Osteogenesis imperfecta and cardiovascular disease. *Annals of Thoracic Surgery* 60:1439–43.

Wood, B. P., Lieberman, E., Landing, B. & Marcus B. (1992). Tuberous sclerosis. *American Journal of Roentgenology* 158:750.

Worthington, S., Colley, A., Fagan, K., Dai, K. & Lipson, A. H. (1997). Anal anomalies: an uncommon feature of velocardiofacial (Shprintzen) syndrome? *Journal of Medical Genetics* 34:79–82.

Wright, C., Healicon, R., English, C. & Burn, J. (1994). Meckel syndrome: what are the minimum diagnostic criteria? *Journal of Medical Genetics* 31:482–5.

Wu, Y. Q., Sutton, V. R., Nickerson, E., Lupski, J. R., Potocki, L., Korenberg, J. R., Greenberg, F., Tassabehji, M. & Shaffer, L. G. (1998). Delineation of the common critical region in Williams syndrome and clinical correlation of growth, heart defects, ethnicity, and parental origin. *American Journal of Medical Genetics* 78:82–9.

Wyse, R. K. H., Al-Mahdawi, H., Burn, J. & Blake, K. (1993). Congenital heart disease in CHARGE association. *Pediatric Cardiology* 14:75–81.

Xu, G., O'Connell, P., Viskochil, D., Cawthon, R., Robertson, M., Culver, M., Dunn, D., Stevens, J., Gesteland, R., White, R. & Weiss R. (1990). The neurofibromatosis type 1 gene encodes a protein related to GAP. *Cell* 62:599–608.

Yagihashi, N., Watanabe, K. & Yagihashi, S. (1995). Transient abnormal myelopoiesis accompanied by hepatic fibrosis in two infants with Down syndrome. *Journal of Clinical Pathology* 48:973–5.

Yamate, T., Kanzaki, S., Tanaka, H., Kubo, T., Moriwake, T., Inoue, M. & Seino, Y. (1993). Growth hormone (GH) treatment in achondroplasia. *Journal of Pediatric Endocrinology* 6:45–52.

Yellon, R. F. (1997). Complications following airway surgery in Noonan syndrome. *Archives of Otolaryngology – Head and Neck Surgery* 123:1341–3.

Yen, I., Khoury, M., Erickson, J., James, L., Waters, G. & Berry, R. (1992). The changing epidemiology of neural tube defects: United States, 1968–1989. *American Journal of Diseases of Children* 146:857–61.

Yoon, P. W., Olney, R. S., Khoury, M. J., Sappenfield, W. M., Chavez, G. F. & Taylor, D. (1996). Contribution of birth defects and genetic diseases to pediatric hospitalizations. A population-based study. *Archives of Pediatric and Adolescent Medicine* 151:1096–103.

Young, I. D. (1988). The Coffin–Lowry syndrome. *Journal of Medical Genetics* 25:344–8.

Young, P. C., Shyr, Y. & Schork, M. A. (1994). The role of the primary care physician in the care of children with serious heart disease. *Pediatrics* 94:284–90.

Zackai, E. H., McDonald-McGinn, D. M., Driscoll, D. A., Emanuel, B. S., Christensen, K. M., Chien, P., Mahboubi, S., Hubbard, A. M., Weinberg, P. & Clark, B. J. III. (1996). Respiratory symptoms may be the first presenting sign of a 22q11.2 deletion: a study of vascular rings. *Proceedings of the Greenwood Genetics Center* 15:49.

Zaunschirm, A. & Muntean, W. (1984). Fetal alcohol syndrome and malignant disease. *European Journal of Pediatrics* 143:160–1.

Zellweger, H. (1987). The cerebro-hepato-renal (Zellweger) syndrome and other peroxisomal disorders. *Developmental Medicine and Child Neurology* 29:821–9.

Zellweger, H. & Schneider, H. J. (1968). Syndrome of hypotonia-hypopigmentia-hypogonadism-obesity (HHHO) or Prader–Willi syndrome. *American Journal of Diseases of Children* 5:588–98.

Zellweger, H. & Soper, R. T. (1979). The Prader–Willi syndrome. *Medical Hygiene* 37:3338–45.

Zimmer-Galler, I. E. & Robertson, D. M. (1995). Long-term observation of retinal lesions in tuberous sclerosis. *American Journal of Ophthalmology* 119:318–24.

Zlotogora, J., Lerer, I., Bar-David, S., Ergaz, Z. & Abeliovich, D. (1995). Homozygosity for Waardenburg syndrome. *American Journal of Human Genetics* 56:1173–8.

Zlotogora, J., Sagi, M., Schuper, A., Leiba, H. & Merin, S. (1992). Variability of Stickler syndrome. *American Journal of Medical Genetics* 42:337–9.

Zonana, J., Rimoin, D. L. & Davis, D. C. (1976). Macrocephaly with multiple lipomas and hemangiomas. *Journal of Pediatrics* 89:600–3.

Index

abdominal CT scan, 427
abdominal ultrasound, 271, 296
absent corpus callosum, 399
absent lacrimal glands, 382
acanthosis nigricans, 224
accelerated aging, 391
accelerated growth, 423
acetaldehyde, 111
achondrogenesis, 249
achondroplasia, complications, 254
achondroplasia, definition, 253
achondroplasia, genetic counseling, 254
achondroplasia, preventive management, 255
acid phosphatase, 251
acidosis, 6, 425, 445, 455
acrocallosal syndrome, 340
acrocephaly, 319
acrocyanosis, 369
activities of daily living, 37
acute monocytic leukemia, 235
acyclovir, 106
adenomatous polyposis coli (APC), 292
ADL scale, 37
adrenal carcinomas, 301
adrenal hyperplasia, 325
adrenal insufficiency, 434
AFP, 64
agenesis of corpus callosum, 435
agenesis of the corpus callosum, 402
aggressive behaviors, 305
Aicardi syndrome, 398
airway obstruction, 322, 334, 424
alanine, 456
Albers–Schonberg syndrome, 251
albinism, 382
alcohol, 114
alcoholic persons, 112
alkaline phosphatase, 250
Alliance of Genetic Support Groups, 142
Alzheimer disease, 150
ambiguous genitalia, 436
amblyopia, 335
American Academy of Pediatrics, 43, 151, 165
amino acid metabolism, 453
amino acid profile, 15
aminoacidopathies, 453

amnion rupture sequence, 80
amniotic band disruptions, 344
amniotic bands, 79, 400
amniotic bands, preventive management, 81
amyoplasia, 400
anesthesia, 225, 227, 306, 325, 397
aneurysm, 366
angiofibromas, 302
angiography, 366
angioid streaks, 360, 369
angiokeratoma, 416
angiokeratoma corporis diffusum universale, 416
angiomyolipomas, 306
angiosarcoma, 295
ankylosis, 400
anophthalmia, 338
anosmia, 252
anticipation, 292
anticipatory guidance, 3, 41
anticoagulant therapy, 366
anticonvulsant medications, 110
anticonvulsant therapy, 115
anticonvulsants, 398
antipyretics, 381
antithrombin III, 434
Antley–Bixler syndrome, 318
aortic aneurysm, 363
aortic regurgitation, 355
aortic root dilatation, 258, 357
Apert syndrome, 319
arachidonic acid, 118
arachnodactyly, 364
Arnold–Chiari malformation, 58, 385
arthralgia, 365
arthritis, 256, 358
arthrochalasis multiplex congenita, 367
arthrogryposes, 393
arthrogryposis, 403
arthrogryposis multiplex congenita, 400
arthrogryposis syndromes, definition, 404
arthrogryposis syndromes, diagnosis, 404
arthrogryposis syndromes, genetic counseling, 405
arthrogryposis syndromes, incidence, 404
arthrogryposis syndromes, preventive
    management, 405
ascorbate, 430

aspartylglucosaminuria, 414
aspirin therapy, 366
Association for Retarded Citizens (ARC), 142
associations, 11
associations, definitions, 11, 85
ataxia, 391
atelosteogenesis, 249
atlantoaxial instability, 150, 252, 336, 339, 424
atrial septal defect, 272
atrophic rhinitis, 381
audiology screening, 43
Austin syndrome, 419
autism, 21, 177
autoimmune disorders, 151, 165
autoimmune thryoiditis, 231
autosomal aneuploidy syndromes, 135
autosomal dominant inheritance, 7
avascular necrosis, 417

baby Doe, 40
baclofen, 57
Baller–Gerold syndrome, 320
Bannayan–Riley–Ruvalcaba syndrome, 289
Barr body, 164
basal cell carcinomas, 223
basal cell nevus syndrome, 292
basal ganglia, 252
basilar impression, 339
basilar skull invagination, 259
Bayley Scales of Infant Development, 53
beaked nose, 392
Beals syndrome, 362
Beckwith–Wiedemann syndrome, 269
Beckwith–Wiedemann syndrome, complications, 275
Beckwith–Wiedemann syndrome, counseling, 274
Beckwith–Wiedemann syndrome, definition, 273
Beckwith–Wiedemann syndrome, differential, 274
Beckwith–Wiedemann syndrome, genetic counseling, 275
Beckwith–Wiedemann syndrome, preventive management, 276
behavioral screening instruments, 43
Bendectin, 103
beneficence, 34
beta-adrenergic blockade, 364
beta-blocker therapy, 364
betaine, 359
bicornuate uterus, 346, 404
biopterin, 454
biotin, 456
biotinidase, 457
biotinidase deficiency, 457
biotinylation, 457
biphosphonates, 259
BKM gene, 223
blastomere analysis before implantation (BABI), 176
bleeding diathesis, 231
blepharitis, 151, 342
blepharophimosis, 324, 357, 401
blindness, 251, 419

Bloch–Sulzberger syndrome, 386
Bloom syndrome, 223
blue sclerae, 257, 355, 369
bone crises, 417
bone fragility, 256
bone marrow transplantation, 251, 425
Bonnevie–Ullrich, 161
Börjeson–Forssman–Lehmann syndrome, 269
botulinum toxin, 57
Brachmann–de Lange syndrome, complications, 233
Brachmann–de Lange syndrome, definition, 232
Brachmann–de Lange syndrome, diagnosis, 233
Brachmann–de Lange syndrome, genetic counseling, 233
Brachmann–de Lange syndrome, incidence, 232
brain imaging, 301
branched chain α-keto acid dehydrogenase, 455
branched chain amino acids, 455
branchial arches, 331
branchial clefts, 331
branchial cysts, 333
branchio-oculo-facial syndrome, 331
branchio-oto-renal (BOR) syndrome, 332
branchio-oto-renal syndrome, 337
breasts, absent, 379
breech presentation, 395
Bright Futures, xiii
broad alveolar ridges, 117
broad thumbs, 345
bronchiectasis, 358
bruisability, 258, 368
Brushfield spots, 147
burden of suffering, 40
burning pain, 417

café-au-lait spots, 298
camptodactyly, 357
carbamazapine, 417
carbohydrate metabolism, disorders, 446
carbohydrate-deficient glycoprotein syndrome, 434
cardiac arrythmia, 429, 451
cardiac septal defects, 117
cardiac valves, 424
cardiomyopathy, 224, 230, 434, 450, 456
Carey, John, MD, v
carnitine, 427, 456
carnitine supplementation, 456
carotid arteries, 358
Carpenter syndrome, 321
cartilage-hair hypoplasia, 247
cataracts, 108, 110, 225, 248, 252, 278, 346, 399, 405
catastrophic illness, 13
caudal regression sequence, 89
CD4 T cell counts, 107
celiac arteries, 360
celiac disease, 151
cell adhesion, 357
cerebellar anomalies, 107
cerebellar hypoplasia, 402

cerebral aneurysm, 258
cerebral dysgenesis, 49
cerebral palsy, 20, 49
cerebral palsy, choreoathetoid, 50
cerebral palsy, coping by families, 58
cerebral palsy, familial, 54
cerebral palsy, implications of diagnosis, 54
cerebral palsy, natural history, 55
cerebral palsy, outcomes, 50
cerebral palsy, parent support group, 54
cerebral palsy, prevalence, 50
cerebral palsy, preventive checklist, 57
cerebral palsy, risk factors, 50
cerebral palsy, services, 55
cerebral palsy, spastic, 55
Cerezyme, 418
cervical spinal cord, 249
cervical spine, 322
cervical spine compression, 253
cervical spine fusion, 320
cervical vertebral fusion, 336
CHARGE association, cardiac anomalies, 93
CHARGE association, complications, 93
CHARGE association, definition, 91
CHARGE association, diagnosis, 92
CHARGE association, differential, 91
CHARGE association, genetic counseling, 93
CHARGE association, incidence, 91
CHARGE association, preventive management, 94
CHARGE syndrome, 91
Charles Darwin, 379
Charlie M syndrome, 344
checklists, compliance, 35
cherry red spot, 416
cherry red spots, 416
cherubism, 230
chest pain, 364
child development clinic, 26
children with special health care needs, 30
choanal atresia, 83, 110, 272, 318, 335
cholesterol metabolism, 435
cholesterol screening, 392
chondrodysplasia, 401
chondrodysplasia punctata, 247, 431
chondrodystrophic myotonia, 401
choreoathetosis, 398
chorioretinal degeneration, 361
chorioretinitis, 105
chorioretinopathy, 271
choristomas, 289
choroidal angioma, 294
choroidemia, 430
chromosomal analysis, 16
chromosomal disorders, 135
chromosomal disorders, complications, 136
chromosomal imbalance, 135
chromosomal inheritance, 9
chromosomal mosaicism, 386
chromosomal region Xp22, 450
chromosome 11p15 region, 274
chromosome 15 region, 384
chromosome analysis, 26

chromosome band 16q12.1, 334
chromosome disorders, parent support groups, 142
chromosome region 17q21, 344
chromosome region 5q32, 335
chromosome region 7p13, 343
chromosome region Xq26, 346
Chronic Condition Management, 27, 28
chronic otitis, 81, 166, 226, 231, 234, 249, 278, 340
chronic rhinorrea, 420
cigarette paper scars, 369
claudication, 360
clavicles, absent, 249
cleft lip and palate, 346
cleft lip/cleft palate, 81, 382
cleft lip/cleft palate, preventive management, 81
cleft palate, 107, 322, 360, 361
cleft palate team, 82
cleft palate, U-shaped, 85
cleidocranial dysplasia, 248
clinodactyly, 147
club feet, 360
coagulation disorder, 271
coarctation of the aorta, 165
cocaine, 105
Cockayne syndrome, 391, 402
coenzyme Q, 429
Coffin–Siris syndrome, 116, 340
cognitive disability, 161
Cohen syndrome, 270
collision sports, 366
coloboma, 84, 335, 385
colon perforation, 366
conductive hearing loss, 321, 339
cone-shaped epiphyses, 334
congenital contractural arachnodactyly, 357
congenital contractures, 395, 403, 405
congenital heart disease, 250
congenital hip dislocation, 117, 424
congenital rubella infection, 107
congenital syphilis, 108
congenital toxoplasmosis, 109
conjunctival aneurysms, 417
connective tissue dysplasia, 355
connective tissue laxity, 359
connective tissue weakness, 355
consanguinity, 8
constipation, 150, 227
contractures, 391
corneal abrasions, 397
corneal clouding, 419, 422
corneal reflex, 397
coronal synostosis, 323
coronary disease, 359
corpus callosum, 278
cortical atrophy, 340
cost-effectiveness, 39
Costello syndrome, 224
costovertebral defects, 399
cranial MRI scan, 107
cranial nerve paralysis, 251
craniofacial surgery team, 83, 317

craniosynostosis, 83, 228, 247, 251
craniosynostosis syndromes, 317
critical embryonic period, 86
Crouzon syndrome, 321
cryptophthalmos, 342
Cryptophthalmos syndrome, 342
cryptorchidism, 117, 144, 228, 230, 250, 271, 321,
    333, 334, 344, 382, 385, 388, 402, 403, 435
curare paralysis, 400
cutis laxa syndromes, 357
cystathionine-β-synthase, 358
cystic hygroma, 229
cystic kidneys, 273, 332, 435
cystic medial necrosis, 355
cytochrome c, 427
cytogenetic notation, 16, 139
cytomegalovirus, 105

dacryocystitis, 331
Dandy–Walker cyst, 342
Dandy–Walker malformation, 331, 342
deafness, 94
deep plantar crease, 147
degenerative course, 402
del(22q11), 92
deletion, 139
demyelination, 432, 456
dental anomalies, 82, 150, 369
dental decay, 397
dental hypoplasia, 379
dental malocclusion, 276
dentinogenesis imperfecta, 258
dermatitis, 391
developmental delay, 6, 26
developmental differences, 19
developmental disabilities, allied health
    professionals, 21
developmental disabilities, causes, 21
developmental disabilites, early intervention
    services, 24
developmental disabilities, epidemiology, 20
developmental disabilities, parental adaptation,
    28
developmental disabilities, parental support, 23
developmental disabilities, people-first language, 29
developmental disabilities, prenatal diagnosis, 23
developmental disabilities, recognition, 22
developmental disabilities, team approach, 42
developmental pediatrician, 26
developmental regression, 26
developmental screening, 19, 25
dextrocardia, 144
diabetes mellitus, 118, 391
diabetic embryopathy, complications, 119
diabetic embryopathy, counseling, 119
diabetic embryopathy, diagnosis, 119
diabetic embryopathy, history, 118
diabetic embryopathy, incidence, 118
diabetic embryopathy,definition, 118
diaphragmatic hernia, 273
diastrophic dwarfism, 249
dichloroacetate, 429

dietary treatment, 445
DiGeorge anomaly, 83, 93, 114
DiGeorge anomaly, preventive management, 83
dihydroxyacetone phosphate acyltransferase, 432
dimpling, 400
diphenylhydantoin, 417
dipyridamol, 359
disability, definition, 37
dislocation of the radial head, 359
disruptions, 80
diverticulae, 358
DNA diagnosis, 15
dolichostenomelia, 357
Donohue syndrome, 224
dorsal rhizotomy, 55
double-jointed, 355
Down syndrome, complications, 149
Down syndrome, definition, 146
Down syndrome, diagnosis, 147
Down syndrome, genetic counseling, 148
Down syndrome, history, 146
Down syndrome, incidence, 147
Down syndrome, preventive management, 150
Duane syndrome, 336
Dubowitz syndrome, 224
duplication, 139
dwarfism, 245
dwarfism, neonatal lethal, 247
dysarthric speech, 398
dysmorphology, 4, 8
dysphagia, 397
dysphonia, 381
dyspnea, 364
dystonia, 398

ear pits, 274
early intervention, 42
early intervention services, 24
ectodermal dysplasias, 379, 417
ectomesenchyme, 331
ectopia lentis, 357, 362
ectrodactyly, 381
ectrodactyly-ectodermal dysplasia-clefting (EEC)
    syndrome, 381
ectropion, 333
eczematoid rash, 387
Ehlers–Danlos syndrome, 366
Ehlers–Danlos syndrome type VII, 367
Ehlers–Danlos syndrome types I–III,
    complications, 369
Ehlers–Danlos syndrome types I–III, genetic
    counseling, 368
Ehlers–Danlos syndrome types I–III, preventive
    management, 369
Ehlers–Danlos syndrome, type IV, 366
Ehlers–Danlos syndrome, type VI, 367
Ehlers–Danlos syndrome, types I–III, definition,
    367
Ehlers–Danlos syndrome, types I–III, incidence,
    367
elastin fibers, 360
electron transfer flavoprotein, 426

Elephant Man, 298
Ellis–van Crevald syndrome, 250
emphysema, 358
enamel hypoplasia, 228, 252, 324
encephalocele, 62, 338
enchondroma, 295
enlarged penis, 346
enzyme assay, 15
enzyme therapy, 418
eosinophilia, 387
epibulbar dermoid, 84
epibulbar dermoid cysts, 336
epicanthal folds, 147
epidermal nevus syndrome, 291
epilepsy, 116
epinephrine response, 397
epiphyseal dysplasia, 269
erythrocyte plasmalogens, 434
estrogen treatment, 166
ETF, 426
Exceptional Parent Magazine, xiv
exposure keratitis, 322
external ophthalmoplegia, 429
extracellular matrix, 357

Fabry disease, 416
facial angiofibromas, 305
facial asymmetry, 291
facioauriculovertebral spectrum, 336
factor IX, 434
FAE, 111
false teeth, 381
familial dysautonomia, 395
Family Support, xiii
family support programs, xiii
Family Village, xiv
Fanconi syndrome, 451
FAP gene, 292
FAS, 111
fatty acid oxidation, 456
fatty acid oxidation disorders, 456
fatty liver, 451
fetal akinesia sequence, 402
fetal alcohol effects, 110
fetal alcohol syndrome, 110
fetal alcohol syndrome, animal models, 111
fetal alcohol syndrome, complications, 113
fetal alcohol syndrome, diagnosis, 111
fetal alcohol syndrome, family support, 113
fetal alcohol syndrome, growth hormone
   secretion, 115
fetal alcohol syndrome, history, 111
fetal alcohol syndrome, incidence, 111
fetal alcohol syndrome, preventive management,
   114
fetal cocaine syndrome, 105
fetal cytomegalovirus syndrome, 105
fetal HIV infection, 106
fetal hydantoin syndrome, 340
fetal hydantoin syndrome, animal models, 116
fetal hydantoin syndrome, complications, 117
fetal hydantoin syndrome, definition, 115

fetal hydantoin syndrome, differential, 116
fetal hydantoin syndrome, history, 115
fetal hydantoin syndrome, incidence, 116
fetal hydantoin syndrome, preventive
   management, 117
fetal hydrops, 247, 403, 421
fetal immobility, 400
fetal movement, 404
fetal rubella syndrome, 107
fetal syphilis syndrome, 108
fetal toluene syndrome, 108
fetal toxoplasmosis syndrome, 109
fetal valproate syndrome, 110
fetal warfarin syndrome, 110
fibrillin-1 locus, 362
fibrillin-2 gene, 357
fibroblast growth factor receptor 2 (FGFR2) gene,
   318
fibroblast growth factor-3 receptor, 255
fibrodysplasia ossificans progressiva, 250
fibroma, 293
fibrosarcoma, 293
fibrous dysplasia, 300
financial issues, 42
first and second branchial arch syndrome, 337
flat feet, 177, 224, 273
flexion contractures, 234
fluorescent DNA probes, 16
focal dermal hypoplasia, 385
folate deficiency, 359, 398
folic acid, 63
foramen magnum, 255
foveal hypoplasia, 382
fractures, 397
fragile X DNA testing, 175
fragile X syndrome, complications, 176
fragile X syndrome, diagnosis, 175
fragile X syndrome, genetic counseling, 175
fragile X syndrome, preventive management,
   177
fragile X testing, 26
Franceschetti–Klein syndrome, 335
Fraser syndrome, 342
Freeman–Sheldon syndrome, 403
frontal encephalocele, 84
frontonasal dysplasia, 84, 337
frontonasal malformation, 84
Fryns syndrome, 343
fucosidosis, 414
full mutation, 176
functional screening, 43

G protein, 298
Gardner syndrome, 289, 292
gastric carcinoma, 292
gastroesophageal reflux, 177, 233
gastrointestinal anomalies, 150
Gaucher disease, 417
genetic diseases, presentations, 4
genetics clinics, 41
genitourinary anomalies, 250
genitourinary defects, 382

genu recurvatum, 369
germinal mosaicism, 257, 324
giant cell astrocytomas, 305
gibbus, 423
glabellar hemangioma, 274, 400
glaucoma, 108
globe rupture, 368
glomerular lesions, 333
glossopalatine ankylosis, 344
glucocerebroside, 417
glucose-6-phosphatase, 451
glucose-6-phosphate, 451
glutaric acid, 426
glutaric acidemia type II, 425, 427
glycogen storage diseases, 14
glycogen storage diseases, definition, 449
glycogen storage diseases, diagnosis, 449
glycogen storage diseases, genetic counseling,
    450
glycogenoses, 450
glycolipid deposition, 417
glycolysis, 451
glycoprotein degradation disorders, 414
glycopyrrolate, 57
glycosaminoglycans, 420
glypican 3 gene, 273
G_{M1} gangliosidosis, 418
G_{M2} gangliosidosis, 414
Goldenhar syndrome, 331
Goldenhar syndrome, complications, 339
Goldenhar syndrome, description, 336
Goldenhar syndrome, diagnosis, 337
Goldenhar syndrome, genetic counseling, 338
Goldenhar syndrome, incidence, 337
Goldenhar syndrome, preventive management,
    339
Goltz–Gorlin syndrome, 385
gonadoblastoma, 165, 343
Gorlin sign, 368
Gorlin syndrome, 292
Greig syndrome, 343
growth failure, 222
growth failure, disproportionate, 221
growth failure, proportionate, 221
growth hormone deficiency, 252
growth hormone therapy, 166, 231, 256, 390
Gs alpha gene, 252
gynecomastia, 270

hair-bulb assay, 384
Hallermann–Streiff syndrome, 225
hamartomas, 289, 295
hamartosis syndromes, 289
handicap, definition, 37
Hanhart syndrome, 344
Hanson, James, MD, v
HARD-E syndrome, 399
Hay–Wells syndrome, 382
head circumference monitoring, 62
head sparing, 221
health care resources, 1
health outcome, 36

health supervision, 150
healthcare "carve-outs", 39
Healthy People 2000, 31
hearing loss, 235, 419
helmets, 83
hemangiomas, 271, 293
hemangiomatous disorders, 379
hematochezia, 306
hemifacial microsomia, 336
hemifacial microsomia/Goldenhar complex, 89
hemihyperplasia, 271, 275, 291
hemihypertrophy, 228
hemiplegia, 49
hepatic adenomas, 451
hepatic cholestasis, 224
hepatic transaminase, 427
hepatoblastoma, 276
hepatocarcinoma, 453
hepatocellular carcinoma, 278
hepatosplenomegaly, 422
hereditary sensory and autonomic neuropathies,
    395
hernias, 358, 365, 369, 401
herpes encephalitis, 106
herpes virus, 106
heteroplasmy, 425
heterotopias, 304, 433
heterozygotes, 178
hexokinase deficiency, 450
high TSH form of hypothyroidism, 150
Himalayan mice, 383
hip dislocation, 114, 435
histamine, 395
HIV testing, 32
HIV-positive children, 107
Hodgkin disease, 247
holocarboxylase synthetase deficiency, 457
holoprosencephaly, 107, 117, 145, 339
homeostasis, 135
homeotic genes, 337
homocystinuria, 359
horseshoe kidney, 385
HSAN, 395
human immunodeficiency virus-1 (HIV-1), 106
human teratogen, criteria, 103
Hunter syndrome, 421
Hurler syndrome, 423
Hurler-like syndrome, 416
Hutchinson–Gilford syndrome, 392
hydrocephalus, 84, 110, 254, 320, 420, 423, 435
hydrocephalus, arrested, 58
hydrocephalus, communicating, 259
hydrocephalus, compensated, 58
hydrocephalus, complications, 61
hydrocephalus, definition, 58
hydrocephalus, diagnosis, 60
hydrocephalus, family support, 60
hydrocephalus, incidence, 58
hydrocephalus, non-communicating, 58
hydrocephalus, parent groups, 61
hydronephrosis, 228, 321, 385
hyperactivity, 112, 177, 305

hyperammonemia, 445, 457
hypercalcemia, 250
hyperinsulinism, 224
hyperlipidemia, 451
hyperphagia, 269
hyperphenylalaninemia, 453
hyperphosphatemia, 252
hyperpigmented lesions, 385
hyperpyrexia, 382
hypertonia, 398
hypertrophic cardiomyopathy, 427
hyperuricemia, 398, 451
hypochondrogenesis, 252
hypochondroplasia, 253
hypoglossia-hypodactylia, 344
hypoglycemia, 6, 274, 445, 452
hypogonadism, 223, 235
hypohidrosis, 417
hypohidrotic ectodermal dysplasia, 379
hypomelanosis of Ito syndrome, 386
hypophosphatasia, 250
hypopigmentation, 382
hypopigmented macules, 302
hypoplastic nails, 250
hypoplastic teeth, 382
hypospadias, 224, 427, 435
hypothyroidism, 146, 252
hypotonia, 25

I-cell disease, 422
ichthyosis, 248, 419
IgM antibodies, 108
imaging studies, 43
impairment, definition, 37
imperforate anus, 319, 321, 339
imprinting, 274
inborn errors of metabolism, 6, 411
incontinentia pigmenti, 386
incontinentia pigmenti achromians, 386
increased intracranial pressure, 320
Individual Family Service Plan (IFSP), 24
Individuals with Disabilities Education Act
    (I.D.E.A.), 42
infantile reflexes, persistence, 53
infantile Refsum syndrome, 431
infantile spasms, 304
infants of diabetic mothers (IDM), 118
infertility, 390
inflammatory bowel disease, 452
inheritance mechanisms, 7
integument, 379
integumentary glands, 379
intestinal atresias, 343
intestinal malrotation, 273
intestinal polyps, 290, 291
intestinal rupture, 366
intracranial bleeding, 233
intracranial calcifications, 105, 106, 294, 304
intracranial hypertension, 305
intracranial pressure, 59
intrauterine growth retardation, 106, 108
intrauterine growth retardation, symmetrical, 221

intravenous gammaglobulin, 107
isochromosome Xp, 162
isotretinoin, 107, 293

Jackson–Weiss syndrome, 322
joint contractures, 400, 401
joint deterioration, 418
joint dislocations, 224
joint fusions, 325
joint hypermobility, 367
joint laxity, 258, 290, 342, 361, 366, 368
juvenile rheumatoid arthritis, 27

Kabuki theater, 225
Kearns–Sayre syndrome, 429
keloid formation, 227
keratitis, 151, 322, 342
keratosis, 392
kernicterus, 50
ketogenic diet, 428
Klinefelter syndrome, definition, 167
Klinefelter syndrome, history, 167
Klinefelter syndrome, incidence, 167
Klippel–Feil anomaly, 84, 114, 336
Klippel–Feil anomaly, complications, 84
Klippel–Trenaunay–Weber syndrome, 293
Krabbe disease, 414
kyphoscoliosis, 357, 364, 403
kyphosis, 255, 296

lactate/pyruvate ratio, 428
lactic acidosis, 427, 451
large anterior fontanelle, 248, 427, 433
large fontanelle, 250
Larsen syndrome, 359
laryngeal hypoplasia, 249
laryngeal stenosis, 343
laryngomalacia, 83, 272, 360
latex allergy, 68
laxatives, 366
learning disabilities, 112
Leber hereditary optic neuropathy (LHON),
    429
Leigh disease, 427
LEOPARD syndrome, 229, 388
leprechaunism, 224
Lesch–Nyhan syndrome, 397
leukemia, 225, 247
limb anomalies, 110, 318
limb bowing, 256
linear sebaceous nevus syndrome, 291
lipodystrophy, 434
lipomas, 290
lipophoresis, 392
Lisch spots, 299
lissencephaly, 49
Little People of America, 254
Little's disease, 49
live viral vaccines, 107
lobster-claw deformity, 381
long philtrum, 232
loose skin, 357

loss of heterozygosity, 298
lower extremity paralysis, 68
lymphangiomas, 296
lymphoma, 247
lysosomal enzyme deficiencies, 414
lysosomal enzymes, 413
lysosome, 414
lysyl oxidase deficiency, 358

macrocephaly, 25, 248, 255, 258, 271, 290, 298, 423, 426
macroglossia, 272, 276
Mafucci syndrome, 295
major anomalies, 10
malignant hyperthermia, 231
malocclusion, 397, 406
management guidelines, rationale, xii
mandibular hypoplasia, 85
mandibular prognathism, 276, 323
mandibulofacial dysostosis, 334, 335
mannose-6-phosphate, 420
mannosidoses, 414
maple syrup urine disease, 455
Marden–Walker syndrome, 401
Marfan syndrome, definition, 362
Marfan syndrome, diagnosis, 363
Marfan syndrome, genetic counseling, 363
Marfan syndrome, incidence, 362
Marfan syndrome, preventive management, 365
Marfanoid habitus, 361
Maroteaux–Lamy disease, 422
Marshall syndrome, 361
Marshall–Smith syndrome, 272
maternal inheritance, 425
maternal PKU, 455
maternal serum alpha-fetoprotein (MSAF), 64
maternal vasculopathy, 118
Meckel syndrome, 344
Medicaid benefits, 42
medium chain coenzyme A dehydrogenase deficiency, 456
medulloblastomas, 293
megaloblastic anemia, 398
megalocornea, 364
melanin pigment, 383
melanin-regulating genes, 382
MELAS, 429
melena, 295
Mendelian inheritance, 3
meningiomas, 296
meningomyelocele, 62
mental retardation, 21
MERRF, 429
Merrick, Joseph, 298
mesomelic shortening, 226
metabolic disorders, 5
metabolic disorders – categories, 14
metabolic disorders – large molecule, 12
metabolic disorders – small molecule, 12
metabolic dysplasias, 411
metachromatic leukodystrophy, 414, 419
Meténier sign, 368

microcephaly, 25, 106, 107, 221, 248, 269, 339, 391, 405, 435
microcornea, 321, 369
microdeletion, chromosome 22, 83, 92
microdontia, 390
micrognathia, 344, 392
microgyria, 321
micropenis, 117, 226, 344
microphthalmia, 107, 108, 386, 402
microstomia, 403
Miller syndrome, 333
Miller–Dieker syndrome, 399
minor anomalies, 6, 10
mitochondrial disease, 427
mitochondrial DNA deletions, 429
mitochondrial encephalopathy with lactic acidemia and strokes, 429
mitochondrial encephalopathy with ragged red fibers, 429
mitochondrial genome, 425
mitochondrial membranes, 425
mitochondrial myopathy, 428
mitochondrial proteins, 425
mitochondrial respiratory function, 425
mitral regurgitation, 364
mitral valve prolapse, 165, 177, 245, 358, 364, 401
Moebius syndrome, 344
monosomy X, 164
Morquio disease, 422
mosaicism, 164
Movement Assessment of Infants (MAI), 53
moya moya disease, 231
MRI scan, 60
mucolipidoses, 414
mucopolysaccharidoses, 414
mucopolysaccharidoses, complications, 423
mucopolysaccharidoses, definition, 421
mucopolysaccharidoses, genetic counseling, 422
mucopolysaccharidoses, incidence, 421
mucopolysaccharidoses, preventive management, 424
multiple congenital anomalies, 6
multiple miscarriages, 4
multiple pterygium syndrome, 402
multiple sulfatase deficiency, 419
myasthenia gravis, 400
myelodysplasia, 62
myeloid malignancy, 145
myelomeningocele, 90
myocardial infarction, 366
myoclonic seizures, 304, 343
myopathies, 400
myopia, 235, 361

NADH dehydrogenase, 428
Naegeli syndrome, 387
Nager syndrome, 334
nail hypoplasia, 117
nasal hypoplasia, 110
nasal saline drops, 151
nasal septum, 322
natural history, 36

neonatal adrenoleukodystrophy, 431
neonatal HIV infection, 106
neonatal polycythemia, 274
neonatal seizures, 51
neonatal vesicles, 106
nephroblastosis, 272
nephrocalcinosis, 251
nephrolithiasis, 398
nephromegaly, 275
nephrotic syndrome, 252
neural crest, 383
neural tube defects, causes, 63
neural tube defects, incidence, 63
neurectoderm, 383
neuroblastoma, 114, 225, 278
neurodegeneration, 413
neurofibromas, 298
neurofibromatosis-1, complications, 300
neurofibromatosis-1, definition, 298
neurofibromatosis-1, diagnosis, 299
neurofibromatosis-1, genetic counseling, 300
neurofibromatosis-1, incidence, 298
neurofibromatosis-1, preventive management, 299
neurofibromatosis-2, 296
neurofibromin, 298
neuronopathic, 417
neurosensory damage, 114
neutropenia, 452
nevoid basal cell carcinoma syndrome, 292
nevus flammeus, 294
Niemann–Pick disease, 414
Niikawa–Kuroki syndrome, 225
nocturnal glucose feeding, 452
Noonan syndrome, 388
Noonan syndrome, complications, 230
Noonan syndrome, definition, 228
Noonan syndrome, diagnosis, 229
Noonan syndrome, differential, 229
Noonan syndrome, genetic counseling, 230
Noonan syndrome, history, 229
Noonan syndrome, incidence, 229
normal variants, 10
Norplant, 151
nystagmus, 382, 385, 386, 427

obesity, 256, 270
obstructive hydrocephalus, 105
obstructive sleep apnea, 225, 319
occipital horn disease, 366
occult blood, 361
ocular albinism, 385
ocular proptosis, 323
oculoauriculovertebral dysplasia, 336
oculocutaneous albinism, 383
odontoid hypoplasia, 423
oligosaccharidoses, 414
omphalocele, 272, 275, 343
opisthotonic posturing, 398
optic atropy, 321
optic disc anomalies, 84
optic gliomas, 300
optic nerve hypoplasia, 399

oral–facial–digital syndromes, 345
orange-peel skin, 360
organellar diseases, 413
organic acid profile, 15
organic acidemias, 456
oromandibular-limb hypogenesis syndromes, 344
oromandibular-limb syndromes, 344
orthopedic treatment, 370
osteodysplastic primordial dwarfism, 228
osteogenesis imperfecta, definition, 256
osteogenesis imperfecta, diagnosis, 257
osteogenesis imperfecta, genetic counseling, 257
osteogenesis imperfecta, incidence, 256
osteogenesis imperfecta, preventive management, 258
osteomas, 292
osteomyelitis, 397
osteopenia, 257, 405
osteopetrosis, 251
osteoporosis, 359
otopalatodigital syndrome, 345
outcome criteria, 36
outcome studies, 38
outcome, interval, 38
outcome, ordinal, 37
outcomes, functional, 37
ovarian failure, 270
ovarian tumors, 224
overbite, 177
overgrowth disorders, 269
oxygen radicals, 118

p, 16
P gene, 384
pain insensitivity, 395
palpitations, 364
pamidronate, 259
pancytopenia, 251
papilledema, 59
papillomas, 224
paradoxical growth retardation, 118
parathormone, 252
parenteral nutrition, 456
paresthesias, 417
parietal foramina, 342
partial chromosome aneuploidies, 135
peau d'orange, 360, 434
pectus deformity, 364
pectus excavatum, 177, 358, 388
pedigree, 6
Pena–Shokeir type I syndrome, 402
Pena–Shokeir type II syndrome, 402
penicillin, 108
penicillin prophylaxis, 418
people-first language, 148
perinatal complications, 19
periventricular leukomalacia, 52
Perlman syndrome, 272
peroxisomal disorders, definition, 431
peroxisomal disorders, diagnosis, 432
peroxisomal disorders, genetic counseling, 432

peroxisomal disorders, incidence, 431
peroxisomal disorders, preventive management, 433
peroxisomes, 248, 430
persistent hyperplastic primary vitreous, 399
Peutz–Jeghers syndrome, 295
Pfeiffer syndrome, 323
pharyngeal muscle hypoplasia, 331
phenylalanine, 453
phenylalanine hydroxylase, 453
phenylketonuria, 453
phosphenolpyruvate carboxykinase, 428
photophobia, 392
physical restraints, 398
phytanic acid, 432
Pierre Robin sequence, 85
pigmentary disorders, 379
pigmentary lesions, 145
pilocarpine, 395
piracetam, 151
pituitary function, 227
PKU, 453
PKU diet, 455
plagiocephaly, 82
plasmalogen, 248
plasmalogens, 431
plastic surgery, 151
platybasia, 245
platyspondyly, 391
Plexiform neuroma, 299
pneumocystis, 107
Poland sequence, 344
policeman's tip, 404
polycystic kidney, 302
polydactyly, 247, 271, 275
polyhydramnios, 247, 275
polyposis, 292
Pompe disease, 450
poor impulse control, 112
popliteal pterygium syndrome, 402
porencephaly, 49
postaxial polydactyly, 343
potassium bromide, 115
Potter sequence, 79, 333
precocious puberty, 62, 301, 305
preconceptional supplementation, 63
prematurity, 369
premutation, 176
prevention, cost-effectiveness, 34
prevention, costs, 45
prevention, disease incidence, 33
prevention, guidelines, 43
prevention, health care systems, 35
prevention, high-risk population, 34
prevention, justification, 40
prevention, physician compliance, 35
prevention, population strategies, 33
prevention, rationale, 40
prevention, scope of disease, 31
prevention, secondary, 32
prevention, tertiary, 32
preventive checklist, 43, 45, 150

primidone, 116
procollagen, 257
Progeria, 392
prolapse of the uterus, 369
propranolol, 365
proprionyl coenzyme A carboxylase, 456
proptosis, 322
protein-losing enteropathy, 294
proteins S and C, 434
Proteus syndrome, 289, 296, 299
pseudoarthrosis, 299
pseudohermaphroditism, 161
pseudo-Hurler polydystrophy, 419
pseudo-hypoparathyroidism, 251
pseudothalidomide syndrome, 346
pseudotumor cerebri, 60
pseudoxanthoma elasticum, 360
psychosocial problems, 41, 368
pterygia, 402
pterygium colli, 84
ptosis, 230, 401
puckered lips, 403
pulmonary artery, 108
pulmonary hypertension, 114
pulmonary hypoplasia, 333, 342, 344, 403, 405
pulmonary stenosis, 358
pulmonic stenosis, 224, 368, 388
punctate calcifications, 248
pyloric stenosis, 433
pyrimethamine, 109
pyruvate, 428
pyruvate carboxylase, 428, 456
pyruvate dehydrogenase deficiency, 428, 455

q, 16
quadriparesis, 259
quality of life measures, 38

rachischisis, 62
radial aplasia, 390
radial ray, 320
radiohumeral synostosis, 319
radioulnar synostosis, 333, 334
ragged red fibers, 427
Rapp–Hodgkin syndrome, 382
rectal prolapse, 368
recurrence risks, 6
recurrent pneumonias, 402
reflux nephropathy, 369
Refsum syndrome, 431
renal agenesis, 79, 332, 333, 343, 433
renal cysts, 427
renal duplication, 382
renal failure, 429
renal sonography, 339, 345
renal tubular acidosis, 429
renal ultrasound, 332
renovascular hypertension, 360
respiratory complex I, 428
respiratory complex IV, 428
retinal detachment, 253, 361, 368, 369, 399
retinal lattice degeneration, 365

retinal pigment epithelium, congenital hypertrophy, 292
retinal pigmentation, 433
retinitis pigmentosa, 391, 429
retinoic acid, 107
retinoic acid embryopathy, 107
retinoic acid embryopathy, preventive management, 107
rib fractures, 257
riboflavin, 427, 429
Riley–Day syndrome, 395
Roberts syndrome, 346
Robertsonian translocation, 147
Robin sequence, 85, 344, 361
Robinow syndrome, 226
Rothmund–Thomson syndrome, 390
rubella syndrome, 108
Rubinstein–Taybi syndrome, 226
Russell–Silver syndrome, 227

sacrococcygeal dysgenesis, 89
Saethre–Chotzen syndrome, 323
salivary gland hypoplasia, 338
Sandhoff disease, 414
Sandifer syndrome, 82
sarcomas, 390
Scheie syndrome, 424
school issues, 42
Schwartz–Jampel syndrome, 401
scoliosis, 114, 224, 226, 248, 272, 300, 367, 369, 386, 397, 399, 400, 401
screening by history, 44
Seckel syndrome, 228
SED, 252
see-saw winking, 345
seizures, 27, 177, 226, 259, 294, 304, 340, 429, 445, 457
self-esteem, 166
self-mutilation, 395, 398
sensorineural deafness, 108, 250, 255, 259, 339, 360, 385
sensorineural hearing loss, 115, 297, 333, 334, 336, 392
sensory impairments, 27
septum pellucidum, 273
sequence, 11, 79
serum alpha-fetoprotein, 276
sex chromosome aneuploidies, 161
sex chromosome imbalance, 161
sex reversal, 435
sexually transmitted diseases, 108
shagreen patch, 302
short limbs, 248
short nose, 248
short stature, 256
Shprintzen syndrome, 93
sialidoses, 414
Siamese cats, 383
simplified pinna, 338
Simpson–Golabi–Behmel syndrome, 272
single anomalies, 9, 79
single palmar creases, 147

sinusitis, 151, 379
skeletal dysplasias, 245
skeletal myopathy, 456
skin fragility, 355, 368
skin rashes, 454
sleep apnea, 81, 150, 322, 397
sleep difficulties, 278
Smith–Lemli–Opitz syndrome, 435
social security law, 42
somatic chromosomal mosaicism, 387
Sotos syndrome, complications, 278
Sotos syndrome, definition, 277
Sotos syndrome, genetic counseling, 277
Sotos syndrome, incidence, 277
Sotos syndrome, preventive management, 279
sparse hair, 379
spastic quadriplegia, 56
spatial reasoning, 166
spatial visualization, 164
special education services, 20
spina bifida, 385
Spina Bifida Association of America, 67
spina bifida occulta, 249
spina bifida, cognitive abilities, 69
spina bifida, complications, 67
spina bifida, definition, 62
spina bifida, family support, 65
spina bifida, foster care, 65
spina bifida, history, 62
spina bifida, intellectual outcomes, 67
spina bifida, level of lesion, 64
spina bifida, management, 65
spina bifida, prenatal diagnosis, 64
spina bifida, preventive checklist, 69
spina bifida, school performance, 68
spina bifida, selection of cases for surgery, 62
spinal compression, 255
spinal cord lipomas, 63
spinal fusion, 278, 370
spiramycin, 109
splenectomy, 418
split hand, 381
spondyloepiphyseal dysplasia congenita, 252
stapedial foot plate, 320
Steinberg, Joel, MD, v
Stickler syndrome, 85, 361
stippled epiphyses, 110, 114, 248
stool guaiac, 390
storage diseases, 15, 413
strabismus, 110, 150, 225, 230, 278, 296, 335, 344, 364, 369, 382, 386, 401, 427
stretch marks, 355
Sturge–Weber syndrome, 294
subependymal nodules, 303
subluxation, 367
submucous cleft palate, 224
sudden death, 363
sulfate transporter, 249
sulfatide lipidosis, 419
sunscreen, 384
supernumerary bones, 360
supernumerary teeth, 292, 323, 390

Supplemental Security Income (SSI), 53
supraorbital ridges, 335
sweat pores, 379
sweat testing, 379
syndactyly, 317
syndromes, 9, 11
synophrys, 232
syringomyelia, 249, 338
systolic click, 364

tactile defensiveness, 177
Taybi syndrome, 345
Tay–Sachs disease, 414
tear flow, 395
telangiectases, 385
telangiectasia, 223, 417
temporomandibular joint, 369
teratogens, 103
terminus, 139
testicular atrophy, 398
tethered cord, 52, 68, 119
tethered cord (spinal dysraphism), 90
tetralogy of Fallot, 93, 144, 321, 338, 435
thalidomide, 104
thanatophoric dwarfism, 247
thanatophoric dysplasia, 253
thiamine, 456
thoracic dysplasia, 250
thrombocytopenia, 347
thromboembolism, 359
thrombotic complications, 359
thumb anomalies, 250, 333
thymic aplasia, 107
thyroid cancer, 292
thyroxine-binding globulin, 276
Title V, 42
Title XIX, 42
toluene, 108
tongue hypoplasia, 339, 344
tongue-tie, 344
TORCH acronym, 104
torticollis, 82, 273
Townes–Brocks syndrome, 334
tracheo-esophageal fistula, 337
tracheomalacia, 249
transcription factor, 391
transferrin, 434
transient myeloid proliferation, 149
translocation, 144
Treacher Collins syndrome, 333, 334, 335
triangular facies, 227
triglyceride synthesis, 451
trigonocephaly, 110, 324
triphalangeal thumbs, 334
triplet repeat expansion, 17
triplet repeats, 176
trisomy 13/18, complications, 143, 145
trisomy 13/18, definitions, 142
trisomy 13/18, diagnosis, 143
trisomy 13/18, genetic counseling, 144
trisomy 13/18, preventive management, 146
TSC1 gene, 302

tuberous sclerosis, definition, 302
tuberous sclerosis, diagnosis, 303
tuberous sclerosis, genetic counseling, 304
tuberous sclerosis, preventive management, 305
Turner syndrome, complications, 165
Turner syndrome, definition, 161
Turner syndrome, diagnosis, 163
Turner syndrome, genetic counseling, 164
Turner syndrome, history, 162
Turner syndrome, incidence, 162
Turner syndrome, preventive management, 165
type I collagen, 367
type II collagen gene, 252, 361
tyrosinase gene, 383
tyrosine, 454

Ullrich–Turner syndrome, 161
ultrasound screening, 276
ultraviolet light, 392
ungual fibromas, 302
unusual distribution of body fat, 434
unusual movements, 27
upslanting palpebral fissures, 147
urinary tract anomalies, 146
urinary tract infections, 227
urine mucopolysaccharide screen, 422
urogenital anomalies, 226, 405
uterine fibroids, 255

VACTERL association, 86
vaginal atresia, 319
varicella, 247
vascular accidents, 79
vascular fragility, 366
VATER association, 86, 120
VATER association, complications, 90
VATER association, definition, 86
VATER association, diagnosis, 89
VATER association, differential, 87
VATER association, etiology, 87
VATER association, genetic counseling, 90
VATER association, history, 87
VATER association, incidence, 87
VATER association, preventive management, 90
velo–cardio–facial syndrome, 83
velopalatine insufficiency, 361
ventricular septal defect, 333
ventriculomegaly, 60
ventriculoperitoneal (VP) shunt, 60
vestibular schwannomas, 297
vidarabine, 106
visceromegaly, 6, 274, 418, 419
vitamin A (retinol), 107
vitamin D-deficient rickets, 250
vitamin K, 110, 429
vitamin supplements, 151
vitreoretinal degeneration, 361

Wagner syndrome, 361
Walker–Warburg syndrome, 399
Warfarin, 248
Watson syndrome, 229

webbed neck, 402
WeeFIM scale, 38
Weissenbacher–Zweymüller syndrome, 361
Werdnig–Hoffman disease, 404
whistling face syndrome, 403
Wildervanck syndrome, 84, 336
Wilms tumor, 235, 276, 292, 298, 301
windvane fingers, 403
Wood's lamp, 303
Wormian bones, 248
WT-1 Wilms tumor gene, 274

X chromosome, 161
xeroderma pigmentosum, 391
X-linked adrenoleukodystrophy, 430
X-linked inheritance, 7

Y chromosome, 161

Zellweger syndrome, 430
zinc, 118
zygomatic process, 335

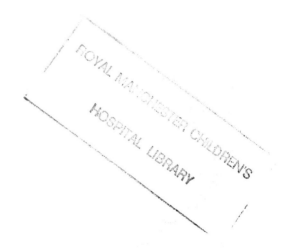